A conserver 1 an à compter
du 24/11/92

AF754523

REVIEW COPY

We would appreciate your sending two copies of your review.

HANDBOOK OF NATURAL TOXINS
VOLUME 7: FOOD POISONING

EDITED BY ANTHONY T. TU

PUBLISHED 1992 656 PAGES, BOUND, ILLUSTRATED

$185.00

PRICE IS SUBJECT TO CHANGE WITHOUT NOTICE.

marcel dekker, inc.
270 MADISON AVENUE • NEW YORK, NY 10016 • 212-696-9000

Food Poisoning

Handbook of Natural Toxins
volume 7

HANDBOOK OF NATURAL TOXINS

Series Editor

Anthony T. Tu
Department of Biochemistry
Colorado State University
Fort Collins, Colorado

1. Plant and Fungal Toxins, *edited by Richard F. Keeler and Anthony T. Tu*
2. Insect Poisons, Allergens, and Other Invertebrate Venoms, *edited by Anthony T. Tu*
3. Marine Toxins and Venoms, *edited by Anthony T. Tu*
4. Bacterial Toxins, *edited by M. Carolyn Hardegree and Anthony T. Tu*
5. Reptile Venoms and Toxins, *edited by Anthony T. Tu*
6. Toxicology of Plant and Fungal Compounds, *edited by Richard F. Keeler and Anthony T. Tu*
7. Food Poisoning, *edited by Anthony T. Tu*

ADDITIONAL VOLUMES IN PREPARATION

Food Poisoning

Handbook of Natural Toxins
volume 7

edited by
Anthony T. Tu
Department of Biochemistry
Colorado State University
Fort Collins, Colorado

Marcel Dekker, Inc. New York • Basel • Hong Kong

Library of Congress Cataloging-in-Publication Data

Food poisoning / edited by Anthony T. Tu.
p. cm. -- (Handbook of natural toxins ; v. 7)
Includes bibliographical references and index.
ISBN 0-8247-8652-1 (alk. paper)
1. Food poisoning. I. Tu, Anthony T. II. Series.
[DNLM: 1. Food Poisoning. QW 630 H236 1983 v. 7]
RC143.F66 1992
615.9'54--dc20
DNLM/DLC
for Library of Congress 92-14624
CIP

This book is printed on acid-free paper.

MARCEL DEKKER, INC.
270 Madison Avenue, New York, New York 10016

Current printing (last digit):
10 9 8 7 6 5 4 3 2 1

PRINTED IN THE UNITED STATES OF AMERICA

Preface to the Handbook

Natural toxins are unique toxins which possess some common properties, whether they are obtained from plants, microorganisms, or animals. One common characteristic is that they exert a pronounced effect on the metabolism and biological functions of the intoxicated animals with just a minute quantity. Since ancient times human beings have pondered the physiological effects of various toxins and venoms. How do these natural poisons work? Despite possessing some common nature, each toxin, however, has its unique mode of action and its own characteristic structure.

Drugs are compounds that have specific beneficial effects with a minute quantity. Usually, natural toxins also have very specific effects. Therefore, it is not surprising that many natural toxins are potentially good drugs.

Heretofore, the study of each field of toxins has been taking an independent pathway. Scientists in a specific toxin field are often unaware of the activity in other toxin fields. It is thus desirable to have a primary source of information on all natural toxins so that scientists in a specific discipline of toxin research can easily obtain useful information from other toxin researchers.

This handbook of toxins includes the following volumes:

1. *Plant and Fungal Toxins*
2. *Insect Poisons, Allergens, and Other Invertebrate Venoms*
3. *Marine Toxins and Venoms*
4. *Bacterial Toxins*
5. *Reptile Venoms and Toxins*
6. *Toxicology of Plant and Fungal Compounds*
7. *Food Poisoning*

The editor expresses sincere thanks to Maurits Dekker for initiating this project.

Anthony T. Tu

Preface to Volume 7

Since I started the first volume of *Handbook of Natural Toxins* with Dr. Richard F. Keeler on *Plant and Fungal Toxins* in 1979, there has been considerable progress in this series. Volume 2, *Insect Poisons, Allergens, and Other Invertebrate Venoms,* was published in 1984. Both Volume 3, *Marine Toxins and Venoms,* and Volume 4, *Bacterial Toxins,* were published in 1988. The most recent publications were Volumes 5 and 6, *Reptile Venoms and Toxins* and *Toxicology of Plant and Fungal Compounds*; both appeared in 1991.

Volume 7 deals with food poisoning. Food is obtained from many sources, hence poisoning associated with food also originates from many sources. In this volume, the first chapter, written by distinguished food scientist Dr. Frank L. Bryan, summarizes the serious problem of food poisoning from a public health viewpoint. Other chapters were subdivided according to the sources of poisoning, such as bacteria, plant, and fungus. This division is not absolute but rather for convenience. Allergic reaction is a different phenomenon from ordinary food poisoning; it is, therefore, treated separately in Part IV. Part V comprises two chapters related to seafood. The other parts cover special topics.

With the addition of Volume 7, *Food Poisoning*, the *Handbook of Natural Toxins* series has become a much more complete set, covering a wider range of topics.

It is my hope that this volume will be a useful reference book for food scientists as well as for practical use by persons dealing with food manufacturing and processing. Further, it is hoped that it will be useful to anyone concerned with the quality of food, as everyone has to take food as part of one's daily activities.

Anthony T. Tu

Contents

Contributors

J. Stan Bailey Department of Microbiological Safety, Russell Research Center, Agricultural Research Service, United States Department of Agriculture, Athens, Georgia

Tracy J. Bargman* Department of Food Science and Technology, University of Nebraska, Lincoln, Nebraska

Merlin S. Bergdoll Food Research Institute, University of Wisconsin, Madison, Wisconsin

Frank L. Bryan Food Safety Consultation and Training, Lithonia, Georgia

Suchitra Changchawalit Department of Bacteriology and Molecular Genetics, Armed Forces Research Institute of Medical Sciences, Bangkok, Thailand

Nelson A. Cox Russell Research Center, Agricultural Research Service, United States Department of Agriculture, Athens, Georgia

Suresh S. Dhumal† Department of Nutrition and Food Science, Utah State University, Logan, Utah

Peter Echeverria Department of Bacteriology and Molecular Genetics, Armed Forces Research Institute of Medical Sciences, Bangkok, Thailand

---

**Present affiliation*: General Mills, Inc., Minneapolis, Minnesota
†*Present affiliation*: Kalyani Agro Corporation, Pune (Maharashtra), India

Heinz Faulstich Max-Planck-Institut für Medizinische Forschung, Heidelberg, Germany

Richard K. Gast Southeast Poultry Research Laboratory, Agricultural Research Service, United States Department of Agriculture, Athens, Georgia

Richard J. Gilbert PHLS Food Hygiene Laboratory, Central Public Health Laboratory, London, United Kingdom

James M. Hungerford Seafood Products Research Center, United States Food and Drug Administration, Bothell, Washington

Ryan J. Huxtable Department of Pharmacology, College of Medicine, University of Arizona, Tucson, Arizona

Werner G. Jaffé Department of Cell Biology, School of Biology, Faculty of Sciences, Universidad Central de Venezuela, Caracas, Venezuela

Charles A. Kaysner Seafood Products Research Center, United States Food and Drug Administration, Bothell, Washington

John M. Kramer PHLS Food Hygiene Laboratory, Central Public Health Laboratory, London, United Kingdom

Ronald G. Labbé Department of Food Science, University of Massachusetts, Amherst, Massachusetts

Pavel Langer Institute of Experimental Endocrinology, Slovak Academy of Sciences, Bratislava, Czech and Slovak Federal Republic

Klaus Lorenz Department of Food Science and Human Nutrition, Colorado State University, Fort Collins, Colorado

Nikolaj Michajlovskij Institute of Experimental Endocrinology, Slovak Academy of Sciences, Bratislava, Czech and Slovak Federal Republic

John H. Rupnow Department of Food Science and Technology, University of Nebraska, Lincoln, Nebraska

Dattajirao K. Salunkhe Department of Nutrition and Food Science, Utah State University, Logan, Utah

James L. Schardein Reproductive and Developmental Toxicology Division, International Research and Development Corporation, Mattawan, Michigan

Dinah S. Seidl Department of Cell Biology, Faculty of Sciences, Universidad Central de Venezuela, Caracas, Venezuela

Nrisinha P. Sen Food Research Division, Bureau of Chemical Safety, Food Directorate, Health Protection Branch, Health and Welfare Canada, Ottawa, Ontario, Canada

Oralak Serichantalergs Department of Bacteriology, Armed Forces Research Institute of Medical Sciences, Bangkok, Thailand

Orntipa Sethabutr Department of Bacteriology, Armed Forces Research Institute of Medical Sciences, Bangkok, Thailand

Irtaza H. Siddique Department of Microbiology, School of Veterinary Medicine, Tuskegee University, Tuskegee, Alabama

Joseph I. Smith* Department of Laboratory Medicine, U.S. Army Medical Research Institute of Infectious Diseases, Fort Detrick, Frederick, Maryland

John N. Sofos Department of Animal Sciences, and Food Science and Human Nutrition, Colorado State University, Fort Collins, Colorado

Steve L. Taylor Department of Food Science and Technology, University of Nebraska, Lincoln, Nebraska

Anthony T. Tu Department of Biochemistry, Colorado State University, Fort Collins, Colorado

Marleen M. Wekell Seafood Products Research Center, United States Food and Drug Administration, Bothell, Washington

Theodor Wieland Max-Planck-Institut für Medizinische Forschung, Heidelberg, Germany

**Present affiliation*: Department of Pathology and Area Laboratory Services, Brooke Army Medical Center, Fort Sam, Houston, Texas

Contents of Previous Volumes

Volume I: Plant and Fungal Toxins

I

PUBLIC HEALTH PROBLEMS

1

Public Health Problems of Foodborne Diseases and Their Prevention

Frank L. Bryan

Food Safety Consultation and Training, Lithonia, Georgia

I. INTRODUCTION

Foodborne diseases are syndromes that are acquired as a result of ingesting foods that contain either an infectious or a toxigenic microorganism or a poisonous substance. For convenience they are classified into three categories.

These are (1) infections, (2) toxin-mediated infections, and (3) poisonings or intoxications. The infections occur when microorganisms (e.g., pathogenic bacteria, viruses, parasites) invade and multiply in the intestinal mucosa or other tissues. The toxin-mediated infections are caused by certain pathogenic bacteria that produce enterotoxins (substances that affect water, glucose, and electrolyte transfer) during their colonization and growth in the intestine tract. The poisonings or intoxications follow ingestion of either poisonous chemicals, radionuclides, or toxins produced by microorganisms (e.g., marine plankton, bacteria). Hence, food poisoning is a misnomer, because illnesses result from mechanisms other than poisonings. The term, however, is often used in a general way to refer to illness resulting from the ingestion of foods or otherwise foodborne diseases.

This chapter introduces the foodborne disease problem by giving examples of the status of foodborne diseases in the United States. It also describes means by which these diseases can be prevented and controlled. The following chapters describe specific foodborne diseases and the measures for their control in more detail.

II. STATUS OF FOODBORNE DISEASES

Foodborne diseases are a continuing and nagging problem in all countries. Reports of foodborne diseases in the developed countries where surveillance is practiced are usually sporadic and quite incomplete. Yet, the sparse data suggests that the problem causes considerable morbidity and economic consequences. In developing countries, a significant proportion of deaths and illnesses attributed to gastroenteritis are foodborne, but the specific amount is unknown because of lack of investigations and surveillance records.

A foodborne disease *outbreak* is defined (with exceptions) as an incident in which two or more persons experience a similar illness, usually gastrointestinal, after ingestion of a common food, and epidemiological analysis indicates that food is the source of the etiological agents. The exceptions are a single case of botulism, a plant or chemical poisoning where ingestion is the mode of transmission, or any situation where ingestion of a food invariably leads to illness. A *case* is a person who shows signs or feels symptoms as a result of eating a contaminated food.

A. Incidence

Table 1 illustrates trends of annual reported outbreaks and cases of foodborne diseases over a period of 50 years. These indicate that there is no decline in the reported incidence despite improvements in sanitation, physical facilities where foods are processed and prepared, standards of living, and education of the populace. From 400 to 600 outbreaks of usually between 10,000 and 30,000 cases are reported annually. Large decreases in the reported number of outbreaks usually indicate a change in responsibility for foodborne disease surveillance or a gap in summarizing the data and a corresponding loss of reporting by

Table 1 Foodborne Outbreaks and Cases Reported in the United States, 1938–1987

Year	Number of outbreaks	Number of cases	Year	Number of outbreaks	Number of cases
1938[a]	81	2,247	1963	369	16,370
1939	155	3,770	1964	206	8,208
1940	230	5,588	1965	91	6,699
1941	241	6,070	1966	182	7,960
1942	254	11,420	1967	263	22,171
1943	294	13,938	1968	341	17,567
1944	310	14,558	1969	356	28,563
1945	278	11,547	1970	356	23,448
1946	301	12,526	1971	317	13,453
1947	324	12,536	1972	301	
1948	331	9,962	1973	307	12,447
1949	369	9,043	1974	456	15,489
1950[b]	351	10,174	1975	497	18,260
1951	256	7,182	1976	438	12,463
1952	153	6,828	1977	436	9,896
1953	200	9,914	1978	481	10,639
1954	234	11,704	1979	460	13,207
1955	196	9,633	1980	612	13,791
1956	212	11,133	1981	568	14,432
1957	254	11,085	1982	666	
1958	239	9,925	1983	505	14,898
1959	225	10,595	1984	543	16,420
1960	184	7,434	1985	495	31,079
1961[c]	197	7,972	1986	467	12,781
1962	215	10,919	1987	387	16,500

[a]Data compiled by Milk and Food Section, Sanitary Engineering Division, United States Public Health Service.
[b]Data compiled by the National Office of Vital Statistics, U.S. Public Health Service.
[c]Data compiled by the Centers for Disease Control (formerly called the Communicable Disease Center), U.S. Public Health Service.
Source: Based on Bryan, 1972, adjusted through 1970; updated with surveillance reports from the CDC without adjustments.

state health agencies. Major changes are noted by footnotes. Variation in annual reported cases relate to whether large outbreaks were detected.

It does not take much experience with surveillance of foodborne diseases to realize that the reports are woefully inadequate. Some of the reasons are that some persons have gastroenteritis and never realize that food was the vehicle ("It's the flu or something.") and others suffer their syndrome without seeking medical attention or complaining to health authorities. They may not, however, return to the place or eat the same type of food they feel made them ill for a long time. Physicians often do not seek causes of illness, but just treat the patient for their discomfort. Laboratories may use the wrong tests or fail to recover pathogens when specimens are submitted. When local health departments are alerted, an investigation may not be made, or only a superficial one may be done. If an investigation is made, the investigative data may be kept on file and not submitted through the surveillance channels. States may not forward all of the reports that are received. Distribution of reported data show that some cities and states do not submit reports frequently. It is usually a lack of priority for foodborne diseases rather than the absence of incidents of foodborne disease that accounts for this problem. To compensate for this state of affairs, various scientists who have an interest in disease surveillance have made estimates of the incidence of foodborne disease (Hauschild and Bryan, 1980; Archer and Kvenberg, 1985; Bennett et al., 1987). These estimates put the number of cases in the millions rather than the tens of thousands. Each estimator made assumptions to compensate for incomplete data.

Table 2 gives a breakdown of outbreaks by disease etiology that occurred in the United States from 1973 to 1987. These data show that bacterial foodborne diseases are of prime importance. Viral foodborne diseases are emerging in importance, while trichinosis is declining. Salmonellosis, staphylococcal food poisoning, *Clostridium perfringens* enteritis, botulism, ciguatera, histamine (scombroid) poisoning, hepatitis A, and shigellosis were frequently responsible for outbreaks of foodborne diseases. Cases were often associated with outbreaks of salmonellosis, staphylococcal food poisoning, *C. perfringens* enteritis, shigellosis, and Norwalk-like gastroenteritis. The diseases of unknown etiology appear to have been caused by many of the same agents that are commonly reported. The incubation-period data (Table 3) suggest that *Bacillus cereus*, *C. perfringens*, staphylococcal enterotoxin, enteric bacteria, and Norwalk-like viruses may be even more common etiological agents than reports indicate.

Deaths directly attributed to foodborne diseases are not common, but they do occur. Table 4 shows that botulism and listeriosis have high case fatality rates.

B. Place of Mishandling

Although data on place of mishandling have not been kept for the past decade, previous information showed that the place where foods were mishandled or mistreated was usually food service establishments (Table 5). Since that time, there has probably been little change. It is obvious from individual reports that food service establishments are often involved. One reason for eliminating this information from summary reports is that there may be multiple points of mishandling and mistreatment. For example, a turkey may be (1) inadequately cooked, (2) subjected to cross-contamination from the raw product by contact with equipment (e.g., a cutting board) used for both raw and cooked items, and (3) left at room temperature for several hours in a restaurant. Salmonellae, however, were on the product initially and either survived the cooking or the source of the cross-contamination. Hence, producers and processors are responsible for initial contamination and perhaps increase of the contaminants. Furthermore, some very large-scale outbreaks have been associated with processed foods. For example, pasteurized milk contaminated by raw milk was responsible for 16,000 confirmed and an estimated 200,000 cases of salmonellosis (Linnan et al., 1988). Nearly 150 cases and 47 deaths due to listeriosis

Table 2 Foodborne Disease and Cases of Known Etiology, United States, 1973–1987

	Number		Percent	
Etiological agent	Outbreaks	Cases	Outbreaks	Cases
Bacteria				
Salmonella	790	55,864	28	45
Staphylococcus aureus	367	17,248	13	14
Clostridium botulinum	231	494	8	<1
Histamine (scombroid)	202	1,216	7	1
Clostridium perfringens	190	12,234	7	10
Shigella	104	14,399	4	12
Bacillus cereus	58	1,123	2	1
Campylobacter	53	1,549	2	1
Vibrio parahaemolyticus	23	535	1	<1
Streptococcus, group A	12	1,917	<1	2
Escherichia coli	10	1,187	<1	1
Streptococcus, other groups	7	248	<1	<1
Vibrio cholerae	6	916	<1	1
Yersinia enterocolitica	5	767	<1	1
Brucella	4	43	<1	<1
Vibrio cholerae, non-O1	2	11	<1	<1
Other bacteria (including *Listeria monocytogenes*)	7	373	<1	<1
Total bacteria	2,071	109,952	73	88
Viruses				
Hepatitis A virus	110	3,133	4	3
Norwalk virus	15	6,474	1	5
Other viruses	10	1,023	<1	1
Total viruses	135	10,630	5	9
Parasites				
Trichinella spiralis	128	843	5	<1
Giardia	5	131	<1	<1
Other parasites	7	30	<1	<1
Total parasites	140	1,004	5	1
Algae and Marine Plankton				
Ciguatoxin	234	1,052	8	1
Paralytic shellfish poison	21	160	1	<1
Total algae/plankton	255	1,212	9	1
Toxic plants				
Mushrooms	61	169	2	1
Chemicals				
Heavy metals	46	752	2	1
Monosodium glutamate	18	58	1	<1
Total chemicals	64	810	3	1
Other toxicants (plants and chemicals)	115	1,046	4	1
Total	2,841	124,994	100	100

Source: Adapted from Bean and Griffin, 1991.

Table 3 Distribution of Median Incubation Periods for Foodborne Disease Outbreaks of Unknown Etiology, United States, 1973–1987

Incubation periods	Outbreaks	Percent vomiting[a]	Possible agents
<1 hour	159	81	Chemical poisonings *B. cereus*
1–7 hours	1632	63	*S. aureus, B. cereus*
8–14 hours	1042	39	*C. perfringens, B. cereus*
15–23 hours	223	36	*Salmonella, Shigella, E. coli, Yersinia, Campylobacter*
24–47 hours	900	50	As above, Norwalk virus
48–95 hours	61	33	Bacterial infections, Viral infections
≥96 hours	11	25	As above
Unknown	589	54	Unknown, but probably many of the above
Total	4617		

[a]Percentage of outbreaks in which 50% or more persons reported vomiting.
Source: Adapted from Bean and Griffin, 1991.

resulted from ingestion of Mexican-style cheese (Ryan et al., 1987). Additional abuse may occur in the hands of the final preparer. There are also reporting biases for this sort of data. Outbreaks that stem from mishandling in homes are not as likely to be reported as those that result from eating in food service establishments. It is rather difficult to identify outbreaks from processed foods because people eat processed foods at different times and places. Hence, getting reports at one place for analysis and making epidemiological associations becomes more difficult.

C. Implicated Foods

Throughout the years certain foods have been important vehicles of foodborne disease surveillance. In the 1940s and 1950s, cream-filled pastries were the most commonly identified vehicle (Bryan, 1976). In the mid-1960s to mid-1970s, roast beef, turkey, and ham became the three most commonly reported vehicles (Bryan, 1975, 1980). From 1977 to 1984 (Table 6), fin fish, roast beef, pork (mostly ham), salads (including potato, chicken, macaroni, turkey, tuna,

Table 4 Number of Deaths and Death-to-Case Ratio for Bacterial Pathogens in Foodborne Disease Outbreaks, United States, 1973–1987

Etiological agent	No. deaths	Death-to-1000 cases ratio (when outcomes of cases are known)
Bacillus cereus	0	0
Brucella	1	23
Campylobacter	2	2
Clostridium botulinum	47	192
C. perfringens	12	1
Escherichia coli	4	3
Listeria monocytogenes	70	317
Salmonella	88	2
Shigella	4	1
Staphylococcus aureus	4	<1
Streptococcus, Group A	0	0
Streptococcus, other Groups	3	15
Vibrio cholerae	12	13
V. cholerae, non-01	0	0
V. parahaemolyticus	0	0
Yersinia enterocolitica	0	0
Other bacteria	0	0

Source: Bean and Griffin, 1991.

egg), shellfish (e.g., clams and oysters), turkey, chicken, Chinese foods (mostly fried rice), vegetables, Mexican-style foods (includes ground and shredded meats and beans), raw milk, and cheeses were the major vehicles (Bryan, 1988a). The fish category is high because many single-case and few-case outbreaks of ciguatera and outbreaks of scombroid poisoning were reported. Few classical foodborne disease outbreaks were associated with fish products. An epidemic of Norwalk-like illnesses in the Northeast, which peaked in 1982, accounted for the high number of outbreaks attributed to shellfish. These declined greatly in later years.

Table 5 Foodborne Disease Outbreaks Classified by Place of Mishandling or Mistreatment of Foods, United States, 1974–1978

Place of mishandling or mistreatment	Number of outbreaks	Percentage of known places
Food service establishments	1285	77
Homes	327	20
Food-processing plants	52	3
Other/unknown/unspecified	615	—
Total	2279	100

Table 6 Vehicles Associated with Outbreaks of Foodborne Diseases, United States, 1977–1984

Food	Number	Percentage
Fish (many one- or few-case outbreaks due to ciguatera)	232	14.9
Beef (mostly roast beef, excluding ground meat)	181	11.7
Pork (mostly ham)	152	9.8
Salads (includes potato, chicken, macaroni, turkey, tuna, egg)	140	9.0
Shellfish (e.g., clams and oysters)	128	8.2
Turkey (+ includes salads)	86 + 10	5.5 (5.9)
Chicken (+ includes salads)	69 + 20	4.4 (5.5)
Chinese foods (mostly fried rice)	78	5.0
Vegetables	78	5.0
Mexican-style foods (includes ground and shredded meats and beans)	77	5.0
Milk and milk products (mostly raw milk, cheese; + ice cream with eggs)	66 + 16	4.2 (5.0)
Baked goods (includes cream-filled pastry and unspecified, which may also be cream-filled)	53	3.4
Eggs (+ including ice cream containing eggs)	35 + 7	2.3 (2.6)
Beverages (many carbonated which back-flowed into copper pipes)	36	2.3
Mushrooms	34	2.2
Pasta (+ includes salads)	17 + 12	1.1 (1.8)
Crustaceans (e.g., shrimp and crabs)	25	1.6
Ground meat (+ includes tacos and other foods containing ground meat)	9 + 14	0.6 (1.4)
Fruits	20	1.3
Food mixtures and others	37	2.4
Total	1553 + 79	99.9

Source: Bryan, 1988a.

D. Factors That Contribute to Causation of Outbreaks

Table 7 lists factors that contributed to outbreaks of foodborne diseases reported in the United States from 1961 to 1982 (Bryan, 1978, 1988b) and England and Wales from 1970 to 1982 (Roberts, 1982, 1986). Inadequate cooling—either leaving foods at room or warm outside temperatures or storing them in large containers while being refrigerated—was associated with most of the outbreaks. Percentages in these tables exceed 100% because multiple factors usually contribute to single outbreaks. To emphasize the relative importance of these factors, the listing has been divided into three categories: vital (high-risk) factors, which ought to be given the greatest attention in preventive actions; intermediate-risk factors, which should be given appropriate attention; and low-risk factors, which should be noted and watched for increasing risks. Ranking of all factors has changed little over four periods of review.

The three most frequently identified factors that contributed to: (1) salmonellosis were improper cooling, contaminated raw products, and inadequate heating; (2) staphylococcal food poisoning were colonized persons handling cooked foods, lapse of 12 or more hours between preparing and eating, and improper cooling; (3) botulism were inadequate heat processing, improper fermentations, improper room temperature holding; (4) *C. perfringens* enteritis were improper cooling, lapse of 12 or more hours between preparing and eating, and inadequate reheating (followed closely by improper hot holding); (5) shigellosis were colonized persons handling implicated foods, improper cooling, and lapse of 12 or more hours between preparing and eating; (6) *Vibrio parahaemolyticus* gastroenteritis were contaminated raw ingredients, improper cooling, and cross-contamination; (7) typhoid fever were colonized persons handling implicated foods, lapse of 12 or more hours between preparing and eating, and several time-temperature factors tied for third; (8) *B. cereus* gastroenteritis were improper cooling, lapse of 12 or more hours between preparing and eating, and improper hot holding (Bryan, 1988b).

The principal factors associated with outbreaks stemming from foods prepared in food service establishments were improper cooling, lapse of 12 or more hours between preparing and eating, colonized persons handling implicated foods, inadequate reheating, and improper hot holding. Important factors that contributed to outbreaks in homes were contaminated raw foods, inadequate cooking, unsafe source, improper cooling, and lapse of 12 or more hours between preparing and eating. Major contributing factors associated with operations in food-processing plants were inadequate heat processing, contaminated raw ingredients, improper cooling, colonized persons handling implicated foods, improper cleaning of equipment, and improper fermentation (Bryan, 1988b).

E. Economic Impact

Some investigators have made attempts to equilibrate disease incidence with costs (e.g., Todd, 1985a,b, 1989; Bennett et al., 1987; Garthright et al., 1988; Roberts, 1989). These estimates consider (1) medical-associated cost and loss of productivity to the patient or family resulting from the illness or sequelae; (2) cost to the food processor or preparer, including legal settlements; and (3) cost to the agency investigating the incident. Estimated cost per case varies with the disease under investigation (e.g., over \$1,000 for a case of salmonellosis, over \$10,000 for a case of listeriosis). In reality, these costs vary from nothing to perhaps the upper range of the estimated cost because some persons neither seek medical attention nor use medicine; others are hospitalized, and yet others die. The cost to the national economy may total billions of dollars per year when estimated incidence is combined with the estimated cost.

III. APPROACHES FOR PREVENTION AND CONTROL

Measures used to prevent and control foodborne infections and intoxications can be classified into surveillance and educational activities. There is

Table 7 Factors That Contributed to the Occurrence of 1918 Outbreaks of Foodborne Disease, United States, 1961–1982, and 1479 Outbreaks of Foodborne Diseases in England and Wales, 1970–1982

Contributory factor	United States		England/Wales		Total	
	Number	Percentage[a]	Number	Percentage	Number	Percentage
Vital factors						
Improper cooling	839	43.7	1,034	69.9	1,873	55.1
Storage at ambient temperature	405	21.1	566	38.3	971	28.6
Inadequate coooling	378	19.7	468	31.6	846	24.9
Lapse of ≥12 hours between preparation and serving	434	22.6	844	57.1	1,278	37.6
Inadequate reheating	203	10.6	391	26.4	594	17.5
Inadequate cooking/canning/heat processing	298	15.5	223	15.8	521	15.3
Colonized person handled implicated food	348	18.1	65	4.4	413	12.2
Incorporating contaminated raw food/ingredient into foods that received no further cooking	303	15.8	93	6.3	396	11.7
Improper hot holding	255	13.3	77	5.2	332	9.8
Contaminated processed food (source unidentified)			246	16.6	246	7.2
Cross-contamination	104	5.4	94	6.4	198	5.8
Obtaining food from unsafe source	192	10.0			192	5.7
Intermediate factors						
Use of leftovers[b]	66	3.3	62	4.2	128	3.8
Improper cleaning of equipment/utensils	103	5.4			103	3.0
Inadequate/improper thawing	7	0.4	95	6.4	102	3.0
Toxic containers/pipelines	61	3.2			61	1.8
Extra-large quantities prepared			48	3.2	48	1.4
Intentional additives	46	2.4			46	1.4
Mistaken for edible varieties	33	1.7			33	1.0
Improper fermentation	25	1.3			25	0.7
Incidental additives	24	1.3			24	0.7

Trivial factors						
Inadequate acidification	5	0.3			5	0.1
Poor dry storage practices	5	0.3			5	0.1
Contaminated water	4	0.2			4	0.1
Postprocessing contamination	3	0.2			3	0.1
Slow/inadequate drying	2	0.1			2	0.06
Misbranding	2	0.1			2	0.06
Faulty sealing	1	0.05			1	0.03
Soaking time too short	1	0.05			1	0.03
Growth during seed germination	1	0.05			1	0.03
Improper preservation	1	0.05			1	0.03
Inadequate dish washing (contamination afterwards)	1	0.05			1	0.03
Contamination by fertilizer or soil	1	0.05			1	0.03
Flies on foods	1	0.05			1	0.03

[a]Percentage exceeds 100 because multiple factors contribute to single outbreaks.
[b]Also lapse of 12 or more hours.
Source: Bryan 1988b; Roberts, 1982, 1986.

surveillance of (1) diseases, (2) foods, (3) food-establishment workers, (4) facilities in which foods are processed, transported, stored, and prepared, (5) equipment on which foods are processed and prepared, and (6) operations (practices, procedures, or processes) to which foods are exposed. Furthermore, professional public health, regulatory, and quality-control personnel must be trained in matters related to surveillance and control of foodborne diseases. In addition, food-industry managers and supervisors, food-establishment workers, and the public must be educated about hazards associated with foodborne diseases and their prevention.

A. Surveillance of Diseases

Surveillance of diseases is an indispensable part of every successful disease-control program, yet foodborne-disease surveillance is either nonexistent or ineffective in many jurisdictions. It consists of (1) seeking notification of illness, (2) identifying and investigating outbreaks, (3) interpreting investigative data, and (4) disseminating findings (Bryan et al., 1987). The primary purpose of surveillance is to provide a basis for taking rational actions that will control continuing outbreaks and prevent the ocurrence of others.

Notification of outbreaks of diseases alleged to be foodborne and reports of sporadic cases of enteric illnesses can be improved by health agencies establishing rapport with community physicians, with personnel in hospital emergency rooms or poison control centers, and with personnel in institutions (e.g., schools, nursing homes). These persons should be encouraged to alert the agency responsible for disease surveillance of any unusual occurrence, such as clustering in respect to time of onset of cases of enteric illness. School and industrial records of absenteeism can be reviewed for indication of either increases in incidence or outbreaks of diarrheal illnesses. Arrangements should be made with hospital and other laboratories to report all isolations of enteric pathogens, such as *Campylobacter, Salmonella, Shigella*, or other agents that might be foodborne. The public should be given information about where to report enteric illnesses and should be encouraged to make such reports. All reported outbreaks should be investigated and all sporadic cases of enteric disease interviewed. Names of suspected foods and places where ill persons have eaten up to 72 hours before the onset of their illnesses should be obtained and recorded on a log sheet. This log should be reviewed periodically for association among the cases.

Investigations consist of (1) taking steps to verify diagnosis (including getting case histories and collecting specimens), (2) making time, place, and person associations of cases, and (3) reviewing operations at the establishment where foods were likely to have been mishandled. The last step consists of interviewing managers and workers, collecting samples, tracing routes of contamination to their source (if possible), examining workers, and identifying operations that contributed to the outbreak. This crucial phase of the investigation must account for contamination of the implicated food, survival of pathogens or toxins during heat processes (if applicable), and multiplication of foodborne pathogenic bacteria to such an extent that would create either cells or toxins in quantities sufficient to cause illness. Once a food is implicated, its sale must be stopped, products already sold recalled, and safeguards established and monitored. Data disclosed during the investigation must be collated, analyzed, and interpreted by making appropriate calculations and illustrations. Salient features of the outbreak should be summarized and a report submitted through appropriate channels to the agency responsible for disease surveillance at the national level.

Information about the factors contributing to an outbreak should be used to either select or devise and institute control and preventive measures in the implicated establishment (Bryan, 1988a,b). Inspectional data about similar establishments should be examined, or surveys initiated, to determine operations similar to those that contributed to the outbreak elsewhere. If such practices are found, education or enforcement efforts (whichever is most appropriate, or in appropriate combinations) should be intensified to decrease the hazards. In time, surveillance data become bases for determining the predominant foodborne diseases in a community, for indicating principal vehicles, and for identifying the primary factors that contribute to the occurrence of outbreaks of foodborne disease (see Table 7). Food-safety program activities and priorities must be related to contemporary foodborne-disease problems in the community.

B. Surveillance of Food-Establishment Workers

Several approaches to detect infected food workers and to take action to prevent them from contaminating foods have been carried out by some health and food regulatory agencies throughout the years. These include medical histories, physical examinations, blood tests, x-rays, examination of feces for parasites or bacterial pathogens (e.g., *Salmonella* and *Shigella*). There has been some public pressure to return to these practices primarily because of the concern about transmission of AIDS. There are significant limitations, however, to each of these practices (WHO, 1989).

Medical histories may suggest previous illnesses in which a carrier state may still exist and a disease condition may be diagnosed. A pathogen may be isolated or a sign of infection detected from a specimen. These are positive attributes of such examinations. The state of health, however, is transitory. A medical or laboratory examination can only indicate a condition at the moment of either the physical examination or collection of a specimen. Persons free of infections on the day of an examination, who are in the incubation phase of a disease, or who have mild, abortive, or atypical illnesses, will be missed. Furthermore, infections may be acquired and terminated between examinations. These examinations can never be scheduled at a frequency that would produce information certain to identify carriers.

Blood tests are usually done to detect venereal diseases, and skin tests and x-ray examinations are done to detect evidence of tubercular infections. Neither type of infection (including AIDS) are transmitted by persons while processing or preparing foods.

Fecal smears may be examined for parasites. This is a rather simple test to perform, and infected persons may undergo a regiment of treatment. After persons are treated for parasites, however, they can readily become reinfected unless they change their personal hygiene practices and improve the sanitation of their home and its environs.

Other than in regions where certain bacterial pathogens are highly prevalent, routine examinations of stools for pathogens frequently would be negative and give variable results. Epidemiological data show that salmonellae usually come from raw foods of animal origin rather than persons who excrete salmonellae. A food handler who is identified as infected during an investigation is more likely to be a victim, as are others who eat epidemiologically implicated foods, rather than the source. The role of asymptomatic carriers is of secondary importance in transmission of salmonellae, and screening for carriers has a high cost-to-benefit ratio.

A health card based on physical examinations or negative cultures, unfortunately, conveys to the public, the worker, food establishment managers, and even some personnel in health agencies the erroneous notion that the worker is incapable of transmitting foodborne pathogens—that if they touch foods or otherwise mishandle or mistreat foods, the outcome will be insignificant, which is not the case. Furthermore, a food-handler examination program by a public health agency or an industry that seldom reveals a carrier or positive stool culture often gives administrators the unjustified feeling that they are protecting the public or safeguarding the food supply. Instead, it should alert them to the inadequacies of the approach and lead them to seek alternative ways to protect foods from contamination.

Many microorganisms sometimes transmitted by foods—*Staphylococcus aureus, C. perfringens, Clostridium botulinum, B. cereus, Vibrio cholerae*, non-O1 vibrios, *Vibrio parahaemolyticus*, pathogenic *Escherichia coli* (enteroinvasive, enterotoxigenic, and hemorrhagic strains), *Campylobacter jejuni, Yersinia enterocolitica*, intestinal viruses (such as Norwalk, Norwalk-like, rota, calici, astro, entero, coxsackie, ECHO, hepatitis A, and adeno)—are seldom if ever sought during routine examination of specimens from food workers. Of those listed, *C. jejuni* and *Y. enterocolitica* are almost always of animal or environmental origin. *Bacillus cereus, C. botulinum*, and *V. parahaemolyticus* are derived from raw foods and the environment (e.g., soil and water) rather than from human carriers. *Staphylococcus aureus* resides in the nose and on the skin of healthy persons. *Clostridium perfringens*, although present in human intestines, is also in the intestines of other animals and in soil, and it is a common contaminant of raw foods. Even if *S. aureus* and *C. perfringens* were eliminated through a regimen of treatment, they would reestablish in their niches within a few days to 2 weeks. Pathogenic *E. coli* may come from human excreters, but it is also present in animal feces and can readily multiply on surfaces of equipment in food establishments. Viruses may come from a human carrier, but they can also reach water-grown foods from sewage-polluted water.

C. Surveillance of Foods

The laboratory is an essential resource for any food-safety program. Foods may be sampled at ports of entry, at harvest, during storage, at critical stages of processing, and after processing in processing plants, in retail stores, at markets, or in food-service establishments and tested for either foodborne pathogens or indicator organisms, as appropriate to the situation (Speck, 1984; Subcommittee, 1985). Isolation of some pathogens (e.g., *Salmonella*) or significant numbers of other pathogens (e.g., 10^6 of *C. perfringens*) indicates a high health risk. High numbers of mesophilic aerobic bacteria in processed foods indicate either gross contamination or bacterial growth, but not health risks. The finding of coliforms, *E. coli, Enterobacteriaceae* in heat-processed foods usually indicates postprocess contamination. Not finding these organisms or high numbers from a small number of samples, however, does not indicate that the food is safe, which many persons seeing the results tend to assume. There are several reasons for this. Contaminants are not always uniformly distributed in a batch or lot of foods; this is particularly true when low numbers of contaminants are present. Hence, the absence of finding contaminated items during sampling can give a false sense of security. When no positive samples are found, this only means that the contaminants were not detected in the number of samples collected and tested, not that the lot was free of contaminants.

Testing only identifies defects and rarely indicates where in the process that contamination occurred or where the process failed. Furthermore, microbiological testing usually requires a few days. By the time results are available, foods under investigation have often been either eaten or shipped to other premises. Microbiological testing is expensive. End-product testing is inadequate when used alone for evaluating the safety of products.

Whenever microbiological criteria are contemplated, they should contain the following information: (1) a description of the food; (2) the organisms for which tests are to be done; (3) analytical methods for their detection or enumeration; (4) a sampling plan that defines the number (n) of sample units to be taken and the size of the unit to be taken and tested; (5) the microbiological limits (m and M) considered appropriate for the organisms in the foods; and (6) the proportion (c) of the sample units that can deviate from the limits (Codex Alimentarius Commission, 1980). Action to take if the lot being sampled fails to comply with the criteria should also be given.

There are statistical limitations of any sampling plan (ICMSF, 1986). Such plans become more stringent: (1) when a large number of samples are taken, (2) when large amounts of sample are tested, (3) when multiple media are used during examinations, (4) when multiple criteria are used in the limits (e.g., three-class plan), (5) when limits are set low, and (6) when tolerances are low or absent.

D. Surveillance of Food-Processing and -Preparation Environments

Potable running water, plumbing systems free from cross-connections and from back-siphoning potentials, toilet facilities, lavatory facilities, and safe sewage-disposal systems are essential for minimizing contamination or promoting personal hygiene of workers in food establishments. Today, in the United States, few outbreaks implicate deficiencies in these facilities. Potential problems, however, must be guarded against because breakdowns of these facilities can permit contamination of foods.

The practice of reviewing plans of new facilities, remolded facilities, and businesses that change hands can detect hazards that are inherent in the operations. Furthermore, such reviews can determine the availability of facilities to promote personal hygiene of workers and to improve sanitation. Equipment should be designed and so arranged in food establishments to reduce the possibilities of cross-contamination.

Traditionally, the emphasis in food-protection programs has been put on inspection. Inspections, however, can be done neither often enough nor thoroughly enough to provide the degree of food safety that is desired by processors and preparers of foods and the public. Furthermore, inspections may be done at times when either high-risk foods are not being prepared or critical processes are not being done; hence, factors critical to food safety may be overlooked. Some inspectors fail to distinguish between factors critical to food safety and those that are purely aesthetic or trivial. Laws and regulations often contain vague terms concerning compliance and seldom suggest relative importance of specific items, and, hence, many interpretations are left to the discretion of an inspector. According to present disease surveillance data, traditional efforts for control have not solved the foodborne disease problem. Hence, a new approach must be sought.

It is not dirty floors, walls, ceilings, or dishes or even the presence of flies or cockroaches in food establishments that lead to outbreaks of foodborne diseases; it is the factors listed in Table 7. Therefore, to ensure quality control and food safety, the emphasis should not be on physical facilities or even on health status of workers, but on processes to which foods are exposed.

E. Surveillance of Food-Processing and -Preparation Operations

The best way to assure food safety is by continued surveillance of operations in food-processing and food-service operations. Emphasis must be put on (1) hazards associated with sources of contamination to which foods are exposed, modes of contamination, and changing the process to decrease the level of that contamination, (2) the probability of microorganisms or toxic substances surviving processing or process failure, and (3) the chances of bacteria or molds multiplying during processing or storage.

A rational and contemporary approach to these concerns is known as the Hazard Analysis Critical Control Point (HACCP) system, (ICMSF, 1988), which consists of:

1. Identification of hazards (contamination, survival of pathogens and toxins, and multiplication of microbes) and assessment of the severity of the hazards and the risks that they pose.
2. Determination of critical control points required to prevent or control identified hazard(s). A critical control point is an operation (practice, procedure, process, or location) at or by which preventive or control

measures can be exercised that will eliminate, prevent, or minimize a hazard or hazards.
3. Implementation of effective preventive and control measures and specification of criteria that indicate whether an operation is under control.
4. Monitoring of each critical control point to evaluate whether it is under control. This involves systematic observations and measurements; recording of these is prudent when practicable.
5. Taking appropriate and immediate corrective action whenever the monitoring results indicate that criteria established for safety at a critical control point are not met—thus, that the operation is out of control.
6. Verification by reviewing the system and using either supplemental tests or reviewing records to determine (1) whether the HACCP system is in place, (2) that appropriate critical control points have been designated, (3) that they are being effectively and properly monitored, and (4) that appropriate action is taken whenever criteria are not within specified limits. Hence, verification evaluates whether the HACCP system is functioning as planned.

The HACCP approach has application for foods during harvesting, during distribution while held in storage, during processing, while on display at retail establishments, during preparation, and while holding before serving. It offers a high level of assurance of food safety to persons concerned with food control, to those who process and prepare foods, and to the public. Hence, it is a desirable alternative to the more traditional control options, which are not always effective or efficient.

Conducting hazard analysis and determining critical control points requires input by trained specialists who are supported by adequate laboratory services. Furthermore, monitoring of critical control points and verification may require specialized equipment such as time-temperature recording devices, pH meters, and hygrometers.

F. Training of Persons Who Handle Foods and Supervise Its Safety and Quality

Food-hygiene and food-safety professions must understand the epidemiology of foodborne diseases and the microbial ecology of foods so that measures to prevent these diseases and food spoilage can be either selected from known measures or devised and given appropriate priority. They must have the skills to investigate outbreaks of foodborne diseases and use the data gathered in their preventive programs to set program priorities. The scientifically and technically trained professionals must be prepared to either develop or verify a HACCP system.

Food-establishment managers have the primary responsibility for preventing conditions within their establishments that can lead to outbreaks of foodborne disease. They have daily supervisory control of operations. They must, therefore, be aware of the kinds of operations that can lead to outbreaks and insist that appropriate preventive measures be practiced and monitored routinely during or before operations. During training, the factors that contribute to foodborne disease outbreaks in the segment of the food industry of which they are a part should be brought to their attention, with strong emphasis put on those most frequently encountered. Also, specific procedures to prevent the occurrence of these factors and to monitor critical points should be taught so that the managers can convey this information to their workers. This training should be related to common situations in the work environment.

For effective foodborne-disease prevention and quality control in food establishments, managers must train the workers who process, prepare, store, or otherwise handle foods, or who maintain the environment where foods are processed or prepared. If this is not feasible, they should provide training for the workers by an outside agency. If industry does not assume its responsibility, agencies responsible for food safety may have to assist industry or even initiate training of food handlers. After the training from whatever source, managers must supervise their personnel to ensure that the information and skills are being applied. Food-establishment workers need to know how to do their jobs properly so that they will not contribute to contamination of foods and so that microbial contaminants that do get into foods are either killed or their multiplication inhibited. Hence, they need skill in monitoring critical control points.

An alternative to clinical examination of food workers or the testing of specimens from them is training and perhaps even testing of their understanding of safe food-handling practices. A health card based on such understanding would give a far greater assurance of food safety than one based on clinical or specimen examinations. Certain communities have such testing and certification programs, and a test is available from a national testing service.

G. Education of the Public About Food Safety

Education of the public ought to start with teachers and students who are preparing to teach and extend to pupils in primary and secondary schools. Children should become more knowledgeable about food-safety practices, which will prepare them in case they enter the food industry work force or become homemakers.

More immediately, adults must be educated so that they become aware of the important hazards associated with the foods they purchase and prepare as well as of safe food preparation and storage practices. To this end, appropriate educational materials must be developed and educational efforts conducted. These may take many forms: (1) preparing and presenting educational films, leaflets, posters, and radio and television short announcements and documentaries; (2) communications by extension specialists, health officials, and food scientists, and (3) informative food-safety information on labels and packages.

REFERENCES

Archer, D. L., and Kvenberg, J. E. (1985). Incidence and cost of foodborne diarrheal disease in the United States. *J. Food Prot. 48*: 887–894.

Bean, N. H., and Griffin, P. M. (1991). Foodborne disease outbreaks in the United States, 1973–1987: Pathogens, vehicles, and trends. *J. Food Prot. 53*: 804–817.

Bennett, J. V., Holmberg, S. D., Rogers, M. F., and Solomon, S. L. (1987). Infectious and parasitic diseases, In *Closing the Gap: The Burden of Unnecessary Illness*, R. W. Amler and H. B. Dull, eds. Oxford University Press, New York, pp. 102–114.

Bryan, F. L. (1975). Status of foodborne disease in the United States. *J. Environ. Health 38*: 74–83.

Bryan, F. L. (1976). Public health aspects of cream-filled pastries. A review. *J. Milk Food Technol. 39*: 289–296.

Bryan, F. L. (1978). Factors that contribute to outbreaks of foodborne diseases. *J. Food Prot. 41*: 818–827.

Bryan, F. L. (1980). Foodborne diseases in the United States associated with meat and poultry. *J. Food Prot. 43*: 140–150.

Bryan, F. L. (1988a). Risk associated with vehicles of foodborne pathogens and toxins. *J. Food Prot. 51*: 498–508.

Bryan, F. L. (1988b). Risks associated with practices, procedures and processes that lead to outbreaks of foodborne diseases. *J. Food Prot. 51*: 663–673.

Bryan, F. L., Anderson, H. W., Cook, O. D., Guzewich, J., Lewis, K. H., Swanson, R. C., and Todd, E. C. D. (1987). *Procedures to Investigate Foodborne Illness*, 4th ed. International Association of Milk, Food, and Environmental Sanitarians, Ames, IA.

Codex Alimentarius Commission. (1980). General Principles for the Establishment and Application of Microbiological Criteria for Foods, Appendix II on Report of the 17th Session of the Committee on Food Hygiene. Food and Agriculture Organization, Rome.

Garthright, W. E., Archer, D. L., and Kvenberg, J. E. (1988). Estimates of incidence and costs of intestinal infections diseases in the United States. *Public Health Rept. 103*: 107–115.

Hauschild, A. H. W., and Bryan, F. L. (1980). Estimate of cases of food- and water-borne illness in Canada and the United States. *J. Food Prot. 43*: 435–440.

ICMSF (International Commission on Microbiological Specifications for Foods). (1986). *Micro-organisms in Foods 2. Sampling for Microbiological Analysis: Principles and Specific Applications*, 2nd ed. University of Toronto Press, Toronto.

ICMSF (International Commission on Microbiological Specifications for Foods). (1988). *Microorganisms in Foods 4. Application of the Hazard Analysis Critical Control Point (HACCP) System to Ensure Microbiological Safety and Quality*. Blackwell Scientific Publications, Ltd., Oxford.

Linnan, M. J., Mascola, L., Lou, X. D., Goulet, V., May, S., Salminen, C., Hird, D. W., Yonekura, L., Hayes, P., Weaver, R., Audurier, A., Plikaytis, B. D., Fannin, S. L., Kleks, A., and Broome, C. V. (1988). Epidemic listeriosis associated with Mexican-style cheese. *N. Engl. J. Med. 319*: 823–828.

Roberts, D. (1982). Factors contributing to outbreaks of food poisoning in England and Wales 1970–1980. *J. Hyg. 89*: 491–498.

Roberts, D. (1986). Factors contributing to outbreaks of foodborne infection and intoxication in England and Wales 1970–1982. *Proc. 2nd World Congress Foodborne Infections and Intoxications*, Vol. 1. Institute of Veterinary Medicine—Robert von Ostertag Institute, Berlin (West).

Roberts, T. (1989). Human illness costs of foodborne bacteria. *Am. J. Agric. Econ. 71*: 468–474.

Ryan, C. A., Nickels, M. K., Hargrett-Bean, M. E., Potter, M. E., Endo, T., Mayer, L., Langkop, C. W., Gibson, C., McDonald, R. C., Kenney, R. T., Phur, N. D., McDonnell, P. J., Martin, R. J., Cohen, M. L., and Blake, P. A. (1987). Massive outbreak of antimicrobial-resistant salmonellosis traced to pasteurized milk. *JAMA 258*: 3269–3274.

Speck, M. L. (ed.). (1984). *Compendium of Methods for the Microbiological Examination of Foods*, 2nd ed. American Public Health Association, Washington, DC.

Subcommittee (Subcommittee on Microbiological Criteria for Foods and Food Ingredients, Committee in Food Protection, Food and Nutrition Board, National Research Council). (1985). *An Evaluation of the Role of Microbiological Criteria for Foods and Food Ingredients*. National Academy Press, Washington, DC.

Todd, E. C. D. (1985a). Economic loss from foodborne disease and non-related recalls because of mishandling by food processors. *J. Food Prot. 48*: 621–633.

Todd, E. C. D. (1985b). Economic loss from foodborne disease outbreaks associated with foodservice establishments. *J. Food Prot. 48*: 169–180.

Todd, E. C. D. (1989). Preliminary estimates of costs of foodborne disease in the United States. *J. Food Prot. 52*: 595–601.

WHO (World Health Organization). (1989). Health surveillance and management procedures for food-handling personnel. Technical Report Series 785. World Health Organization, Geneva.

II

BACTERIAL ORIGIN

2

Staphylococcal Intoxication in Mass Feeding

Merlin S. Bergdoll

University of Wisconsin–Madison, Madison, Wisconsin

I. INTRODUCTION

Staphylococcal food poisoning is one of the most common types of foodborne disease and probably occurs in every country of the world, although records of the milder foodborne diseases are not kept in most countries. The illness is due to the ingestion of enterotoxins present in the food as a result of enterotoxigenic staphylococci growing in the food. Recovery is rapid, hence, in most cases individuals do not consult a doctor but conclude it was something they ate. It is not a reportable disease because of its relative mildness, however, enough identifiable outbreaks are reported to the Centers for Disease Control (CDC) to result in its listing as one of the leading foodborne disease in the United States. Many cases of foodborne illness with symptoms similar to those of staphylococcal food poisoning are reported to the CDC, but are not classified because of inadequate information about the presence of staphylococci or enterotoxin in the foods involved (Table 1).

Most staphylococcal food-poisoning incidents involve a relatively small number of people, such as a family group or even only one individual, which accounts for many outbreaks never being reported. There have been very large outbreaks, such as one involving over 1300 people attending a picnic in Indiana. An even larger outbreak occurred in Japan when 1500 people became ill after eating contaminated rice balls contained in lunch boxes prepared at one location. The latter two outbreaks are the type that will be considered here, as the food was prepared in one location for serving to a large number of individuals. Also, outbreaks that result from foods prepared at one location, such as by a food processor, for mass distribution will be considered. One example of this was corned beef produced in Brazil for distribution to other countries, such as England, where many people became ill after consuming it (Mansfield et al., 1983). Another example was a butter outbreak among individuals eating at restaurants serving whipped butter prepared by one manufacturer (CDC, 1977c).

A. Determination as Staphylococcal Food Poisoning

1. *Symptoms of the Disease*

The major symptoms of staphylococcal food poisoning, i.e., vomiting and diarrhea, occur within 1–6 h after the ingestion of food containing enterotoxin.

Table 1 Guidelines for Confirmation of Staphylococcal Food Outbreaks[a]

Clinical syndrome
a) Incubation period 30 min–8 h (usually 2–4 h).
b) Gastrointestinal syndrome—majority of cases with vomiting.
Laboratory, clinical, and epidemiologic criteria for confirmation
a) Detection of enterotoxin in epidemiologically implicated food.
or
b) Organisms with same phage type in stools or vomitus of ill individuals; isolation from epidemiologically implicated food/or skin or nose of food handler is supportive evidence.
or
c) Isolation of $>10^5$ organisms/g in epidemiologically implicated food.

[a]At least two individuals must be involved. The clinical syndrome must be confirmed by adequate laboratory information.

A representative set of symptoms observed in 122 cases of illness that occurred among high school students after they had eaten cream puffs was described by Dennison (1936) (Table 2). He describes the typical symptoms as follows:

> Within 2-4 hours after eating there was first noticed a feeling of nausea. Severe abdominal cramps developed and were quickly followed by vomiting which was severe and continued at 5-21 minute intervals for 1-8 hours. The vomitus was blood streaked in 13% of the cases. A diarrhea of 1-7 liquid stools usually began with the vomiting of several hours after its onset. Blood, not infrequently, was present in the stool. During the acute stage the temperature was normal or subnormal, the pulse noticeably increased, there was cold sweats, prostration was severe, and the patients were very definitely in a state of shock. Headache was mild and of a short duration. Muscular cramping, usually of the flexors of the legs, was present in the majority. Dehydration was marked in some.

While the acute symptoms usually lasted only 1-8 hours, complete recovery, because of prostration, was delayed for 1-2 days. During this time temperatures of 100° were not uncommon. Three cases were hospitalized. There were no fatalities. He summarized the symptoms with their variations as follows:

> The most common interval between eating and the onset of illness was 3 hours. Eighty percent were ill by the fourth hour, while in a small number the onset was delayed for 6, 7, and 8 hours. Twenty-one percent were ill only for the short period of 1-4 hours while in 36%, recovery was delayed for 25-48 h. Vomiting was the most pronounced symptom, and 50% were described as 'continuous'. In the majority of cases (92%), however, vomiting had ceased within 5-8 hours. There was severe vomiting in 78.2%, severe abdominal pain in 62.5%, mild diarrhea (1-7 stools) in 72.8%, mild and usually transient headache in 58%, mild muscular cramps in 51.3% and sweating in 67%. Prostration, dehydration and the degree of shock varied accordingly.

The frequency of the various symptoms is given in Table 2.

Ninety-five (57%) of the 165 students who ate the cream puffs became ill, whereas none of those who did not eat them became ill. This is typical of outbreaks involving a large number of people. The average onset time in the outbreak was also normal for large outbreaks with a few having earlier onset times, usually because of consumption of large amounts of toxin or increased sensitivity of some individuals, and a few that have delayed onset times of

Table 2 Symptoms of Staphylococcal Food Poisoning from 122 Cases[a]

Symptom	Cases[b]	No reaction	Mild reaction	Severe reaction
Vomiting	122	15	12	95
Pains in abdomen	122	6	40	76
Diarrhea	103	13	75	15
Headache	101	29	59	13
Muscular cramping	113	41	58	14

[a]Includes 94 students, 8 lunchroom supervisors who took some home and 20 from cream puffs sold at 3 cafes and from the bakery truck.
[b]Cases from which this information was available.
Source: Dennison, 1936.

7–8 h. Although vomiting is the symptom most frequently observed, some individuals may have other symptoms such as diarrhea without vomiting. Diarrhea may not be observed in milder cases, whereas vomiting usually is. Changes in temperature and blood pressure are not common, particularly with milder cases, although it is known that in experimental cases a change in temperature can occur, either up or down; a drastic lowering of blood pressure may occur also.

Death is uncommon with this type of food poisoning, but deaths have occurred. The deaths reported have been in children or older individuals, often with other complications. Weed et al. (1943) reported the deaths of two children, 3 and 4 years of age, who died within 24 h after each drank 125 ml of milk from a goat with staphylococcal mastitis. The deaths of the children and the results of the autopsy indicated that the children received a relatively large amount of enterotoxin in the milk they drank.

Several deaths of older people who consumed food containing enterotoxin have been reported (CDC, 1969; Anon., 1971, 1975; Currier et al., 1973); the deaths usually occurred after severe vomiting and diarrhea. One elderly woman died of acute vascular collapse secondary to fulminating gastroenteritis in an outbreak of staphylococcal food poisoning that occurred in Wisconsin in 1968 (CDC, 1969). The illness developed $1^1/_4$–3 h after eating. Twenty-eight people were known to have become ill with symptoms characterized by vomiting, diarrhea, and severe prostration; of these, six individuals required hospitalization. Baked ham obtained from a food store was the vehicle of infection. The sliced ham was kept in a roaster at 120°F awaiting sale. *Staphylococcus aureus* cultures from the implicated ham slices, the wood block cutting table, and a nasal swab from the food handler produced enterotoxin A (SEA).

A 57-year-old woman reported to have been in excellent health died in shock within a few hours of the onset of illness after eating a cold plate lunch at a restaurant in Montgomery, Alabama (Currier et al., 1973). Three other individuals developed severe gastroenteritis after eating plate lunches at the same restaurant. SEA-producing staphylococci of phage type 83A/85 were cultured from sliced ham and from the chronically infected thumbnails of the cook who had baked and hand-sliced it.

2. *Detection of Enterotoxin in Food*

The detection of enterotoxin in a food implicated in food poisoning is acceptable proof of staphylococcal food poisoning. The methods for detection of the enterotoxin in foods are borderline for detection of the small amounts of enterotoxin that may be present (0.5 ng/g); hence, the detection of any amount of enterotoxin is considered adequate proof of food poisoning. This was demonstrated in the food-poisoning outbreak from chocolate milk which contained as little as 0.4 ng/ml of milk (Evenson et al., 1988). The symptoms of the illness were those of staphylococcal food poisoning, but no staphylococci could be isolated from the milk. The method used for analysis of the milk was an enzyme-linked immunosorbent assay (ELISA) (Freed et al., 1982). Commercial ELISA kits are available for this purpose.

3. *Determination of Contamination Source*

Phage typing of staphylococci has been used for many years as an epidemiological tool in tracing the source of contamination in food-poisoning outbreaks. In many instances the phage-typing data can pinpoint the source of an outbreak; however, this is not always the case. For example, in one food-poisoning outbreak, two food handlers carried in their throats staphylococci of the same phage pattern as staphylococci isolated from the suspect food, but organisms from only one of the individuals produced enterotoxins. Checking food-poisoning–associated staphylococcal isolates for enterotoxin production is as important as phage typing. It is not always possible to trace the source of the organism by determining enterotoxin production alone, because sometimes organisms isolated from different food handlers may produce the same enterotoxin. In this case the combination of phage typing and enterotoxin type produced is very important. In at least one food-poisoning case, the enterotoxin type was very important because the organism located from the food was not phage typable. There was no question about the source in this case because the enterotoxin produced was E (SEE), which is infrequently involved in food-poisoning outbreaks.

B. Amount of Enterotoxin Required for Illness

Normally, the amount of enterotoxin present in foods is relatively small, usually 5–10 ng/g of food, hence the amount of enterotoxin required to result in death would seldom be present. Results of the examination of food implicated in food-poisoning outbreaks for the presence of enterotoxin have indicated that considerably less than 1 μg of toxin (as little as 100 ng) may be sufficient to produce symptoms in sensitive individuals (Reiser et al., 1974). However, it was not until the fall of 1985 that an opportunity was presented to obtain a good estimate of the amount necessary to produce illness in sensitive individuals. This occurred when more than 850 school children became ill with typical staphylococcal food-poisoning symptoms after drinking 2% chocolate milk (Evenson et al., 1988). Analysis of 12 $^1/_2$-pint cartons of the 2% chocolate milk revealed an average of 144 ng of SEA per carton, with a range of 94–187 ng/carton (Table 3). Most of those who became ill had drunk only one carton of the milk.

C. The Enterotoxins

The enterotoxins are a series of low molecular weight proteins (27,000–29,000 daltons) that are similar in their reactivity and composition but are identified as separate proteins because of their antigenic differences (Bergdoll, 1989). On this basis they are labeled enterotoxins A (SEA), B (SEB), C (SEC), etc. (Casman et al., 1963), with each reacting with a different antibody. They are classed as enterotoxins because of the emetic and diarrheal reaction they elicit when taken intragastrically. Seven enterotoxins have been identified, purified, and characterized, but this is not an integral part of the discussion here except to identify the chemical nature of the enterotoxins that are responsible for the rather violent reactions sometimes seen in humans.

Table 3 Enterotoxin Analysis in 2% Chocolate Milk

Sample	Enterotoxin A (ng/ml)	Enterotoxin A (ng/½ pint)
1	0.40	94
2	0.73	172
3	0.48	113
4	0.63	149
5	0.78	184
6	0.65	153
Average	0.61	144

Source: Evenson et al., 1988.

II. EPIDEMIOLOGY

It is necessary for enterotoxigenic staphylococci to grow and produce enterotoxin in foods before food poisoning can occur; however, certain conditions are necessary for this to take place: (1) the food must be a good medium for growth of staphylococci; (2) enterotoxigenic staphylococci must be present in the food; and (3) adequate conditions must exist for the staphylococci to grow and produce enterotoxin (sufficient time at a warm temperature).

A. Foods Involved in Outbreaks

Many foods provide a good medium for the growth of the staphylococci. Examples include dairy products, various types of salads, and cooked meats such as baked ham.

1. *Dairy Products*

Milk is rarely involved in staphylococcal food poisoning in the United States, however, the outbreak from chocolate milk among school children in Kentucky in 1985 was exceptional (Evenson et al., 1988). SEA was detected in the milk even though staphylococci could not be isolated from the milk. Accidently, warm instead of cold water had been circulated in the milk holding tank for 4–5 h before the milk was pasteurized, during which time the staphylococci grew and produced enterotoxin. Unfortunately, enterotoxin is not inactivated by pasteurization.

In more recent times food-poisoning outbreaks from cream-filled bakery goods such as the one from eclairs used as an example of a typical mass-feeding outbreak are infrequent, probably because greater care is taken in handling such foods, particularly during the warmer months. Apparently this is not true in some countries, as chocolate eclairs were implicated in illnesses on an airplane flight in 1976 from Rio de Janeiro to New York City; approximately half of the 153 passengers served the eclairs became ill 2–3 h following the meal at which the eclairs were served (CDC, 1976c). The eclairs had been left unrefrigerated from 8:30 a.m. until

10:30 p.m., when they were placed on the plane, *S. aureus* (10^9/g) that produced enterotoxin D (SED) was isolated from the eclairs, and SED was detected in the eclairs.

Cream-filled cakes have been implicated in several staphylococcal food-poisoning outbreaks. A relatively large outbreak resulting from the consumption of cream-filled coffee cakes occurred in Wisconsin in 1970; this outbreak is used later to illustrate the importance of refrigeration in prevention of this type of food poisoning. An outbreak occurred in Spain from Easter cakes with a cream filling that were widely distributed. They were the suspected cause of 1800 illnesses with typical staphylococcal food-poisoning symptoms. The cream filling contained more than 5×10^6 staphylococci/g, which produced SEA. The source of the staphylococci was not determined as the only human staphylococci isolate obtained produced SEB.

Many outbreaks have occurred from the consumption of cheese, although with the advent of the use of pasteurized milk in cheese manufacture, fewer problems have been encountered. However, a number of people became ill from eating cheese that had been manufactured in a plant that was using pasteurized milk (Zehren and Zehren, 1968). In this case the pasteurized milk had become recontaminated with staphylococci through a leaky valve. The staphylococci isolated from the valve and the cheese produced SEA; SEA was detected in the cheese. Even so, there would have been no problem except that a starter culture failure allowed the staphylococci to grow in the vat and produce the SEA.

Ice cream is frequently involved in staphylococcal food poisoning in other countries, but has not been the cause of food poisoning in the United States. However, a staphylococcal food-poisoning outbreak did occur in the eastern part of the United States in which ice cream prepared commercially was implicated. The ice cream was distributed over a rather wide area, and illnesses were reported from several different locations. Enterotoxin was not detectable in the ice cream; it is not known whether it was present in any of the ingredients as none was available for analysis.

Many episodes of illness with features compatible with staphylococcal food poisoning were reported in Pennsylvania and nearby states in 1974 (CDC, 1974). In nine episodes involving at least 43 individuals, food histories implicated milkshakes purchased in several restaurants, all of which used a liquid milkshake mix made by a dairy in eastern Pennsylvania. The dairy voluntarily recalled the suspect lots of mix. A few weeks later, 37 episodes of illness, involving about 120 people, in which a liquid milkshake mix manufactured by a second Pennsylvania dairy was implicated. This dairy recalled all of its milkshake mixes and ceased production of milkshake mix. Whey powder from a single distributer was used in the mixes manufactured by both dairies. Cultures from the whey obtained from one of the dairies yielded enterotoxigenic staphylococci. The long onset time (5–6 h) for the appearance of the symptoms indicates a very low level of contamination in the milkshake mixes. Such a low level of contamination would be expected if an ingredient rather than postcontamination of a finished product was involved because of the dilution of the ingredient.

Butter is an unlikely food to be involved in food poisoning, primarily because of the small amount eaten at any one time; however, an outbreak occurred in 1977 when over 100 customers of pancake houses in the Midwest were made ill from whipped butter (CDC, 1977c). Staphylococci was found in relatively large numbers (up to 10^7) in some packages of the whipped butter. Some of the isolates produced SEA and others were nonenterotoxigenic (by monkey-feeding tests) indicating that the contamination was not of a common origin. SEA was found in small amounts in two packages of butter (70 and 150 ng/100 g), which is generally considered too little to cause food poisoning unless a large amount of the food was consumed. In the package with the smaller amount of SEA, the nonenterotoxigenic staphylococci outnumbered the enterotoxigenic staphylococci by 10–15 to 1. Considerable variation existed from package to package in the staphylococci present, both in numbers and type; hence, it could be concluded that the packages involved in the illnesses contained larger numbers of enterotoxigenic staphylococci than those examined in the Food Research Institute. The cream used to prepare the butter was pasteurized, but it apparently was recontaminated in some manner by the incoming cream during processing. The butter was distributed also to steak houses, but no one eating at these restaurants became ill, indicating that it is possible to consume enterotoxin in small amounts without becoming ill. This was the second outbreak in which butter was the implicated food. The other outbreak involved whipped butter that had been prepared from commercial butter that contained enterotoxin, apparently from the whey cream used in its manufacture (CDC, 1970).

2. *Salads*

Different types of salads—ham, chicken (CDC, 1968a, 1976b), tuna (CDC, 1968b), macaroni (CDC, 1973b), and potato (CDC, 1973a, 1980)—have been involved in staphylococcal food poisoning from time to time. Salad dressing has been suggested as a cause of staphylococcal food-poisoning outbreaks, but this is highly unlikely because salad dressing by itself does not support the growth of staphylococci. Actually, staphylococci cannot survive in salad dressing due to its low pH. The food from which the salads are made provide the nutrients for growth of the staphylococci, and mixing the main ingredients of the salad with the salad dressing moderates the pH of the salad dressing, hence, allowing growth of the staphylococci.

One outbreak occurred when 600 of 1000 high school girls who were attending a meeting in Crawfordsville, Indiana, became ill after eating ham salad sandwiches. The ham used to make the sandwiches had been baked, ground, and held at room temperature at least one day before making the sandwiches. Such large outbreaks occurring in small towns pose a considerable problem as the facilities for caring for those becoming ill is inadequate. In this case because of inadequate hospital facilities, beds were set up in the school gymnasium. Many of the young women became ill in transit to their homes or after they arrived home. The staphylococci isolated from the ham salad was not examined for staphylococcal enterotoxin because the outbreak occurred in 1958 before adequate information was available to analyze for enterotoxin.

One of the largest outbreaks of staphylococcal food poisoning to occur in the United States resulted from chicken salad consumed by school children in Laredo, Texas (CDC, 1968a). A total of 1364 of 5824 children who ate lunch in elementary school cafeterias became ill with abdominal cramps, vomiting, and diarrhea in 1–9 h; about half of those ill required treatment at a hospital. Food histories implicated the chicken salad. The chicken was prepared in a central kitchen and distributed to the various elementary schools. The day before the outbreak, the chickens were boiled for 3 h, cooled and deboned, ground into small pieces, placed in 12-inch-deep aluminum pans, and stored overnight in a cooler which was maintained at 42–45°F. The following morning, pickles, pimento, and mayonnaise were added to the chicken, and the mixture was blended in an electric mixer. The food was placed in thermal carriers and transported to the schools by trucks. The schools had no facilities for refrigerating food; the salad was kept at room temperature until it was served between 11:30 a.m. and noon. March 21 was a cold day in Laredo, and the heating systems were operating in all class-rooms. At some of the schools, the food arrived at 9:14 a.m., and at others, at 10:30 a.m. The schools that received the food at the earlier time had a significantly higher attack rate (32.6%) than those which received the food at 10:30 (18.4%). *S. aureus* was isolated from the chicken salad, from a nasal culture of one food handler, and from throat cultures of two food handlers. No staphylococcal infections were noted in any of the food handlers. Further testing of the staphylococcal isolates were not reported.

Seventeen of 33 students and teachers attending a graduation banquet in West Virginia became ill with vomiting and diarrhea from eating potato salad (CDC, 1980). The attack rate was 79% among those who had eaten potato salad and zero among those who did not. The *S. aureus* isolated from the potato salad (3×10^8/g), chocolate pie (1×10^5/g), the deviled eggs (1.8×10^5/g), from the lesions on the two food handlers' hands, and the feces of one patient all belonged to phage type 83A/85. The potato salad and other foods had been stored for $4^1/_2$–12 h at room temperature before being served.

3. *Meats*

Many outbreaks involving large numbers of people have resulted from eating baked ham, primarily at picnics. One of the largest outbreaks ever recorded in the United States involved 1300 individuals attending a company picnic in Indiana. The signs and symptoms of ill individuals included vomiting and diarrhea, which occurred within 2–3 h after eating the baked ham. Large numbers of SEA-producing staphylococci were isolated from the ham, but it was impossible to trace the source of contamination because the food handlers who prepared the baked ham refused to cooperate.

Several outbreaks of staphylococcal food poisoning from salami, particularly Genoa salami, occurred in the 1970s (CDC, 1971a,b,c, 1975b, 1979a). This particular salami is made from raw meat, which is usually contaminated with staphylococci; it is fermented without heating, usually with use of a starter culture. Experiments at the Food Research Institute showed that sufficient growth of staphylococci can occur in the first 24 h before adequate acid is produced by the starter culture to prevent the growth of the staphylococci (unpublished data). Large numbers of staphylococci were often found in the salami involved, and both SEA and SEC were found in some sticks of salami. Apparently the problem has been resolved, because no more outbreaks from this type of salami have been reported.

4. Pasta

Occasionally other types of foods are involved in staphylococcal food-poisoning outbreaks, such as those that occurred in England, Wales, Italy, and Luxembourg in 1985 from dried lasagna prepared in Italy (Woolway et al., 1986). High counts of SEA-producing *S. aureus* (up to 2×10^8/g) were present in some packets of lasagna; SEA was detected in the lasagna at levels of 1–10 μg/100 g. Apparently the contamination originated with liquid egg that was inadequately pasteurized. The early stages of the pasta manufacture, when the dough containing egg is mixed, shaped or extruded, and then dried slowly, provided a suitable environment for growth of the organisms. Prolonged holding of unrefrigerated raw pasta dough would have permitted prolific growth of the staphylococci.

5. Easter Eggs

An estimated 300 out of 850 children who had participated in an Easter egg hunt in California became ill with staphylococcal food poisoning (Merrill et al., 1984). Enterotoxigenic staphylococci isolated from the eggs were identical to those isolated from a nasal culture from the individual who had prepared the eggs. The cook stated that he had had a cut on his hand at the time of preparing the eggs. SEB was produced by both cultures and was present in the eggs. The eggs had been prepared 3–5 days prior to the Easter egg hunt and were stored at room temperature because of inadequate refrigeration facilities at the school where the eggs were prepared. The eggs were boiled for 10–12 min and were dyed while still hot. After the dyeing they were cooled in tap water. Prior to this outbreak, four small outbreaks occurred in Wisconsin from consuming Easter eggs. Boiled eggs are an unlikely food to be involved in food poisoning, however, it has been shown that staphylococci can penetrate the egg shell during the cooling process (Harbrecht and Bergdoll, 1980). In this outbreak, the cooling water was undoubtedly contaminated with the staphylococci from the cook's hand.

6. Mushrooms

Four confirmed and three suspected outbreaks of staphylococcal food poisoning associated with consumption of canned mushrooms from the People's Republic of China were reported in the United States during February–April, 1989 (CDC, 1989). At least 102 persons in the confirmed outbreaks became ill with nausea, vomiting, diarrhea, and abdominal cramps, and 16 were hospitalized. The mushrooms had been served with omelets, hamburgers, pizza, and at a salad bar in cafeterias or restaurants. Staphylococcal enterotoxin A was detected in unopened cans of mushrooms from the same lot at all four sites and in samples of the implicated mushrooms at three sites. All cans in these outbreaks were large, institutional-sized cans of pieces and stems.

B. Source of Contamination

Staphylococcal food poisoning results from enterotoxigenic staphylococci growing and producing enterotoxin in foods. The number of organisms necessary to produce enterotoxin is not known, but the best estimate is 10^6–10^7 per gram of food (Noleto and Bergdoll, 1980); however, it is not unusual to find 10^8–10^9 organisms per gram of foods that have been involved in food poisoning.

1. Inoculum Size

The size of the inoculum can vary considerably, from a cough or sneeze by a food handler who happens to carry enterotoxigenic staphylococci in his or her nose or throat, to contamination by a food handler with some type of staphylococcal infection, such as an infected cut on the hands. The smaller the inoculum, the longer it is necessary to hold the food at a warm temperature before problems are encountered. This can be demonstrated from an outbreak in which sliced ham was packaged by an individual who carried the same enterotoxigenic staphylococci in her throat that was isolated in relatively large numbers from the implicated ham. The ham was packaged on a Saturday morning and sold throughout the day without any of the purchasers becoming ill. The leftover ham was packed into a relatively deep pan, and although it was refrigerated, cooling would have been quite slow. On Sunday morning, the ham was removed from the refrigerator and warmed before being sold late in the morning. Those who purchased the ham on Sunday became ill with typical symptoms of staphylococcal food poisoning. SEA was isolated from the leftover ham.

This is in contrast to an outbreak from sliced baked ham at a postal employees picnic in Ohio; the individuals who ate the ham became ill even though it had been held only a few hours at a warm temperature before it was eaten. In this case, enterotoxigenic staphylococci isolated from the ham were identical to those isolated from lesions on the face of an individual who had sliced the ham at the location where it was baked. The hams were baked overnight and early in the morning of the following day were deboned, sliced, and placed in a warm oven (74°C) until it was removed at 2 p.m. and taken to the picnic grounds, arriving there at 3 p.m. It was a warm day (32°C) and the ham was not refrigerated. The ham was served at about 6 p.m.; people became very ill with vomiting and diarrhea at about the time they were leaving the picnic grounds. Those who prepared the ham sandwiches during the afternoon ate some of the ham and became ill, whereas those who deboned and sliced the ham remained unaffected. The ham was well inoculated because the individual with the facial lesions frequently wiped his face with his hands during the slicing operation.

2. Food Handlers

Staphylococci are ubiquitous, although their major reservoirs are humans and animals. The percentage of healthy humans who carry staphylococci at any one time varies from 30 to 50%, with 15–35% being persistent carriers (Williams, 1963). Hospitalized humans have an even higher carriage rate, ranging up to 60% (Munch-Peterson, 1961). At least two reports on the carriage of staphylococci by food handlers have been published. Untermann (Untermann, 1972) isolated *S. aureus* from the nares and/or throats of 99 (36.9%) of 268 food handlers in Germany. Mori et al. (1977) isolated *S. aureus* at least at one out of four times during the year from the nasal cavities, pharynx, hair, fingers, or feces of 74 of the 100 food handlers they examined in Japan. Staphylococci were detected in only 12 individuals at each of the four times the examinations were done. Nineteen (19%) of the German strains produced enterotoxin (only examined for SEA, SEB, and SEC), whereas 50 (50%) of the Japanese strains produced enterotoxin (examined for all enterotoxins) (Table 4). Food-poisoning outbreaks do occur from foods that have been contaminated by healthy staphylococcal carriers such as the outbreak from packaged ham.

However, more frequently, outbreaks result from contamination by food handlers with some type of staphylococcal infection, such as an infected cut on the hands. This is illustrated by the Easter egg outbreak in California; the source of contamination was undoubtedly an infected lesion on the hands of the individual at the time he prepared the eggs (Merrill et al., 1984). Both the *S. aureus* isolated from the eggs and the cook's nose were of the same phage type and produced SEB. The enterotoxigenicity of staphylococci isolated from human sources has been reported by several investigators; some results are listed in Table 4.

3. *Animals*

It is well known that animals also develop staphylococcal infections; mastitis is a typical example of a staphylococcal disease occurring in animals, particularly cows (Olson et al., 1970), sheep (Guitierrez et al., 1982), and goats (De Buyser et al., 1987). In addition to infections, most animal species carry staphylococci in their nares. Animal carriers are of less importance than human carriers because most food-poisoning outbreaks result from contamination by food handlers. Most outbreaks result from staphylococci growing in foods after the food has been heated. Heat treatment generally will destroy any staphylococci present before there is adequate growth for enterotoxin production. Enterotoxin is produced in the food by staphylococci introduced onto the food after heating. The major possibility for enterotoxin production in food by staphylococci from animal sources is in milk from mastitic animals, such as occurred with the deaths of two children after drinking milk from a goat with

Table 4 Enterotoxigenicity of Staphylococcal Isolates from Human Carriers

Source	No. of staphyloccocal isolates	No. of isolates producing enterotoxin	% of enterotoxin producing isolates
Healthy students	117	18	15.4
Healthy children	70	28	40.0
Food handlers	73	32	43.8
Food handlers	249	135	54.2

Source: Mori et al. (1977), Untermann (1972).

mastitis (Weed et al., 1943). It is possible that before the use of pasteurized milk in cheese making became common practice, staphylococcal food-poisoning outbreaks from cheese could have been due to staphylococci from the cows.

Raw meats are usually contaminated with staphylococci, but these organisms usually are destroyed when the meat is processed or heated before eating. Furthermore, even though raw foods such as uncooked meat and unpasteurized milk may be contaminated with staphylococci, these foods also are contaminated with other organisms that inhibit the growth of the staphylococci; the staphylococci are not good microbial competitors. The only time that unpasteurized milk is likely to be involved in food poisoning is when the milk contains a large inoculum, which can occur if it comes from a mastitic animal.

C. Temperature and Time

The food-poisoning outbreaks described above illustrate the conditions favorable for staphylococcal growth and enterotoxin production. In the case of the Ohio picnic, the ham was held at a warm temperature (32°C) for not more than 3–4 h before it was eaten by the individuals who became ill. However, a much longer period of time was required for enterotoxin to be produced in the packaged ham outbreak, partly because of a low inoculum and partly because of a lower incubation temperature (probably around 24°C). In general, the lower the temperature, the longer the time required for enterotoxin to be produced.

The inoculum in the California Easter egg outbreak would have been quite small also because it was necessary for the organisms to pass through the egg shells during the cooling process. The eggs (3600) were prepared 3–5 days in advance and were kept at room temperature because adequate refrigerated storage space was not available (Merrill et al., 1984). The time was more than adequate for the staphylococci to grow and produce enterotoxin.

III. LOCATION OF OUTBREAKS

A. General Public Eating Places

1. *Restaurants*

Eighty-one persons became ill after eating chicken salad at a luncheon in a restaurant. Staphylococci that produced SEA were isolated from the chicken salad and from an open lesion on the thumb of the cook who prepared the salad (CDC, 1975a). Organisms from both sources were of the same phage type. Inadequate refrigeration of both the cooked chicken and the chicken salad allowed the staphylococci to grow sufficiently to produce enough enterotoxin to cause the illness.

2. *Fast-Food Outlets*

A diabetic woman and two children became ill with staphylococcal food poisoning after eating hot dogs at a fast-food restaurant (CDC, 1977b). Coagulase-positive staphylococci were isolated from a rectal swab and vomitus specimens from the ill women, from a hot dog from the restaurant's serving line, and from an opened, but not from an unopened, box of refrigerated frankfurters. All isolates produced SEA. Employees at the restaurant had adopted the practice of removing frankfurters from refrigerated storage and holding them for extended periods on a warming tray at 120–140°F. They were then heated further by steaming as orders were received.

3. Vending Machines

In Denver 11 employees became violently ill with nausea and vomiting after eating Greek spaghetti from a food vending machine (CDC, 1977a). Investigation revealed that three other persons had become ill after eating Greek spaghetti from other vending machines supplied by the same firm. In addition, two employees of the catering firm, who had eaten Greek spaghetti the previous evening became ill. *S. aureus*, phage type 85, was isolated from the stools of two hospitalized patients, from the hands of one food handler, and meat used to prepare the spaghetti. All *S. aureus* isolates of phage type 85 produced SEA, whereas SED was found in samples of spaghetti and in chili samples from the food preparation area of the vending machine company. An employee with lesions on his hands had helped to portion cooked meat onto the spaghetti. The central commissary refrigerator at the vending machine firm was found to be inadequate; many hot food items remained at temperatures favoring growth of staphylococci for up to 8 h after being placed in the refrigerator. The widespread finding of *S. aureus* phage type 85 indicates extensive cross-contamination as a result of poor food-handling practices. The original SED-producing organism apparently had been overgrown by other strains. Something appears to be lacking in the investigation as the explanation that the staphylococcal strain producing SED found in the food was overgrown by the SEA-producing strain is inadequate. Adequate examination of the staphylococci isolated from the food should have revealed the presence of the organisms producing SED because they should have been present in relatively large numbers. It is possible that SEA was present in the food but below detectable levels by the methods in use at that time for detection of enterotoxins in foods.

B. Semi-Private Eating Places

1. Conferences

More than 80 of 230 participants at a literary conference in California became ill 3–14 hours after eating cheese tortellini prepared by a single food handler (Bryant et al., 1988). The day before the meal, 50 lb of tortellini had been boiled, allowed to cool for 3–4 hours, layered in plastic bags, and stored in a small refrigerator. The following morning the pasta was mixed by hand with a cheese sauce, packed in shallow pans, transported to the conference site, and reheated in large ovens. The tortellini before reheating had an *S. aureus* count of 6×10^7 cfu/g; the reheated pasta had a count of 1.0×10^6 cfu/g. Isolates from the tortellini and from the hands and nares of the food handler produced SEA and SEC. The reheated tortellini contained SEA at a concentration of 0.9 μg/100 g; SEC was not detected.

2. Hospitals

An outbreak of food poisoning occurred on September 3, 1968, in Ponce, Puerto Rico, among doctors, nurses, student nurses, and employees of the Ponce District hospital (CDC, 1968c). The illnesses followed a luncheon in the hospital cafeteria. Of 446 employees eligible to eat at the noon meal, as many as 143 individuals may have become ill with an attack rate of 32%. The symptoms were those of staphylococcal food poisoning. Ham was implicated as the vehicle of infection. The ham was prepared by a catering service on the day of the outbreak and delivered to the cafeteria. *S. aureus* was isolated from leftover ham, vomitus from patients, and from the nose and throat of the food handlers at the catering service. Inspection of the caterer's kitchen facilities revealed violations of recommended sanitary practices.

3. Picnics and Outings

Some of the largest outbreaks have occurred at picnics, due primarily to baked ham sandwiches. Two outbreaks, the Ohio and Indiana outbreaks, are used to illustrate other aspects of staphylococcal food poisoning. In a school outing in England, 30 children and 5 adults developed stomach pains, copious vomiting, and severe diarrhea after eating the school lunch prepared by the school kitchen staff (Communicable Disease Surveillance Centre, 1984). Large numbers of *S. aureus* were isolated from the egg (3.5×10^9/g) and meat (6.5×10^7/g) sandwiches. The sandwiches were prepared the day before the outing and were placed in large tins for overnight cooling. The tins containing the egg sandwiches were placed on a larder cold slab, and the tins containing the meat sandwiches were placed in the refrigerator. The temperature in the kitchen larder fluctuated between 15 and 27°C and the temperature in the refrigerator was 9°C. Apparently the ingredients of the sandwiches were contaminated during preparation, but no cultures were taken from the kitchen staff.

4. Wedding Receptions

Chicken salad was identified as the vehicle in an outbreak of staphylococcal food poisoning affecting 64 of 107 guests at a wedding reception in Delaware (CDC, 1979b). *S. aureus* phage type 95 was isolated from the salad, a food grinder used in its preparation, and a nasal swab from the person who prepared it. The chicken was cooked, deboned, and refrigerated in a large plastic washtub 2 days before the reception. The next day the chicken was ground with celery and onions, mixed with mayonnaise, and again refrigerated in the same tub. On the day of the reception the salad was held unrefrigerated for a total of 7 h.

5. Schools

A number of outbreaks have occurred in schools, such as the chocolate milk outbreak in Kentucky (Evenson et al., 1988) and the chicken salad outbreak in Texas (CDC, 1968a). In most of these outbreaks the food was prepared in a central location and distributed to the various schools in the area, such as was the case with the chicken salad. Transport of the food from the central preparation place and the storage of the food after delivery often allows time at nonrefrigeration temperatures for staphylococci to grow and produce enterotoxin. In addition, much larger numbers of children are exposed than if each school prepared its own food.

6. Senior Citizens Center

Forty-three of 87 senior citizens at the Senior Citizen Center in Kenosha, Wisconsin, became ill with classic symptoms of staphylococcal food poisoning after eating potato salad. The eggs, the presumptive vehicle, had been cooked, sliced, and cooled in very large vats in the refrigerator overnight. The next day the potato salad was made and the eggs added. The staphylococci isolated from the potato salad produced SED, the second most common enterotoxin to be involved in food poisoning. The concentration of the organisms in the salad was 5.7×10^7/g salad.

7. Military

A large outbreak of staphylococcal food poisoning caused by SEE occurred among soldiers on a march in England (Morris et al., 1972). Of 200 soldiers, 100 became ill after eating ham sandwiches and sausage rolls which had been kept for 30 hours at room temperature. Staphylococci, phage type 85, that produced SEE were isolated from fecal samples and from the ham (9×10^9/g) and the sausage (1.25×10^7/g).

C. Private Eating Places

1. Nursing Homes

Several residents of a nursing home became ill with vomiting and diarrhea after eating chicken salad sandwiches. None of the implicated chicken was available for testing. One of the food handlers who had manually mixed the chicken salad had lesions on her hands. Staphylococci were isolated from her nares and the hand lesions as well as from the stools of two of the nursing home residents who became ill. The culture from the food handler's nares produced SEA, and the culture from the lesions on her hands produced SEA and SEB. The culture from one of the stool samples produced SEA; one culture from the other stool sample produced SEA and another culture from the same stool produced SEA and SEB. This showed that the chicken salad was contaminated with both cultures from the food handler. Although the chicken salad was refrigerated, it was placed in a very large container, thus giving the organisms time to grow and produce enterotoxin before adequate cooling took place.

2. Jails

Seventeen of 19 inmates at a jail in Wisconsin became ill with vomiting and diarrhea 4 hours after eating ham sandwiches at lunch. Attack rate tables implicated the ham sandwiches as the likely food item involved. The leftover ham contained a count of 2.1×10^7 *S. aureus* organisms/g that produced SEA and the toxic shock syndrome toxin (TSST). Also, staphylococci that produced SEA and TSST were isolated from the stool samples from several of those who became ill. A nasalpharyngeal isolate from one of the food handlers produced SEA and TSST.

D. Public Transportation

1. Airplanes

Many smaller outbreaks following the consumption of baked ham have been reported including one that occurred on a Japanese airplane en route from Tokyo to Paris with intermediate stops in Anchorage, Alaska, and Copenhagen, Denmark (Eisenberg et al., 1975). The 344 passengers were served a breakfast of ham and omelette (prepared in Anchorage) during their flight to Copenhagen. Passengers began experiencing symptoms of vomiting and diarrhea shortly before they arrived in Copenhagen and about 1 h after the breakfast was served. One-hundred and ninety-six (57%) of the 344 passengers and one steward became ill, with 143 needing hospitalization in Copenhagen. About half of these patients had temperatures above 38°C; 14 had systolic blood pressure readings below 100 mm Hg; and 9 had bloody diarrhea. Two patients, previously in good health, had severe complications. A 52-year-old man developed shock and anuria, and a 64-year-old woman had a transitory cerebral ischemia with hemiparesis. The source of illness was the ham that was prepared by a cook who had lesions on his hand from which enterotoxigenic staphylococci were isolated. Enterotoxin was detected in the leftover ham. Only those who ate the ham handled by the cook with the lesions were ill (86%), whereas none of those who ate ham prepared by another cook became ill. The ham had been held at room temperature for about 6 hours during preparation of the meal and for another 8 hours in the plane's galleys before being served, with an interval of $14^1/_2$ hours at 10°C between the two periods at room temperature.

This outbreak and two others (CDC, 1973c, 1976c) that occurred on airplanes are of considerable concern. It cannot be overemphasized that foods for airplane passengers be prepared under careful supervision as an outbreak during a long-distance flight could be a serious matter. Food for the airlines is prepared in many cities around the world, some in countries where little attention is paid to proper handling of foods. Problems are more apt to arise in the developing countries where little attention is paid to staphylococcal food poisoning. This type of food poisoning is of greater concern than other types of food poisoning on planes because of its short incubation period. Only by chance did the cockpit crew on the Japanese flight eat a different meal from that served the passengers. It is urged that individual members of a cockpit crew each eat a different meal prepared by different cooks.

2. Trains

The illness of about 200 passengers on an excursion train traveling through Kentucky, Tennessee, and North and South Carolina was traced to box lunches served during a stop at a restaurant in Tennessee (CDC, 1976a). At least 55 victims were hospitalized. At various stages during preparation, the hams had been stored in a walk-in refrigerator which at one point registered a temperature of 57°F. Staphylococci of one phage type that produced SEA were isolated from ham samples, a stool specimen, and a fingernail culture from a food handler. Ham samples contained SEA.

3. Cruise Ships

Cream pastries served at two separate meals were the suspected vehicle in an outbreak of staphylococcal food poisoning aboard a Caribbean cruise ship sailing from a U.S. port (CDC, 1983). Food histories implicated the pastries served at both meals. No pastries from these meals were available for culturing, but *S. aureus* phage type 85/+ was isolated from patients' stools and from a perirectal swab, a culture from the anterior nares, and a swab of a forearm lesion from three of seven crew members who had prepared the pastry. No deficiencies in food handling were revealed in an investigation of the ship's pastry kitchen.

E. Commercial Foods

1. Canned Foods

There have been several food-poisoning outbreaks following the consumption of canned foods of various kinds. Most frequently, the problem arises from larger cans that have defective seams, which allows the staphylococci to enter the cans during the cooling process. Sometimes the enterotoxin is present in the food at the time of the canning operation and is not completely destroyed during the processing. This appeared to be the case in some of the cans of mushrooms from China (CDC, 1989).

A series of outbreaks occurred in 1979 in four different countries from canned corned beef processed in five different countries. Most of the cases occurred in England from corned beef canned in Brazil (Mansfield et al., 1983) with a few cases from corned beef from Argentina and Malta (Communicable Disease Surveillance Centre, 1979a, 1979b). One outbreak occurred in Virginia from Argentinean corned beef (Anon., 1979) and another outbreak in Canada reportedly due to corned beef from Australia. The other outbreak was in France from corned beef processed in Europe. Most of the outbreaks were linked to corned beef packaged in 6-lb cans; faulty seams which allowed staphylococci to enter the cans during the cooling process apparently were the cause of the problem (Mansfield et al., 1983). SEA-producing staphylococci were isolated from the corned beef processed in Brazil, Argentina, and Malta. No staphylococci could be isolated from the European corned beef, but SEA and TNase were detected in the corned beef. Two other outbreaks of staphylococcal food poisoning occurring in Great Britain during 1973 were traced to commercially canned rice pudding and salmon (Anon., 1973).

2. Bakery Foods

An outbreak occurred from eating chocolate eclairs and "Boston Creme Pie" made by the same bakery in Ohio. Staphylococcal isolates from these food items were of the same phage type, and all produced SEA. A culture from one of the food handlers was of the same phage type but was negative for enterotoxin. This shows that not all cultures of the same phage type are identical. The food items involved stood at room temperature for several hours, again showing the importance of refrigeration.

IV. PREVENTION

A. Refrigeration

The only satisfactory control of staphylococcal food poisoning is refrigeration of susceptible foods except when they are being prepared and during serving. The lower the temperature, the slower the growth of the staphylococci, with little or no growth at refrigeration temperatures. An excellent example of the effect of refrigeration is the outbreak from cream-filled coffee cake that occurred in Wisconsin in 1970. Approximately 50 people became ill after eating the cake with different degrees of symptoms, depending on the length of time the cake stood unrefrigerated before being eaten. The cakes were made by a bakery and delivered to several stores at 5:30 a.m. on a warm Saturday morning; the cakes were not refrigerated at the stores. Purchases were made all day Saturday and on Sunday morning. Many who bought the cakes on Saturday did not eat them until Sunday morning, but in most cases the cakes were refrigerated by the purchasers. One family who bought a cake relatively early on Saturday morning and refrigerated it but did not eat it until Sunday morning did not become ill. No one who ate cakes purchased at the bakery became ill because the cakes were refrigerated at the bakery. The source of the staphylococci was from the throat of the food handler who had placed the cream filling into the cakes with his hands. The organisms isolated from his throat and the cakes produced SEE; not many staphylococci produce this enterotoxin, and its involvement in food poisoning is rare.

Some of the largest outbreaks of staphylococcal food poisoning have occurred at picnics, a number of these from baked ham sandwiches. This food item is an excellent medium for growth of staphylococci, which is not always appreciated because it is a cooked food. However, if the ham is recontaminated after the baking as was the case in the Ohio picnic outbreak, the results could be tragic. Providing refrigeration for such a large quantity of food is difficult at a large picnic and normally the food will be at the picnic for a number of hours before being consumed. In cases such as this, every effort should be made to provide refrigeration for the food at the picnic grounds or not transport it to the grounds until shortly before it is to be served.

One error that is frequently made is to place the food in large containers to conserve space before it is placed in the refrigerator. Under these conditions, cooling is very slow and allows sufficient time for the staphylococci to grow and produce enterotoxin. A staphylococcal food poisoning outbreak, in which 104 of 231 inmates in a county jail in New York became ill, resulted from macaroni salad being inadequately refrigerated (CDC, 1979c). The macaroni salad had been prepared the day before it was served and had been stored overnight in 2 large, deep containers in a walk-in cooler. Isolation of over 10^7 staphylococci/g from the macaroni salad indicated inadequate cooling.

B. Food-Handling Practices

In the jail outbreak it was ascertained that the food was prepared by inmates who were inadequately trained and not well supervised (CDC, 1979c). Many food-poisoning outbreaks are a result of inadequate training and supervision of the individuals preparing the food. The major conclusion from both the First and Second National Conferences for Food Protection held in Denver, Colorado, in 1971 and in Washington, D.C., in 1984 was the need for educating the food handler as well as the consumer on food safety. Unfortunately, very little has been done in this area.

C. Food Handlers' Infections

One method for preventing staphylococcal food-poisoning outbreaks is to prohibit food handlers with infections from handling foods. In some countries food handlers who are staphylococcal carriers are not allowed to handle foods as long as they are carriers. In England an assistant cook who carried the same staphylococcal organism in her nose as the one isolated from lemon snow pudding (Communicable Disease Surveillance Centre, 1978) involved in the illness of six adults and 101 children in a primary school was excluded from work until the organisms were eradicated by treatment with gentamicin cream. The pudding contained large numbers of staphylococci, 1.5×10^8/g, that produced SEA and SED, as did the staphylococci isolated from the nose of the assistant cook. Although it was feasible to exclude the cook in this case, usually it is difficult to bar workers who are carriers of staphylococci in their noses or throats from handling foods because approximately 50% of the population are carriers. On the other hand, food handlers with any type of infection should not be permitted to handle foods, particularly if the food is for mass feeding. The only viable solution to this problem is proper refrigeration of vulnerable foods between preparation and consumption.

REFERENCES

Anonymous. (1971). Death from staphylococcal food poisoning. *Br. Med. J. 4*: 244.

Anonymous. (1973). Food poisoning from canned food. *Br. Med. J. 3*: 461.

Anonymous. (1975). Staphylococcal infections: II. Food poisoning. *Br. Med. J. 4*: 293.

Anonymous (1979). Food poisoning outbreak traced to Argentina corned beef. *Food Chem. News xx*: 28.

Bergdoll, M. S. (1989). *Staphylococcus aureus*. In *Foodborne Bacterial Pathogens*, M. P. Doyle, ed. Marcel Dekker, New York, pp. 463–523.

Bryant, R. G., Jarvis, J., and Guibert, G. (1988). Selective enterotoxin production by a *Staphylococcus aureus* strain implicated in a foodborne outbreak. *J. Food Protect. 51*: 130–131.

Casman, E. P., Bergdoll, M. S., and Robinson, J. (1963). Designation of staphylococcal enterotoxins. *J. Bacteriol. 94*: 715–716.

Centers for Disease Control. (1968a). Food poisoning—Laredo, Texas. *MMWR 17*: 109–110.

Centers for Disease Control. (1968b). Food poisoning—Morton, Mississippi. *MMWR 17*: 348–349.

Centers for Disease Control. (1968c). Staphylococcal food poisoning—Ponce, Puerto Rico. *MMWR 17*: 377–378.

Centers for Disease Control. (1969). Staphylococcal food poisoning—Waukesha County, Wisconsin. *MMWR 18*: 21.

Centers for Disease Control. (1970). Staphylococcal food poisoning traced to butter. *MMWR 19*: 271.

Centers for Disease Control. (1971a). Staphylococcal gastroenteritis associated with salami—United States. *MMWR 20*: 253, 258.

Centers for Disease Control. (1971b). Gastroenteritis associated with Genoa salami—United States. *MMWR 20*: 261, 266.

Centers for Disease Control. (1971c). Gastroenteritis attributed to Hormel San Remo stick Genoa salami—Maryland. *MMWR 20*: 370.

Centers for Disease Control. (1973a). Staphylococcal foodborne disease—Tennessee. *MMWR 22*: 141.

Centers for Disease Control. (1973b). Type C staphylococcal enterotoxin gastroenteritis—Tennessee. *MMWR 22*: 285–286.

Centers for Disease Control. (1973c). Staphylococcal food poisoning aloft—Pennsylvania, Puerto Rico, New York. *MMWR 22*: 381–382.

Centers for Disease Control. (1974). Probable staphylococcal enterotoxin contamination of commercially produced milkshake mixes—Maryland, New Jersey, Pennsylvania, West Virginia. *MMWR 23*: 155–156.

Centers for Disease Control. (1975a). Staphylococcal food poisoning—Georgia. *MMWR 24*: 350.

Centers for Disease Control. (1975b). Staphylococcal food poisoning associated with Italian dry salami—California. *MMWR 24*: 374–379.

Centers for Disease Control. (1976a). Staphylococcal foodborne illness—Tennessee, North Carolina, South Carolina. *MMWR 25*: 49–50.

Centers for Disease Control. (1976b). Staphylococcal food poisoning—Florida. *MMWR 25*: 131–132.

Centers for Disease Control. (1976c). Outbreak of staphylococcal poisoning aboard an aircraft. *MMWR 25*: 317–318.

Centers for Disease Control. (1977a). Staphylococcal food poisoning—Colorado. *MMWR 26*: 22, 27.

Centers for Disease Control. (1977b). Staphylococcal food poisoning—Wisconsin. *MMWR 26*: 226, 231.

Centers for Disease Control. (1977c). Presumed staphylococcal food poisoning associated with whipped butter. *MMWR 26*: 268.

Centers for Disease Control. (1979a). Staphylococcal food poisoning associated with Genoa and hard salami—United States. *MMWR 28*: 179–180.

Centers for Disease Control. (1979b). Staphylococcal food poisoning—Delaware. *MMWR 28*: 445–446.

Centers for Disease Control. (1979c). Staphylococcal food poisoning—New York. *MMWR 28*: 45.

Centers for Disease Control. (1980). Staphylococcal food poisoning—West Virginia. *MMWR 29*: 367–368.

Centers for Disease Control. (1983). Staphylococcal food poisoning on a cruise ship. *MMWR 32*: 294–295.

Centers for Disease Control. (1989). Multiple outbreaks of staphylococcal food poisoning caused by canned mushrooms. *MMWR 38*: 417–418.

Communicable Disease Surveillance Centre (England). (1978). An outbreak of staphylococcal food poisoning. *Commun. Dis. Rep. 78*: No. 38.

Communicable Disease Surveillance Centre (England). (1979a). Canned corned beef from Malta. *Commun. Dis. Rep. 79*: No. 38.
Communicable Disease Surveillance Centre (England). (1979b). Corned beef—Argentina Establishment 1. *Commun. Dis. Rep. 79*: No. 48.
Communicable Disease Surveillance Centre (England). (1984). Staphylococcal food poisoning on a junior school outing. *Commun. Dis. Rep. 84*: No. 06.
Currier, R. W., II, Taylor, A., Jr., Wolf, F. S., and Warr, M. (1973). Fatal staphylococcal food poisoning. *South. Med. J. 66*: 703–705.
Dennison, G. A. (1936). Epidemiology and symptomatology of staphylococcus food poisoning. *Am. J. Public Health 26*: 1168–1175.
De Buyser, M. L., Dilasser, F., Hummel, R., and Bergdoll, M. S. (1987). Enterotoxin and toxic shock syndrome toxin-1 production by staphylococci isolated from goat's milk. *Int. J. Food Microbiol. 5*: 301–309.
Eisenberg, M. S., Gaarslev, K., Brown, W., Horwitz, M., and Hill, D. (1975). Staphylococcal food poisoning aboard a commercial aircraft. *Lancet ii*: 595–599.
Evenson, M. L., Hinds, M. W., Bernstein, R. S., and Bergdoll, M. S. (1988). Estimation of human dose of staphylococcal enterotoxin A from a large outbreak of staphylococcal food poisoning involving chocolate milk. *Int. J. Food Microbiol. 7*: 311–316.
Freed, R. C., Evenson, M. L., Reiser, R. F., and Bergdoll, M. S. (1982). Enzyme-linked immunosorbent assay for detection of staphylococcal enterotoxins in foods. *Appl. Environ. Microbiol. 44*: 1349–1355.
Harbrecht, D. F., and Bergdoll, M. S. (1980). Staphylococcal enterotoxin B production in hard-boiled eggs. *J. Food Sci. 45*: 307–309.
Guitierrez, L. M., Menes, I., Garcia, M. L., Moreno, B., and Bergdoll, M. S. (1982). Characterization and enterotoxigenicity of staphylococci isolated from mastitic ovine milk in Spain. *J. Food Protect. 45*: 1282–1286.
Mansfield, J. M., Farkas, G., Wieneke, A. A., and Gilberg, R. J. (1983). Studies on the growth and survival of *Staphylococcus aureus* in corned beef. *J. Hyg.* (Camb.) *91*: 467–478.
Merrill, A., Werner, S. B., Bryant, R. G., Fredson, D., and Kelly, K. (1984). Staphylococcal food poisoning associated with an Easter egg hunt. *JAMA 252*: 1019–1022.
Mori, M., Kato, E., and Hamada, S. (1977). Distribution of enterotoxigenic staphylococci in healthy food handlers and biological properties of isolates. *Jap. J. Bacteriol. 32*: 501–508.
Morris, C. A., Conway, H. D., and Everall, P. H. (1972). Food poisoning due to staphylococcal enterotoxin E. *Lancet 2*: 1375–1376.
Munch-Peterson, E. (1961). Staphylococcal carriage in man. An attempt at a quantitative survey. *Bull. WHO 24*: 761–769.
Noleto, A. L., and Bergdoll, M. S. (1980). Staphylococcal enterotoxin production in the presence of non-enterotoxigenic staphylococci. *Appl. Environ. Microbiol. 39*: 1167–1171.
Olson, J. C., Jr., Casman, E. P., Baer, E. F., and Stone, J. E. (1970). Enterotoxigenicity of *Staphylococcus aureus* cultures isolated from acute cases of bovine mastitis. *Appl. Microbiol. 20*: 605–607.
Reiser, R., Conaway, D., and Bergdoll, M. S. (1974). Detection of staphylococcal enterotoxin in foods. *Appl. Microbiol. 27*: 83–85.
Untermann, F. (1972). Contribution to the occurrence of enterotoxin producing staphylococci in man. *Zbl. Bakt. Abt. I Orig. A222*: 18–26.
Weed, L. A., Michael, A. C., and Harger, R. N. (1943). Fatal staphylococcus intoxication from goat milk. *Am. J. Public Health 33*: 1314–1318.
Williams, R. E. O. (1963). Healthy carriage of *Staphylococcus aureus*: Its prevalence and importance. *Bacteriol. Rev. 27*: 56–71.

Woolway, M. C., Bartlett, C. L. R., Wieneke, A. A., Gilbert, R. J., Murrell, H. C., and Aureli, P. (1986). International outbreak of staphylococcal food poisoning caused by contaminated lasagne. *J. Hyg. 96*: 67–73.

Zehren, V. L., and Zehren, V. F. (1968). Relation of acid development during cheesemaking to development of staphylococcal enterotoxin A. *J. Dairy Sci. 51*: 645–649.

3

Salmonellae in Eggs

Richard K. Gast, Nelson A. Cox and J. Stan Bailey

United States Department of Agriculture, Athens, Georgia

I. INTRODUCTION

Salmonellae are widely distributed in nature and are frequently associated with both wild and domestic animals. Present technology and processing methods do not result in raw beef, pork, poultry, seafood, eggs, or vegetables that are assured of being free of salmonellae. In this chapter, we will discuss *Salmonella* in eggs. This will include a discussion of *Salmonella enteritidis* and the table egg, which have received so much publicity since 1988. In addition, this chapter will discuss *Salmonella* contamination of fertile hatching eggs and the impact of that on the contamination of raw poultry meat.

II. HISTORY AND EPIDEMIOLOGY OF EGGBORNE *SALMONELLA ENTERITIDIS* INFECTIONS

A. United States

Egg-associated outbreaks of salmonellosis, generally attributed to either bulk egg products or cracked shell eggs, occurred frequently before enactment of the 1970 Egg Products Inspection Act (Philbrook et al., 1960; Sanders et al., 1963). Considerably fewer egg-associated salmonellosis outbreaks were reported after implementation of this legislation, which mandated the pasteurization of all bulk egg products and instituted federally supervised inspection to eliminate the retail sale of cracked shell eggs (Cohen and Blake, 1977).

In 1987, the Centers for Disease Control (CDC) presented evidence of a fivefold increase in the isolation rate of *Salmonella enteritidis* (SE) in the northeastern and middle Atlantic states between 1976 and 1985, whereas the isolation rate for all other serotypes increased by a factor of only 1.7. By 1985, SE had replaced *S. typhimurium* as the most commonly isolated serotype in several states in that region (CDC, 1987a). In 1989, 20% of all *Salmonella* isolations from humans in the United States were SE, surpassed only by *S. typhimurium* (CDC, 1990b).

The geographic range of involvement in the SE problem has been continually expanding. By 1987, an increase in reported SE isolations was evident in the south Atlantic states (CDC, 1988). Between 1985 and 1989, SE outbreaks were reported in 17 states and territories (Madden, 1990), and the proportion of SE outbreaks occurring outside the northeastern and middle Atlantic states rose from 5 to 43% (CDC, 1990a).

Another CDC investigation indicated that at least 6 of 10 northeastern SE outbreaks during 1986–87 for which a vehicle of transmission was identified could be linked directly to the consumption of raw or undercooked eggs (CDC, 1987b). The overall percentage of *Salmonella* outbreaks in the United States with known vehicles of transmission that were associated with eggs increased from less than 5% to more than 15% between 1973 and 1987 (Bean and Griffin, 1990). From 1985 to 1989, 244 SE outbreaks involved 8607 illnesses and 44 deaths (CDC, 1990b). Of 109 SE outbreaks during this period for which a food source was implicated, 89 (82%) were attributed to eggs. During the first 10 months of 1990 there were 49 SE outbreaks with 1646 cases (CDC, 1990b).

A highly publicized 1988 paper written by CDC epidemiologists (St. Louis et al., 1988) reported that, of 35 SE outbreaks in the northeast between 1985 and 1987 for which a food vehicle was identified, 27 (72%) were associated with foods consisting of or containing Grade A shell eggs. SE, moreover, was recovered in environmental samples from farms implicated in producing contaminated eggs. Furthermore, 10% of samples of bulk raw eggs from the Northeast (but none from other regions) were found to contain SE. Between 1973 and 1984, 44% of the human SE outbreaks were determined to be egg-associated, as contrasted with only 15% of the outbreaks caused by other serotypes (St. Louis et al., 1988).

A 1987 nosocomial outbreak at a New York hospital, traced to the use of raw eggs in the preparation of mayonnaise (Telzak et al., 1990), was illustrative of the epidemiology of eggborne SE infections. Phage type 8 SE was isolated from patients, pooled samples of implicated eggs, and a large percentage of ovaries of spent hens from the implicated flock. The percentage of egg-associated foodborne disease outbreaks ascribed to commercial or institutional establishments increased from 67% in 1973–75 to 100% in 1985–87 (Bean and Griffin, 1990).

The incidence of SE outbreaks (1973–87) has been particularly high in the warm summer months, when the opportunity for bacterial multiplication during handling, storage, and use is greatest (CDC, 1988). Some outbreaks, nevertheless, have been associated with no apparent breakdowns in proper food-handling techniques (CDC, 1988), and foods with as few as one raw egg have been implicated (CDC, 1990a). Even healthy adults have been infected with fatal consequences (CDC, 1990a).

The official response to the SE crisis has included a U.S. Department of Agriculture (USDA) testing program to identify infected poultry houses or flocks and to restrict eggs from these chickens for use only in pasteurized or boiled egg products (USDA, 1991). In addition, the Food and Drug Administration (FDA) has classified eggs as a "potentially hazardous food" and provided recommendations that eggs be properly refrigerated, not used raw or pooled for holding, and cooked and held at adequate temperatures.

B. United Kingdom

In recent years, SE infections have reached epidemic proportions in the United Kingdom, with human isolations in England and Wales jumping from 2071 in 1981 to 6858 in 1987 (Coyle et al., 1988). In 1988, public health officials reported a high correlation between phage type 4 SE infections and the consumption of foods containing shell eggs in four Welsh outbreaks (Coyle et al., 1988). Examination of data from 160 cases of phage type 4 SE in England, during a 2-month period in 1988, revealed that infected individuals were significantly more likely to have eaten foods containing raw or lightly cooked eggs than were uninfected control subjects (Cowden et al., 1989b). An SE outbreak in the United Kingdom that affected 173 people, some of whom became ill after an incubation period of less than 3 hours, was traced to eggs imported from Denmark (Stevens et al., 1989). In two SE outbreaks, one involving homemade ice cream and the other involving a dessert prepared by hotel cooks using raw egg white and lightly cooked yolk, phage type 4 SE was isolated from environmental samples taken from both farms responsible for producing the implicated eggs (Cowden et al., 1989a).

By 1988, eggs had become the most common source of *Salmonella* food-poisoning outbreaks reported to the U.K. Public Health Laboratory Service in which a food vehicle was identified (Bartlett et al., 1989). Eggs have also emerged as a principal source of salmonellosis in Western Europe (Perales and Audicana, 1989). Only 4% of the *Salmonella* isolates identified by the Division of Enteric Pathogens in the United Kingdom in 1981 were phage type 4 SE, but by 1988 this figure had risen to 46% (Bartlett et al., 1989). Nearly all (81%) of the SE isolates in the United Kingdom have been phage type 4 (Bartlett et al., 1989). In the United States, on the other hand, a variety of phage types (including 8, 13a, and 14b) have been involved and phage type 4 has not been epidemiologically important. Recent egg-associated outbreaks involving several *S. typhimurium* phage types have also been reported in the United Kingdom (Chapman et al., 1988; Mitchell et al., 1989).

A remark by a Deputy Health Minister that most eggs in the United Kingdom were contaminated with *Salmonella* had a devastating effect on the British egg industry as egg sales plummeted (Phelps, 1988). Broiler chickens in the United Kingdom were also shown to be infected with SE. In one survey, phage type 4 SE was isolated from 58% of broiler carcasses condemned because of gross signs of pericarditis and from 40% of fresh chilled chickens on retail sale (Rampling et al., 1989). As in the United States, efforts to control SE in the United Kingdom have relied on testing poultry to detect SE infections, with the subsequent elimination of infected birds. Recommendations regarding proper refrigeration and cooking of eggs have also been issued to protect consumers (Humphrey, 1990b).

III. IDENTIFICATION AND DIFFERENTIATION OF *S. ENTERITIDIS*

Explaining the high rate of isolation of SE in recent years and the frequent association of some SE strains with eggs requires an understanding of the attributes that distinguish epidemiologically important strains from other SE strains and from other serotypes. More than 2000 *Salmonella* serotypes have been identified, each characterized by a unique set of expressed somatic and flagellar antigens. *Salmonella* serotype *enteritidis*, based on somatic (O) antigen composition, is classified as a member of group D (Krieg and Holt, 1984). This group also includes *S. gallinarum* and *S. pullorum*, host-adapted serotypes that cause vertically transmissible systemic diseases in poultry (Pomeroy, 1984; Snoeyenbos, 1984). Unlike *S. pullorum* and *S. gallinarum*, however, SE is a motile organism and cannot be differentiated from other paratyphoid serotypes by any unique biochemical reactions (Ewing, 1986).

Phage typing, based on susceptibility to lysis by particular combinations of bacteriophages, has been useful for establishing epidemiological relationships in the United Kingdom and Western Europe, where most outbreaks have been caused by phage type 4 (Bartlett et al., 1989). An explanation for the prevalence of this single phage type is not yet available, although phage type 4 has been observed to be more invasive for chicks than phage types 7, 8, or 13a (Hinton et al., 1990). Loss of the ability of strains of phage type 4 to synthesize lipopolysaccharide was found to both alter the phage type (to 7) and reduce the virulence of the strain for mice (Chart et al., 1989a).

In the United States, no single phage type has been responsible for a preponderance of the outbreaks, although phage types 8, 13a, 14b, and 23 have been isolated most often. Phage typing was valuable for establishing an epidemiological linkage between SE isolates from patients, eggs, and laying hens in a 1987 hospital outbreak (Telzak et al., 1990).

The phage types of SE strains can be influenced, in some instances, by the presence of plasmids. Acquisition of certain drug-resistance plasmids, for example, was observed to convert a phage type 4 SE strain to phage type 24 (Frost et al., 1989). In a recent outbreak in a hospital in the Central African Republic, SE isolates were distinguished from U.S. and European isolates by extensive drug resistance and a unique phage susceptibility pattern (Georges-Courbot et al., 1990).

Plasmids have been evaluated as potential sources of virulence factors responsible for the eggborne transmission of some SE strains. Specific plasmids have been associated with virulence properties of several *Salmonella* serotypes (Helmuth et al., 1985; Poppe and Gyles, 1987). Full expression of virulence for mice by phage type 4 SE has been found to depend on the possession of a 38-megadalton plasmid (Chart et al., 1989b). Plasmid profiles have also been useful as markers for determining epidemiological relationships of SE isolates (Sorum et al., 1990; Telzak et al., 1990). A comparison of the differentiation of SE strains by plasmid profile typing and phage typing showed that greater discrimination was obtained by phage typing, but that plasmid profiles provided a useful adjunct (Threlfall et al., 1989).

IV. *S. ENTERITIDIS* INFECTIONS OF CHICKENS

A. Pathogenesis and Consequences

A thorough understanding of the dynamics of SE infections in poultry is essential to the formulation of an effective strategy to interrupt the eggborne transmission of SE from laying hens to human consumers. Salmonellae cause disease by colonizing and invading the intestinal epithelium. In some cases, *Salmonella* penetration through the intestinal mucosa to the bloodstream is followed by widespread dissemination and systemic disease. SE is an invasive serotype in chicks (Popiel and Turnbull, 1985), but has not exhibited a level of pathogenicity for chicks that is markedly different from that of other paratyphoid *Salmonella* serotypes (Henderson et al., 1960). Chicks can be readily infected, involving both intestinal colonization and invasion to reach internal tissues such as the liver, with SE from contaminated feed (Hinton et al., 1989). Variations in the ability to invade to the livers of young chicks have been observed between phage types of SE, with phage type 4 doing so more frequently than phage types 7, 8, or 13a (Hinton et al., 1990).

Experimental infections of adult hens with some SE strains have led to intestinal colonization that persisted for several months (Gast and

Beard, 1990a), although in studies with other SE strains the duration of fecal shedding has been considerably shorter (Shivaprasad et al., 1990). In one study, intravenously infected birds shed SE for a longer period than did orally infected birds (Shivaprasad et al., 1990).

S. pullorum and *S. gallinarum* are host-adapted serotypes that cause systemic diseases in chickens involving dissemination to numerous internal tissues, including the ovary. Both diseases have been responsible for substantial morbidity and mortality losses to the poultry industry (Pomeroy, 1984; Snoeyenbos, 1984). Other (paratyphoid) serotypes, in contrast, have generally been found to lack consequential invasive ability in adult chickens (Cox et al., 1973). In a few instances, however, several paratyphoid serotypes (including SE) have been isolated from the peritoneum and ovary of mature chickens (Snoeyenbos et al., 1969).

In the United Kingdom, phage type 4 SE has been isolated from the ovaries of commercial laying hens (Hopper and Mawer, 1988), broiler breeders (Lister, 1988), and broilers (Rampling et al., 1989). Experimental infection of hens with phage type 4 SE by oral inoculation has confirmed that SE can reach a wide range of target organs (Timoney et al., 1989; Humphrey et al., 1989a). In the United States, experimental infections with phage types 8 and 13a have also resulted in dissemination of SE to a number of internal organs, including the liver, spleen, heart blood, ovary, oviduct, and peritoneum (Gast and Beard, 1990c; Shivaprasad et al., 1990). SE has been isolated from the internal organs of experimentally infected hens for as long as 22 weeks postinoculation (Gast and Beard, 1990c).

The isolation of SE from the organs of chickens is playing an important epidemiological role as an indicator that a flock is infected with an invasive strain of SE. In the testing program administered by the USDA, for example, final confirmation that a flock is indeed SE-positive is based on the results of organ culturing (USDA, 1991). Among 555 ovaries of spent hens from a flock implicated as responsible for a New York SE outbreak, 383 (69%) were found to be positive for group D *Salmonella* (Telzak et al., 1990).

The effects of SE infection on the overall rate of egg production by infected hens have varied with different SE strains. Large doses of some SE strains have significantly reduced the total egg production of experimentally infected hens (Gast and Beard, 1990a; Shivaprasad et al., 1990), whereas other SE strains have not demonstrably affected the egg production of infected hens (Timoney et al., 1989).

B. Detection

Thorough implementation of programs to reduce the spread of SE into poultry flocks from feed, equipment, pests, other flocks, and human workers is essential for controlling the incidence of SE in chickens (McIlroy et al., 1989). Reducing the eggborne transmission of SE to humans, however, additionally requires efficient and accurate detection of infected poultry flocks (O'Brien, 1990). Both bacteriological and serological approaches to SE detection have been investigated and applied.

Cloacal swabs do not consistently identify SE-infected birds, and thus do not reliably detect positive flocks (Cooper et al., 1989; Shivaprasad et al., 1990). Persistent fecal shedding of SE by infected birds (Gast and Beard, 1990a), however, suggests that bacteriological monitoring of the environment should be a sensitive indicator of the status of a flock. The USDA testing program, accordingly, relies principally on environmental testing for SE by a drag-swab technique (Mallinson et al., 1989) as a primary screening method, with organ culturing providing the final confirmation that a flock is infected (USDA, 1991).

The SE testing program also makes use of serological testing as an adjunct screening method (USDA, 1991). Serological detection of specific circulating antibodies was very useful in identifying infected birds as part of the control program implemented to eradicate *S. pullorum* in chickens (Snoeyenbos, 1984). Information regarding the serological response to SE, however, has not incontrovertibly established the usefulness of this approach for detecting SE-infected flocks.

Paratyphoid *Salmonella* infections, often involving minimal invasion and no systemic disease phase, can generally be detected serologically only by highly sensitive tests such as the microantiglobulin assay (Williams and Whittemore, 1979). Humphrey et al. (1989a) found no anti-SE antibodies in sera from experimentally infected hens, a few of which produced contaminated eggs. Cooper et al. (1989) observed, in a study of flocks with a history of natural SE infection, that antibodies could be consistently detected only by highly sensitive ELISA and microantiglobulin tests and that the presence of antibodies in particular birds did not correlate well with the isolation of SE from internal organs.

Hopper and Mawer (1988), on the other hand, reported that the presence of antibodies in the blood correlated strongly with subsequent postmortem isolation of SE from internal organs. Chart et al. (1990a) detected antibodies to SE lipopolysaccharide in a high percentage of serum samples from chickens in two naturally infected flocks. An ELISA assay using SE lipopolysaccharide as the antigen, however, identified infected birds less effectively than a whole blood agglutination assay (Chart et al., 1990b). Both agglutination and ELISA assays have detected significant antibody levels in flocks that are culture-negative for SE (Chart et al., 1990b). In experimentally infected hens, SE antigens were found to be more sensitive than commercially available *S. pullorum* antigens (another group D serotype) in rapid serum plate tests. Antibodies were detected in orally, intravenously, and intracloacally infected hens (Shivaprasad et al., 1990). Gast and Beard (1990b) experimentally infected hens of three different ages with large doses of SE. Plate, tube, and microplate agglutination tests all detected antibodies in a high percentage of inoculated hens, with antibody titers peaking within 2 weeks postinoculation and remaining at detectable levels for at least 10 weeks. Variations in antigen sensitivity were observed between antigens made from different SE strains, and between commercially prepared *S. pullorum* antigens. Hens horizontally infected by contact transmission of SE also gradually became seropositive.

The need to enter poultry houses to collect blood samples, potentially compromising biosecurity and stressing the birds, can be avoided by taking advantage of maternal antibodies that are deposited in the yolk of eggs. Detectable antibodies to SE have been found in egg yolk by ELISA (Dadrast et al., 1990) and microantiglobulin (Gast and Beard, 1991) methods.

The immunological response to SE may also offer opportunities for developing vaccines to protect birds against infection. Early results have shown that vaccines may have some potential for reducing the incidence of SE infections and the frequency of production of contaminated eggs in exposed flocks (Barrow et al., 1990; Cooper et al., 1990; Timms et al., 1990).

V. *S. ENTERITIDIS* IN EGGS

A. Production of Contaminated Eggs

Egg-associated salmonellosis outbreaks have occurred sporadically in the past in association with serotypes other than SE (Blaser et al., 1981) and in some instances have been traced to infected laying flocks (Philbrook et al., 1960). The mechanisms by which eggs become contaminated have always been the subject of considerable debate. Differentiation of transovarian contamination of egg contents before oviposition from penetration of *Salmonella* through the shell after the egg is laid is not easily accomplished. For one thing, gaining access to the egg contents for sampling without contamination by the shell is logistically complicated (Board, 1966). Penetration of the shell by *Salmonella*, furthermore, can occur very rapidly (Williams et al., 1968), even in the absence of a high moisture level (Padron, 1990).

Even before the 1970 Egg Products Inspection Act eliminated cracked and dirty eggs from the table egg market, the numbers of *Salmonella* that could be found in the contents of eggs was not especially high (Garibaldi et al., 1969). A survey of egg shells in 1980 found only 0.2% to be contaminated by *Salmonella* (Baker et al., 1980b).

Information gained from experimentally infected hens has not clearly identified any particular mechanism of contamination of eggs. When pullets were inoculated with six *Salmonella* serotypes, salmonellae were recovered from feces and shells, but not from the contents, of 1728 eggs (Mundt and Tugwell, 1958). In another experiment, no *Salmonella* were recovered from either the shells or contents of eggs laid by hens orally inoculated with *S. typhimurium* (Baker et al., 1980a). Forsythe et al. (1967) observed that even direct ovarian inoculation with *S. anatum* did not result in the production of contaminated eggs, although egg contamination did result after hens were inoculated with *S. pullorum*. Gordon and Tucker (1965), on the other hand, found that *S. menston* could be recovered from both the eggs and hatched chicks of infected hens.

Hopper and Mawer (1988) reported that phage type 4 SE was present in small numbers in some yolks and albumens produced by systemically infected laying hens. Mawer et al. (1989) found SE in the yolks or albumens of only 5 of 360 (1.4%) eggs from an implicated small flock in the United Kingdom. In contrast, Paul and Batchelor (1988) recovered SE from the contents of 5 of 10 eggs from another implicated British flock. Humphrey et al. (1989b) sampled 1119 eggs from two small naturally infected flocks in the United Kingdom and determined that only 11 (1%) had SE-contaminated contents. Contaminated eggs were produced by less than one third of these hens and the production of contaminated eggs was observed to occur in intermittent clusters.

Experimental infections have yielded similarly equivocal results, although valuable information about the dynamics of production of SE-contaminated eggs has been gained. Humphrey et al. (1989a) challenged 52-week-old hens with an oral inoculation of phage type 4 SE and observed that none of 255 eggs contained SE. A similar challenge of 18-week-old hens resulted in 4 of 375 (1%) of the eggs containing SE in the contents during a period of more than 3 months after inoculation. In another study involving experimental phage type 4 infections, SE was found in the contents of up to 15% of the yolks or albumens produced on particular days during the first 2 weeks postinoculation (Timoney et al., 1989). Shivaprasad et al. (1990) observed that hens infected with two of the three phage type 8 SE strains laid eggs with contaminated contents. When birds were orally inoculated with one of these strains, 3% of the eggs produced during the first 42 days postinoculation had contaminated contents and about 1% had contaminated shells; no contaminated eggs were detected after 14 days postinoculation.

Gast and Beard (1990a) infected hens of three age groups with a phage type 13a SE strain and sampled 845 eggs. Contaminated eggs were produced at a relatively high frequency, by both orally inoculated and horizontally contact-exposed hens, for a short period after exposure (up to 23 days postinoculation). SE was recovered from both whole yolks and albumens, but not from the contents of the yolks (free of yolk membrane). Far fewer shells were SE-contaminated, none after 12 days postinoculation, suggesting that shell penetration was unlikely to have been exclusively responsible for SE contamination of the egg contents.

B. Growth of *S. enteritidis* in Contaminated Eggs

Although very little definitive information is available, most evidence at the present time indicates that the numbers of SE in contaminated eggs are generally quite small. Gast and Beard (1990a) observed an increase in the frequency of recovery of SE from the contents of eggs laid by experimentally infected hens when the samples were incubated for 48 hours instead of 24 hours, indirectly suggesting that the initial levels of contamination were very low. Sampling eggs from naturally infected flocks similarly indicated that all contaminated eggs contained fewer than 10 SE cells (Humphrey et al., 1989b). Highly sensitive ELISA assays might be useful for detecting such small *Salmonella* numbers (Lee et al., 1989).

Any increase from this initially low level of contamination, as a result of bacterial multiplication during storage, is heavily dependent on temperature. Kim et al. (1989) artificially contaminated eggs by injection of SE into the albumen. When the egg contents were cultured after incubation at 4°C, a minimal increase in the number of SE was observed, whereas the extent of multiplication of SE during storage increased as the storage temperature rose above 4°C. Bradshaw et al. (1990) noted that the generation time of SE inoculated into egg yolk increased from 25 minutes at 37°C to 3.5 hours at 15.5°C, and growth ceased altogether at 7°C. Humphrey (1990a) inoculated SE phage types 4, 8, and 13a into egg yolks and observed no growth at 8°C, slow or no growth at 10°C, and relatively rapid growth at 12°C or above. In albumen, however, no growth was observed at any temperature. Baker (1990) likewise noted that SE strains survived and grew in yolk, but survived only a few days in albumen. Antibacterial components, including lysozyme and ovotransferrin, may make albumen an unsatisfactory medium for supporting extensive bacterial growth (Stadelman and Cotterill, 1986). Specific antibodies in yolk, however, have not been observed to have any inhibitory effects on the growth of SE (Bradshaw et al., 1990).

C. Eliminating *S. enteritidis* from Eggs and Egg Products

The effectiveness of various methods of destroying SE in eggs and egg products has become a topic of increasing importance to public health authorities and the egg industry. Such information is vitally needed in order to provide instructions to consumers and commercial or institutional users of eggs regarding safe preparation of egg-containing foods. Baker (1990) observed that the time/temperature requirements for destroying SE in eggs by various cooking methods did not differ significantly from similar requirements previously determined for *S. typhimurium* (Baker et al., 1983). Humphrey et al. (1989c) found that strains of phage type 4 SE, *S. typhimurium*, and *S. senftenberg*, when inoculated into egg yolk, could survive forms of cooking in which some of the yolk remained liquid. Moreover, when eggs were stored at room temperature for 2 days after inoculation, the SE population grew to such a high level in the yolk that no standard cooking method completely eliminated the *Salmonella*. Storage of SE cultures at refrigerator temperatures, on the other hand, has been found to increase their sensitivity to heat (Humphrey, 1990c). In another study, SE phage type 4 in homogenized whole egg was determined to be more heat resistant than phage types 8 or 13a and *S. typhimurium*, but less than the highly heat-resistant *S. senftenberg* strain 775W. All *Salmonella* strains tested were more heat resistant in yolk than in whole egg or albumen (Humphrey et al., 1990).

The elimination of SE in the preparation of commercial egg products has also been examined. Humphrey et al. (1990) concluded that SE phage type 4 should not survive pasteurization. Baker (1990) observed that pasteurization at 60°C for 3.5 minutes provided at least a 7-decimal reduction in the numbers of all but one SE strain tested. Radiation has also been proposed as a means of reducing the microbial loads in egg products. Thermoradiation has been reported to effectively inactivate SE in liquid whole egg (Schaffner et al., 1989), and gamma irradiation was found to effect a significant reduction in *Salmonella* levels in powdered eggs (Matic et al., 1990). The need to consider interactive effects of various treatments for reducing *Salmonella* levels in egg products is illustrated by the observation of Perales and Garcia (1990) that the antibacterial effectiveness of acidulants used in mayonnaise production was lower at refrigerator temperatures than under warmer conditions.

The FDA has recently classified eggs as a "potentially hazardous food," and recommended several general steps to minimize the chances of eggborne transmission of salmonellosis. The first of these recommendations is to maintain shell eggs at a storage temperature of 70°C (45°F) or lower until the eggs are sold or used. Second, the use of raw eggs should be avoided. Instead, FDA recommends the substitution of commercially pasteurized egg products in menu items (such as Caesar salad, sauces, and homemade mayonnaise, ice cream, or eggnog) that require uncooked eggs. Third, the pooling of raw eggs for holding before cooking should be avoided; raw eggs should be cooked immediately or replaced with pasteurized egg products. The final FDA recommendation is to always cook eggs adequately (to 60°C or 140°F) and to hold them at hot temperatures until they are served.

The importance of proper handling of eggs, particularly in institutional of commercial kitchens, is illustrated by two documented outbreak investigations. Telzak et al. (1990) reported that a hospital outbreak could be attributed to product abuse in the kitchen, wherein mayonnaise was made from raw eggs, added to a tuna-macaroni salad, and allowed to sit unrefrigerated for 5 hours before being served. Lin et al. (1988) discussed an outbreak that could be traced back to a restaurant breakfast bar, on which incompletely cooked scrambled eggs were placed and expected to continue cooking slowly at the maintenance temperature of the bar.

VI. SUMMARY

The incidence of *S. enteritidis* (SE) infections in humans has risen dramatically in recent years in the United States, the United Kingdom, and several regions in Eastern and Western Europe. Much of this increase has been attributed to the eggborne transmission of SE from poultry flocks to human consumers. SE causes a systemic infection of chickens, which can be detected by both bacteriological and serological techniques. Infected hens can produce eggs with contaminated contents, although such eggs are apparently produced infrequently and generally contain very small numbers of SE. Improper storage, handling, and preparation of raw eggs can permit multiplication of SE to highly dangerous levels. Effective disruption of the chain of transmission of SE from eggs to humans will require stringent sanitation efforts by poultry farmers to reduce the incidence of SE in chickens, accurate detection of infected flocks to prevent their eggs from reaching market channels, more thorough control over the conditions under which shell eggs are stored and handled prior to retail sale, and extensive education of home, commercial, and institutional users of eggs regarding safe and practical methods for preparing eggs for consumption.

VII. SALMONELLAE CONTAMINATION OF BROILER CHICKENS

When most people think of salmonellae and eggs they think about *Salmonella enteritidis* and table eggs. However, because more human salmonellosis can be traced to broiler carcasses than to eggs, the many other paratyphoid *Salmonella* serotypes and their penetration of fertile hatching eggs may possibly be of more importance to human health. The presence of salmonellae in hatching eggs has been identified as a critical control point in the control of salmonellae colonization of chickens.

The understanding of the problem has improved with the realization that the association of salmonellae with poultry is extremely complex and touches all levels of the integrated poultry operation. An international conference on salmonellae held in New Orleans, Louisiana, in 1984, ended with very pessimistic conclusions regarding the control or reduction of salmonellae due in large part to the reality that when contaminated chickens are presented for slaughter, the opportunity for spread of foodborne bacterial pathogens during processing is substantial, even under the best of conditions. Once the pathogens become attached to carcasses and fresh meat products, there are no acceptable chemical or physical means that can effectively eliminate them. If the means could be developed to substantially reduce or eliminate the intestinal colonization of chickens by salmonellae, then salmonellae-free chickens could be delivered to the processing plant, thereby eliminating or at least reducing the prevalence and levels of salmonellae on processed broilers.

To date, the most effective approach to prevent the colonization of live poultry by salmonellae has been competitive exclusion (CE). First reported by Nurmi and Rantala (1973), CE involves the oral introduction of intestinal microflora from salmonellae-free adult birds into newly hatched chicks. The CE concept was summarized by Pivnick and Nurmi (1982) as follows: (1) newly hatched chicks may be infected by a single cell of *Salmonella*, (2) older birds are resistant to infection because of the autochthonous (normal flora) microbiota of the gut, (3) the introduction of flora from an adult bird into a day-old chick speeds the maturation process of the gut microflora and increases the resistance of most chicks to salmonellae colonization. The CE concept has been conclusively shown in many laboratories around the world to be an effective approach (Nurmi and Rantala, 1973; Snoeyenbos et al., 1978; Rigby and Pettit, 1980; Pivnick et al., 1981; Bailey et al., 1988), but large-scale field trials have shown mixed results (Huttner et al., 1981; Goren et al., 1988). One reason for this is that commercial hatcheries and hatchery environments have been shown to be highly contaminated with salmonellae (Cox and Bailey, 1990) and this hatchery contamination can limit the effectiveness of CE (Goren et al., 1988; Nurmi, personal communication).

Therefore, hatchery contamination must be addressed and eliminated. In the interim, innovative means of applying CE that circumvent the present contamination must be sought. The presence and persistence of salmonellae contamination in the commercial broiler hatcheries suggest that the day-of-hatch chick may be at greater colonization risk from salmonellae in the hatchery environment than at subsequent times during grow-out. Contamination and penetration of the shell of fresh and incubating hatching eggs perhaps constitute the most important link (or critical control point) in the transmission of salmonellae to young birds and, as such, should be a primary target for any intervention procedure.

The probable mode of natural bacterial contamination of hatching eggs is the cooling of moist, freshly laid eggs from body temperature of the hen to air temperature in the presence of contaminating organisms. The hen brings soil and feces into the nest and these materials have been shown to contain microorganisms, including salmonellae. Eggs laid in wet, dirty nests will very likely be contaminated. It has been known for over 100 years that salmonellae could penetrate egg shells, and since that time, numerous studies have demonstrated the penetration and multiplication of salmonellae within the contents of both chicken and turkey hatching eggs. There exists significant variability in salmonellae penetration between eggs (Stokes et al., 1956). Shell quality (Sauter and Petersen, 1974), pH (Sauter et al., 1977), number of pores on an egg shell (Walden et al., 1956), temperature (Graves and Maclaury, 1962), humidity (Gregory, 1948), and vapor pressure (Graves and Maclaury, 1962) are some of the factors that can have an effect on bacterial penetration of eggs. The outer and inner shell membranes of an egg do offer some protection against bacterial penetration (Baker, 1974), but in spite of this several researchers have demonstrated rapid and deep penetration of the egg by various bacteria, including salmonellae. MacClaury and Moran (1959) demonstrated bacterial penetration beneath the inner membrane in 25–60% of the eggs tested on the day of contamination and albumen contamination in 10–15% of the inoculated eggs on the first day. Williams et al. (1968) demonstrated that salmonellae penetration of the cuticle and shell occurred almost immediately in some eggs. In fact, in one egg, penetration below both membranes was detected as early as 6 minutes following shell exposure.

Once organisms get past the membranes of hatching eggs, there is no way to prevent their further invasion of the egg contents or developing embryo. In addition, the warm temperature of incubation enhances the multiplication of salmonellae. Rizk et al. (1966b) demonstrated that the numbers of salmonellae that have penetrated an egg will greatly increase as the temperature of storage increases and that the conditions that exist during the incubation of a hatching egg tend to favor the proliferation of salmonellae. Hatching egg–sanitizing programs can only be effective if applied at the breeder farm level (Brown, 1989). Williams and Dillard (1973) demonstrated with *S. typhimurium* that a 90-minute penetration period on the egg shell prior to exposure to a chemical treatment allowed the organism to reach substance areas within the egg that were adequately protected from the germicidal action of disinfectant solution. This indicates that if a disinfectant is to be effectively employed to decontaminate a hatching egg, it must be applied almost immediately after the egg is laid. At present, most poultry companies gather eggs from breeder hens every 4–6 hours, and in some instances this may be 12–24 hours.

The idea of dipping or washing hatching eggs in disinfectant has been around for a long time (Pritsker, 1941), and a large number of chemicals and protocols of use have been tested in years past. However, the information generated in these earlier studies may be of limited value because inadequate methods were often used to recover sublethally injured cells of salmonellae. Also, when a chemical or chemicals were shown to be ineffective, too much time had often transpired prior to chemical treatment. For example, 30 minutes (Bierer et al., 1961a,b; Rizk et al., 1966a), 60 minutes (Frank and Wright, 1956), 3 hours (Gordon et al., 1956), 2 days (Mellor and Banwart, 1965), and

1–5 days (Lancaster and Crabb, 1953) were the time intervals between inoculation and application of treatment. We know from the later work of Williams and Dillard (1973) that these time intervals are too long.

Each year in the United States, the poultry industry processes about 7.5 billion hatching eggs through incubating facilities (Brown, 1989). Usually, the invading bacteria do not cause extensive decomposition of the egg, and the chick hatches from the contaminated egg (Maclaury and Moran, 1959). This results in the establishment of extensive bacterial reservoirs in the commercial hatcheries. Wright et al. (1959) analyzed more than 1000 samples from 120 commercial hatcheries and found high microbial populations. In recent years, commercial hatcheries have been switching from one chemical or chemical application method to another believing that the answer lies in either correct choice of chemical or how often or how much to apply. In general, chemicals have had little effect on salmonellae of hatching eggs as many researchers have demonstrated the presence of salmonellae in commercial hatcheries. Goren et al. (1988) isolated salmonellae from three commercial hatcheries in Europe and demonstrated that the *Salmonella* serotypes originating from the hatchery could subsequently be found on the final product (processed broiler carcass skin). Cox and Bailey (1990) isolated salmonellae from over 75% of the samples taken in several commercial hatcheries. It has been demonstrated that salmonellae organisms have the ability to persist for long periods of time in commercial hatcheries. Muira et al. (1964) found that over 50% of chick fluff samples in commercial hatcheries were contaminated with salmonellae and that hatcher fluff kept 4 years at room temperature still had 1,000–1,000,000 viable *Salmonella* cells per gram. That this situation exists even when fumigants and disinfectants recommended for hatchery sanitation are used suggests a review of the efficacy of many such recommendations.

The first approach to assure reduced salmonellae in the hatchery and in newly hatched chicks is to chemically disinfect hatching eggs. First, a sensitive method for recovering low levels of sublethally injured salmonellae from hatching eggs was developed. This was necessary so that various chemical treatments can be accurately assessed or evaluated.

Using this method, optimum chemical treatment(s) to disinfect hatching eggs are being evaluated. Chemicals are being applied at different concentrations, in different forms (e.g., dip, spray, foam, fog), at different temperatures, and within minutes and hours after *Salmonella* inoculation of the egg. Hatchability and livability of chicks following treatment of hatching eggs must also be determined to assure no adverse effects.

A second approach has been taken to circumvent any contamination which may get into the hatchery prior to exposure of the newly hatched chick to salmonellae. A novel technique for introducing CE into the digestive tract of the bird was developed (Bailey and Cox, 1990). The method involves the administration of CE to the air cell between the outer membranes or beneath the inner membranes of an 18-day-old incubating embryo. Early CE in ovo experiments produced treated chicks that were resistant to being colonized by high-level challenges of *Salmonella*, while the untreated animals were readily colonized with low levels of *Salmonella*. Refinements are required to optimize technology so that larger experiments (field trials) can be conducted to determine if in ovo is a feasible and effective method of administering CE in commercial operations.

To assure reduction of paratyphoid salmonellosis associated with the consumption of undercooked or mishandled chicken, salmonellae-free chickens should be grown and delivered to the processing plant. An effective method, CE, of preventing environmentally introduced salmonellae from colonizing the gut of chickens has been developed. For CE to be most effective, the salmonellae on fertile hatching eggs and in the hatchery will have to be controlled. Chemical disinfection of newly layed eggs and in ovo introduction of CE are approaches that offer opportunities to make the production of salmonellae-free chicks a reality.

REFERENCES

Bailey, J. S., and Cox, N. A. (1990). U.S. Patent Application Serial No. 07/362,635.

Bailey, J. S., Blankenship, L. C., Stern, N. J., Cox, N. A., and McHan, F. (1988). Effect of anticoccidial and antimicrobial feed additives on prevention of *Salmonella* colonization chicks of treated with anaerobic culture of chicken feces. *Avian Dis. 32*: 324–329.

Baker, R. C. (1974). Microbiology of eggs. *J. Milk Food Technol. 37*: 265–268.

Baker, R. C. (1990). Survival of *Salmonella enteritidis* on and in shelled eggs, liquid eggs, and cooked egg products. *Dairy Food Environ. Sanitation 10*:273–275.

Baker, R. C., Goff, J. P., and Mulnix, E. J. (1980a). Salmonellae recovery following oral and intravenous inoculation of laying hens. *Poultry Sci. 59*:1067–1072.

Baker, R. C., Goff, J. P., and Timoney, J. F. (1980b). Prevalence of salmonellae on eggs from poultry farms in New York State. *Poultry Sci. 59*:289–292.

Baker, R. C., Hogarty, S., Poon, W., and Vadehra, D. V. (1983). Survival of *Salmonella typhimurium* and *Staphylococcus aureus* in eggs cooked by different methods. *Poultry Sci. 62*: 1211–1216.

Barrow, P. A., Lovell, M. A., and Berchieri, A. (1990). Immunisation of laying hens against *Salmonella enteritidis* with live attenuated vaccines. *Vet. Rec. 126*: 241–242.

Bartlett, C. L. R., Davies, J. R., Gilbert, R. J., Roberts, C., Rowe, B., Smith, J. W. G. (1989). Memorandum of evidence to the agriculture committee inquiry on *Salmonella* in eggs. *PHLS Microbiology Digest 6*: 1–9.

Bean, N. H., and Griffin, P. M. (1990). Foodborne disease outbreaks in the United States, 1973–1987: pathogens, vehicles, and trends. *J. Food Protect. 53*: 804–817.

Bierer, B. W., Barnett, B. D., and Valentine, H. D. (1961a). Experimentally killing *Salmonella typhimurium* on egg shells by washing. *Poultry Sci. 40*: 1009–1014.

Bierer, B. W., Valentine, H. D., Barnett, B. D., and Rhodes, W. H. (1961b). Germicidal efficiency of egg washing compounds on eggs artificially contaminated with *Salmonella typhimurium*. *Poultry Sci. 40*: 148–152.

Blaser, M. J., Rafuse, E. M., Wells, J. G., Pollard, R. A., and Feldman, R. A. (1981). An outbreak of salmonellosis involving multiple vehicles. *Am. J. Epidemiol. 114*: 663–670.

Board, R. G. (1966). The course of microbial infection of the hen's egg. *J. Appl. Bacteriol. 29*: 319–341.

Bradshaw, J. G., Shah, D. B., Forney, E., and Madden, J. M. (1990). Growth of *Salmonella enteritidis* in yolk of shell eggs from normal and seropositive hens. *J. Food Protect. 53*: 1033–1036.

Brown, M. (1989). The scientists tell me . . . Glutaraldehyde tested as an alternative sanitizer for egg disinfectant. *Dairy Food Environ. San. 9*: 256.

Centers for Disease Control. (1987a). Increasing rate of *Salmonella enteritidis* infections in the northeastern United States. *MMWR 36*: 10–11.

Centers for Disease Control. (1987b). Update: *Salmonella enteritidis* infections in the northeastern United States. *MMWR 36*: 204–205.

Centers for Disease Control. (1988). Update: *Salmonella enteritidis* infections and Grade A shell eggs—United States. *MMWR 37*: 490, 495–496.

Centers for Disease Control. (1990a). Update: *Salmonella enteritidis* infections and Grade A shell eggs-United States, 1989. *MMWR 38*: 877–880.

Centers for Disease Control. (1990b). Update: *Salmonella enteritidis* infections and shell eggs—United States, 1990. *MMWR 39*: 909–912.

Chapman, P. A., Rhodes, P., and Rylands, W. (1988). *Salmonella typhimurium* phage type 141 infections in Sheffield during 1984 and 1985: Association with hens' eggs. *Epidemiol. Infect. 101*: 75–82.

Chart, H., Rowe, B., Baskerville, A., and Humphrey, T. J. (1990a). Serological response of chickens to *Salmonella enteritidis* infection. *Epidemiol. Infect. 104*: 63–71.

Chart, H., Rowe, B., Baskerville, A., and Humphrey, T. J. (1990b). Serological analysis of chicken flocks for antibodies to *Salmonella enteritidis*. *Vet. Rec. 127*: 501–502.

Chart, H., Rowe, B., Baskerville, A., and Humphrey, T. J. (1990a). Serological response of chickens to *Salmonella enteritidis* infection. *Epidemiol. Infect. 104*: 63–71.

Chart, H., Rowe, B., Threlfall, E. J., and Ward, L. R. (1989a). Conversion of *Salmonella enteritidis* phage type 4 to phage type 7 involves loss of lipopolysaccharide with concomitant loss of virulence. *FEMS Microbiol. Lett. 60*: 37–40.

Chart, H., Threlfall, E. J., and Rowe, B. (1989b). Virulence of *Salmonella enteritidis* phage type 4 is related to the possession of a 38 MDa plasmid. *FEMS Microbiol. Lett. 58*: 299–304.

Cohen, M. L., and Blake, P. A. (1977). Trends in foodborne salmonellosis outbreaks: 1963–1975. *J. Food Prot. 40*: 798–800.

Cooper, G. L., Nicholas, R. A. J., Cullen, G. A., and Hormaeche, C. E. (1990). Vaccination of chickens with a *Salmonella enteritidis aro A* live oral salmonella vaccine. *Microbiol Pathogenesis 9*: 255–265.

Cooper, G. L., Nicholas, R. A., Bracewell, C. D. (1989). Serological and bacteriological investigations of chickens from flocks naturally infected with *Salmonella enteritidis*. *Vet. Rec. 125*: 567–572.

Cowden, J. M., Chisholm, D., O'Mahony, M., Lynch, D., Mawer, S. L., Spain, G. E., Ward, L., and Rose, B. (1989a). Two outbreaks of *Salmonella enteritidis* phage type 4 infection associated with the consumption of fresh shell-egg products. *Epidemiol. Infect. 103*: 47–52.

Cowden, J. M., Lynch, D., Joseph, C. A., O'Mahony, M., Mawer, S. L., Rowe, B., and Bartlett, C. L. R. (1989b). Case-control study of infections with *Salmonella enteritidis* phage type 4 in England. *Brit. Med. J. 299*: 771–773.

Cox, N. A., and Bailey, J. S. (1990). Presence and impact of salmonellae contamination in the commercial integrated broiler hatchery. *Poultry Sci. 69*: 1606–1609.

Cox, N. A., Davis, B. H., Watts, A. B., and Colmer, A. R. (1973). *Salmonella* in the laying hen. 1. *Salmonella* recovery from viscera, feces and eggs following oral inoculation. *Poultry Sci. 52*: 661–666.

Coyle, E. F., Ribeiro, C. D., Howard, A. J., Palmer, S. R., Jones, H. I., Ward, L., and Rowe, B. (1988). *Salmonella enteritidis* phage type 4 infection: association with hens' eggs. *Lancet 2*: 1295–1297.

Dadrast, H., Hesketh, R., and Taylor, D. J. (1990). Egg yolk antibody detection in identification of salmonella infected poultry. *Vet. Rec. 126*: 219.

Ewing, W. H. (1986). *Edwards and Ewing's Identification of Enterobacteriaceae*, 4th ed. Elsevier Science Publishing Co., New York.

FDA. (1990). *Retail Food Protection Information Manual*. U.S. Department of Health and Human Services, Food and Drug Administration, Rockville, MD.

Forsythe, R. H., Ross, W. J., and Ayres, J. C. (1967). *Salmonellae* recovery following gastro-intestinal and ovarian inoculation in the domestic fowl. *Poultry Sci. 46*: 849–855.

Frank, J. F., and Wright, G. W. (1956). The disinfection of eggs contaminated with *Salmonella typhimurium. Can. J. Comp. Med. 20*: 406–410.

Frost, J. A., Ward, L. R., and Rowe, B. (1989). Acquisition of a drug resistance plasmid converts *Salmonella enteritidis* phage type 4 to phage type 24. *Epidemiol. Infect. 103*: 243–248.

Garibaldi, J. A., Lineweaver, H., and Ijichi, K. (1969). Number of salmonellae in commercially broken eggs before pasteurization. *Poultry Sci. 48*: 1096–1101.

Gast, R. K., and Beard, C. W. (1990a). Production of *Salmonella enteritidis*-contaminated eggs by experimentally infected hens. *Avian Dis. 34*: 438–446.

Gast, R. K., and Beard, C. W. (1990b). Serological detection of experimental *Salmonella enteritidis* infections in laying hens. *Avian Dis. 34*: 721–728.

Gast, R. K., and Beard, C. W. (1990c). Isolation of *Salmonella enteritidis* from internal organs of experimentally infected hens. *Avian Dis. 34*: 991–993.

Gast, R. K., and Beard, C. W. (1991). Detection of *Salmonella* serogroup D-specific antibodies in the yolks of eggs laid by hens infected with *S. enteritidis. Poultry Sci. 70*: 1269–1272.

Georges-Courbot, M. C., Wachsmuth, I. K., Bouquety, J. C., Siopathis, M. R., Cameron, D. N., and Georges, A. J. (1990). Cluster of antibiotic-resistant *Salmonella enteritidis* infections in the Central African Republic. *J. Clin. Microbiol. 28*: 771–773.

Gordon, R. F., and Tucker, J. F. (1965). The epizootiology of *Salmonella menston* infection of fowls and the effect of feeding poultry food artificially infected with salmonella. *Br. Poultry Sci. 6*: 251–264.

Gordon, R. F., Harry, E. G., and Tucker, J. F. (1956). The use of germicidal dips in the control of bacterial contamination of the shells of hatching eggs. *Vet. Rec. 68*: 33–38.

Goren, E., deJong, W. A., Doornenbal, P., Bolder, N. M., Mulder, R. W. A. W., and Jansen, A. (1988). Reduction of salmonellae infection of broilers by spray application of intestinal microflora: a longitudinal study. *Vet. Quart. 10*: 249–255.

Graves, R. C., and Maclaury, D. W. (1962). The effects of temperature, vapor pressure, and absolute humidity on bacterial contamination of shell eggs. *Poultry Sci. 41*: 1219–1225.

Gregory, D. W. (1948). *Salmonella* infections of turkey eggs. *Poultry Sci. 27*: 359–366.

Helmuth, R., Stephan, R., Bunge, C., Hoog, B., Steinbeck, A., and Bulling, E. (1985). Epidemiology of virulence-associated plasmids and outer membrane protein patterns within seven common *Salmonella* serotypes. *Infect. Immun. 48*: 175–182.

Henderson, W., Ostendorf, J., Jr., and Morehouse, G. L. (1960). The relative pathogenicity of some Salmonella serotypes for chicks. *Avian Dis. 4*: 103–109.

Hinton, M., Pearson, G. R., Threlfall, E. J., Rowe, B., Woodward, M., and Wray, C. (1989). Experimental *Salmonella enteritidis* infection in chicks. *Vet. Rec. 124*: 223.

Hinton, M., Threlfall, E. J., and Rowe, B. (1990). The invasive potential of *Salmonella enteritidis* phage types for young chickens. *Lett. Appl. Microbiol. 10*: 237–239.

Hopper, S. A., and Mawer, S. (1988). *Salmonella enteritidis* in a commercial layer flock, *Vet. Rec. 123*: 351.

Humphrey, T. J. (1990a). Growth of salmonellas in intact egg shells: Influence of storage temperature. *Vet. Rec. 126*: 292.

Humphrey, T. J. (1990b). Public health implication of the infection of egg-laying hens with *Salmonella enteritidis* phage type 4. *World's Poultry Sci. J. 46*: 5–13.

Humphrey, T. J. (1990c). Heat resistance in *Salmonella enteritidis* phage type 4: the influence of storage temperatures before heating. *J. Appl. Bacteriol. 69*: 493–497.

Humphrey, T. J., Baskerville, A., Chart, H., and Rowe, B. (1989a). Infection of egg-laying hens with *Salmonella enteritidis* PT4 by oral inoculation. *Vet. Rec. 125*: 531–532.

Humphrey, T. J., Baskerville, A., Mawer, S., Rowe, B., and Hopper, S. (1989b). *Salmonella enteritidis* phage type 4 from the contents of intact eggs: A study involving naturally infected hens. *Epidemiol. Infect. 103*: 415–423.

Humphrey, T. J., Chapman, P. A., Rowe, B., and Gilbert, R. J. (1990). A comparative study of the heat resistance of salmonellas in homogenized whole egg, egg yolk or albumen. *Epidemiol. Infect. 104*: 237–241.

Humphrey, T. J., Greenwood, M., Gilbert, R. J., Rowe, B., and Chapman, P. A. (1989c). The survival of salmonellas in shell eggs cooked under simulated domestic conditions. *Epidemiol. Infect. 103*: 35–45.

Huttner, B., Landgraf, H., and Vielitz, E. (1981). Kontrolle der Salmonelleninfectionen in Mastelterntier-Bestanden durch Verabreichung von SPF-Darmflora an Eintagskuken. *Dtsch. Tieraerztl. Wochenschr. 88*: 529–532.

Kim, C. J., Emery, D. A., Rinke, H., Nagaraja, K. V., and Halvorson, D. A. (1989). Effect of time and temperature on growth of *Salmonella enteritidis* in experimentally inoculated eggs. *Avian Dis. 33*: 735–742.

Krieg, N. R., and Holt, J. G., eds. (1984). *Bergey's Manual of Systematic Bacteriology*, Vol. 1. Williams and Wilkins, Baltimore, MD.

Lancaster, J. E., and Crabb, W. E. (1953). Studies on disinfection of eggs and incubators. I. The survival of *Salmonella pullorum, thompson*, and *typhimurium* on the surface of the hens' egg and on incubator debris. *Br. Vet. J. 109*: 139–148.

Lee, H. A., Wyatt, G. M., Bramham, S., and Morgan, M. R. A. (1989). Rapid enzyme-linked immunosorbent assays for the detection of *Salmonella enteritidis* in eggs. *Food Agr. Immunol. 1*: 89–99.

Lin, F.-Y., Morris, J. G., Jr., Trump, D., Tilghman, D., Wood, P. K., Jackman, N., Israel, E., and Libonati, J. P. (1988). Investigation of an outbreak of *Salmonella enteritidis* gastroenteritis associated with consumption of eggs in a restaurant chain in Maryland. *Am. J. Epidemiol. 128*: 839–844.

Lister, S. A. (1988). *Salmonella enteritidis* infection in broilers and broiler breeders. *Vet. Rec. 123*: 350.

Maclaury, D. W., and Moran, A. B. (1959). Bacterial contamination of hatching eggs. *Ky. Agr. Exp. Sta. Bul.* 665.

Madden, J. M. (1990). *Salmonella enteritidis* contamination of whole chicken eggs. *Dairy Food Environ. Sanitation 10*: 268–270.

Mallinson, E. T., Tate, C. R., Miller, R. G., Bennett, B., and Russek-Cohen, E. (1989). Monitoring poultry farms for *Salmonella* by drag-swab sampling and antigen-capture immunoassay. *Avian Dis. 33*: 684–690.

Matic, S., Mihokovic, V., Katusin-Razem, B., and Razem, D. (1990). The eradication of *Salmonella* in egg powder by gamma irradiation. *J. Food Protect. 53*: 111–114.

Mawer, S. L., Spain, G. E., and Rowe, B. (1989). *Salmonella enteritidis* phage type 4 and hens' eggs. *Lancet 1*: 280–281.

McIlroy, S. G., McCracken, R. M., Neill, S. D., O'Brien, J. J. (1989). Control, prevention and eradication of *Salmonella enteritidis* infection in broiler and broiler breeder flocks. *Vet. Rec. 125*: 545–548.

Mellor, D. B., and Banwart, G. H. (1965). Recovery of *Salmonella derby* from inoculated egg shell surfaces following sanitizing. *Poultry Sci. 44*: 1244–1248.

Mitchell, E., O'Mahony, M., Lynch, D., Ward, L. R., Rowe, B., Uttley, A., Rogers, T., Cunningham, D. G., and Watson, R. (1989). Large outbreak of food poisoning caused by *Salmonella typhimurium* definitive type 49 in mayonnaise. *Br. Med. J . 298*: 99–101.

Muira, S., Sato, G., and Miyamae, T. (1964). Occurrence and survival of *Salmonella* organisms in hatcher chick fluff from commercial hatcheries. *Avian Dis. 8*: 546–554.

Mundt, J. O., and Tugwell, R. L. (1958). The relationship of the chicken egg to selected paratyphoids. *Poultry Sci. 37*: 415–420.

Nurmi, E., and Rantala, M. (1973). New aspects of *Salmonella* infection in broiler production. *Nature 241*: 210–211.

O'Brien, J. D. P. (1990). Aspects of *Salmonella enteritidis* control in poultry. *World's Poultry Sci. J. 46*: 119–124.

Padron, M. N. (1990). Salmonella typhimurium penetration through the eggshell of hatching eggs. *Avian Dis. 34*: 463–465.

Paul, J., and Batchelor, B. (1988). Salmonella enteritidis phage type 4 and hens' eggs. *Lancet 2*: 1421.

Perales, I., and Audicana, A. (1989). The role of hens' eggs in outbreaks of salmonellosis in north Spain. *Int. J. Food Microbiol. 8*: 175–180.

Perales, I., and Garcia, M. I. (1990). The influence of pH and temperature on the behavior of *Salmonella enteritidis* phage type 4 in home-made mayonnaise. *Lett. Appl. Microbiol. 10*: 19–22.

Phelps, A. (1988). *Salmonella* scare in Britain could halve U.K. laying flock: Egg sales plummet 60%. *Feedstuffs, Dec. 19*: 3.

Philbrook, F. R., MacCready, R. A., Van Roekel, H., Anderson, E. S., Smyser, C. F., Sanen, F. J., and Groton, W. M. (1960). Salmonellosis spread by a dietary supplement of avian source. *N. Engl. J. Med. 263*: 713–718.

Pivnick, H., and Nurmi, E. (1982). The Nurmi concept and its role in the control of salmonella in poultry. In *Developments in Food Microbiology*, R. Davies, ed. Appl. Sci. Publ. Ltd., Essex, England, pp. 41–70.

Pivnick, H., Blanchfield, B., and D'Aoust, J. Y. (1981). Prevention of *Salmonella* infection in chicks by treatment with fecal cultures from mature chickens (Nurmi cultures). *J. Food Prot. 44*: 909–916.

Pomeroy, B. S. (1984). Fowl typhoid. In *Diseases of Poultry*, 8th ed. M. S. Hofstad, H. J. Barnes, B. W. Calnek, W. M. Reid, and H. W. Yoder, Jr., eds. Iowa State University Press, Ames, IA, pp. 79–91.

Popiel, I., and Turnbull, P. C. B. (1985). Passage of *Salmonella enteritidis* and *Salmonella thompson* through chick ileocecal mucosa. *Infect. Immun. 47*: 786–792.

Poppe, C., and Gyles, C. L. (1987). Relation of plasmids to virulence and other properties of Salmonellae from avian sources. *Avian Dis. 31*: 844–854.

Pritsker, I. Y. (1941). Researches on the hatching qualities of eggs. Disinfection of egg shell under increased pressure within the egg. *Poultry Sci. 20*: 102–103.

Rampling, A., Upson, R., Ward, L. R., Anderson, J. R., Peters, E., and Rowe, B. (1989). Salmonella enteritidis phage type 4 infection of broiler chickens: A hazard to public health. *Lancet 2*: 436–438.

Rigby, C. E., and Pettit, J. R. (1980). Observations on competitive exclusion in chickens. *Avian Dis. 24*: 604–615.

Rizk, S. S., Ayres, J. C., and Kraft, A. A. (1966a). Disinfection of eggs artificially inoculated with salmonellae. I. Application of several disinfectants. *Poultry Sci. 45*: 764–769.

Rizk, S. S., Ayres, J. C., and Kraft, A. A. (1966b). Effect of holding condition on the development of salmonellae in artificially inoculated hen's eggs. *Poultry Sci. 45*: 825–829.

Sanders, E., Sweeney, F. J., Jr., Friedman, E. A., Boring, J. R., Randall, E. L., and Polk, L. D. (1963). An outbreak of hospital-associated infections due to *Salmonella derby*. *J. Am. Med. Assoc. 186*: 984–986.

Sauter, E. A., and Petersen, C. F. (1974). The effect of egg shell quality on penetration by various salmonellae. *Poultry Sci. 53*: 2159–2162.

Sauter, E. A., Peterson, C. F., Parkinson, J. F., and Steele, E. E. (1977). Effect of pH on egg shell penetration by salmonellae. *Poultry Sci. 56*: 1754–1755.

Schaffner, D. F., Hamdy, M. K., Toledo, R. T., and Tift, M. L. (1989). *Salmonella* inactivation in liquid whole egg by thermoradiation. *J. Food Sci. 54*: 902–905.

Shivaprasad, H. L., Timoney, J. F., Morales, S., Lucio, B., and Baker, R. C. (1990). Pathogenesis of *Salmonella enteritidis* infection in laying chickens. I. Studies on egg transmission, clinical signs, fecal shedding, and serologic responses. *Avian Dis. 34*: 548–557.

Snoeyenbos, G. H. (1984). Pullorum disease. In *Diseases of Poultry*, 8th ed., M. S. Hofstad, H. J. Barnes, B. W. Calnek, W. M. Reid, and H. W. Yoder, Jr., eds. Iowa State University Press, Ames, IA, pp. 66–79.

Snoeyenbos, G. H., Weinak, O. M., and Smyser, C. F. (1978). Protecting chicks and poultry from salmonellae by oral administration of "normal" gut microflora. *Avian Dis. 22*: 273–287.

Snoeyenbos, G. H., Smyser, C. F., and Van Roekel, H. (1969). Salmonella infections of the ovary and peritoneum of chickens. *Avian Dis. 13*: 668–670.

Sorum, H., Bovre, K., Bukholm, G., Lassen, J., and Olsvik, O. (1990). A unique plasmid profile characterizing *Salmonella enteritidis* isolates from patients and employees in a hospital. *Acta Pathol. Microbiol. Immunol. Scand. 98*: 25–29.

St. Louis, M. E., Morse, D. L., Potter, M. E., DeMelfi, T. M., Guzewich, J. J., Tauxe, R. V., and Blake, P. A. (1988). The emergence of Grade A eggs as a major source of *Salmonella enteritidis* infections: New implications for the control of salmonellosis. *JAMA 259*: 2103–2107.

Stadelman, W. J., and Cotterill, O. J. (1986). *Egg Science and Technology*, 3rd ed. AVI Publishing Co., Westport, CT.

Stevens, A., Joseph, C., Bruce, J., Fenton, D., O'Mahony, M., Cunningham, D., O'Connor, B., and Rowe, B. (1969). A large outbreak of *Salmonella enteritidis* phage type 4 associated with eggs from overseas. *Epidemiol. Infect. 103*: 425–433.

Stokes, J. L., Osborne, W. W., and Bayne, H. G. (1956). Penetration and growth of *Salmonella* in shell eggs. *Food Res. 21*: 510–518.

Telzak, E. E., Budnick, L. D., Greenberg, M. S. Z., Blum, S., Shayegani, M., Benson, C. E., and Schultz, S. (1990). A nosocomial outbreak of *Salmonella enteritidis* infection due to the consumption of raw eggs. *N. Engl. J. Med. 323*: 394–397.

Threlfall, E. J., Rowe, B., and Ward, L. R. (1989). Subdivision of *Salmonella enteritidis* phage types by plasmid profile typing. *Epidemiol. Infect. 102*: 459–465.

Timms, L. M., Marshall, R. M., and Breslin, M. F. (1990). Laboratory assessment of protection given by an experimental *Salmonella enteritidis* PT4 inactivated, adjuvant vaccine. *Vet. Rec. 127*: 611–614.

Timoney, J. F., Shivaprasad, H. L., Baker, R. C., and Rowe, B. (1989). Egg transmission after inspection of hens with *Salmonella enteritidis* phage type 4. *Vet. Rec. 125*: 600–601.

USDA (1991). Rules and regulations: Chickens affected by *Salmonella enteritidis*. *Federal Register 56*: 3730–3743.

Walden, C. C., Allen, I. V. F., and Trussell, P. C. (1956). The role of the egg shell and shell membranes in restraining the entry of microorganisms. *Poultry Sci. 35*: 1190–1196.

Williams, J. E., and Dillard, J. H. (1973). The effect of external shell treatments on salmonella penetration of chicken eggs. *Poultry Sci. 52*: 1084–1089.
Williams, J. E., and Whittemore, A. D. (1979). Serological response of chickens to *Salmonella thompson* and *Salmonella pullorum* infections. *J. Clin. Microbiol. 9*: 108–114.
Williams, J. E., Dillard, L. H., and Hall, G. O. (1968). The penetration patterns of *Salmonella typhimurium* through the outer structures of chicken eggs. *Avian Dis. 12*: 445–466.
Wright, M. L., Anderson, G. W., and Epps, N. A. (1959). Hatchery sanitation. *Avian Dis. 3*: 486.

4

Escherichia coli Gastroenteritis: Food and Waterborne Infections

Peter Echeverria, Oralak Serichantalergs, Suchitra Changchawalit, and Orntipa Sethabutr

Armed Forces Research Institute of Medical Sciences, Bangkok, Thailand

I. INTRODUCTION

Escherichia coli are ubiquitous, being one of the major constituents of the intestinal tract of man and most animals. It was, therefore, believed that these bacteria produced no gastrointestinal disease. However, epidemiologic studies in Germany in the 1920s (Adam, 1923) and in England in the 1940s (Bray, 1945) suggested a role of certain *E. coli* strains in institutional epidemics of enteritis in infants. This thesis could not be adequately documented because methods for the identification of individual isolates were unsatisfactory. Not until the currently employed antigen classification system was introduced by Kauffman (1947) in the 1940s was it recognized that certain *E. coli* strains were associated with diarrheal disease (Kauffmann and DuPont, 1950). *E. coli* strains that cause diarrhea are now classified into four major categories: enterotoxigenic, enteroinvasive, enteropathogenic, and enterohemorrhagic *E. coli* (ETEC, EIEC, EPEC, and EHEC, respectively) (Levine, 1987). These strains cause diarrhea by one or more identified pathogenic mechanisms: enterotoxin production, enteroinvasion, attachment and effacement, and cytotoxin production (La Brec et al., 1964; Konowalchuk et al., 1985; Knutton et al., 1987; Levine, 1987). Many of these virulence determinants are encoded by extra chromosomal genetic elements (either plasmids or phages). Genes coding for these determinants have been cloned, and specific probes to identify these *E. coli* have been constructed (Echeverria et al., 1990). Recent investigations suggest that attachment of EPEC is plasmid mediated (Nataro et al., 1985a), while genes causing effacement (intimate attachment, destruction of microvilli, and disruption of the enterocyte cytoskeleton) are chromosomally encoded (Knutton et al., 1987). In this chapter, these four groups of *E. coli* will be described and their transmission from food and water discussed. Lastly, a newer technique to identify these *E. coli* strains in food and water will be described.

II. BACKGROUND

A. Enterotoxigenic *E. coli*

ETEC is one of the most common causes of diarrhea in young children in tropical developing countries (Ryder et al., 1976a; Echeverria et al., 1978b; Black et al., 1980) and is one of the leading causes of diarrhea in travelers (Merson et al., 1976; Echeverria et al., 1981). In order to cause diarrhea, ETEC require two virulence determinants: colonization adhesins and enterotoxin production. First, ETEC must adhere to the proximal small bowel. Intestinal adhesin is mediated by surface fimbriae. A number of adhesins have been recognized including colonization factor antigen (CFA) and *E. coli* surface (CS) fimbriae. The ETEC adhesins that have been recognized include CFA I (Evans et al., 1975), CS1, CS2, CS3, CS4, CS5, CS6 (Cravioto et al., 1982; Smyth, 1982; McConnell et al., 1985), and PCF 0159:H44 (Tacket et al., 1987). CS1, CS2, and CS3 in various combinations have been reported as CFA II (Cravioto, 1982; Smyth, 1982), and CS4, CS5, and CS6 as PCF 8775 (McConnell et al., 1985), now called CFA IV (McConnell et al., 1988). Genes coding for CFA I and CFA II are plasmid-encoded and are closely associated with genes coding for heat-stable toxin Ib (Echeverria et al., 1986). Additional colonization factors have been described, but it is not clear from the published data whether they are distinct from described adhesins (these include CFA II, presumably CS6 (Darfeuille et al., 1983; Darfeuille-Michaud et al., 1986) and CFA V, presumably CS5 (Manning et al., 1987)). Many ETEC have been isolated that do not have any of these adhesins.

Additional adhesins presumably exist and remain to be identified. These adhesins are the logical target proteins to which vaccines against ETEC could be directed.

The second virulence factor is enterotoxin, which causes fluid and electrolyte secretion. ETEC produce heat-labile, heat-stable enterotoxin (LT, ST) or both (Sack, 1975). The LT form is immunogenic and is composed of an A subunit of 25,000 daltons and five B subunits of 11,500 daltons each (Dallas and Falkow, 1979; Kunkel and Robertson, 1979; Clements et al., 1980). The A subunit of LT acts on small intestinal cells by stimulating adenyl cyclase with a resultant increase in intracellular cAMP (Moss and Richardson, 1978) and net secretion of electrolytes and water (Gill and Richardson, 1980). The B subunit of LT that attaches to ganglioside receptors on intestinal epithelial cells is involved in the binding of the toxin to intestinal cells and the delivery of the enzymatically active A subunit into the cell cytosol. LT produced by strains of *E. coli* from humans (LT-H) and pigs (LT-P) have common and unique antigenic determinants (Honda et al., 1981; Tsuji et al., 1982; Holmes et al., 1983). Antibodies to *V. cholerae* toxin (CT) neutralize LT-H and LT-P. These toxins have been designated LT-I (Pickett et al., 1986). LT-H ETEC strains have been isolated primarily from humans, and LT-P ETEC strains have been isolated primarily from pigs. LT-II originally described in *E. coli* SA 53 isolated from a water buffalo in Thailand (Green et al., 1983) resembles LT-I with respect to several of its biological properties, but is not neutralized by antibodies to CT, LT-H, or LT-P (Green et al., 1983). Two different types of LT-II have been identified serologically: LT-IIa from *E. coli* SA 53 and LT-IIb from *E. coli* 41 isolated from beef in Brazil (Holmes et al., 1983; Green et al., 1983; Guth et al., 1986a,b).

ST is thermostable, nonimmunogenic, and has a MW $< 5{,}000$ (Alderete and Robertson, 1978). One form of ST, ST-I, is soluble in methanol (Burgess et al., 1978), acts by stimulating guanylate cyclase (Field et al., 1978; Hughes et al., 1978) and causes distension of suckling mouse intestine (Dean et al., 1972). There are several forms of ST-I (Kapitany et al., 1979; So and McCarty, 1980; Moseley et al., 1982, 1983a); ETEC strains that produce ST-Ia have been isolated primarily from pigs and cows (So and McCarty, 1980; Utomporn et al., 1983). An *E. coli* strain that produces a second ST-I, designated ST-Ib, was originally isolated from a person with diarrhea in Bangladesh (Moseley et al., 1980). Almost all ETEC strains that produce ST-Ib are isolated from humans (Fig. 1), and ST-Ia ETEC strains from animals or food of animal origin (Table 1). A foodborne epidemic of ST Ia ETEC has been traced to cheese (MacDonald et al., 1985). Genes coding for ST-Ib are often associated with plasmids coding for CFA I and II (Echeverria et al., 1986). ST-II is a methanol-insoluble toxin that is active only in piglet jejunal loops (Burgess et al., 1978) and is negative in the suckling mouse assay (Dean et al., 1972). ST II ETEC do not appear to be a cause of diarrhea in man (Echeverria et al., 1984b, 1985a). ETEC have been described that contain genes coding for LT-I, ST-Ia, ST-Ib, and ST-II in different combinations (Moseley et al., 1983b; Echeverria et al., 1984b, 1985a, 1987a).

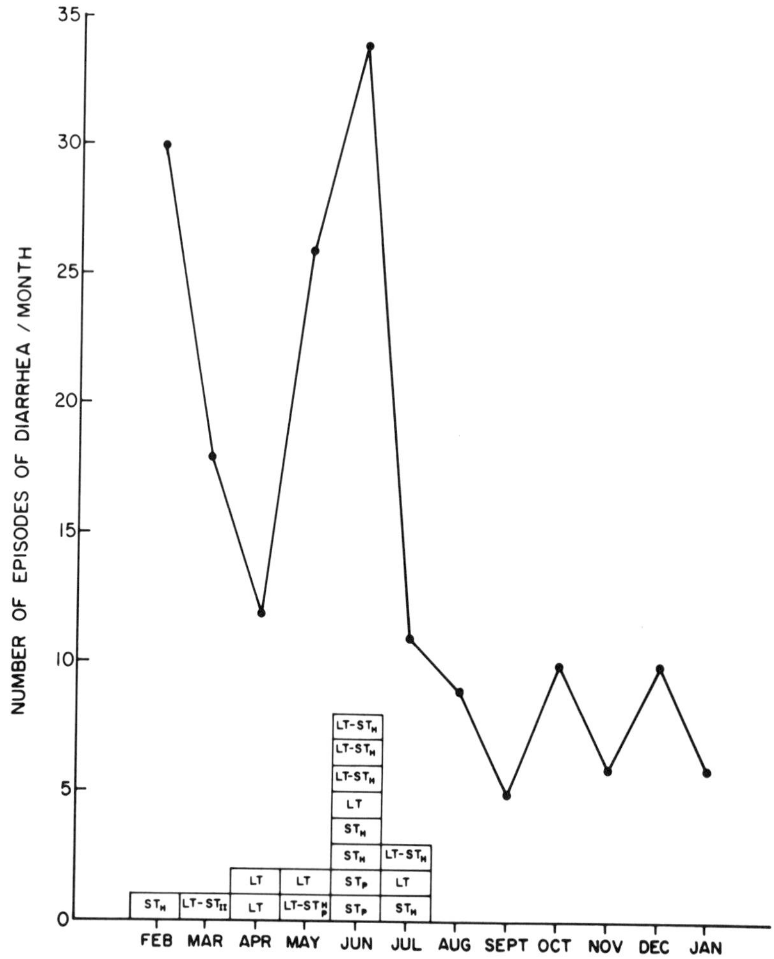

Figure 1 Number of episodes of diarrhea and those associated with ETEC infections in the villages of Nongsano and Sra Preng from February 1982 to January 1983. LT, STH (ST Ib), STP (ST Ia), and STII refer to the genes identified by DNA hybridization in *E. coli* in stools during episodes of diarrhea.

B. Enteroinvasive *E. coli*

EIEC cause dysentery by invading epithelial cells of the colon (Hale et al., 1983). Similar to *Shigella*, as many as half of the patients infected with EIEC present with watery diarrhea (Taylor et al., 1986, 1988a). Some EIEC strains have identical somatic antigens as *Shigella* (Formal and Hornick, 1987), EIEC 0124:H30 strains agglutinate in *S. dysenteriae* three antisera and may be mistaken for *Shigella*. EIEC are often nonmotile, slow, or non–lactose fermenting, fail to produce gas from glucose, or to decarboxylate lysine (Silva et al., 1980; Toledo and Trabulsi, 1983). EIEC belong to a relatively small number of O groups: 028, 029, 112, 124, 136, 143, 144, 147, 152, and 167 (Silva et al., 1980;

Table 1 Enterotoxigenic *E. coli* Identified in Pigs by DNA Hybridization in 87 Litters of Pigs with Diarrhea at 10 Farms in Thailand in 1981

Farm (month)	Number of pigs	Number of litters with ETEC/number of litters examined	Number of litters with type of ETEC infections
A (Jan.)	12	3/3	3 ST Ia
B (Feb.)	5	2/2	2 ST Ia
C (Feb.)	25	4/4	4 ST Ia
D (Feb.)	24	2/3	2 ST Ia
E (Mar.)	133	2/17	2 LT I ST Ia
F (Apr.)	144	6/15	1 LT I ST Ia, 2 LT I, 3 ST Ia
G (Apr.)	103	2/7	2 ST Ia
B (Apr.)	95	2/7	2 ST Ia
H (Apr.)	64	1/8	1 ST Ia
I (Jun.)	72	2/5	2 ST Ia
H (Aug.)	37	0/7	—
I (Sep.)	29	0/3	—
J (Mar.)	50	2/5	1 LT 1 ST Ia, 1 ST Ia
I (Oct.)	10	0/1	—

Toledo and Trabulsi, 1983). EIEC and *Shigella* produce keratoconjunctivitis when inoculated into the conjunctivae of guinea pigs (Fig. 2). This assay, the Sereny test (Sereny, 1955), is the definitive laboratory test for EIEC. Because most clinical laboratories do not have guinea pigs and EIEC O antisera is not usually available, EIEC are rarely identified.

The genetics of the virulence of *Shigella* and EIEC are similar (Sansonetti et al., 1982, 1983; Hale et al., 1983). Both *Shigella* and EIEC contain plasmids in the range of 120–140 megadaltons. A 17 kilobase *EcoR*I digestion fragment of pWR100, the 140 megadalton plasmid of *S. flexneri* 5 (M90T) has been used as a specific probe to identify EIEC and *Shigella* (Boileau et al., 1984; Sethabutr et al., 1985a,b). In a study of the etiology of childhood dysentery in Thailand, EIEC was isolated from 5% of 200 children with dysentery (Taylor et al., 1986). EIEC was a less common cause of dysentery than *Shigella* (5% vs. 44%) but was as likely as *S. flexneri* to result in hospitalization (20% vs. 18%). EIEC was identified in 4% of 410 children with diarrhea and 1% of age-matched controls without diarrhea in Bangkok (Taylor et al., 1988a). The isolation rates of both *Shigella* and EIEC increased with age, and the isolation rate was highest in children 36 to 54 months of age from whom *S. flexneri* was isolated from 24%, *S. sonnei* from 14%, and EIEC from 9% (Fig. 3). EIEC have been isolated from 2% of 328 Westerners with diarrhea seen at two medical clinics in Nepal (Taylor et al., 1988b) and from 5% of travelers with diarrhea in Mexico (Wanger et al., 1988). In Thailand, EIEC were relatively rare in children less than 6 months of age (Taylor et al., 1988a).

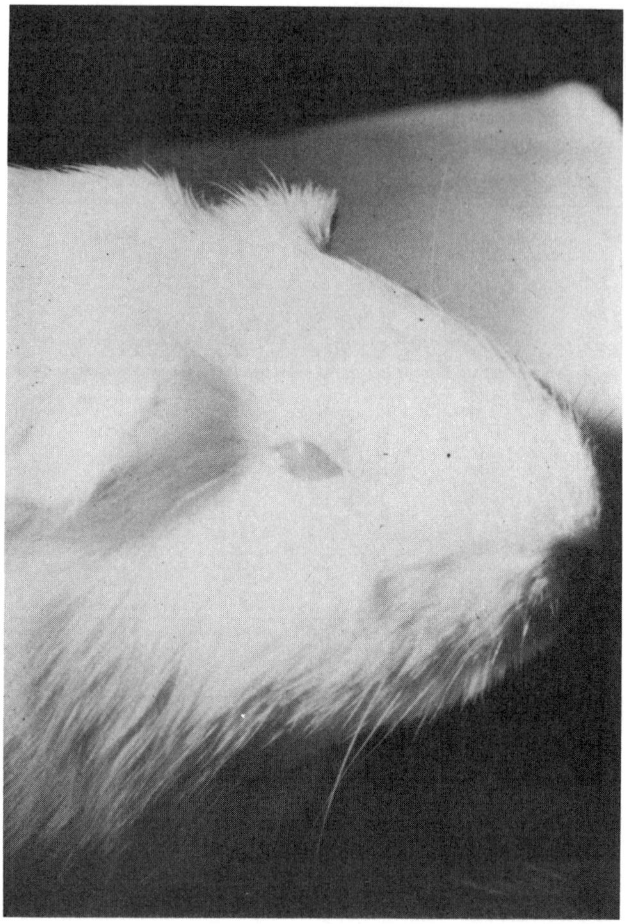

Figure 2 An example of a Sereny test with enteroinvasive *E. coli* 028:H-.

C. Enteropathogenic *E. coli*

Certain serotypes of *E. coli* termed EPEC by Neter et al. (1955) were recognized as a cause of epidemic and sporadic infantile diarrhea in the 1940s and 1950s (Bray, 1945, Taylor et al., 1949; Kauffmann and DuPont, 1950). Most EPEC strains isolated in the 1970s and a few isolated in the 1950s that were available for testing did not produce LT or ST or cause *Shigella*-like enteroinvasion (Goldschmidt and DuPont, 1976; Gross et al., 1976; Gurwith et al., 1977). Some felt that EPEC strains were not pathogenic because they lacked these virulence determinants. They hypothesized that these strains may have originally contained plasmids coding for enterotoxin when initially isolated, but had lost them upon storage (Sack, 1976; Gangarosa and Merson, 1977). This observation led to the abandonment of serogrouping *E. coli* in most

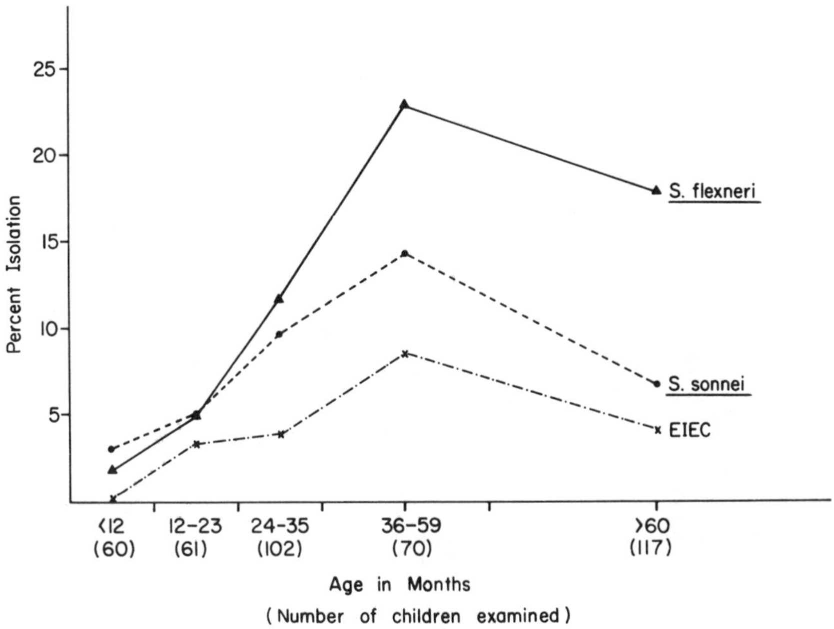

Figure 3 Age-specific isolation rates of *Shigella flexneri, S. sonnei*, and enteroinvasive *E. coli* (EIEC) from children with diarrhea in Bangkok, Thailand, January to June, 1985.

hospital laboratories (Gangarosa and Merson, 1977). Nevertheless, the capacity of several EPEC strains to cause diarrhea was demonstrated in adult challenge studies (Ferguson and June, 1952; June et al., 1953; Koya et al., 1954; Wentworth et al., 1956).

Since 1977, considerable progress has been made in defining the pathogenesis of EPEC. Polotsky et al. (1977) reported that EPEC 0111:H2 adhered to the mucosa of rabbit intestine causing localized destruction of microvilli. These EPEC strains were seen to indent the outer enterocyte membrane (Fig. 4). Similar lesions were described by Moon et al. (1983) in pigs and rabbits infected with EPEC. They coined the term "attaching and effacing *E. coli*" for those strains with the ability to cause these attaching effacing (AE) membrane lesions. Cravioto et al. (1979) reported that a higher proportion of EPEC strains isolated from outbreaks of diarrheal disease adhered to HEp-2 cells than did non-EPEC strains. Ultrastructural studies showed that an accumulation of cytoplasmic fibrils, subsequently identified as cytoskeletal actin, was present at the site of adherence of EPEC to HEp-2 cells (Knutton et al., 1987). The detection of the AE lesion on tissue culture cells has been facilitated by Knutton et al. (1989) through the development of the fluorescence actin-staining (FAS) assay. This assay utilized fluorescein isothiocyanate–labeled phallodin to detect actin filaments that are concentrated at the site of bacterial attachment in the AE lesion (Knutton et al., 1989) (Fig. 5).

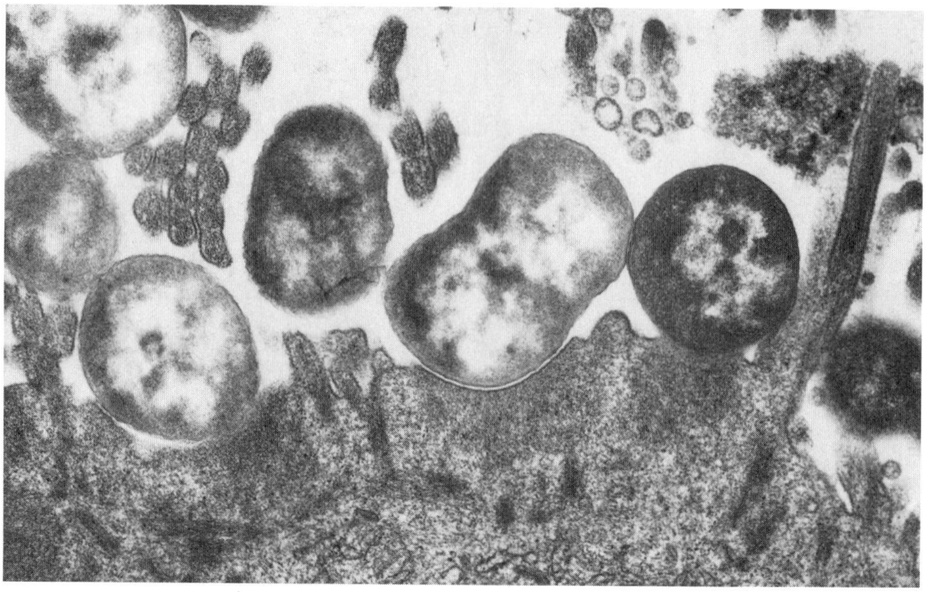

Figure 4 A transmission electromicrograph demonstrating an attachment and effacement lesion in human intestinal mucosa infected with EPEC 055:H7 (×20,000).

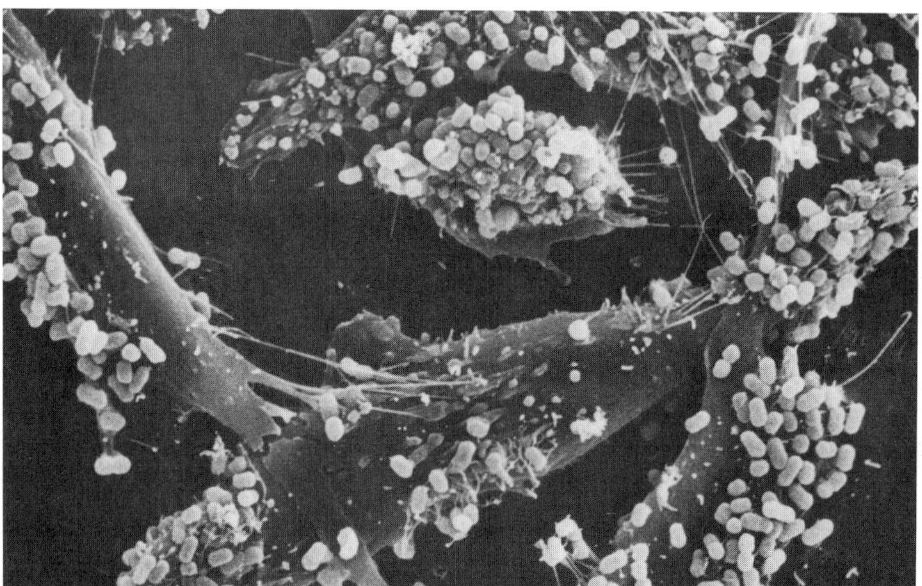

Figure 5 Fluorescence micrography of an actin-staining preparation showing adherence and fluorescence actin staining of EPEC 055:H- to HEp-2 cells after 6 h incubation (×4000).

A DNA probe to identify *E. coli* that adhere in a localized pattern to tissue culture cells has been constructed from a 1 kilobase fragment of a 60-megadalton plasmid of an adherent EPEC strain (Nataro et al., 1985a). This probe that detects genes coding for an adhesin, called the EPEC adherence factor (EAF), hybridized with EPEC of certain serotypes frequently incriminated in infantile diarrhea (Nataro et al., 1985b; Levine, 1988; Gomes et al., 1989). Adult volunteers developed diarrhea after challenge with EPEC 0127:H6 that adhered to HEp-2 cells in a localized pattern (Levine et al., 1985). This strain was subsequently shown by Knutton et al. (1987) to cause an AE lesion in human intestinal mucosa. *Shigella*-like toxin (SLT) produced in low amounts has also been identified as a possible virulence determinant of some EPEC serotypes (O'Brien et al., 1982). EPEC 0119, 0111, and 0127 isolated from children with chronic diarrhea were shown by examining intestinal biopsies of infected children to cause AE lesions in the small intestine (Ulshen and Rollo, 1980; Rothbaum et al., 1982; Clausen and Christie, 1982).

EPEC include O serogroups 018, 026, 044, 055, 086, 111, 0112, 114, 119, 125, 126, 127, 128, 142, and 158 with 026, 055, 111, 119, 125, 126, 127, and 128 occurring most commonly (Rowe, 1979). O and H serotyping remains the standard diagnostic test for EPEC, although there is some debate between investigators as to which O:H types to consider as classical EPEC serotypes. O and H serotyping is both time consuming and expensive, and most laboratories rely solely on commercial EPEC antisera to identify O antigens. Many *E. coli* selected using these pools are not subsequently identified as EPEC O and H serotypes (Echeverria et al., 1987b). There is a need for a more accurate diagnostic test for EPEC based on specific virulence properties of EPEC.

In a recent study of diarrhea in children less than 6 months of age in Thailand, the only *E. coli* strains associated with diarrhea were classical EPEC O and H serotypes—0124:H2, 0119:H6, 0125ac:H21, 0127:H6, and 0142:H6—that hybridized with the EAF probe and caused an AE lesion as detected in the fluorescence actin-staining test (Echeverria et al., 1991). These EPEC strains were only isolated from 3% of 509 children with diarrhea, but children infected with these EPEC strains were hospitalized more often than children infected with rotavirus, *C. jejuni*, or enteric adenovirus, the other enteric pathogens associated with diarrhea in this population.

D. Enterohemorrhagic *E. coli*

EHEC or Shiga-like toxin (SLT) (or verocytoxin) producing *E. coli* have been associated with persons with hemorrhagic colitis and hemolytic uremic syndrome worldwide (Karmali et al., 1983, 1985; O'Brien et al., 1984; Smith et al., 1988). EHEC produce antigenically distinct toxins SLT I, SLT II, and SLT II variant (Strockbine et al., 1986; Marques et al., 1987). Other cytotoxins that are antigenically related to SLT may exist. SLT I and SLT II are encoded on two distinct bacteriophages, 933J and 933W (Strockbine et al., 1986). EHEC was initially identified by testing culture filtrates for cytotoxicity to Vero cells (Konowalchuk et al., 1985). The genes for SLT I and SLT II have subsequently been cloned, and DNA probes specific for each have been constructed (Newland

and Neill, 1988). These probes have been used to identify EHEC in patients with diarrhea (Brown et al., 1988; Smith et al., 1988). EHEC also possess plasmid-encoded fimbriae that promote attachment to intestinal epithelial cells in tissue culture (Karch et al., 1987). A DNA probe consisting of a cryptic fragment of the 60-megadalton plasmid found in *E. coli* 0157:H7 was used, prior to the constructions of DNA probes to detect genes coding for SLT I and II, to search for EHEC (Levine et al., 1987). This probe hybridized with 80% of EHEC isolates from patients with hemolytic uremic syndrome or hemorrhagic colitis. Subsequently when SLT-producing *E. coli* isolates from environmental cultures and patients who did not have hemorrhagic colitis or develop hemolytic uremic syndrome were examined, only 60% of SLT-producing *E. coli* hybridized with this probe, and *E. coli* that hybridized with this probe, but did not contain genes coding for SLT were found (Brown et al., 1988; Suthienkul et al., 1990).

A total of 5415 patients with diarrhea in Canada were examined for SLT-producing *E. coli* and other enteric pathogens (Pai et al., 1988). SLT-producing *E. coli* was isolated from 3% and was found more often than *Salmonella* (2.6%) and *Campylobacter* (1.9%). SLT-producing *E. coli* was isolated more often from children 0–4 years and adults greater than 60 years of age. In Canada, the frequency of SLT-producing *E. coli* infection has been shown to be higher among certain groups of patients. The isolation rate of SLT-producing *E. coli* was 3% in patients with diarrhea (Pai et al., 1988), 15–37% in patients with bloody diarrhea (Riley et al., 1983; Pai et al., 1984, 1988; Riley, 1987), and increased to 75% in patients with hemolytic uremic syndrome (Karmali et al., 1985). Verocytotoxin-producing *E. coli* was identified with DNA probes in 39% of fecal specimens collected from patients with hemorrhagic colitis in Great Britain (Smith et al., 1988). The percent of probe-positive colonies in these specimens ranged from <1 to 100%. In Bangkok, specific DNA probes were used to identify SLT-producing *E. coli* in children <5 years of age with bloody diarrhea, in infants with diarrhea, and controls without diarrhea (Brown et al., 1988). At one hospital, SLT-producing *E. coli* was identified in 7% of 54 children with bloody diarrhea in whom other enteric pathogens were not identified and from 6% of 50 children without diarrhea. At another hospital SLT-producing *E. coli* was not identified in 113 infants with diarrhea and 119 controls without diarrhea. None of the EPEC strains isolated in Thailand that were examined hybridized with the SLT probes (Seriwatana et al., 1988a).

III. FOODBORNE AND WATERBORNE INFECTIONS WITH *E. COLI*

Numerous foodborne outbreaks of diarrhea occur every year in developed countries. It is generally recognized that the number of reported outbreaks and cases substantially underestimate the true magnitude of the problem because of restrictive definitions of food and waterborne epidemics, a failure of sick individuals to seek medical case, and a failure of the responsible authorities to investigate suspected outbreaks especially if they are small and are not known to cause severe disease or deaths. In the United States, two or more people must experience a similar illness after ingestion of a common food, and the food must be implicated as the source of illness before a foodborne outbreak is declared (MacDonald and Griffin, 1986). Clearly, an episode of foodborne diarrhea in single-member household could not be an outbreak by this definition. It has been estimated that actual food and waterborne cases may be 25–100 times more frequent than reported cases (Hauschild and Bryan, 1980; NRC, 1969).

The proportion of diarrhea that is food- and waterborne may be lower in developing than in developed countries because of the more varied and frequent opportunities for other modes of transmission. The actual rates of food and waterborne cases, however, are likely to be higher than in developed countries. Small epidemics in isolated villages, especially within the home, are even more likely not to come to the attention of public health authorities than in developed countries. Most information on food and waterborne *E. coli* infections in developing countries has come from prospective studies of villages or investigations of homes of patients with diarrhea seen at the hospital rather than from point source epidemics. The difficulty with these investigations is that foods that may have been the sources of the infections are frequently not available for culture. In developing countries, diarrhea occurs frequently so small epidemics are not brought to the attention of public health authorities. Hopefully as public health surveillance improves in developing countries, more food- and waterborne epidemics will be investigated.

As reviewed by Bryan (1979), *E. coli* is commonly isolated from hands of workers in the food industry in developed countries. *E. coli* was isolated from 4% of 500 healthy persons in England and from the hands of 12% of 110 workers after they left a meat line in a large processing plant. In food distribution centers, *E. coli* was frequently isolated from foods including salads, fruits, vegetables, meats, and poultry. *E. coli* of serotypes frequently found in animals are isolated from foods served in hospitals and patients in hospitals.

In Thailand, *E. coli* was isolated from approximately 10% of children's hands, sources of drinking water (Fig. 6), and foods (Fig. 7) in the home throughout the year (Fig. 8) (Echeverria et al., 1984a, 1985a,b, 1987a). *E. coli* was isolated in high concentrations from 45% of 289 samples of food prepared in kitchens at the airport in Bangkok in 1971 (Vadhanasin et al., 1976). The percent isolation of *E. coli* from 2741 samples of the 10 most common foods (vegetables, fish, powdered milk, pork, etc.) collected in homes of children in Bangkok in 1983 ranged from 8 to 25% (Echeverria et al., 1987a) (Table 2). A total of 130 specimens of each of four types of food were collected in 10 markets in Bangkok. *E. coli* was isolated from 85% of pork, 83% of chicken intestines, 78% of beef, and 12% of vegetables samples collected (Rasrinaul et al., 1988). High concentrations of fecal coliforms were found in foods obtained in Mexico (Wood et al., 1983a) and Gambia (Barrett and Rowland, 1979). Foods were identified as an important source of enteric pathogens, primarily ETEC, for American students who developed diarrhea in Mexico (Wood et al., 1983).

A. Enterotoxigenic *E. coli*

Although ETEC is a leading cause of diarrhea in children in tropical developing countries and travelers who visit these countries, most epidemics of ETEC

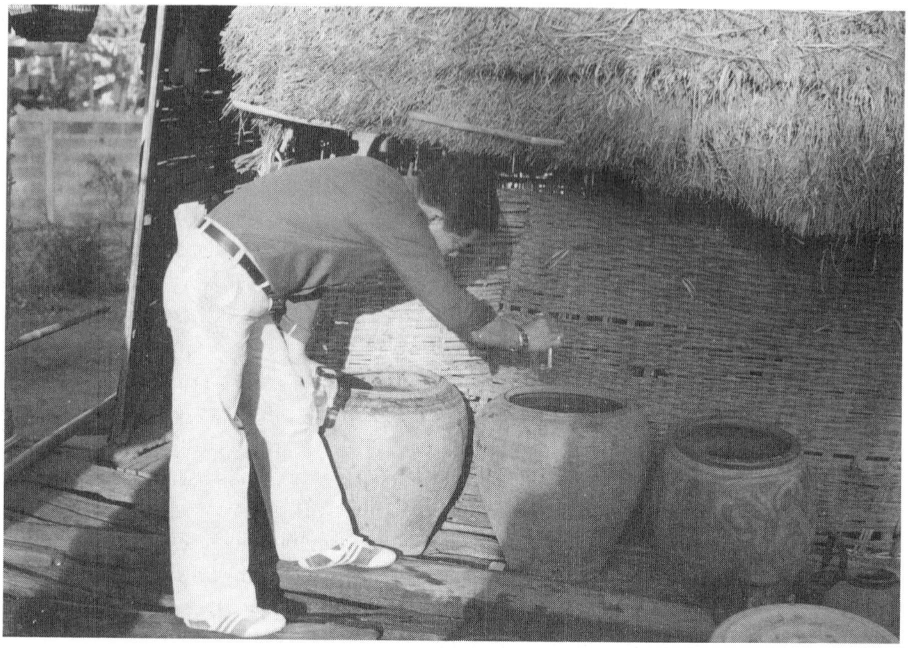

Figure 6 Collecting a sample of drinking water from a jar at a home in rural Thailand.

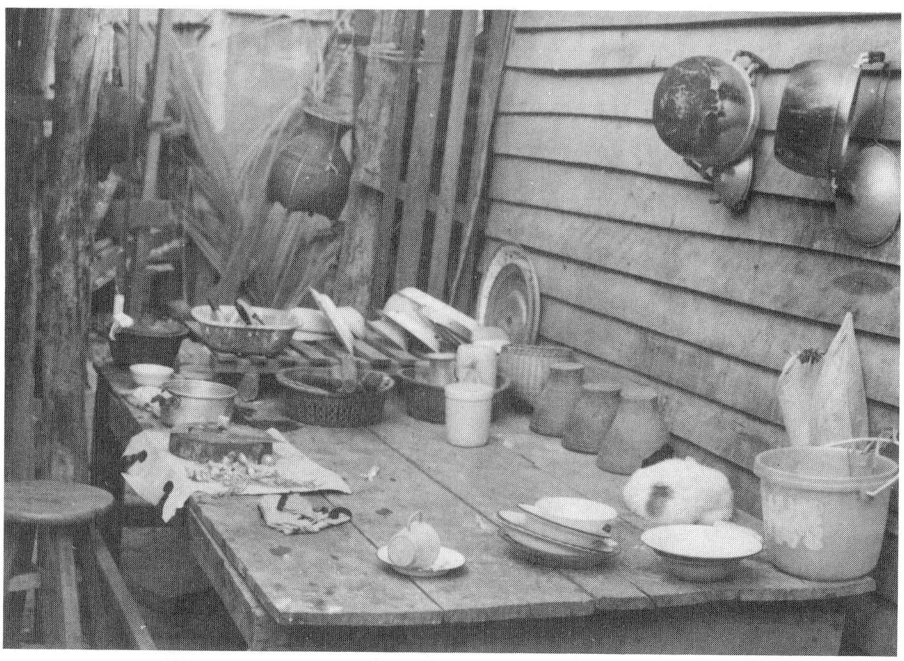

Figure 7 Food at a home in rural Thailand.

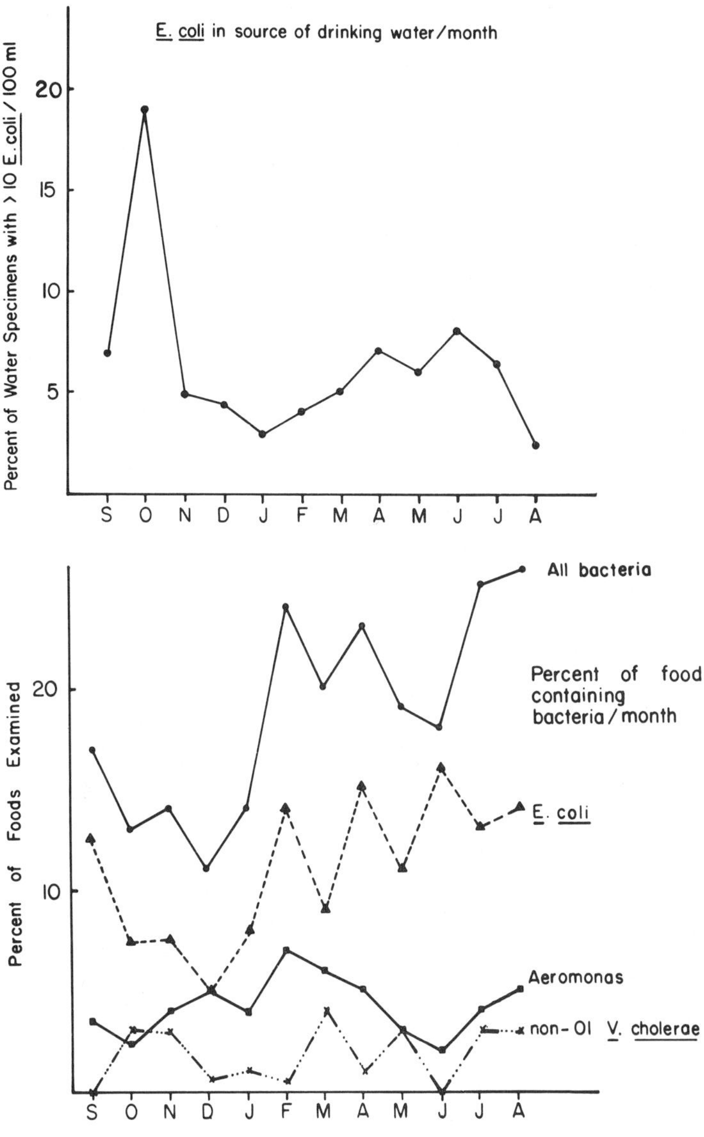

Figure 8 Percentage of drinking water samples containing more than 10 *E. coli*/100 ml and of food specimens containing more than 10 *E. coli*/g collected in homes of children in Bangkok between September 1982 and August 1983.

have been reported in developed countries where diarrheal disease is less common and epidemics of diarrhea come to the attention of public health authorities. The first epidemics of food- and waterborne ETEC were reported in restaurants in Japan in 1977 (Kudoh et al., 1977). Outbreaks of ETEC have subsequently been described in the United States and England. In an epidemic of ST ETEC 078:H12 in a special care nursery of a large children's hospital, the

Table 2 Isolation of *E. coli* from the 10 Most Common Foods Collected in Homes of Children with Diarrhea and Their Neighbors' Homes in Bangkok

Food item[a]	No. examined	No. with *E. coli* isolates
Vegetables	914	112 (12)[b]
Fish	603	55 (9)
Powdered milk	433	55 (13)
Pork	321	24 (7)
Rice	149	25 (17)
Egg	127	17 (13)
Chicken	90	16 (18)
Sweets	52	4 (8)
Noodles	31	8 (25)
Fruits	21	2 (9)

[a]Most foods contained more than one item, e.g., pork and vegetables, egg, and rice, etc.
[b]Figures in parentheses are percentages.
Source: Echeverria et al., 1987a.

epidemic strain was isolated from 18 of 25 infants with diarrhea and formula fed to infants in the nursery. Of the potential risk factors examined, only oral consumption of formula was associated with illness and isolation of the epidemic strain from infants (Ryder et al., 1976b). LTST ETEC 06:H16 was isolated from persons with diarrhea who ate at a single restaurant in the United States. The incubation period ranged from 3 to 166 h with a median of 44 ± 28 h. The overall attack rate was estimated to be at least 16%. Diarrhea lasted a median of 7 days and six persons had diarrhea for more than 14 days. The secondary attack rate in family contacts was low, 2 of 122 family contacts becoming infected with ETEC. ETEC infections were epidemiologically related to eating Mexican food at a restaurant (Taylor et al., 1982). In a foodborne ETEC epidemic in England, LTST ETEC 06:H16 and ST ETEC 027:H20 was isolated from the staff of a school and their guests who developed diarrhea after a social function (Riordan et al., 1985). Eight persons were infected with both strains. The mean incubation period was 36 h with a range of 12 to 66 h. Eating curried turkey mayonnaise was associated with infection, but food samples were not available for examination. Brie cheese was implicated in a multistate outbreak of ST Ia ETEC 027:H20 in the United States (MacDonald et al., 1985). ETEC was not isolated from cheese; however, in one cheese specimen organisms that bound antisera to *E. coli* 027 were detected by solid-phase RIA at a concentration of 10^4 organisms/g. On two successive 4-day cruises, LT ETEC 025:H- was isolated from 83% of 35 ill passengers (CDC, 1976; Lumish et al., 1980). Passengers on one cruise were asked about food and water consumption during their first 24 h of the cruise. Analysis revealed an association between diarrhea and eating crabmeat cocktail ($p < 0.001$). Consumption of one or more glasses of water per day was also associated with illness ($p < 0.05$). On the other cruise, no association between ship's water or ice and illness could be demonstrated, but crabmeat cocktail was again implicated of a source of ETEC infections. An environmental survey revealed numerous deficiencies in food-handling practices in the galley of the ship.

LT ETEC 025:H- was also associated with eating at a large cafeteria in Texas (Wood et al., 1983b). Foodborne epidemics of ETEC involving more than one serotype and other enteric pathogens have been reported (Birkelman et al., 1983). Common source epidemics in developed countries have been relatively rare presumably because an inoculum of 10^8 is required to induce illness in healthy American volunteers (DuPont et al., 1971; Levine et al., 1977) and ETEC has a low prevalence (Echeverria et al., 1975; Back et al., 1977; Brunton et al., 1980). ETEC was a common cause of diarrhea on an Arizona Indian reservation where sanitary conditions were substandard (Sack et al., 1975). Foodborne epidemics of ETEC reported in developed countries have involved travelers eating in tropical countries (Haiti or Mexico) and passengers on cruise ships. However, in at least three epidemics of ETEC in the United States, one waterborne (Rosenberg et al., 1979) and two foodborne (Ryder et al., 1976b; Taylor et al., 1982), no obvious connection with a tropical country was identified.

The situation is somewhat different in tropical developing countries where ETEC are more prevalent (Echeverria et al., 1978a; Black et al., 1980). Food- and waterborne epidemics of ETEC have been difficult to identify because in most tropical countries where refrigeration does not exist, foods thought to be sources of infections are seldom available for culture and epidemics are rarely investigated. Foods have been identified as a vehicle of ETEC in travelers' diarrhea in Mexico (Wood et al., 1983a), but ETEC isolated from foods collected in markets in Bangkok were different from those ETEC strains infecting children (Rasrinaul et al., 1988). LT ETEC strains isolated from foods often contained genes coding for LT II, but LT II ETEC are rarely isolated from people with diarrhea (Seriwatana et al., 1988b). In a study to identify potential sources of ETEC in homes of children with diarrhea in Thailand, *E. coli* was isolated as often from foods collected in homes of children with diarrhea as in homes of their neighbors who did not have diarrhea (Echeverria et al., 1987a). ETEC was identified in 8% (10/130) of inhabitants of 42 homes of children with ETEC diarrhea and 6% (8/137) of their neighbors. ETEC was not isolated from any food or water collected in 42 homes of children with ETEC associated diarrhea (Table 3). Either ETEC were not acquired from food, or the food which was a source of ETEC was not examined. In another study in Bangkok (Echeverria et al., 1984a), food in the home was implicated in only one of 30 homes of children infected with ETEC. ST ETEC 017:H45 was isolated from an 11-month-old boy with diarrhea and from a can of powdered milk in his home.

In Thailand as in Bangladesh, ETEC was isolated from family contacts and food/water samples more often in homes of persons with ETEC diarrhea than in homes not associated with ETEC-infected persons (Black et al., 1981; Echeverria et al., 1984a, 1985a,b, 1987a). Attempts to identify the source of ETEC within the homes in endemic situations have not been very successful. In Thailand in over 100 homes of children with ETEC-associated diarrhea, ETEC was isolated from only two foods (powdered milk and dried fish) and two drinking water sources (Echeverria et al., 1984a, 1985a,b, 1987a). In

Table 3 Enterotoxigenic *E. coli* Detected by DNA Hybridization in Environmental Specimens from Homes of Children with ETEC Diarrhea, Their Neighbors, and Homes Not Associated with ETEC Infections

	Number of positive specimens/number examined		
Specimen	42 homes of children with ETEC diarrhea	42 homes of neighbors	866 homes not associated with ETEC diarrhea
Source of drinking water	1/38	0/33	0/529
Drinking water in home	0/41	0/42	1/866
Food	0/84	0/84	2/1732
Mothers' hands	6/42	0/42	2/866
Children's hands	5/37	0/43	01/966

Source: Echeverria et al., 1987a.

Bangladesh (Black et al., 1981) ETEC of the same serotype as the index case was found in 9% of water sources used by the index household and in a small number of food and drinking water specimens collected in the index home. The proportion of a child's food samples that contained *E. coli* was significantly related to the children's incidence of ETEC diarrhea (Black et al., 1982).

B. Enteroinvasive *E. coli*

Most epidemics of EIEC that have been described were foodborne. This is presumably because a large inoculum is required to cause disease. An inoculum of 10^8 EIEC was required to cause illness in healthy adult volunteers (DuPont et al., 1971). Several foodborne epidemics of diarrhea caused by EIEC have been described. The first and largest recognized EIEC outbreak in the United States occurred in 1971. Between November 12 and 26, 20 separate outbreaks of gastroenteritis were reported involving at least 111 people who became ill 24–48 h after eating imported French Camembert or Brie cheese (Schnurrenberger et al., 1971). On November 28, 28 of 37 persons developed dysentery 24–48 h after eating Camembert cheese at a party in Washington, D.C. EIEC 0124 was isolated from the cheese eaten at the party, and stools were collected from nine individuals who became ill (Tulloch et al., 1973). By early December, the number of cases had risen to 227 in 96 separate outbreaks. *E. coli* 0124 was recovered from some cases, and *E. coli* 0124 was again isolated from samples of imported French cheese (Barnard and Callahan, 1972).

More recently, EIEC ONT:NM was isolated from 7 of 10 passengers who developed diarrhea during a 5-day ocean cruise (Snyder et al., 1984). Eating cold buffets on the ship, specifically potato salad, was significantly associated with illness. Forty-seven persons reported having had diarrhea during the cruise: Other symptoms among those with diarrhea included nausea (72%), abdominal cramps (68%), headache (68%), chills (60%), dizziness (53%), myalgia (43%), subjective fever (36%), and vomiting (26%). The median duration of symptoms was 3 days. No evidence of secondary spread of illness in household contacts of ill persons was found.

In 1984, a foodborne epidemic of EIEC 028:H- occurred at a primary school in Beijing. EIEC was isolated from children with diarrhea and a meal of eggs eaten by the children. The same strain was isolated from cooking utensils in the school children (Report from Dr. Zheng Shi Yang, 1987). An outbreak of EIEC in a mental institution suggested that person-to-person transmission may be more important than previously considered (Harris et al., 1985). A large waterborne epidemic of EIEC has been reported from Hungary (Lanyai et al., 1959). EIEC 0124 was isolated from 19 people. Epidemiological evidence incriminated well-water.

In Thailand, EIEC has been isolated from 4–5% of children with diarrhea (Taylor et al., 1986, 1988a). Since there is presently no information on environmental sources or routes of transmission of EIEC in tropical developing countries, we are currently performing a study of homes of children >3 years of age with diarrhea in Bangkok. To date, the percent isolation of *Shigella* is 43% and EIEC is 6% in 266 children with diarrhea. Cultures have been collected in 17 homes of children with EIEC diarrhea and 114 homes of children with shigellosis. *Shigella* was isolated from 4% and EIEC from 5% of family members of infected cases. *Shigella* and EIEC have not been identified in food and drinking water in these homes, although one water filtrate of a sample of bathing water collected in a home of a child infected with *S. sonnei* hybridized with the EIEC/*Shigella* probe. *Shigella* and EIEC were not isolated from vegetables and foods of animal origin in markets in Bangkok (Rasrinaul et al., 1988). This preliminary data suggests that *Shigella* and EIEC are acquired in an endemic situation primarily by person-to-person transmission, although in developed countries epidemics of food- and waterborne infections have been reported.

C. Enteropathogenic *E. coli*

From volunteer studies in adults the infective dose of EPEC is high (10^8) suggesting that EPEC is most likely transmitted by food or water (Ferguson and June, 1952; June et al., 1953; Koya et al., 1954; Wentworth et al., 1956). Most of the observations on the epidemiology of EPEC infections come from experiences in the 1940s and 1950s when large epidemics of EPEC occurred in young children in North America and Europe. As mentioned in a review of enteritis due to EPEC by Neter (1959), a number of authors have reported that bottle-fed babies are more susceptible to EPEC-associated enteritis than breast-fed infants, and the potential danger of nonsterilized milk in milk banks was demonstrated in Europe in the 1950s. EPEC has been isolated from unheated cows' milk, and Thomson et al. (1956) suggested that summer epidemics of EPEC that occurred early in this century may have been milkborne.

The epidemiology of EPEC in Great Britain, reviewed by Rowe (1979), exemplifies the situation that occurred in industrial countries. Up until the 1930s annual outbreaks of "summer diarrhea," often associated with a high mortality, occurred in poor and crowded industrial areas. An association with bottle feeding was observed; with improvement in living conditions and hygiene in the 1940s, the summer outbreaks were overshadowed by epidemics affecting infants in hospitals and nurseries. These outbreaks predominated during the cold season. Still, bottle-fed babies were at particular risk, with mortality rates of over 50%. Today, the incidence and mortality from EPEC infections is much lower, although reports from Canada (Gurwith et al., 1978), Finland (Maki et al., 1980), and Brazil (Toledo et al., 1983) still describe EPEC as the most common bacterial enteropathogen among young children.

Hinton and MacGregor (1958) described an explosive outbreak of EPEC-associated diarrhea in a local nursery upon transfer from another hospital of a child who has been treated for gastroenteritis. Transfer of EPEC diarrhea from one institution to another has been studied extensively (Thomson et al., 1956; Stock and Shuman, 1956). Stools containing a large number of EPEC are most likely the main sources for the spread of this pathogen. EPEC has been isolated from fecally soiled hands, gowns, and formites (Rodgers and Koegler, 1951). EPEC survive for many days or weeks in dust and on furniture (Hutchinson, 1957). EPEC strains have been isolated from the pharynx and upper respiratory tract of infants even in the absence of vomiting (Neter and Shamsay, 1950), and an airborne spread of infection has been suggested (Laurell et al., 1951). The most likely sequence of events is that children with EPEC diarrhea shed large numbers of these organisms which are transferred via milk or water to other infants. Direct transfer from one infant to another seems unlikely because of the large inoculum required to cause disease in adult volunteers.

EPEC outbreaks of gastroenteritis in adults that were either water- or foodborne have been reported from Romania (Costin et al., 1964), Sweden (Bengtsson et al., 1966), and the United States (Schroeder et al., 1968). The Romanian outbreak was traced to a substitute coffee drink. Ten of 30 adults who drank the coffee drink developed diarrhea. EPEC 086 was isolated from the drink and stools of ill persons. EPEC 0111, 026, and 0128 were isolated both from the well water and stools of individuals of all ages involved in a waterborne outbreak of gastritis in Sweden. An outbreak of gastroenteritis traced to a contaminated water supply occurred at a conference center near Washington, D.C. *E. coli* 0111 was isolated from both the water supply for the center and from 14 participants with diarrhea.

D. Enterohemorrhagic *E. coli*

In 1982, two separate outbreaks in the United States led to the discovery of a particular serotype of *E. coli*, 0157:H7, as an etiologic agent of hemorrhagic colitis (Riley et al., 1983). This disease was distinguished by a natural progression from watery to bloody diarrhea over the course of a few days and a relative lack of the usual signs of inflammation such as fever and large number of leukocytes in the stool. This newly discovered organism was initially isolated from hamburger (Riley et al., 1983) and then from cattle (Borczyk et al., 1987) and subsequently from dairy products (Martin et al., 1986). Animals have been identified as a common source of *E. coli* 0157:H7 and other serotypes of SLT producing *E. coli* (Riley, 1987). Since these organisms are spread mainly through processed food, it was originally thought that the relative absence of EHEC in some developing countries, in spite of poor sanitation, was due to the lack of processed foods. This assumption is probably not correct since EHEC and hemolytic uremic syndrome, which frequently follow EHEC infections, are common in Argentina, and evidence of SLT *E. coli* infections has been found in a high proportion of Argentine children who developed hemolytic uremic syndrome (Lopez et al., 1990).

Although ingestion of uncooked food products of animal origin seems the likely route of transmission in most cases of human EHEC infection, there is strong evidence that EHEC can be acquired by person-to-person transmission (Riley, 1987). In a daycare center outbreak, no common food source was identified, and the sequential movement of illness from class to class was consistent with person-to-person transmission. In a large outbreak of EHEC 0157:H7 infection in a nursing home (Carter et al., 1987) affecting 55 elderly residents and 18 staff members, the epidemic curve was biphasic. The first phase, which included the majority of the affected residents, was consistent with a point source infection presumed to be from ingestion of contaminated sandwiches. The second phase, which involved many of the staff who cared for the sick patients, suggested person-to-person transmission. In an outbreak among kindergarten children (Duncan et al., 1987) who probably acquired their infection after drinking raw milk at a farm, the occurrence of secondary cases among family members of some of the children suggested intrafamily spread of infection.

IV. A NEW METHOD OF IDENTIFYING *E. COLI* STRAINS THAT CAUSE DIARRHEA IN FOOD AND WATER

DNA probes to identify ETEC in food and water have been used extensively in our laboratory to identify sources of this organism in Thailand. These methods have recently been reviewed (Echeverria et al., 1990). This technique was shown to be 5 logs more sensitive in identifying ETEC than testing 10 *E. coli* isolates from a water specimen for enterotoxin production (Table 4). Recovering the actual *E. coli* for serotyping purposes can be difficult if the *E. coli* is only present in low concentrations (Echeverria et al., 1987a). When the concentration of *E. coli* in food specimens is high, dilutions that contain only approximately 300 colonies can be probed. By using a replicate plate arrangement (Echeverria et al., 1989), it is not difficult to recover the *E. coli* strain in question for further characterization. With this technique, it is possible to process many more food and water specimens. Nonradioactive probes have been developed to make this technology safer for untrained technicians and not dependent on frequent shipments of radioisotopes (Sethabutr et al., 1985b; Seriwatana et al., 1987). A procedure for amplifying specific DNA sequences within a sample by using a pair of primers and DNA polymerase has been developed (Saiki et al., 1988). In this procedure, specific primers are added that bind on either end of the nucleotide sequence to be amplified. On addition of heat-resistant DNA polymerase, the target sequence is replicated first in one direction from one primer and then in the other direction from the opposite primer making multiple copies of the DNA sequence. This procedure has been used to identify LT ETEC in stools (Oliver, 1989), and we are currently evaluating this technique in the identification of *Shigella* and EIEC infections by Thailand. By extracting DNA from food and water, augmenting the DNA sequence of interest with a specific primer and DNA polymerase, it should be possible to increase the amount of target cell DNA of *E. coli* in food and water. This increased ability to identify diarrheogenic *E. coli* in food and water needs to be used in carefully designed epidemiological studies in both developed and developing countries.

V. CONCLUSION

The epidemiology of *E. coli* that cause diarrhea suggest that most infections are acquired from food and water. The high inoculum of *E. coli* (10^8) required to induce diarrhea in healthy volunteers supports this observation. Animals (cattle and pigs) are frequently infected with *E. coli* that cause diarrhea in man. Animals and foods of animal origin have been incriminated in ETEC, EIEC, EPEC, and EHEC infections (Fig. 9).

The application of molecular genetic techniques will enable investigators to trace the spread of these *E. coli* strains from their source to humans. A hypothetical explanation given to the inhabitants of Nongsano, a village in northeastern Thailand, serves to illustrate how complex tracing the epidemiology of these organisms in a developing country can be (Fig. 10). Prompt identification of outbreaks and well-designed epidemiological studies with

Table 4 Comparison of Identification of Enterotoxigenic *E. coli* by Testing 10 Lactose-Fermenting Colonies for Enterotoxin Production Versus Probing Filtrates of 100 ml of Water with Radiolabeled Enterotoxin Gene Probes

LT 1 ST Ib ETEC/ml of canal water[a]	Testing 10 colonies for enterotoxin production[b]	Hybridization of filtrates with enterotoxin gene probe[c]
10^8	+	+
10^7	+	+
10^6	+	+
10^5	+	+
10^4	−	+
10^3	−	+
10^2	−	+
10	−	−
0	−	−

[a]Canal water contained 5.4×10^5 *A. hydrophila*, 5×10^4 non-ETEC, 2×10^4 *E. agglomerans*, and 1×10^2 *Klebsiella pneumoniae*.
[b]As identified with the Y-1 adrenal and suckling mouse assays.
[c]Enterotoxin gene probes are radiolabeled polynucleotide probes coding for LT I and ST Ib.

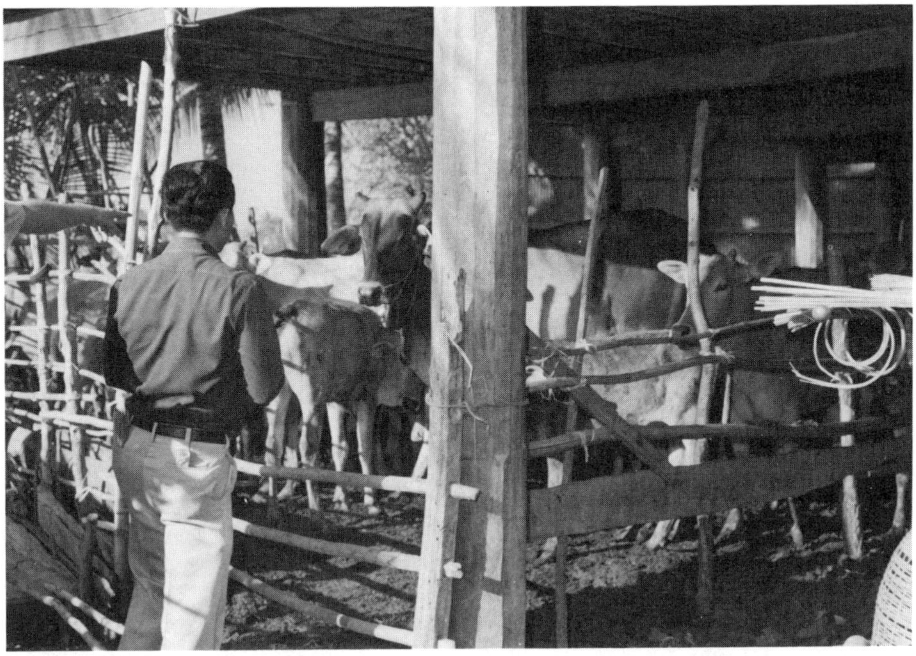

Figure 9 Animals kept under the house in a village in rural Thailand.

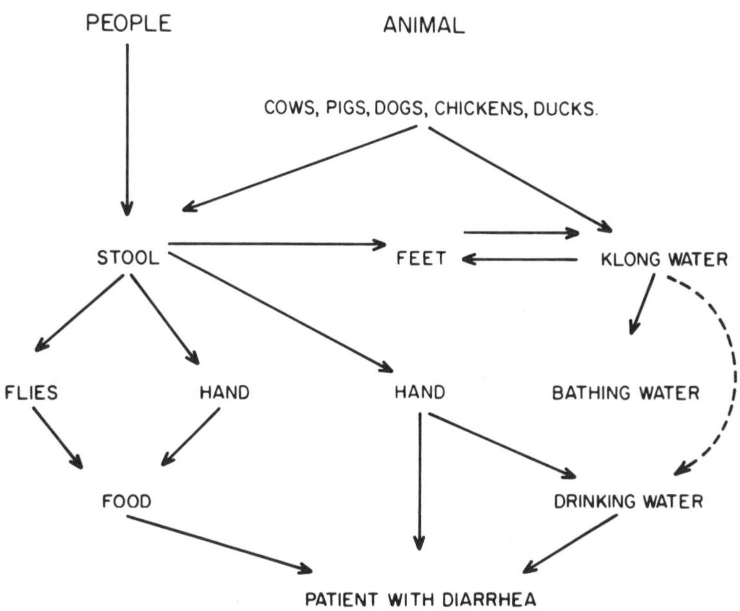

Figure 10 Explanation of possible routes of transmission of enteric pathogens given to the inhabitants of Nongsano in Soongnern district after the completion of a study of their village.

recently developed molecular genetic techniques will increase our knowledge of food- and waterborne *E. coli* gastroenteritis in both developed and developing countries.

REFERENCES

Adam, A. (1923). Über die Biologie der Dyspepsiecoli und Ihre Beziehungen zur Pathogese der Dyspepsie und Intoxikation. *Jahrbuch für Kinderheilkunde 51*: 295–315.

Alderete, J. F., and Robertson, D. C. (1978). Purification and chemical characterization of the heat-stable enterotoxin produced by porcine strains of enterotoxigenic *Escherichia coli. Infect. Immun. 19*: 1021–1030.

Back, E., Blomberg, S., and Wadstrom, T. (1977). Enterotoxigenic *Escherichia coli* in Sweden. *Infection 5*: 2–5.

Barnard, R., and Callahan, W. (1972). Follow-up gastroenteritis attributed to imported French cheese. *MMWR 20*: 445.

Barrett, R. A. E., and Rowland, M. G. M. (1979). Infant food as a potential source of diarrhoeal illness in rural West Africa. *Trans. Roy. Soc. Trop. Med. Hyg. 73*: 85–90.

Bengtsson, S., Berg, R., Danielsson, D., Lundmark, K-M., Norbring, F., and Sandler, O. (1966). En vattenburen epidemi med enteropatogena *Escherichia coli. Lakartidningen 63*: 4499–4506.

Birkelman, R. L., Cohen, M. L., Yashuk, J., Barrett, T., Wells, J. G., and Blake, P. A. (1983). Traveler's diarrhea at sea: Two multiple-pathogen outbreaks caused by food eaten on shore visits. *Am. J. Public Health 73*: 770–772.

Black, R. E., Merson, M. H., Rahman, A. S. M. M., Yunnus, M., Alim, A. R. M. A., Huq, I., Yolken, E. H., Curlin, G. T. (1980). A two-year study of bacterial, viral, and parasitic agents associated with dirrhea in rural Bangladesh. *J. Infect. Dis. 142*: 660–664.

Black, R. E., Merson, M. H., Rowe, B., Taylor, P. R., Alim, A. R. M. A., and Gross, R., and Sack, D. A. (1981). Enterotoxigenic *Escherichia coli* diarrhea: Acquired immunity and transmission in an endemic area. *Bull. WHO 59*: 263–268.

Black, R. E., Brown, K. H., Becker, S., Alim, A. R. M. A., and Merson, M. H. (1982). Contamination of weaning foods and transmission of enterotoxigenic *Escherichia coli* diarrhea in children in rural Bangladesh. *Trans. Roy. Soc. Trop. Med. Hyg. 76*: 259–264.

Boileau, C. R., d'Hauteville, H. M., and Sansonetti, P. J. (1984). DNA hybridization techniques to detect *Shigella* species and enteroinvasive *Escherichia coli. J. Clin. Microbiol. 20*: 959–961.

Borczyk, A. A., Karmali, M. A., Lior, H., and Duncan, M. C. (1987). Bovine reservoir for verotoxin-producing *Escherichia coli* 0157:H7. *Lancet 1*: 98.

Bray, J. (1945). Isolation of antigenically homogenous strains of *Bact coli neapolitanum* from summer diarrhea of infants. *J. Pathol. Bacteriol. 57*: 239–247.

Brown, J. E., Echeverria, P., Taylor, D. N., Seriwatana, J., Vanapruks, V., Lexomboon, U., Neill, R. N., and Newland, J. W. (1988). Determination by DNA hybridization of Shiga-like toxin producing *Escherichia coli* in children with diarrhea in Thailand. *J. Clin. Microbiol. 27*: 291–294.

Brunton, J., Hinde, D., Langston, C., Gross, R., Rowe, B., and Gurwith, M. (1980). Enterotoxigenic *Escherichia coli* in central Canada. *J. Clin. Microbiol. 11*: 343–348.

Bryan, F. L. (1979). Infections and Intoxications caused by other bacteria. In *Food-borne Infections and Intoxications*, H. Riemann and F. L. Bryan, eds. Academic Press, New York, pp. 212–298.

Burgess, N. M., Bywater, R. J., Cowley, C. M., Mullan, N. A., and Newsome, P. M. (1978). Biological evaluation of a methanol-soluble, heat-stable *Escherichia coli* enterotoxin in infant mice, pigs, rabbits, and calves. *Infect. Immun. 21*: 526–531.

Carter, A. O., Borcyk, A. A., Carlson, J. A. K., Harvey, B., Hockin, J. C., Karmali, M. A., Krishnan, C., Korn, D. A., and Lior, H. (1987). A severe outbreak of *Escherichia coli* 0157:H7 associated hemorrhagic colitis in a nursing home. *N. Engl. J. Med. 317*: 1496–1500.

Centers for Disease Control (CDC). (1976). Diarrheal illness on a cruise ship caused by enterotoxigenic *Escherichia coli. MMWR 25*: 229.

Clausen, C. R., and Christie, D. L. (1982). Chronic diarrhea in infants caused by adherent enteropathogenic *Escherichia coli. J. Pediatr. 100*: 358–361.

Clements, J. D., Yancey, R. J., and Finkelstein, R. A. (1980). Properties of homogenous heat-labile enterotoxins from *Escherichia coli. Infect. Immun. 29*: 91–97.

Costin, I. D., Voiculescu, D., and Gorcea, V. (1964). An outbreak of food poisoning in adults associated with *Escherichia coli* serotype 86:B7:H34. *Patho. Microbiol. 27*: 68–78.

Cravioto, A., Gross, R. J., Scotland, S. M., and Rowe, B. (1979). An adhesive factor found in strains of *Escherichia coli* belonging to the traditional infantile enteropathogenic serotypes. *Curr. Microbiol. 3*: 95–99.

Cravioto, A., Scotland, S. M., and Rowe, B. (1982). Hemagglutination activity and colonization factor antigens I and II in enterotoxigenic and non-enterotoxigenic strains of *Escherichia coli* isolated from humans. *Infect. Immun. 36*: 189–197.

Dallas, W. S., and Falkow, S. (1979). The molecular nature of heat-labile enterotoxin (LT) of *Escherichia coli. Nature* (London) *277*: 406–407.

Darfeuille, A., Lafeville, B., Joly, B., and Cluzel, R. (1983). A new colonization factor antigen (CFA/III) produced by enteropathogenic *Escherichia coli* 0128:B12. *Ann. Microbiol.* (Paris) *134A*: 53–64.

Darfeuille-Michaud, A., Forcester, C., Joly, B., Cluzel, R. (1986). Identification of a non-fimbrial adhesive factor of an enterotoxigenic *Escherichia coli* strain. *Infect. Immun. 52*: 468–475.

Dean, A. G., Ching, Y. C., Williams, R. G., and Harden, L. B. (1972). Test for *Escherichia coli* enterotoxin using infant mice: Application in a study of diarrhea in children in Honolulu. *J. Infect. Dis. 125*: 407–411.

Duncan, L., Mai, V., Carter, A., Carlson, J. A. K., Borczyk, A., and Karmali, M. A. (1987). Outbreak of gastrointestinal disease in Ontario. *Canada Dis. Weekly Report 13*: 5–8.

DuPont, H. L., Formal, S. B., Hornick, R. B., Snyder, M. J., Libonati, J. P., Sheahan, B. G., La Brec, E. H., and Kalas, J. P. (1971). Pathogenesis of *Escherichia coli* diarrhea. *N. Engl. J. Med. 285*: 1–9.

Echeverria, P., Blacklow, N. R., and Smith, D. H. (1975). The role of heat-labile enterotoxigenic *Escherichia coli* and reovirus-like agent in diarrhea in Boston children. *Lancet 2*: 1113–1115.

Echeverria, P., Verhaert, L., Basaca-Sevilla, V., Banson, T., and Cross, J. H. (1978a). Prevalence of heat-labile enterotoxigenic *Escherichia coli* in humans, livestock, food, and water in a community in the Philippines. *J. Infect. Dis. 138*: 87–89.

Echeverria, P., Blacklow, N. R., Vollet, J. L., Uylangco, C. V., Cukor, G., Soriano, V. B., DuPont, H. L., Cross, J. H., Orskov, F., and Orskov, I. (1978b). Reovirus-like agent and enterotoxigenic *Escherichia coli* infections in pediatric diarrhea in the Philippines. *J. Infect. Dis. 138*: 326–332.

Echeverria, P., Blacklow, N. R., Sanaford, L. B., Cukor, G. G. (1981). Traveler's diarrhea among American Peace Corps volunteers in rural Thailand. *J. Infect. Dis. 143*: 767–771.

Echeverria, P., Seriwatana, J., Leksomboon, U., Tirapat, C., Chaicumpa, W., and Rowe, B. (1984a). Identification by DNA hybridization of enterotoxigenic *Escherichia coli* in homes of children with diarrhea. *Lancet 1*: 63–65.

Echeverria, P., Seriwatana, J., Patamaroj, U., Moseley, S. L., McFarland, A., Chityothin, O., and Chaicumpa, W. (1984b). Prevalence of heat-stable II enterotoxigenic *Escherichia coli* in pigs, water, and people at farms in Thailand as determined by DNA hybridization. *J. Clin. Microbiol. 19*: 489–491.

Echeverria, P., Seriwatana, J., Taylor, D. N., Tirapat, C., Chaicumpa, W., and Rowe, B. (1985a). Identification by DNA hybridization of enterotoxigenic *Escherichia coli* in a longitudinal study of villages in Thailand. *J. Infect. Dis. 151*: 124–130.

Echeverria, P., Seriwatana, J., Taylor, D. N., Yanggratoke, S., and Tirapat, C. (1985b). A comparative study of enterotoxigenic *Escherichia coli, Shigella, Aeromonas*, and *Vibrio* as etiologies of diarrhea in northeastern Thailand. *Am. J. Trop. Med. Hyg. 34*: 547–554.

Echeverria, P., Seriwatana, J., Taylor, D. N., Changchawalit, S., Smyth, C. J., Twohig, J., and Rowe, B. (1986). Plasmids coding for colonization factors antigens I and II, LT and STA-2 in *Escherichia coli. Infect. Immun. 51*: 626–630.

Echeverria, P., Taylor, D. N., Seriwatana, J., Leksomboon, U., Chaicumpa, W., Tirapat, C., and Rowe, B. (1987a). Potential sources of enterotoxigenic *Escherichia coli* in homes of children with diarrhea in Thailand. *Bull. WHO 65*: 207–215.

Echeverria, P., Taylor, D. N., Bettelheim, K. A., Chatkaeomorakot, A., Thongcharoen, A., and Leksomboon, U. (1987b). HeLa cell adherent enteropathogenic *Escherichia coli* in children under one year of age in Thailand. *J. Clin. Microbiol. 25*: 1472–1475.

Echeverria, P., Taylor, D. N., Seriwatana, J., Brown, J. E., and Lexomboon, U. (1989). Examination of colonies and stool blots for the detection of enteropathogens by DNA hybridization with eight DNA probes. *J. Clin. Microbiol. 27*: 331–334.

Echeverria, P., Seriwatana, J., Sethabutr, O., and Chatkaeomorakot, A. (1990). Detection of diarrheogenic *Escherichia coli* using nucleotide probes. In *Gene Probes for Bacteria*, A. J. L. Macario and E. Conway de Macario, eds. Academic Press, San Diego, CA, pp. 95–141.

Echeverria, P., Orskov, F., Orskov, I., Knutton, S., Scheutz, F., Brown, J. E., and Lexomboon, U. (1991). Attaching and effacing *Escherichia coli* as a cause of infantile diarrhea in Thailand. (submitted for publication)

Evans, D. G., Silver, R. D., Evans, D. J., Chase, D. G., and Gorbach, S. L. (1975). Plasmid-controlled colonization factor associated with virulence in *Escherichia coli* enterotoxigenic in humans. *Infect. Immun. 12*: 656–667.

Ferguson, W. W., and June, R. C. (1952). Experiments on feeding adult volunteers with *Escherichia coli* 0111, B4, a coliform organism associated with infant diarrhea. *Amer. J. Hyg. 55*: 155–169.

Field, M., Graf, L. H., Laird, W. J., and Smith, P. L. (1978). Heat-stable enterotoxin of *Escherichia coli*: *In-vitro* effects on guanylate cyclase activity, cyclic AMP concentration, and ion transport in the small intestine. *Proc. Natl. Acad. Sci. USA 75*: 2800–2804.

Formal, S. B., and Hornick, R. B. (1987). Invasive *Escherichia coli. J. Infect. Dis. 137*: 641–644.

Gangarosa, E. J., and Merson, M. H. (1977). Epidemiologic assessment of the relevance of the so-called enteropathogenic serogroups of *Escherichia coli* in diarrhea. *N. Engl. J. Med. 296*: 1210–1213.

Gill, D. M., and Richardson, S. H. (1980). Adenosine diphosphate-ribosylation of adenylate cyclase catalyzed by heat-labile enterotoxin of *Escherichia coli*: Comparison with cholera toxin. *J. Infect. Dis. 141*: 64–70.

Goldschmidt, M. C., and DuPont, H. L. (1976). Enteropathogenic *Escherichia coli*: Lack of correlation of serotype with pathogenicity. *J. Infect. Dis. 133*: 153–156.

Gomes, T. A. T., Vieira, M. A. M., Wachsmuth, I. K., Blake, P. A., Trabulsi, L. R. (1989). Serotype-specific prevalence of *Escherichia coli* strains with EPEC adherence factor genes in infants with and without diarrhea in Sao Paulo, Brazil. *J. Infect. Dis. 160*: 131–135.

Green, B. A., Neill, R. J., Ruyechan, W. T., and Holmes, R. K. (1983). Evidence that a new enterotoxin which activates adenyl cyclase in eucaryotic target cells is not plasmid mediated. *Infect. Immun. 41*: 383–390.

Gross, R. J., Scotland, S. M., and Rowe, B. (1976). Enterotoxin testing of *Escherichia coli* causing epidemic infantile enteritis in the UK. *Lancet i*: 629–632.

Gurwith, M. J., Wiseman, D. A., and Chow, P. (1977). Clinical and laboratory assessment of the pathogenicity of serotyped *Escherichia coli. J. Infect. Dis. 135*: 736–743.

Gurwith, M. J., Hinde, D., Gross, R., and Rowe, B. (1978). A prospective study of enteropathogenic *Escherichia coli* in endemic diarrheal disease. *J. Infect. Dis. 137*: 292–297.

Guth, B. E. C., Pickett, C. L., Twiddy, E. M., Holmes, R. K., Gomes, T. A. T., Lima, A. A. M., Guerrant, R. L., Franco, B. D. G. M., and Trabulsi, L. R. (1986a). Production of type II heat-labile enterotoxin by *Escherichia coli* isolated from food and human feces. *Infect. Immun. 54*: 587–589.

Guth, B. E. C., Twiddy, E. M., Trabulsi, L. R., and Holmes, R. K. (1986b). Variations in chemical properties and antigenic determinants among type II heat-labile enterotoxins of *Escherichia coli. Infect. Immun. 54*: 529–536.

Hale, T. L., Sansonetti, P. J., Schad, D. A., Austin, S., and Formal, S. B. (1983). Characterization of virulence plasmids and plasmid-associated outer membrane proteins in *Shigella flexneri, Shigella sonnei*, and *Escherichia coli. Infect. Immun. 40*: 340–350.

Harris, J. R., Mariano, J., Wells, J. G., Payne, B. J., Donnell, H. D., and Cohen, M. L. (1985). Person-to-person transmission in an outbreak of enteroinvasive *Escherichia coli. Am. J. Epidemiol. 122*: 245–252.

Hauschild, A. H. W., and Bryan, F. L. (1980). Estimate of cases of food and waterborne illness in Canada and the United States. *J. Food Protection 43*: 435–440.

Hinton, N. A., and MacGregor, R. R. (1958). A study of infections due to pathogenic serogroups of *Escherichia coli. Can. Med. Assoc. J. 79*: 359–364.

Holmes, R. K., Twiddy, E. M., and Bramucci, M. G. (1983). Antigenic heterogeneity among heat-labile toxins from *Escherichia coli*. In *Advances in Research on Cholera and Related Diarrhea*, Vol. 1, S. Kuwahara and N. F. Pierce, eds. Martinus Nihoff Publishers, Boston, pp. 293–300.

Honda, T., Tsuji, T., Takeda, Y., and Miwatani, T. (1981). Immunological non-identity of heat-labile enterotoxins from human and porcine enterotoxigenic *Escherichia coli. Infect. Immun. 34*: 337–340.

Hughes, J. M., Murad, F., Chang, B., and Guerrant, R. L. (1978). Role of cyclic GMP in the action of heat-stable enterotoxin of *Escherichia coli. Nature* (London) *271*: 755–756.

Hutchinson, R. I. (1957). *Escherichia coli* (O types 111, 55, and 26) and their association with infantile diarrhea. A five year study. *J. Hyg.* (Camb) *55*: 27–44.

June, R. C., Ferguson, W. W., and Worfel, M. T. (1953). Experiments in feeding adult volunteers with *Escherichia coli* 55, B5, a coliform organism associated with infantile diarrhea. *Am. J. Hyg. 57*: 222–236.

Kapitany, R. A., Scott, A., Forsyth, G. W., McKenzie, S. L., and Worthington, R. W. (1979). Evidence for two heat-stable enterotoxins produced by enterotoxigenic *Escherichia coli. Infect. Immun. 24*: 965–966.

Karch, H., Hessemann, J., Laufs, R., O'Brien, A. D., Tackett, C. O., and Levine, M. M. (1987). A plasmid of enterohemorrhagic *Escherichia coli* 0157:H7 is required for expression of a new fimbrial antigen and for adhesion to epithelial cells. *Infect. Immun. 55*: 455–461.

Karmali, M. A., Petric, M., Lim, C., Fleming, P. C., and Steele, B. T. (1983). *Escherichia coli* cytotoxin hemolytic-uremic syndrome and hemorrhagic colitis. *Lancet 2*: 1299–1300.

Karmali, M. A., Petric, M., Lim, C., Flemming, P. C., Arbus, G. S., and Lior, H. (1985). The association between idiopathic hemolytic uremic syndrome and infection by verocytotoxin-producing *Escherichia coli. J. Infect. Dis. 151*: 775–782.

Kauffman, F. (1947). The serology of the coli group. *J. Immunol. 57*: 71–100.

Kauffman, F., and DuPont, A. (1950). Escherichia strains from infantile epidemic gastroenteritis. *Acta Pathol. Microbiol. Scand. 27*: 552–564.

Knutton, S., Baldini, M. M., Kaper, J. B., and McNeisch, A. S. (1987). Role of a plasmid-encoded adhesion of enteropathogenic *Escherichia coli* to HEp-2 cells. *Infect. Immun. 55*: 78–85.

Knutton, S., Balwin, T., Williams, P. H., McNeish, A. S. (1989). Actin accumulation sites of bacterial adhesion to tissue culture cells basis of a new diagnostic test for enteropathogenic and enterohemorrhagic *Escherichia coli. Infect. Immun. 57*: 1290–1298.

Konowalchuk, J. J., Speirs, J. I., Stavric, S. (1985). Vero response to a cytotoxin of *Escherichia coli. Infect. Immun. 18*: 775–779.

Koya, G., Kosakai, N., Kono, M., Mori, M., and Fusakawa, Y. (1954). Observations on the multiplication of *Escherichia coli* 0111, B4 in the intestinal tract of adult volunteers in feeding experiments: Intubation study with Miller-Abbott's double lumen tube. *Jpn. Med. Sci. Biol. 7*: 197–201.

Kudoh, Y., Zen-Yoji, H., Matsushita, S., Sakai, S., and Maruyama, T. (1977). Outbreaks of acute enteritis due to heat-stable enterotoxin-producing strains of *Escherichia coli. Microbiol. Immunol. 21*: 175–178.

Kunkel, S. L., and Robertson, D. C. (1979). Purification and chemical characterization of the heat-labile enterotoxin produced by enterotoxigenic *Escherichia coli. Infect. Immun. 25*: 586–596.

LaBrec, E. H., Schneider, H., Maghani, T. J., and Formal, S. P. (1964). Epithelial cell penetration is an essential step in the pathogenesis of bacillary dysentery. *J. Bacteriol. 88*: 1503–1518.

Lanyai, B., Szita, J., Ringelhann, B., and Kovach, K. (1959). A waterborne outbreak of enteritis associated with *Escherichia coli* serotype. *Acta Sci. Hung. 6*: 77–84.

Laurell, G., Magnusson, J. H., Frisell, E., and Werner, B. (1951). Epidemic infantile diarrhea and vomiting. *Acta Paediatar. Scand. 40*: 302–437.

Levine, M. M. (1987). *Escherichia coli* that cause diarrhea: Enterotoxigenic, enteropathogenic, enteroinvasive, enterohemorrhagic, and enteroadherent. *J. Infect. Dis. 155*: 377–389.

Levine, M. M., Caplan, E. S., Waterman, D., Cash, R. A., Hornick, R. B., and Snyder, M. I. (1977). Diarrhea caused by *Escherichia coli* that produce only heat-stable enterotoxin. *Infect. Immun. 17*: 78–82.

Levine, M. M., Nataro, J. P., Karch, H., Baldini, M. M., Karch, J. B., Black, R. E., Clements, M. L., and O'Brien, A. D. (1985). The diarrheal response of humans to some classical serotypes of enteropathogenic *Escherichia coli* is dependent on a plasmid encoding an enteroadhesive factor. *J. Infect. Dis. 152*: 550–559.

Levine, M. M., Xu, J-G., Kaper, J. B., Lior, H., Prado, V., Tall, B., Nataro, J., Karch, H., and Wachsmuth, K. (1987). A DNA probe to identify enterohemorrhagic *Escherichia coli* of 0157:H7 and other serotype that caused hemorrhagic colitis and hemolytic uremic syndrome. *J. Infect. Dis. 156*: 175–182.

Levine, M. M., Prado, V., Robins-Browne, R. M., Lior, H., Kaper, J. B., Moseley, S. L., Gicquelais, K., Nataro, J. P., Vial, P., and Tall, B. (1988). Use of DNA probes and HEp-2 cell adherence assay to detect diarrheogenic *E. coli. J. Infect. Dis. 158*: 224–227.

Lopez, E. L., Diaz, M., Grinstein, J., Devota, S., Mendilaharza, F., Murray, B. E., Ashkenazi, S., Rubeglio, E., Woloj, M., Vasquez, M., Turco, M., Pickering, L. K., and Cleary, T. G. (1990). Hemolytic uremic syndrome and diarrhea in Argentine children: The role of Shiga-like toxins. *J. Infect. Dis. 160*: 469–475.

Lumish, R. M., Ryder, R. W., Anderson, D. C., Wells, J. G., and Puhr, N. D. (1980). Heat-labile enterotoxigenic *Escherichia coli* induced diarrhea aboard a Miami-based service ship. *Am. J. Epidemiol. 111*: 432–436.

MacDonald, K. L., and Griffin, P. M. (1986). Foodborne disease outbreaks, annual summary, 1982. *MMWR 35(ISS)*: 7SS–16SS.

MacDonald, K. L., Eidson, M., Strohmeyer, C., Levy, M. E., Wells, J. G., Puhr, N. D., Wachsmuth, K., Hargrett, N. T., and Cohen, M. L. (1985). A multi-state outbreak of gastrointestinal illness caused by enterotoxigenic *Escherichia coli* in imported semi-soft cheese. *J. Infect. Dis. 151*: 716–720.

Maki, M., Vesikari, T., and Gronroos, P. (1980). Enterotoxigenic and enteroinvasive *Escherichia coli* as a cause of childhood diarrhoea in Finland. *Acta Paediatr. Scand. 69*: 219–224.

Manning, P. A., Higgins, G. D., Lump, R., and Lanser, J. A. (1987). Colonization factor antigens and a new fimbrial type (CFA/V) on 0115:H4 and H-strains of enterotoxigenic *Escherichia coli* in central Australia. *J. Infect. Dis. 156*: 841–844.

Martin, M. L., Shipman, L. D., Potter, M. E., Wachsmuth, I. K., Wells, J. G., Hedberg, K., Tauxe, R. V., Davis, J. P., Arnoldi, J., and Tilleli, J. (1986). Isolation of *Escherichia coli* 0157:H7 from dairy cattle associated with two cases of haemolytic uremic syndrome. *Lancet 2*: 1043.

Marques, L. R. M., Peiris, J. S. M., Cryz, S. J., and O'Brien, A. D. (1987). *Escherichia coli* strains isolated from pigs with edema disease produce a variant of Shiga-like toxin II. *FEMS Microbiol. Lett. 44*: 33–38.

McConnell, M. M., Thomas, L. V., Day, N. P., and Rowe, B. (1985). Enzyme-linked immunosorbent assays for the detection of adhesion factor antigens of enterotoxigenic *Escherichia coli. J. Infect. Dis. 152*: 1220–1227.

McConnell, M. M., Thomas, L. V., Willshaw, G. A., Smith, H. B., and Rowe, B. (1988). Genetic control and properties of coli surface of colonization factor antigen IV (PCF 8775) of enterotoxigenic *Escherichia coli. Infect. Immun. 56*: 1974–1980.

Merson, M. H., Morris, G. K., Sack, D. A., Wells, J. C., Feeley, R. B., Sack, R. B., Creech, W. B., Kapikian, A. Z., and Gangarosa, E. J. (1976). Travelers' diarrhea in Mexico: A prospective study of physicians and family members attending a congress. *N. Engl. J. Med. 294*: 1299–1305.

Moon, H. W., Whipp, S. C., Argenzio, R. A., Levine, M. M., and Gianella, R. A. (1983). Attaching and effacing activities of rabbit and human enteropathogenic *Escherichia coli* in pig and rabbit intestines. *Infect. Immun. 41*: 1340–1351.

Moseley, S. L., Huq, I., Alim, A. R. M. A., So, M., Samadpour-Motalebi, M., and Falkow, S. (1980). Detection of enterotoxigenic *Escherichia coli* by DNA colony hybridization. *J. Infect. Dis. 142*: 892–898.

Moseley, S. L., Echeverria, P., Seriwatana, J., Tirapat, C., Chaicumpa, W., Sakuldaipeara, T., and Falkow, S. (1982). Identification of enterotoxigenic *Escherichia coli* using three enterotoxin gene probes. *J. Infect. Dis. 145*: 863–869.

Moseley, S. L., Hardy, J. N., Huq, M. I., Echeverria, P., and Falkow, S. (1983a). Isolation and nucleotide sequence determinations of a gene encoding a heat-stable enterotoxin of *Escherichia coli. Infect. Immun. 39*: 1167–1174.

Moseley, S. L., Smadpour-Motalebi, M., and Falkow, S. (1983b). Plasmid association of nucleotide sequence relationship of two genes encoding heat-stable enterotoxin production in *Escherichia coli* H10407. *J. Bacteriol. 156*: 441–443.

Moss, J., and Richardson, S. H. (1978). Activation of adenylate cyclase by heat-labile *Escherichia coli* enterotoxin: Evidence for ADP-ribosyl transferase activity similar to that of choleragen. *J. Clin. Invest. 62*: 281–285.

Nataro, J. P., Scaletsky, I. C. A., Kaper, J. B., Levine, M. M., and Trabulsi, L. R. (1985a). Plasmid-mediated factors conferring diffuse and localized adherence of enteropathogenic *Escherichia coli. Infect. Immun. 48*: 378–383.

Nataro, J. P., Baldini, M. M., Kaper, J. P., Black, R. E., Bravo, N., Levine, M. M. (1985b). Detection of an adherence factor of enteropathogenic *Escherichia coli* with a DNA probe. *J. Infect. Dis. 152*: 560–565.

National Research Council Committee on *Salmonella*. (1969). *An Evaluation of the* Salmonella *Problem*. National Academy of Science, Washington, D.C.

Neter, E. (1959). Enteritis due to enteropathogenic *Escherichia coli*: Present-day status and unsolved problems. *J. Pediatr. 55*: 223–239.

Neter, E., and Shamsay, C. N. (1950). Serotype D433: Occurrence in intestinal and respiratory tracts, cultural characteristics, pathogenicity, sensitivity to antibiotics. *Proc. Soc. Exper. Biol. and Med. 75*: 504–507.

Neter, E., Westphal, O., Luderitz, O., Gino, R. M., and Gorzynski, L. A. (1955). Demonstration of antibodies against enteropathogenic *Escherichia coli* in sera of children of various ages. *Pediatr. 16*: 801–808.

Newland, J. W., and Neill, R. J. (1988). DNA probes for Shiga-like toxin I and II and for toxin converting bacteriophages. *J. Clin. Microbiol. 26*: 958–967.

O'Brien, A. D., LaVeck, G. D., Thompson, M. R., and Formal, S. B. (1982). Production of *Shigella dysenteriae* type 1-like cytotoxin by *Escherichia coli. J. Infect. Dis. 146*: 763–769.

O'Brien, A. D., Newland, J. W., Miller, S. F., Holmes, R. K., Smith H. W., and Formal, S. B. (1984). Shiga-like toxin converting phages from *Escherichia coli* strains that cause hemorrhagic colitis or infantile diarrhea. *Science 226*: 694–696.

Olive, D. M. (1989). Detection of enterotoxigenic *Escherichia coli* after polymerase chain reaction amplification with a thermostable DNA polymerase. *J. Clin. Microbiol. 27*: 261–265.

Pai, C. H., Gordon, R., Sims, H. V., and Bryan, L. E. (1984). Sporadic cases of hemorrhagic colitis associated with *Escherichia coli* 0157:H7 clinical epidemiological and bacteriologic features. *Ann. Intern. Med. 101*: 738–742.

Pai, C. H., Ahmed, N., Lior, H., Johnson, W. M., Sims, H. V., and Woods, D. E. (1988). Epidemiology of sporadic diarrhea due to verocytotoxin-producing *Escherichia coli*: A two year prospective study. *J. Infect. Dis. 157*: 1054–1057.

Pickett, C. L., Twiddy, E. M., Belisle, B. W., and Holmes, R. K. (1986). Cloning of genes that encode a new heat-labile enterotoxin of *Escherichia coli. J. Bacteriol. 165*: 348–352.

Polotsky, Y. E., Dragunskaya, E. M., Seliverstova, V. G., Audeeva, T. A., Chakhutinskaya, M. G., Keyti, I., Vertenyi, A., Ralovich, B., Emody, L., Malovics, L., Safonova, Y. V., Snigirevskaya, E. S., and Karyagina, E. I. (1977). Pathogenic effect of enterotoxigenic *Escherichia coli* and *Escherichia coli* causing infantile diarrhea. *Acta Microbiol. Acad. Sci. Hung. 24*: 221–236.

Rasrinaul, L., Suthienkul, O., Echeverria, P., Taylor, D. N., Seriwatana, J., Bangtrakulnonth, A., and Lexomboon, U. (1988). Foods as a source of enteropathogens causing childhood diarrhea in Thailand. *Am. J. Trop. Med. Hyg. 39*: 97–102.

Report from Dr. Zheng Shi Yang. (1987). National Institute for the Central of Pharmaceutical and Biological Products, Ministry of Health, Beijing, China.

Riley, L. W. (1987). The epidemiologic, clinical, and microbiological features of hemorrhagic colitis. *Annu. Rev. Microbiol. 41*: 383–407.

Riley, L. W., Remis, R. S., Helgerson, S. D., McGee, H. B. N., Wells, J. G., Davis, B. R., Herbert, R. J., Olcott, E. S., Johnson, L. M., Hargrett, N. T., Blake, P. A., and Cohen, M. L. (1983). Hemorrhagic colitis associated with a rare *Escherichia coli* serotype. *N. Engl. J. Med. 308*: 681–685.

Riordan, T., Gross, R. J., Rowe, B., Scotland, S. M., and Johnson, S. M. (1985). An outbreak of food-borne enterotoxigenic *Escherichia coli* diarrhoea in England. *J. Infect. 11*: 167–171.

Rodgers, K. B., and Koegler, S. J. (1951). Inter-hospital cross-infection of epidemic infantile gastroenteritis associated with type strains of *Bacterium coli. J. Hyg.* (Camb) *49*: 152–161.

Rosenberg, M. L., Koplan, J. P., Wachsmuth, I. K., Wells, J. G., Gangarosa, E. J., Guerrant, R. L., and Sack, D. A. (1979). Epidemic diarrhea at Crater lake from enterotoxigenic *Escherichia coli. Ann. Intern. Med. 86*: 714–718.

Rothbaum, R., McAdams, A. J., Gianella, R., and Partin, J. C. (1982). A clinicopathologic study of enterocyte-adherent *Escherichia coli*: A cause of protracted diarrhea in infants. *Gastroenterol 83*: 441–454.

Rowe, B. (1979). The role of *Escherichia coli* in gastroenteritis. *Clin. Gastroenterol. 8*: 625–644.

Ryder, R. W., Sack, D. A., Kapikian, A. Z., McLaughlin, J., Chakraborty, J., Rahman, R. J. M. M., Merson, M. H., Wells, J. G. (1976a). Enterotoxigenic *Escherichia coli* and reovirus-like agent in rural Bangladesh. *Lancet 1*: 659–662.

Ryder, R. W., Wachsmuth, I. K., Buxton, A. E., Evans, O. G., DuPont, H. L., Mason, E., and Barrett, F. F. (1976b). Infantile diarrhea produced by heat-stable enterotoxigenic *Escherichia coli. N. Engl. J. Med. 295*: 849–853.

Sack, R. B. (1975). Human diarrheal disease caused by enterotoxigenic *Escherichia coli. Annu. Rev. Microbiol. 29*: 333–353.

Sack, R. B. (1976). Serotyping of *E. coli. Lancet 1*: 1132.

Sack, R. B., Hirschhorn, N., Brownlee, I., Cach, R. A., Woodward, W. E., and Sack, D. A. (1975). Enterotoxigenic *Escherichia coli*-associated diarrheal disease in Apache children. *N. Engl. J. Med. 292*: 1041–1045.

Saiki, R. K., Gelfand, D. H., Stoffel, S., Scharf, S. I., Higuchi, R., Horn, G. T., Mullis, K. B., and Erlich, H. A. (1988). Primer-directed enzymatic amplification of DNA with a thermostable DNA polymerase. *Science 239*: 487–491.

Sansonetti, P. J., d'Hauteville, H., Formal, S. B., and Toucas, M. (1982). Plasmid-mediated invasiveness of *Shigella*-like *Escherichia coli. Ann. Microbiol.* (Paris) *132A*: 351–355.

Sansonetti, P. J., Kopecko, D. J., and Formal, S. B. (1983). Involvement of a plasmid in the invasive ability of *Shigella flexneri. Infect. Immun. 35*: 852–860.

Schnurrenberger, L. W., Beck, R., and Pate, J. (1971). Gastroenteritis attributed to imported French cheese. *MMWR 20*: 427–428.

Schroeder, S. A., Caldwell, J. R., Vernon, T. M., White, P. C., Granger, S. I., and Bennett, J. V. (1968). A waterborne outbreak of gastroenteritis in adults associated with *Escherichia coli. Lancet 1*: 737–740.

Sereny, B. (1955). Experimental *Shigella* conjunctivitis. *Acta Microbiol. Acad. Sci. Hung. 2*: 293–296.

Seriwatana, J., Echeverria, P., Taylor, D. N., Sakuldaipeara, T., Changchawalit, S., and Chivoratanond, O. (1987). Identification of enterotoxigenic *Escherichia coli* with synthetic alkaline phosphatase conjugated oligonucleotide DNA probes. *J. Clin. Microbiol. 25*: 1438–1441.

Seriwatana, J., Brown, J. E., Echeverria, P., Taylor, D. N., Suthienkul, O., and Newland, J. (1988a). DNA probes to identify Shiga-like toxin I and II producing enteric bacterial pathogens isolated from patients with diarrhea in Thailand. *J. Clin. Microbiol. 26*: 1614–1615.

Seriwatana, J., Echeverria, P., Taylor, D. N., Rasrinaul, L., Brown, J. E., and Peiris, J. S. M. (1988b). Type II heat-labile enterotoxin producing *Escherichia coli* isolated from animals and humans. *Infect. Immun. 56*: 1158–1161.

Sethabutr, O., Echeverria, P., Taylor, D. N., Pal, T., and Rowe, B. (1985a). DNA hybridization in the identification of enteroinvasive *Escherichia coli* and *Shigella* in children with dysentery. In *Infectious Diarrhea in the Young*, S. Tzipori, eds. Elsevier, Amsterdam, pp. 350–356.

Sethabutr, O., Hanchalay, S., Echeverria, P., Taylor, D. N., and Leksomboon, U. (1985b). A non-radioactive DNA probe to identify *Shigella* and enteroinvasive *Escherichia coli* in stools of children with diarrhea. *Lancet 2*: 1095–1097.

Silva, R. M., Toledo, M. R. F., and Trabulsi, L. R. (1980). Biochemical and cultural characteristics of invasive *Escherichia coli*. *J. Clin. Microbiol. 11*: 441–444.

Smith, H. R., Rowe, B., Gross, R. J., Fry, N. K., and Scotland, S. M. (1988). Hemorrhagic colitis and vero cytotoxin-producing *Escherichia coli* in England and Wales. *Lancet 1*: 1062–1065.

Smyth, C. J. (1982). Two mannose-resistant hemagglutinations on enterotoxigenic *Escherichia coli* of serotype 06:K15:H16 or H- isolated from travelers' and infantile diarrhea. *J. Gen. Microbiol. 128*: 2081–2096.

Snyder, J. D., Wells, J. G., Yashuk, J., Puhr, N., and Blake, P. A. (1984). Outbreak of invasive *Escherichia coli* gastroenteritis on a cruise ship. *Am. J. Trop. Med. Hyg. 32*: 281–284.

So, M., and McCarty, B. J. (1980). Nucleotide sequence of the bacterial transposon Tn 1681 encoding a heat-stable (ST) toxin and its identification in enterotoxigenic *Escherichia coli* strains. *Proc. Natl. Acad. Sci. USA 77*: 4011–4015.

Stock, A. H., and Shuman, M. E. (1956). Gastroenteritis in infants associated with specific serotypes of *Escherichia coli* II. An epidemic of *Escherichia coli* 0111:B4 gastroenteritis involving multiple institutions. *Pediat. 17*: 196–203.

Strockbine, N. A., Marques, L. R. M., Newland, J. W., Smith, H. W., Holmes, R. K., and O'Brien, A. D. (1986). Two toxin converting phages from strain 933 encoded antigenically distinct toxins with similar biological activities. *Infect. Immun. 53*: 135–140.

Suthienkul, O., Brown, J. E., Seriwatana, J., Tienthongdee, S., Sastravaha, S., and Echeverria, P. (1990). Shiga-like toxin producing *Escherichia coli* in retail meats and cattle in Thailand. *J. Clin. Microbiol. 56*: 1135–1139.

Tacket, C. O., Maneval, D. R., and Levine, M. M. (1987). A new fimbrial putative colonization factor of enterotoxigenic *Escherichia coli* serotype 0159:H4, purification, morphology and genetics. *Infect. Immun. 55*: 1063–1069.

Taylor, J., Powell, B. W., and Wright, J. (1949). Infantile diarrhea and vomiting: A clinical and bacteriological investigation. *Br. Med. J. 2*: 117–141.

Taylor, W. R., Schell, W. L., Wells, J. G., Choi, K., Kinnunen, D. E., Heiser, P. T., and Helstad, A. G. (1982). A foodborne outbreak of enterotoxigenic *Escherichia coli* diarrhea. *N. Engl. J. Med. 306*: 1093–1095.

Taylor, D. N., Echeverria, P., Pal, T., Sethabutr, O., Wankitcharoen, S., Sricharmorn, S., Rowe, B., and Cross, J. H. (1986). The role of *Shigella* spp. enteroinvasive *Escherichia coli* and other enteropathogens as causes of childhood dysentery in Thailand. *J. Infect. Dis. 153*: 1132–1138.

Taylor, D. N., Echeverria, P., Sethabutr, O., Pitarangsi, C., Leksomboon, U., Blacklow, N. R., Rowe, B., Gross, R., and Cross, J. (1988a). Clinical and microbiological features of *Shigella* and enteroinvasive *Escherichia coli* infections detected by DNA hybridization. *J. Clin. Microbiol. 26*: 1362–1366.

Taylor, D. N., Houston, R., Shlim, D. R., Bhaibulaya, M., Ungar, B. L. P., and Echeverria, P. (1988b). Etiology of diarrhea among travelers and foreign residents in Nepal. *JAMA 260*: 1245–1248.

Thomson, S., Watkins, A. G., and Gray, P. O. (1956). *Escherichia coli* gastroenteritis. *Arch. Dis. Childhood 31*: 340–345.

Toledo, M. R. F., and Trabulsi, L. R. (1983). Correlation between biochemical and serological characteristics of *Escherichia coli* and results of the Sereny test. *J. Clin. Microbiol. 17*: 419–421.

Toledo, M. R. F., Alvariza, M. C. B., Murahovschi, J., Ramos, S. R. T. S., and Trabulsi, L. R. (1983). Enteropathogenic *Escherichia coli* serotypes and endemic diarrhea in infants. *Infect. Immun. 39*: 586–589.

Tsuji, T., Taga, S., Honda, T., Takeda, Y., and Miwatani, T. (1982). Molecular heterogeneity of heat-labile enterotoxins from humans and porcine enterotoxigenic *Escherichia coli. Infect. Immun. 38*: 444–448.

Tulloch, E. F., Ryan, K. J., Formal, S. B., and Franklin, F. A. (1973). Invasive enteropathogenic *Escherichia coli* dysentery: An outbreak in 28 adults. *Ann. Intern. Med. 79*: 13–17.

Ulshen, M. H., and Rollo, J. L. (1980). Pathogenesis of *Escherichia coli* gastroenteritis in man—another mechanism. *N. Engl. J. Med. 302*: 99–101.

Utomporn, P., Seriwatana, J., and Echeverria, P. (1983). Identification of enterotoxigenic *Escherichia coli* isolated from swine with diarrhea in Thailand by colony hybridization using three enterotoxin gene probes. *J. Clin. Microbiol. 18*: 1424–1431.

Vadhanasin, S., Poomchatra, A., Ratanasuda, M. L., Foopanichpuck, C., and Thudsri, P. (1976). A bacteriological survey of foods from the flight and restaurant kitchens serving Bangkok International Airport. *J. Med. Assoc. Thailand 59*: 156–161.

Wanger, A. R., Murray, B. E., Echeverria, P., Mathewson, J. S., and DuPont, H. L. (1988). Enteroinvasive *Escherichia coli* in travelers with diarrhea. *J. Infect. Dis. 158*: 640–642.

Wentworth, F. H., Brock, D. W., Stulberg, C. S., and Doge, R. H. (1956). Clinical, bacteriological, and serological observations on two human volunteers following ingestation of *Escherichia coli* 0127:138. *Proc. Soc. Exp. Biol. Med. 91*: 586–588.

Wood, L. V., Ferguson, L. E., Hogan, P., Thurman, D., Morgan, D. R., DuPont, H. L., and Ericsson, C. D. (1983a). Incidence of bacterial enteropathogens in foods from Mexico. *Appl. Environ. Microbiol. 46*: 328–332.

Wood, L. V., Wolfe, W. H., Ruiz-Palacios, G., Fushce, W. S., Corman, L. I., and McCleskey, F., Wright, J. A., and DuPont, H. L. (1983b). An outbreak of gastroenteritis due to a heat-labile enterotoxin-producing strain of *Escherichia coli. Infect. Immun. 41*: 931–934.

5

Clostridium perfringens Gastroenteritis

Ronald G. Labbé

University of Massachusetts, Amherst, Massachusetts

I. INTRODUCTION

Historically, *Clostridium perfringens* is best known for its role as a causative agent for gas gangrene (clostridial myonecrosis) especially due to wound infections. The advent of antibiotics has reduced the incidence and severity of such infections, which were especially common in warfare. More recently isolated reports have linked *C. perfringens* with antibiotic-associated diarrhea (Boriello et al., 1984), infantile diarrhea (Luzzi et al., 1986), and sudden infant death syndrome (SIDS) (Murrell et al., 1987). This chapter describes the association of this organism with a type of human food poisoning. To be discussed are the characteristics of the organism, the illness, and the responsible toxin.

Compared to other types of bacteria foodborne gastroenteritis, such as those caused by *Staphylococcus aureus* and *Salmonella*, that due to *C. perfringens* is relatively recently described. The basic aspects of the illness, isolation and identification of the organism, and purification of the responsible toxin occurred in the 1960s and early 1970s. Not surprisingly, this was accompanied by a dramatic increase in the number of reported cases. Previously such incidents would have been diagnosed as due to "unknown etiology." (It should be noted that the vast majority of foodborne disease outbreaks by whatever etiology remain unreported.)

II. CHARACTERISTICS OF THE ILLNESS

Gastroenteritis due to *C. perfringens* type A is characterized by diarrhea and severe abdominal pain 8–24 h following ingestion of food containing large numbers of the organism. Nausea is less common, and fever and vomiting are unusual. Death is uncommon, usually occurring in debilitated or institutionalized individuals, especially the elderly. The severity of the symptoms diminish within 24 h, although mild aspects can continue somewhat longer. Immunity to future episodes is not conferred.

Since the organism is often found (in meat and poultry) in the spore state, it can survive a cooking step and resume (vegetative) cell growth if the food is improperly cooled. The illness occurs when temperature-abused food in which large numbers of cells have grown is ingested. The cells sporulate in the small intestine and produce an intracellular enterotoxin, which is released into the intestine when the mother cell lyses to release the mature spore.

A more severe type of illness occurs among natives of the New Guinea Highlands. It is classified as a necrotizing, hemorrhagic jejunitis, commonly called Pig-Bel, and is caused by type C strains of the organism, which produce β toxin. The illness, which follows traditional pig feasting, is rare in Western countries (Walker, 1985; Lawrence, 1986). It will not be described further here.

III. CHARACTERISTICS OF THE ORGANISM

A. Classification

C. perfringens is a gram-positive, spore-forming rod. Its shape varies with the stage of growth as well as the nutritional composition of the medium. Unlike other pathogenic clostridia, *C. perfringens* is nonmotile. It does not produce many spores in ordinary media. Special media must be used to demonstrate sporulation (see below).

Strains of *C. perfringens* produce at least 12 different extracellular enzymes or toxins. (The enterotoxin, an intracellular protein, is not one of these.) Details of each have been described by Smith and Williams (1984). Strains are classified into five types, A–E, based on the production of four of the extracellular toxins: α, β, ε, and ι. All strains produce α toxin, also known as lecithinase or phospholipase C.

B. Serotyping

Because virtually all food-poisoning outbreaks are caused by type A strains, toxin typing of isolates from outbreaks is not performed. However, one of the laboratory criteria for confirming *C. perfringens* as the causative agent of gastroenteritis involves determining the organism serotype, which is based on the chemical composition of the capsular polysaccharide on the cell's exterior. The procedure for serotyping is described by Stringer et al. (1982).

The first serological typing scheme for *C. perfringens* was developed by Hobbs et al. (1953) using strains associated with eight outbreaks. The number of strains against which antisera were prepared has grown substantially. Nevertheless, Hatheway et al. (1980), using 91 antisera prepared against isolates of *C. perfringens* from various sources, could only serotype 35% of isolates from 163 outbreaks that occurred in the United States. Other attempts at serotyping have yielded success rates of between 60 and 70% (Stringer et al., 1980, 1982). Another drawback of serotyping as an epidemiological tool is the lack of commercially available antisera. Antisera to 13 serotypes is available from Denka Sieken Co., Ltd., Tokyo. It is likely that serotyping will continue to be performed predominantly by a few large, national references laboratories (Gross et al., 1989).

C. Effect of Temperature on Growth

The involvement of *C. perfringens* in foodborne gastroenteritis is invariably associated with its ability to (1) form spores and (2) grow at elevated temperatures. Sporulation of the organism is discussed below. The optimal temperature for growth is generally between 43 and 45°C. Generation times of 10 min or less have been reported (Willardsen et al., 1978) for certain strains.

The maximum and minimum growth temperatures for *C. perfringens* vary depending on the strain, pH, and composition of growth medium used. For example, autoclaved ground beef is a better growth medium than the commonly used glucose-rich laboratory medium, fluid thioglycollate medium (Willardsen et al., 1978). The generally accepted temperature range for growth of *C. perfringens* is 15–50°C. Although growth can occur to a limited extent above 50°C, it is usually accompanied by rapid death (Brown and Twedt, 1972). A temperature of 60°C will readily inactivate vegetative cells of *C. perfringens* in laboratory media. The temperature stability of *C. perfringens* is greater in foods than in culture media, perhaps due to the fat content of the former (Bradshaw et al., 1977).

D. Other Factors Affecting Growth

1. *Oxidation-Reduction Potential (E_h)*

C. perfringens is an anaerobe and will not produce surface colonies on agar exposed to air. Compared to other obligate anaerobes, it will tolerate a brief exposure to air. Cooked foods such as gravies typically have a lowered E_h allowing the organism to initiate growth. The latter is accompanied by the production of reducing compounds further depressing the E_h and thus enhancing the environment for growth of the organism. In the laboratory, commercially available anaerobe chambers can be used with oxygen-removal methods to culture the organisms on agar media. To grow the organism in liquid media, reducing agents such as cysteine and sodium thioglycollate are used. However, the latter can be toxic to some strains (Pearson and Walker, 1976). Low concentrations of agar (0.1–0.3%) are sometimes added to minimize the diffusion of oxygen into media. Steaming liquid media for 15–20 min prior to use also removes dissolved oxygen.

2. *Water Activity*

Water-activity levels are important in preventing the growth of pathogens in intermediate moisture foods. However, compared to *S. aureus, C. perfringens* is not very tolerant to low water activity. The lowest level supporting growth is between 0.97 and 0.95 (Kang et al., 1969; Strong et al., 1970; Bartsch and Walker, 1982).

C. perfringens grows best at pH values between 6.0 and 7.0, the same pH range as many meat and poultry products. In glucose-rich laboratory media the pH typically falls to near 5.0 after overnight incubation. Cells will die at such low pH values. The organism is considerably more stable in meat-containing media such as cooked meat medium in which meat proteins buffer the medium.

Cured meats products are rarely vehicles for outbreaks of *C. perfringens* food poisoning. This is presumably due to a combination of factors including the inhibitory action of the curing agents (sodium chloride and sodium nitrite), the low initial spore load in such products, the heat treatment administered, and the relative sensitivity of the surviving, and perhaps injured, spore population to the curing agents.

IV. SPORULATION AND ENTEROTOXIN FORMATION

Sporulation is an important aspect of *C. perfringens* for several reasons: (1) it is an important factor in classification; (2) spores can survive heating procedures and resume vegetative cell growth if proper conditions are present; and (3) large amounts of enterotoxin are produced during the sporulation stage, which, in the case of gastroenteritis, occurs in the small intestine.

Although sporulation can apparently occur readily in the intestine during cases of gastroenteritis, uniform and reproducible sporulation by *C. perfringens* is quite difficult in the laboratory and is distinctly strain- and medium-dependent. This is an important aspect since the demonstration of enterotoxin-producing ability of a given isolate requires a certain level of sporulation to be achieved in a laboratory medium. A dehydrated cooked-meat medium is commercially available, but it supports only a low level of sporulation and is used primarily for preparing stock cultures.

Many different complex media have been proposed for sporulation of *C. perfringens*, but the formulation proposed by Duncan and Strong (1968) or minor modifications of it (Labbe and Rey, 1979; Harmon and Kautter, 1986) have been most widely adopted. Certain methylxanthines (e.g., caffeine) have also been reported to stimulate sporulation (Sacks and Thompson, 1977), perhaps by affecting nucleic acid metabolism (Labbe and Nolan, 1987). Chemically defined media for sporulation have also been proposed (Sacks and Thompson, 1978; Sacks, 1983) but are tedious to prepare. Nevertheless, some strains do sporulate better in such a medium (Labbe, 1981).

Certain strains (those associated with gastroenteritis) of this organism have the genetic ability to produce an enterotoxin when they sporulate. The sequence of events can be reproduced in the laboratory by growing the cells in a sporulation medium (Fig. 1). Vegetative (nonsporulating) cells are used to inoculate the medium. In the case of human gastroenteritis the "inoculum" is temperature-abused food that contains large numbers of cells, and the sporulation medium is the contents of the lower small intestine. In laboratory media heat-resistant spores appear between 3 and 4 h and increase rapidly, reaching maximum numbers by 7 h, and remain at constant levels for several hours thereafter. Intracellular enterotoxin concentration parallels spore formation but decreases after about 10 h. This coincides with the lysis of the mother cell

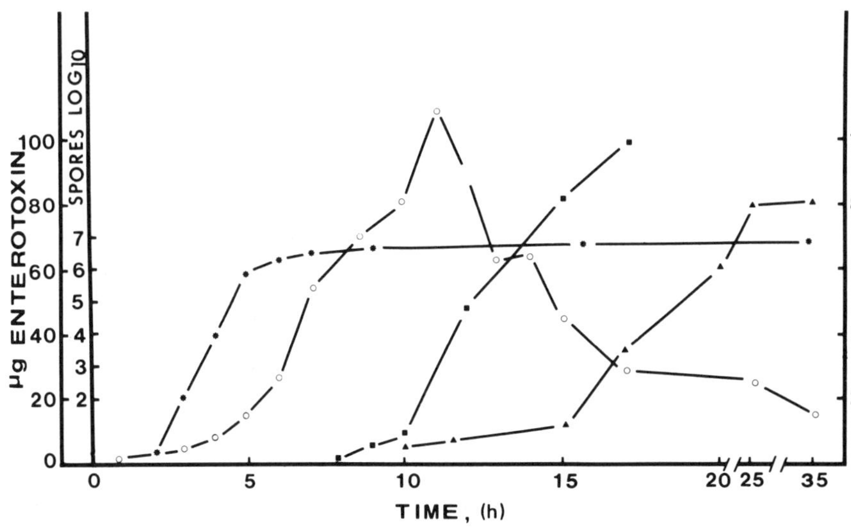

Figure 1 Time course of sporulation and intracellular enterotoxin formation and release by *C. perfringens* type A in a laboratory medium. (○) μg of biologically active enterotoxin/mg of cell protein extract; (■) μg of biologically active enterotoxin/ml of culture supernatant fluid; (✱) heat-resistant spores/ml; (▲) percentage of refractile spores free from sporangium.

and release of the toxin (and spore), which in vivo would then act on human intestinal cells.

An inclusion body is associated with the sporulation of enterotoxin-positive strains (Duncan et al., 1973). The inclusion has been isolated (Loffler and Labbe, 1985); it possesses enterotoxin-like biological activity and is composed of enterotoxin subunits (Loffler and Labbe, 1986). Its role in human illness is unclear.

V. CHARACTERISTICS OF THE ENTEROTOXIN

A. Mode of Action

Gastroenteritis caused by *C. perfringens* is characterized by diarrhea and abdominal cramps. Attempts to determine the mode of action and the responsible enterotoxin initially sought to reproduce the fluid loss using animal models. To this end rabbit and rat ileal loops (sections of the small intestine) were perfused after exposure to enterotoxin to assess the effects of the latter on intestinal transport and surface structure. The result was a net increase in secretion of water, sodium, and chloride. Glucose absorption was inhibited, whereas potassium and bicarbonate absorption was unaffected (McDonel, 1974, 1979; McDonel and Asano, 1975). Histological studies of enterotoxin-treated ileal loops revealed desquamation of intestinal epithelial cells at villous tips (Fig. 2). Brush borders (microvillous membrane) lost their characteristic folded configuration, and large quantities of membrane and cytoplasm were lost to the lumen (McDonel et al., 1978). The brush border of villous tip epithelial cells is the primary site of action of the enterotoxin. In contrast to the effects of cholera toxin and *Escherichia coli* heat-labile enterotoxin, *C. perfringens* enterotoxin does not increase the levels of cyclic AMP in intestinal mucosa that is actively secreting fluid (McDonel, 1979).

More recently, various cell lines have been employed in an attempt to determine the cellular and molecular sites of action of the enterotoxin. Vero (African green monkey kidney) cells are particularly sensitive to the enterotoxin, although rat liver, HeLa, small intestine epithelial, and other cell lines have also been used (Horiguchi et al., 1985). The enterotoxin causes rapid membrane bleb formation in cultured Vero cells, results in changes in permeability for ions, amino acids, and nucleotides, and inhibits macromolecular synthesis. The toxin appears to bind to a 50,000 molecular weight membrane receptor to form a 160,000 molecular weight complex (Wnek and McClane, 1989). In humans the loss of fluid associated with gastroenteritis is the visible manifestation associated with enterotoxin activity on intestinal cells. For a detailed discussion of the action of this toxin, see McClane et al. (1988).

B. Biochemical Characteristics

Amino acid sequence analysis of the enterotoxin has yielded a molecular weight of 34,262 consisting of a single polypeptide of 309 amino acids

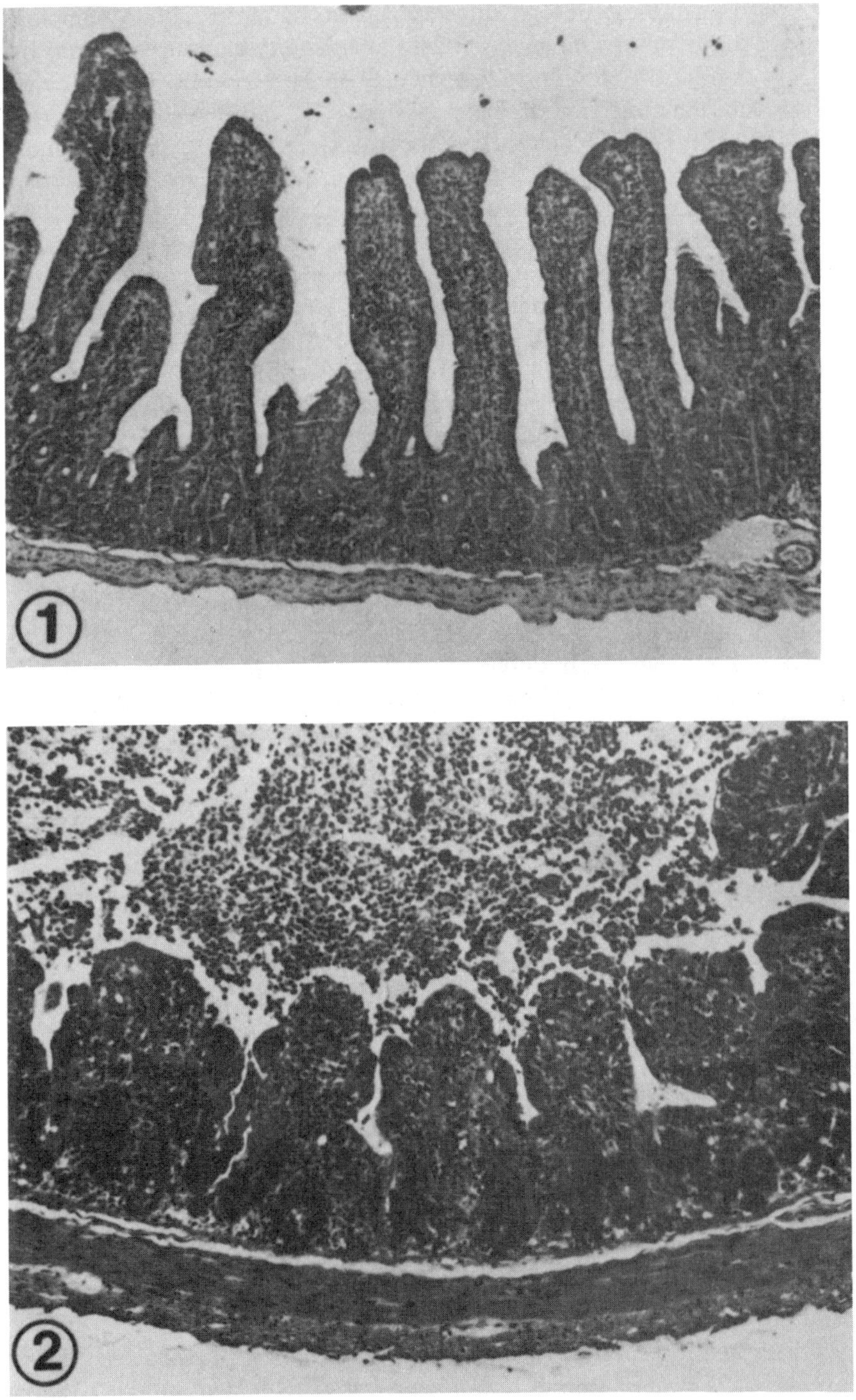

Figure 2 Effect of *C. perfringens* enterotoxin on rabbit ileum. 1, Control showing typical villus morphology. 2, Ileum treated with enterotoxin for 90 min showing shortened villi with tips denuded of epithelial cells. (Reprinted with permission of *Laboratory Investigation*.)

(Richardson and Granum, 1985). The sequence of the toxin has no homology with any other toxin for which sequence data are available, indicating that the enterotoxin represents a unique polypeptide primary structure (Duffy et al., 1982; Richardson and Granum, 1985).

The enterotoxin loses biological activity by treatment with pronase and subtilisin but is insensitive to trypsin, chymotrypsin, bacterial lipase, α-amylase, papain, and neuraminidase (Duncan and Strong, 1969; Hauschild and Hilsheimer, 1971). In fact, trypsinization of the toxin results in a threefold increase in biological activity (Granum, 1982). The latter suggests that there may be some activation of the toxin by proteolysis in the small intestine.

The enterotoxin is heat-labile, with heating in saline at 60°C for 5 min destroying biological activity. At the same temperature 20% of serological activity remains after heating for 20 min (Naik and Duncan, 1978).

Enterotoxin stored at 37°C for 7 days or at –20°C for 28 days loses biological activity but not serological activity (McDonel and McClane, 1981). However, neither biological nor serological activity is affected by storage at 4°C for several weeks (Granum et al., 1981). About 5–10% of the original activity of the toxin is lost each time it is thawed. Lyophilization is the preferred method of storing toxin.

Enterotoxin has also been detected in *C. perfringens* types C and D (Skjelkvale and Duncan, 1975; Uemura and Skjelkvale, 1976), and its properties are similar to those of enterotoxin from type A strains.

C. Purification of Enterotoxin

Early methods for enterotoxin purification were tedious and time-consuming. They involved nuclease treatment and multiple chromatographic steps. A simplified method has become available and widely adopted (Granum and Whitaker, 1980). This procedure involves ammonium sulfate precipitation of sporulating cell extracts followed by gel filtration. Using this basic method, a scaled-up protocol involving 40 L of culture has been described (Reynolds et al., 1986).

Several investigators have reported that some toxin preparations contain a minor band (seen on polyacrylamide gel electrophoresis) after purification. This minor band possesses weak biological and serological activity. This is an artifact due to endogenous protease activity (Park and Labbe, 1990). The use of protease inhibitors, sterilized elution buffers, low temperatures, and pasteurization (or similar heat treatment) of gel filtration media can alleviate this problem.

Many other techniques have been used for enterotoxin purification. These include high-performance liquid chromatography (Uemura et al., 1985), affinity chromatography (Scott and Duncan, 1975; Barnhart et al., 1976; Uemura and Skjelkvale, 1976), and preparative polyacrylamide gel electrophoresis (Enders and Duncan, 1977). None of these has been as widely adopted as the ammonium sulfate–gel filtration method.

D. Enterotoxin Assays

1. Biological Assays

Many biological assays have been developed for detecting *C. perfringens* enterotoxin. The earliest was the rabbit ileal loop (Duncan et al., 1968; Hauschild et al., 1971), which had been used previously for studying cholera toxin. The assay involves the measurement fluid accumulation in ligated intestinal sections in response to the enterotoxin. The procedure is time-consuming, not well suited to multiple assays, and relatively insensitive. Intestinal sections of other animal species have also been used but are even less sensitive than the rabbit model.

Other animal assays include oral inoculation (and subsequent diarrhea) of mice (Tsai and Riemann, 1975), intraperitoneal injection (and subsequent death) of mice (Stark and Duncan, 1971), capillary permeability in the skin of guinea pigs (Stark and Duncan, 1972), and erythemal activity in guinea pigs and rabbits following intradermal injection of enterotoxin (Hauschild, 1970). In the capillary permeability assay animals are injected intradermally with 50-μl samples followed 20 min later by an intravenous injection of blue dye, which allows the measurement of the diameter of a blue zone that develops because of increased capillary permeability caused by the enterotoxin. The diameter of the reaction is proportional to the concentration of injected enterotoxin. Of the proposed biological assays, the erythemal activity test is the most sensitive (1.2–2.5 μg/ml) (Genigeorgis et al., 1973).

2. Serological Assays

The need for speed, sensitivity, and convenience led to the development of several serological assays for *C. perfringens* enterotoxin. All require the preparation of specific antiserum or immunoglobulin G against *C. perfringens* enterotoxin. Early assays used precipitation reactions under an electrical field. These included electroimmunodiffusion (Duncan and Somers, 1972), also known as rocket electrophoresis, and counterimmunoelectrophoresis (CIEP) (Naik and Duncan, 1977). In CIEP serial dilutions of enterotoxin are placed in wells about 5 mm apart from enterotoxin antibody-containing wells. A precipitation reaction (white band) occurs under the influence of an electric field. Sensitivity is approximately 0.2 μg/ml.

ELISA (enzyme-linked immunosorbent assay) procedures have been developed by a number of laboratories for enterotoxin detection with reported detection limits of 1–5 ng/g for feces and even less for aqueous samples (Olsvik et al., 1982; McClane and Strouse, 1984; Notermans et al., 1984; Bartholomew et al., 1985; Jackson et al., 1985; Wimsatt et al., 1986). Each proposed ELISA method differs in speed and sensitivity. Because of their sensitivity, ELISA methods are better than CIEP for detecting enterotoxin in feces, with results from one study indicating that the ELISA procedure detected enterotoxins in 89% of fecal samples compared to 66% by CIEP (Bartholomew et al., 1985).

The only commercially available (Oxoid, Inc.) serological assay for *C. perfringens* enterotoxin is a reversed passive latex agglutination (RPLA) test. Comparative evaluations of ELISA and RPLA have revealed that, in general,

RPLA is similar in sensitivity to the ELISA (Berry et al., 1986, 1988; Harmon and Kautter, 1986), although sensitivity is reduced when the enterotoxin is present in fecal extracts (Harmon and Kautter, 1986). The procedure is simple and involves exposure of antienterotoxin-coated latex beads to serial dilutions of enterotoxin-containing material. After overnight incubation, the agglutination titer is determined. Expensive equipment such as microplate reader (needed for ELISA) is not necessary. On the other hand, for routine use the kit is expensive; cost per assay is $8–9.

A more rapid (1 h) and inexpensive (for large number of assays) slide latex agglutination assay has been described by McClane and Snyder (1987) with a sensitivity limit of 1 μg/g feces. Most recently, dot-blotting procedures have been proposed and used (Mehta et al., 1989; Park and Labbe, 1990). These are ELISA-like assays in which enterotoxin (or unknown samples) is applied to a nitrocellulose membrane followed by immunostaining with, successively, rabbit anti-enterotoxin serum and horseradish peroxidase-conjugated anti-rabbit immunoglobulin. Given the low detection level (0.02 μg of enterotoxin in feces), the technique is unsurpassed in sensitivity and low cost.

3. Tissue Culture Assays

The enterotoxin binds to many different mammalian and human cell lines (Giugliano et al., 1983). Although tissue culture methods have been used mainly to study the mode of action of the enterotoxin, the Vero cell line in particular has been reported to be useful for enterotoxin assay. The technique, described in detail by McDonel and McClane (1981), involves the ability of enterotoxin to prevent growth ("plating efficiency") of Vero cells on tissue culture plates. Although the method can detect a concentration of enterotoxin of 1 ng/ml, severe nonspecific interference occurs from compounds present in fecal extracts.

E. Detection of Enterotoxin in Feces

Gastroenteritis due to *C. perfringens* enterotoxin can be confirmed by detection of enterotoxin in feces of ill individuals (Stringer et al., 1985; Jackson et al., 1986; Birkhead et al., 1988). The time after onset of symptoms at which samples are collected is important. In one study enterotoxin could be detected in fecal extracts if the stool samples were collected within 1 but not 5 days after symptoms began (Itoh et al., 1978). The levels of enterotoxin detected in feces following foodborne outbreaks have ranged from 0.001 to more than 100 μg/g feces (Notermans et al., 1984; Bartholomew et al., 1985; Harmon and Kautter, 1986; Wimsatt et al., 1986; Berry et al., 1988). Specimens from healthy adults contain undetectable amounts of enterotoxin.

In addition to the presence of enterotoxin in feces, an elevated ($\geq 10^6$ spores/g feces) fecal spore count has been proposed to confirm illness due to this organism (Harmon et al., 1986). However, healthy elderly patients may normally carry high numbers of spores of this organism in their intestinal tract (Yamagishi et al., 1976; Stringer et al., 1985). In these instances the elevated fecal spore count has limited usefulness. In one study (Itoh et al., 1978) the only definitive evidence confirming *C. perfringens* as the causative agent in gastroenteritis cases involving elderly patients was the detection of enterotoxin in feces.

F. Molecular Genetics

As with other bacteria, *C. perfringens* carry a number of plasmids. The function for a few have been identified. These include plasmids conferring resistance to the antibiotics tetracycline and chloramphenicol (Abraham and Rood, 1987) and those coding for the production of bacteriocins (Ionesco et al., 1976; Garnier and Cole, 1988). Bacteriocins are low molecular weight, heat-stable proteins which are lethal to other related bacteria.

Analysis of plasmid profiles is increasingly used as an indication of strain relatedness for a number of medically important bacterial species. In the case of *C. perfringens*, 77% of food poisoning isolates (Mahony et al., 1987) and 65% of meat-associated isolates (Phillips-Jones, 1989) were found to contain plasmids. In the latter study 71% of plasmid-carrying strains possessed a 6.2 kb plasmid whose function is unknown. Some loss of plasmids during laboratory storage of this organism has been noted (Phillips-Jones, 1989). In spite of recent work, plasmid profiling analysis is still in its infancy.

Genetic studies involving *C. perfringens* have been hampered by a lack of efficient and rapid techniques for genetic exchange. Electroporation-mediated transformation (exchange of DNA) of this organism with plasmid DNA has recently been reported (Allen and Blaschek, 1988, 1990; Scott and Rood, 1989; Phillips-Jones, 1990). Nevertheless, relatively little is known about the genetics of enterotoxin production except that genes responsible for its synthesis are located on the chromosome. About 6% of isolates from fecal samples of animal origin (non–food poisoning isolates) contain the enterotoxin gene (Van Damme-Jongsten et al., 1989).

A physical map of the genome of this organism has recently been established (Canard and Cole, 1989). In addition the gene encoding for the enterotoxin has been cloned in *E. coli* and sequenced (Iwanejko et al., 1989; Van Damme-Jongsten et al., 1989).

REFERENCES

Abraham, L., and Rood, J. (1987). Identification of Tn 4451 and Tn 4452, chloramphenicol resistance transposons from *Clostridium perfringens*. *J. Bacteriol. 169*: 1579–1584.

Allen, S., and Blaschek, H. (1988). Electroporation-induced transformation of intact cells of *Clostridium perfringens*. *Appl. Environ. Microbiol. 54*: 2322–2324.

Allen, S., and Blaschek, H. (1990). Factors involved in the electroporation induced transformation of *Clostridium perfringens*. *FEMS Microbiol. Lett. 70*: 217–220.

Barnhart, H., Bullerman, L., Ball, E., and Wagner, F. (1976). Isolation and purification of *Clostridium perfringens* enterotoxin by affinity chromatography. *J. Food Sci. 41*: 903–906.

Bartholomew, B., Stringer, M., Watson, G., and Gilbert, R. (1985). Development and application of an enzyme-linked immunosorbent assay for *Clostridium perfringens* type A enterotoxin. *J. Clin. Path. 38*: 222–228.

Bartsch, A., and Walker, H. (1982). Effect of temperature, solute and pH on the tolerance of *Clostridium perfringens* to reduced water activities. *J. Food Sci. 47*: 1754–1755.

Berry, P., Stringer, M., and Uemura, T. (1986). Comparison of latex agglutination and ELISA for the detection of *Clostridium perfringens* Type A enterotoxin in feces. *Letts. Appl. Microbiol. 2*: 101–102.

Berry, P., Rodhouse, J., Hughes, S., Bartholomew, B., and Gilbert, R. (1988). Evaluation of ELISA, RPLA, and Vero cell assays for detecting *Clostridium perfringens* enterotoxin in fecal specimens. *J. Clin. Pathol. 41*: 458–461.

Birkhead, G., Vogt, R., Heun, R., Snyder, J., and McClane, B. (1988). Characterization of an outbreak of *Clostridium perfringens* food poisoning by quantitative fecal culture and fecal enterotoxin measurement. *J. Clin. Microbiol. 26*: 471–474.

Boriello, S., Larson, H., Welch, A., Barclay, F., Stringer, M., and Bartholomew, B. (1984). *Clostridium Perfringens*: A possible cause of antibiotic-associated diarrhea. *Lancet 1*: 305–307.

Bradshaw, J., Peeler, J., and Twedt, R. (1977). Thermal inactivation of ileal-loop reactive *Clostridium perfringens* type A strains in phosphate buffer and beef gravy. *Appl. Environ. Microbiol. 34*: 280–284.

Brown, D., and Twedt, R. (1972). Assessment of the sanitary effectiveness of holding temperatures on beef cooked at low temperature. *Appl. Microbiol. 24*: 599–603.

Canard, B., and Cole, S. (1989). Genome organization of the anaerobic pathogen *Clostridium perfringens. Proc. Natl. Acad. Sci. 86*: 6676–6680.

Craven, S. (1980). Growth and sporulation of *Clostridium perfringens* in foods. *Food Technol. 34*: 80–87.

Duffy, K., McDonel, J., McClane, B., and Kurosky, A. (1982). *Clostridium perfringens* type A enterotoxin: Characterization of the amino terminal region. *Infect. Immun. 38*: 386–388.

Duncan, C., and Somers, E. (1972). Quantitation of *Clostridium perfringens* type A enterotoxin by electroimmunodiffusion. *Appl. Microbiol. 24*: 801–804.

Duncan, C., and Strong, D. (1968). Improved medium for sporulation of *Clostridium perfringens. Appl. Microbiol. 16*: 82–89.

Duncan, C., and Strong, D. (1969). Ileal loop fluid accumulation and production of diarrhea in rabbits by cell-free products of *Clostridium perfringens. J. Bacteriol. 100*: 86–94.

Duncan, C., Sugiyama, H., and Strong, D. (1968). Rabbit ileal loop response to strains of *Clostridium perfringens. J. Bacteriol. 95*: 1560–1566.

Duncan, C., King, G., and Frieben, W. (1973). A paracrystalline inclusion formed during sporulation of enterotoxin-producing *Clostridium perfringens* type A. *J. Bacteriol. 114*: 845–859.

Enders, G., and Duncan, G. (1977). Preparative polyacrylamide gel electrophoresis purification of *Clostridium perfringens* enterotoxin. *Infect. Immun. 17*: 425–429.

Garnier, T., and Cole, S. (1988). Identification and molecular genetic analysis of replication functions of the bacteriocinogenic plasmic pIP404 from *Clostridium perfringens. Plasmid 19*: 151–160.

Genigeorgis, C., Sakaguchi, G., and Riemann, H. (1973). Assay methods for *Clostridium perfringens* type A enterotoxin. *Appl. Microbiol. 26*: 111–115.

Giugliano, L., Stringer, M., and Drasar, B. (1983). Detection of *Clostridium perfringens* enterotoxin by tissue culture and double gel diffusion. *J. Med. Microbiol. 16*: 233–237.

Granum, P. (1982). Inhibition of protein synthesis by a tryptic polypeptide of *Clostridium perfringens* type A enterotoxin. *Biochim. Biophys. Acta 708*: 6–11.

Granum, P., and Whitaker, J. R. (1980). Improved method for purification of enterotoxin from *Clostridium perfringens* type A. *Appl. Environ. Microbiol. 39*: 1120–1122.

Granum, P., Whitaker, J., and Skjelkvale, R. (1981). Trypsin activation of enterotoxin from *Clostridium perfringens* type A. *Biochim. Biophys. Acta 668*: 325–332.

Gross, T., Kamara, L., Hatheway, C., Powers, P., Libonati, J., Harmon, S., and Israel, E. (1989). *Clostridium perfringens* food poisoning: Use of serotyping in an outbreak setting. *J. Clin. Microbiol. 27*: 660–663.

Harmon, S., and Kautter, D. (1986). Evaluation of a reversed passive latex agglutination test kit for *Clostridium perfringens. J. Food Prot. 49*: 523–525.

Harmon, S., Kautter, D., and Hatheway, C. (1986). Enumeration and characterization of *Clostridium perfringens* spores in the feces of food poisoning patients and normal controls. *J. Food Protect. 49*: 23–28.

Hatheway, C., Whaley, D., and Dowell, V. (1980). Epidemiological aspects of *Clostridium perfringens* food-borne illness. *Food Tech. 34*: 77–79.

Hauschild, A. (1970). Erythemal activity of the cellular enteropathogenic factor of *Clostridium perfringens* type A. *Can. J. Microbiol. 16*: 651–654.

Hauschild, A., and Hilsheimer, R. (1971). Purification and characteristics of the enterotoxin of *Clostridium perfringens* type A. *Can. J. Microbiol. 17*: 1425–1433.

Hauschild, A., Hilscheimer, R., and Rogers, C. (1971). Rapid detection of *Clostridium perfringens* enterotoxin by a modified ligated intestinal loop technique. *Can. J. Microbiol. 17*: 1475–1476.

Hobbs, B., Smith, M., Oakley, C., Warrack, and Cruickshank, J. (1953). *Clostridium welchii* food poisoning. *J. Hyg. 51*: 75–101.

Horiguchi, Y., Uemura, T., Kozaki, S., and Sakaguchi, G. (1985). The relationships between cytotoxic effects and binding to mammalian cultured cells of *Clostridium perfringens* enterotoxin. *FEMS Microbiol. Lett. 28*: 131–135.

Ionesco, H., Bieth, G., Dauget, C., and Bouanchaud, D. (1976). Isolement et identification de deux plasmids d'une souch bacteriocingene de *Clostridium perfringens. Ann. Microbiol.* (Inst. Pasteur) *127B*: 283–294.

Itoh, T., Saito, K., Inaba, M., and Saki, S. (1978). Detection of *Clostridium perfringens* enterotoxin from feces of food poisoning cases. In *Symposium on Cholera*, K. Takeya and Y. Zinnaka, eds. Proceedings, 14th Joint Conference U.S.–Japan Cooperative Medical Science Program, Tokyo, Fuji Printing, Tokyo.

Iwanejko, L., Routledge, M., and Stewart, G. (1989). Cloning in *Escherichia coli* of the enterotoxin gene from *Clostridium perfringens* type A. *J. Gen. Microbiol. 135*: 903–909.

Jackson, S., Yip-Chuck, D., and Brodsky, M. (1985). A double antibody sandwich enzyme-immunoassay for *Clostridium perfringens* type A enterotoxin detection in stool specimens. *J. Immunol. Meth. 83*: 141–150.

Jackson, S., Yip-Chuck, D., Clark, J., and Brodsky, M. (1986). Diagnostic importance of *Clostridium perfringens* enterotoxin analysis in recurring enteritis among elderly chronic care psychiatric patients. *J. Clin. Microbiol. 23*: 748–751.

Kang, C., Woodburn, M., Pagenkopf, A., and Cheney, R. (1969). Growth sporulation and germination of *Clostridium perfringens* in media of controlled water activity. *Appl. Microbiol. 18*: 798–805.

Labbe, R. (1981). Enterotoxin formation by *Clostridium perfringens* type A in a defined medium. *Appl. Environ. Microbiol. 41*: 315–317.

Labbe, R., and Nolan, L. (1987). Inhibition of macromolecular synthesis by caffeine in *Clostridium perfringens. Can. J. Microbiol. 33*: 589–592.

Labbe, R., and Rey, D. (1979). Raffinose increases sporulation and enterotoxin production by *Clostridium perfringens* type A. *Appl. Environ. Microbiol. 37*: 1196–1200.

Lawrence, G. (1986). Necrotizing enteritis of *Clostridium perfringens. J. Infect. Dis. 153*: 803–806.

Loffler, A., and Labbe, R. (1985). Isolation of an inclusion body from enterotoxin-positive *Clostridium perfringens. FEMS Microbiol. Lett. 27*: 143–147.

Loffler, A., and Labbe, R. (1986). Characterization of a parasporal inclusion body from sporulating enterotoxin-positive *Clostridium perfringens* type A. *J. Bacteriol. 165*: 542–548.

Luzzi, I., Caprioli, A., Falbo, V., Guarino, A., Capano, G., Alessio, M., Malamisura, B., and Gianfrilli, P. (1986). Detection of clostridial toxins in stools from children with diarrhea. *J. Med. Microbiol. 22*: 29–31.

Mahony, D., Stringer, M., Borriello, S., and Mader, J. (1987). Plasmid analysis as a means of strain differentiation in *Clostridium perfringens. J. Clin. Microbiol. 25*: 1333–1335.

McClane, B., and Snyder, J. (1987). Development and preliminary evaluation of a slide agglutination assay for detection of *Clostridium perfringens* type A enterotoxin. *J. Immunol. Meth. 100*: 131–136.

McClane, B., and Strouse, R. (1984). Rapid detection of *Clostridium perfringens* type A enterotoxin by enzyme-linked immunosorbent assay. *J. Clin. Microbiol. 19*: 112–115.

McClane, B., Hanna, P., and Wnek, A. (1988). *Clostridium perfringens* enterotoxin. *Microbiol. Path. 4*: 317–323.

McDonel, J. (1974). In vivo effects of *Clostridium perfringens* enteropathogenic factors on the rat ileum. *Infect. Immun. 10*: 1156–1162.

McDonel, J. (1979). The molecular mode of action of *Clostridium perfringens* enterotoxin. *Amer. J. Clin. Nutr. 32*: 210–218.

McDonel, J., and Asano, J. (1975). Analysis of unidirectional fluxes of sodium during diarrhea induced by *Clostridium perfringens* enterotoxin in the rat terminal ileum. *Infect. Immun. 11*: 526–529.

McDonel, J., and McClane, B. (1981). Highly sensitive assay for *Clostridium perfringens* enterotoxin that uses inhibition of plating efficiency of Vero cells grown in culture. *J. Clin. Microbiol. 13*: 940–946.

McDonel, J., Chang, L., Pounds, J., and Duncan, C. (1978). The effects of *Clostridium perfringens* enterotoxin on rat and rabbit ileum. *Lab. Invest. 39*: 210–218.

Mehta, R., Narayan, K., and Notermans, S. (1989). DOT-enzyme linked immunosorbent assay for detection of *Clostridium perfringens* type A enterotoxin. *Int. J. Food Microbiol. 9*: 45–50.

Murrell, T., Ingham, B., Moss, J., and Taylor, W. (1987). A hypothesis concerning *Clostridium perfringens* type A enterotoxin and sudden infant death syndrome. *Med. Hypoth. 22*: 401–413.

Naik, H., and Duncan, C. (1977). Rapid detection and quantitation of *Clostridium perfringens* enterotoxin by counterimmunoelectrophoresis. *Appl. Environ. Microbiol. 34*: 125–128.

Naik, H., and Duncan, C. (1978). Thermal inactivation of *Clostridium perfringens* enterotoxin. *J. Food Protect. 41*: 100–103.

Notermans, S., Heuvelman, C., Beckers, H., and Uemura, T. (1984). Evaluation of the ELISA tool in diagnosing *Clostridium perfringens* enterotoxin. *Zentralb. Bakt. Hyg*., I. Abt. Orig. B *179*: 225–239.

Olsvik, O., Granum, P., and Berdal, B. (1982). Detection of *Clostridium perfringens* type A enterotoxin by ELISA. *Acta Pathol. Microbiol. Immunol. Scand*. Sect. B *90*: 445–447.

Park, K., and Labbe, R. (1990). Proteolysis of *Clostridium perfringens* type A enterotoxin during purification. *Infect. Immun. 58*: 1999–2001.

Pearson, C., and Walker, H. (1976). Effect of oxidation-eduction potential upon growth and sporulation of *Clostridium perfringens. J. Milk Food Technol. 39*: 421–425.

Phillips-Jones, M. (1990). Plasmid transformation of *Clostridium perfringens* by electroporation methods. *FEMS Microbiol. Lett. 66*: 221–226.

Phillips-Jones, M., Iwanejko, L., and Longden, M. (1989). Analysis of plasmid profiling as a method for rapid differentiation of food-associated *Clostridium perfringens* strains. *J. Appl. Bacteriol. 67*: 243–254.

Reynolds, D., Tranter, H., and Hambleton, P. (1986). Scaled-up production and purification of *Clostridium perfringens* Type A enterotoxin. *J. Appl. Bacteriol. 60*: 517–525.

Richardson, M., and Granum, P. (1985). The amino sequence of the enterotoxin from *Clostridium perfringens. FEBS Lett. 182*: 479–484.

Sacks, L. (1983). Influence of carbohydrates on growth and sporulation of *Clostridium perfringens* in a defined medium with or without guanosine. *Appl. Environ. Microbiol. 46*: 1169–1175.

Sacks, L., and Thompson, P. (1977). Increased spore yields of *Clostridium perfringens* in the presence of methylxanthines. *Appl. Environ. Microbiol. 34*: 189–193.

Sacks, L., and Thompson, P. (1978). Clear defined medium for the sporulation of *Clostridium perfringens. Appl. Environ. Microbiol. 35*: 405–410.

Scott, V., and Duncan, C. (1975). Affinity chromatography purification of *Clostridium perfringens* enterotoxin. *Infect. Immun. 12*: 536–543.

Scott, P., and Rood, J. (1989). Electroporation-mediated transformation of lysostaphin-treated *Clostridium perfringens. Gene 82*: 327–333.

Skjelkvale, R., and Duncan, C. (1975). Enterotoxin from different toxigenic types of *Clostridium perfringens. Infect. Immun. 11*: 563–575.

Smith, L., and Williams, B. (1984). *The Pathogenic Anaerobic Bacteria.* Charles Thomas, Springfield, IL, pp. 101–134.

Stark, R., and Duncan, C. (1971). Biological characteristics of *Clostridium perfringens* type A enterotoxin. *Infect. Immun. 4*: 89–96.

Stark, R., and Duncan, C. (1972). Transient increase in capillary permeability induced by *Clostridium perfringens* type A enterotoxin. *Infect. Immun. 5*: 147–150.

Stringer, M., Turnbull, P., and Gilbert, R. (1980). Application of serological typing to the investigation of outbreaks of *Clostridium perfringens* food poisoning. *J. Hyg. 84*: 443–456.

Stringer, M., Watson, G., and Gilbert, R. (1982). *Clostridium perfringens* type A: Serological typing and methods for the detection of enterotoxin. In *Isolation and Identification Methods for Food Poisoning Microorganisms*, J. Corry, D. Roberts, and F. Skinner, eds. Academic Press, London, pp. 111–135.

Stringer, M., Watson, G., Gilbert, R., Wallace, J., Hassall, J., Tanner, E., and Webber, P. (1985). Fecal carriage of *Clostridium perfringens. J. Hyg. 95*: 277–288.

Strong, D., Foster, E., and Duncan, C. (1970). Influence of water activity on the growth of *Clostridium perfringens. Appl. Microbiol. 19*: 980–987.

Tsai, C., and Riemann, H. (1975). Food poisoning signs in mice induced orally by *Clostridium perfringens* type A enterotoxin. *J. Formosan Med. Assoc. 74*: 310–315.

Uemura, T., and Skjelkvale, R. (1976). An enterotoxin produced by *Clostridium perfringens* type D. *Acta Pathol. Microbiol. Immunol. Scand.* Sect. B *84*: 414–420.

Uemura, T., Aoi, Y., Horiguchi, Y., Wadano, A., Goshima, N., and Sakaguchi, G. (1985). Purification of *Clostridium perfringens* enterotoxins by high performance liquid chromatography. *FEMS Microbiol. Lett. 29*: 293–297.

Van Damme-Jongsten, M., Wernars, K., and Noterman, S. (1989). Cloning and sequencing of the *Clostridium perfringens* enterotoxin gene. *Ant. van Leeuwen. 56*: 181–190.

Walker, H. (1985). Pig-bel. In *Clostridia in Gastrointestinal Disease*, S. Borriello, ed. CRC Press, Boca Raton, FL.

Willardsen, R., Busta, F., Allen, C., and Smith, L. (1978). Growth and survival of *Clostridium perfringens* during constantly rising temperatures. *J. Food Sci. 43*: 470–475.

Wimsatt, J., Harmon, S., and Shah, D. (1986). Detection of *Clostridium perfringens* enterotoxin in stool specimens and culture supernatants by enzyme-linked immunosorbent assay. *Diagn. Microbiol. Infect. Dis. 4*: 307–313.

Wnek, A., and McClane, B. (1989). Preliminary evidence that *Clostridium perfringens* type A enterotoxin is present in a 160,000-M_r complex in mammalian membranes. *Infect. Immun. 57*: 574–581.

Yamagishi, T., Serikawa, T., Morita, R., Nakamura, S., and Nishida, S. (1976). Persistent high numbers of *Clostridium perfringens* in the intestines of Japanese aged adults. *Jpn. J. Microbiol. 20*: 397–403.

6

Bacillus cereus Gastroenteritis

John M. Kramer and Richard J. Gilbert

PHLS Food Hygiene Laboratory, Central Public Health Laboratory, London, United Kingdom

I. INTRODUCTION

The European literature from the beginning of this century contains numerous accounts of food poisonings caused by *Bacillus cereus* or *B. cereus*-like organisms. One of the earliest recorded episodes appeared in 1906, when Lubenau described a hospital outbreak involving 300 patients and staff who developed symptoms of acute gastroenteritis shortly after eating dinner. The main item on the menu had been meatballs, remnants of which were later found to be grossly contaminated with an aerobic spore-forming bacterium.

Later, Seitz (1913) was to record the isolation of large numbers of *B. cereus*-like microorganisms from the feces of a young man suffering from severe enteritis and diarrhea, and Brekenfeld (1926, 1929) implicated aerobic sporogenic bacilli as the cause of two separate outbreaks involving vanilla sauce and a jellied meat dish.

By current epidemiological standards, early reports of food poisoning associated with *Bacillus* species were somewhat sketchy. Quantitative bacteriology was rarely undertaken, either on suspect foods or clinical specimens, and the nomenclature used to classify the isolates (e.g., *B. subtilis-mesentericus*, anthracoid, or pseudoanthraxlike) became imprecise and inevitably confusing.

This apparent confusion in terminology, reflecting as it did the disorder then prevailing in *Bacillus* taxonomy, contributed to the slow recognition of pathogenicity among members of the genus other than *B. anthracis*. No review of this subject can therefore fail to acknowledge the importance of the contribution made by Smith (1946, 1952) and Gordon and colleagues (1973) in bringing order to *Bacillus* taxonomy, and in providing a foundation of tests and interpretations on which rests our present understanding of this group of microorganisms.

It was against this background in the early 1950s that Hauge finally succeeded in placing *B. cereus* on the map as a recognized food-poisoning organism, following publication of his meticulous investigations into four large outbreaks in Norway (Hauge, 1950, 1955) (see Sec. IV.A).

II. CHARACTERISTICS OF *B. CEREUS*

A. General Classification of *Bacillus* species

Members of the genus *Bacillus* have a ubiquitous environmental distribution. Because of the resistance of their spores and the capacity of the vegetative cell forms to secrete enzymes capable of degrading many organic materials, the genus represents arguably the most commercially important group of bacteria. Nonetheless, it is apparent that most bacteriologists still consider the identification of these organisms too difficult to carry out properly, or even at all.

In contrast to other bacterial genera, the genus *Bacillus* encompasses a great diversity of species and strains. The eighth edition of *Bergey's Manual of Determinative Bacteriology* (Gibson and Gordon, 1974) lists 22 officially recognized species and a further 26 of uncertain status. Most are not difficult to isolate or culture, and the persistence of the endospores assists both the isolation and maintenance of strains in the laboratory.

Of the various identification schemes proposed, that of Gordon et al. (1973) remains preeminent. Following a detailed study of more than a thousand strains, these authors proposed a primary division of the genus into three groups according to their cellular morphology and physiological properties.

Group 1 comprised gram-positive species that formed ellipsoidal or cylindrical spores which did not appreciably distend the sporangia. Organisms of Group 2 and 3 were differentiated on the basis of having swollen sporangia and either ellipsoidal (Group 2) or spherical (Group 3) spores. Members of these latter two groups could be either gram-positive, gram-negative, or variable. Group 1 species were further subdivided according to their vegetative cell dimensions and the presence of lipid globules in the protoplasm. Thus the "large-celled" species (Group 1A), having cell widths greater than 0.9 μm and producing lipid globules, included *B. megaterium, B. cereus*, and the closely related *B. cereus* var. *mycoides, B. thuringiensis*, and *B. anthracis*, while the "small-celled" species (Group 1B) (cell diameter <0.9 μm; lipid globules not formed) included *B. subtilis, B. pumilus, B. licheniformis*, and *B. coagulans*.

This classification, however, is still not entirely satisfactory. Evidence from studies of DNA composition suggests that the genus *Bacillus* is equivalent to some bacterial families (Priest, 1981), a fact that will undoubtably necessitate further rationalization of this genus.

From the public health viewpoint several, in the main Group 1, *Bacillus* species have received particular attention as either suspect or proven pathogens. The majority of *Bacillus* species, however, are apparently harmless saprophytes that have, by virtue of their proteolytic and saccharolytic capabilities, an important role to play in the recycling of nutrients in nature.

B. *B. cereus*: Properties of the Organism

Microscopically, the bacteria may be seen as large, gram-positive rods that are motile by means of peritrichous flagella. Cells are typically 1.0–1.2 μm in diameter by 3.0–5.0 μm in length. Single endospores may be formed in either a central or paracentral position without distention of the sporangium. The organism sporulates freely on many media under well-aerated conditions, although vegetative cells can also grow anaerobically. *B. cereus* is able to utilize glucose, fructose, and trehalose, but not pentoses and many of the sugar alcohols. Certain strains attack sucrose, salicin, maltose, mannose, glycerol, *m*-inositol, and lactose. A small percentage of strains are urease-positive; the majority actively hydrolyze starch, casein, and gelatin (Gordon et al., 1973; Gibson and Gordon, 1974; Gilbert and Taylor, 1976; Gordon, 1977).

A summary of those physiological characteristics of *B. cereus* having direct industrial and public health applications is presented in Table 1. It should be noted that, as with other *Bacillus* species, certain properties of *B. cereus* are subject to extraordinarily wide strain variation, which in many instances remain to be adequately investigated.

The influence of temperature on spore germination, outgrowth, and cell division has been the subject of several studies. Growth and multiplication of vegetative *B. cereus* cells typically occur within the temperature range of 10–50°C (Mol, 1957; Gibson and Gordon, 1974; Johnson et al., 1983), the optimum arising between 28 and 35°C (Gilbert, 1979). However, psychrotrophic variants of *B. cereus* have been identified in raw and pasteurized milk (Larkin and Stokes, 1966; Shehata and Collins, 1971, 1972) capable of

Table 1 Physiological Properties of *B. cereus*

Property	Test parameters	Values reported	Ref.
Spore heat resistance	$D_{95°C}$ (aqu./PB′ suspn.)	1.2–36.2 min	Gilbert et al., 1974; Parry and Gilbert, 1980; Johnson et al., 1982
	$D_{100°C}$ (aqu./PB′ suspn.)	1.2–8.0 min	Molin and Snygg, 1967; Gilbert et al., 1974; Johnson et al., 1982
	$D_{100°C}$ (skimmed milk)	2.7–3.1 min	Mikolajcik, 1970
	$D_{121°C}$ (vegetable oils)	17.5–30.0 min	Molin and Snygg, 1967
	z (aqu./PB′ suspn.)	6.1–9.2°C	Gilbert et al., 1974; Johnson et al., 1982
Spore germination temperatures	Range (laboratory media)[a]	−1°–59°C	Knaysi, 1964
	(cooked rice)	5°–50°C	Mol, 1957; Johnson et al., 1983
	Optimum	30°C	Mol, 1957; Knaysi, 1964; Johnson et al., 1983
Vegetative cell growth			
pH	Lower limits	4.35–4.90	Kim and Goepfert, 1971; Raevuori and Genigeorgis, 1975
	Upper limit	9.30	Fluer and Ezepchuk, 1970
A_w	Minimum range	0.912–0.950	Raevuori and Genigeorgis, 1975; Bryan et al., 1981
temperature	Minimum range	5°–15°C	Mol, 1957; Larkin and Stokes, 1966; Shehata and Collins, 1971, 1972; Johnson et al., 1983
	Maximum range	40°–50°C	Mol, 1957; Johnson et al., 1983
	Optimum range	28°–35°C	Gilbert, 1979
Generation times	Range (laboratory media, 35°C incubation)	18–27 min	Beuchat et al., 1980
	(boiled rice, 30°C incubation)	26–57 min	Lee and Chang, 1980; Johnson et al., 1983

aqu./PB′ suspn. = spores in either aqueous or phosphate buffer (pH 7.0) suspension.
[a]Values apply to initial-stage germination.

growth—and initiation of spoilage—at temperatures as low as 5°C. Under laboratory conditions, "initial-stage" spore germination has been demonstrated within wider limits: −1, 30, and 59°C being, respectively, the minimum, optimum, and maximum temperatures reported (Knaysi, 1964).

Johnson et al. (1983) showed that the germination of *B. cereus* spores in cooked rice and trypticase soy broth occurred between 5 and 50°C and was most rapid at 30°C, findings supported by the results of an earlier study by Mol (1957). Outgrowth and cell division have been observed to take place in cooked rice between 15 and 50°C (Gilbert et al., 1974; Johnson et al., 1983) with generation times from 26 to 57 min being reported for optimum growth temperatures around 30°C (Lee and Chang, 1980; Johnson et al., 1983). Growth of *B. cereus* in cooked rice is enhanced by the addition of proteins (Morita and Woodburn, 1977; Beuchat et al., 1980). Heat activation is not generally considered to be necessary for the maximum recovery of *B. cereus* from rice (Parry and Gilbert, 1980), although "heat shock" has been noted to increase recovery of "slow germinators" in HTST pasteurized milk (Stadhouders et al., 1980).

The heat resistance of *B. cereus* spores is a factor of primary concern to the food and pharmaceutical industries and has received much attention. While *B. cereus* spores on the whole appear to possess unremarkable properties of heat resistance in line with most other mesophilic spore-formers, a number of studies have produced evidence of nonlinear spore survivor curves associated with certain strains. Vas and Proszt (1957) and Franklin (1970) demonstrated that a single spore in a total spore population of 10^6 or greater would show an unusually high degree of heat resistance. Interestingly, Bradshaw et al. (1975) later reported isolating two strains of *B. cereus* from underprocessed canned soups that exhibited $D_{95°C}$ values of 256.7 and 5122.3 min.

For *B. cereus* spores in skimmed milk, a $D_{100°C}$ of 2.7–3.1 min has been reported (Mikolajcik, 1970), while in low acid foods (pH > 4.5), Ingram (1969) has estimated a $D_{100°C}$ of 5 min. Molin and Snygg (1967) demonstrated the protective effect of lipid material in relation to heat resistance, obtaining a $D_{95°C}$ value of 13 min for spores suspended in phosphate buffer and $D_{121°C}$ values of 17.5–30 min for the same spores in olive and soybean oils.

Using aqueous spore suspensions, Gilbert et al. (1974) determined $D_{90°C}$, $D_{95°C}$, and $D_{100°C}$ values for several different strains: from these data z-values ranging from 6.7 to 8.3°C were derived. Later, Parry and Gilbert (1980) demonstrated the greater heat resistance of 10 (serotype H.1) outbreak strains from rice-associated "emetic syndrome" food poisoning ($D_{95°C}$: 22.4–36.2 min) as compared to 9 (random serotype) routine isolates of *B. cereus* from samples of raw rice ($D_{95°C}$: 1.5–6.0 min). Johnson et al. (1982) also studied the heat resistance of outbreak strains from "emetic" and "diarrheal" syndrome food-poisoning episodes. Using phosphate-buffered spore suspensions, both linear and nonlinear survivor curves were observed. Calculated $D_{95°C}$ values ranged from 1.2 to 20.2 min, with an average z-value of 9.2°C.

Thermal injury of *B. cereus* and other spores has been reviewed by Foegeding and Busta (1981). The recovery of thermally injured vegetative cells of *B. cereus* has also been investigated by Rapport and Goepfert (1978).

Data on other growth-inhibition characteristics of *B. cereus* are remarkably scant. The effect of pH, for example, has received little attention. In laboratory media, the minimum and maximum pH permitting growth have been reported as 4.9 and 9.3, respectively (Fluer and Ezepchuk, 1970; Kim and Goepfert, 1971). Raevuori and Genigeorgis (1975) obtained limited growth in meat at pH 4.35 and observed that the inhibitory effects of extreme pH and high NaCl concentration were less marked in foods than in laboratory media.

Other factors that have been shown to exert an inhibitory effect of *B. cereus* growth include 0.2% sorbic acid and 0.4% potassium sorbate (Raevuori, 1976) and garlic extract (Saleem and Al-Delaimy, 1982).

III. CHARACTERISTICS OF FOODBORNE ILLNESS DUE TO *B. CEREUS*

B. cereus is now well established as a significant cause of foodborne illness in man, accounting for approximately 1–23% of outbreaks reported worldwide of known bacterial etiology (Kramer and Gilbert, 1989). Moreover, it is recognized that distinct clinical forms of gastroenteritis can result from the ingestion of foods heavily contaminated with this organism. The so-called diarrheal syndrome, usually associated with proteinaceous foods, vegetables, sauces, and puddings, is characterized by an incubation period within the range of 8–16 h (average 10–12 h) prior to onset of abdominal pain, profuse watery diarrhea, rectal tenesmus, and occasional nausea which seldom results in vomiting. Symptoms generally resolve within 12–24 h.

In contrast, the emetic syndrome form of illness is almost exclusively associated with farinaceous foods, particularly cooked rice, and is characterized by rapid-onset (1–5 h) nausea, vomiting, and malaise, in some cases followed by diarrhea, of between 6–24 h duration. Both syndromes are believed to arise from the activities of separate enterotoxins (see Sect. VI), and interesting parallels can be drawn between *B. cereus*–related illness and the clinical features of *Clostridium perfringens* and *Staphylococcus aureus* food poisoning (Gilbert and Kramer, 1986, 1989) (Table 2).

IV. EPIDEMIOLOGY

A. *B. cereus* Diarrheal-Syndrome Food Poisoning

The first and most comprehensive description of the diarrheal syndrome was provided by Hauge (1950, 1955), who investigated four outbreaks in Norway involving some 600 cases. Since the incidents were similar, only one, involving patients and staff of a hospital, was described in detail. The suspect meal, a Sunday dinner, included chocolate pudding with vanilla sauce for dessert. Both items had been prepared on the previous day and stored in a large container at room temperature. Of the 80 persons who ate the meal, 61 were affected; of the 19 who were not ill, 11 had refused the dessert and 8 had eaten only small quantities. The average incubation period was 10 h for the patients and 12.5 h for 20 staff who ate 2–3 h later. The staff were more severely affected, and their symptoms persisted for longer. The symptoms included abdominal pain,

Table 2 *B. cereus, C. perfringens,* and *S. aureus* Food Poisoning: Comparative Clinical and Epidemiological Data

	C. perfringens	*B. cereus* (diarrheal syndrome)	*B. cereus* (emetic syndrome)	*S. aureus*
Onset of symptoms (h)	8–22	8–16	1–5	2–6
Duration of illness (h)	12–24	12–24	6–24	6–24
Diarrhea, abdominal cramps	Predominant	Predominant	Fairly common	Common
Nausea, vomiting	Rare	Occasional	Predominant	Predominant
Pathogenesis	Toxin-mediated[a]	Toxin-mediated[b]	Toxin-mediated[c]	Toxin-mediated[c]
Principal food vehicles	Cooked meat and poultry	Meat products, soups, vegetables, puddings, sauces	Cooked rice and pasta	Cold cooked meat and poultry, dairy products

[a]Sporulation-associated toxin release in the small intestine.
[b]Toxin may be preformed in food or produced in the small intestine.
[c]Toxin preformed in food.
Source: Kramer and Gilbert, 1989.

profuse watery diarrhea, rectal tenesmus (spasms), and some nausea (seldom accompanied by vomiting); fever was uncommon. In most cases symptoms resolved within 12 h.

Vanilla sauce prepared from similar constituents the day before it was served was also the cause of other outbreaks. Although samples of the sauce contained between 2.5×10^7 and 1.1×10^8 *B. cereus*/ml, there was apparently little change in the odor, taste, or consistency of the product. Numerous spores of *B. cereus*—up to 10^4 cfu/g—were found in the cornstarch used to prepare the sauce.

Since 1950, increasing awareness and recognition of *B. cereus*–associated illness has resulted in a substantial increase in the number of reports of the diarrheal syndrome type of food poisoning, the majority originating from northern and eastern European countries (Kramer and Gilbert, 1989).

The earlier outbreaks have been reviewed in detail by Goepfert et al. (1972), and Gilbert and Taylor (1976), and Gilbert (1979): a notable feature is the diversity of foods implicated—casseroles, sausages, other cooked meat and poultry dishes, raw and cooked vegetables, meat and vegetable soups, various dessert dishes including sauces, and occasionally fish, pasta, milk, and ice cream. The levels of *B. cereus* recovered from these, when recorded, were almost all within the range of 5×10^5 to 9.5×10^8 cfu/g or /ml.

The first well-documented outbreak in the United States occurred in 1969 (Midura et al., 1970). The food vehicle was a meat loaf contaminated with 7×10^6 *B. cereus*/g, and 15 persons developed a typical diarrheal syndrome illness approximately 10 h later. During the following years up until 1981, 37 outbreaks of food poisoning attributed to *B. cereus* and involving 698 cases were reported to CDC, Atlanta (see Gilbert and Kramer, 1986). Many of these, however, are not easily categorized on the basis of the available data. Details of selected published reports of *B. cereus* food poisoning in the United States are given in Table 3.

B. *B. cereus* Emetic-Syndrome Food Poisoning

A new form of *B. cereus* gastroenteritis was identified in the United Kingdom following six incidents associated with the consumption of cooked (usually fried) rice from Chinese restaurants and take-away outlets (Public Health Laboratory Service, 1972; Mortimer and McCann, 1974). Notable features of this form of illness, now referred to as *B. cereus* emetic syndrome food poisoning, included rapid onset (1–5 h) with nausea, vomiting, and malaise as the predominant symptoms, occasionally accompanied by diarrhea some time later (see Table 2).

Between 1971 and 1989, 219 such episodes were recorded in the United Kingdom involving more than 1500 cases (Goepfert et al., 1972; Gilbert, 1979; Kramer and Gilbert, 1989; FHL, unpublished data), the majority of these occurring during the summer months of June to September. However, as this form of illness is relatively mild and of short duration, significant underreporting would seem likely. *B. cereus* gastroenteritis also probably accounts for a

Table 3 Examples of *B. cereus* Food-Poisoning Outbreaks Reported in the United States

Year	Ref.	Incriminated food	*B. cereus* (cfu/g)	Number ill	Symptoms	Incubation period (h)
1969	Midura et al., 1970	Meat loaf	7×10^6	15	N,(V),D,A	10
1975	Yrios et al., 1975	Mashed potatoes	$2–10^7$	2	V,A,D	3–9
1980	Holmes et al., 1981	Macaroni and cheese	$10^8–10^9$	8	N,V,A,(D)	1–3
1985	DeBuono et al., 1988	Beef stew	ND	46	A,D,(N)	2–13

A = abdominal cramps; D = diarrhea; N = nausea; V = vomiting; ND = not determined.

proportion of the outbreaks of unknown etiology reported each year, particularly those in which rice-associated vehicles are implicated.

In a small percentage of episodes, incubation periods markedly shorter (15–30 min) or longer (6–12 h) than average were reported. Abdominal pain occurred in some cases, but diarrhea was reported in only approximately 30% of those affected. Fever was not an associated feature, and recovery was rapid, generally taking from 6 to 24 h (Gilbert, 1979). On occasion, patients have been hospitalized with excessive vomiting, and in at least one case periorbital edema has been reported to be an additional complication (Gutkin, 1975).

Approximately 95% of all emetic syndrome episodes have been associated with the consumption of cooked rice, this being largely Cantonese-style as served by Chinese restaurants and take-aways. However, a small proportion of incidents either involved other ethnic rice dishes (risotto, curries, rice salad) or were not rice-associated. Food vehicles in this latter category included vanilla slices (Pinegar and Buxton, 1977), pasteurized cream, milk pudding, chicken supreme, reconstituted infant formulas, and cooked pasta (Kramer et al., 1982).

Most episodes involving Chinese restaurants are linked with the common practice in these establishments of saving portions of boiled rice from bulk cooking. The boiled rice is allowed to "dry off" at kitchen temperature and, when required, fried quickly with beaten egg. Boiled rice may be stored for periods varying from a few hours to 3 days, but usually it is held overnight. Chinese chefs are reluctant to store boiled rice in a refrigerator as this causes the grains to become sticky and clump. The situation is further exacerbated by the preparation of large bulks of boiled rice that may take several hours to cool (Gilbert et al., 1974; Bryan et al., 1981).

These various practices result in the selection and proliferation of those strains of *B. cereus*, originally present in the raw rice, which are able to produce spores of greater heat resistance (Gilbert and Parry, 1977; Parry and Gilbert, 1980). Vegetative cell growth is rapid in cooked rice held at ambient temperatures (Gilbert et al., 1974) and is stimulated further by additions of egg, beef, or chicken (Morita and Woodburn, 1977). The common usage of these ingredients, together with the additional opportunities for mishandling, account for the predominance of fried rice over boiled rice in emetic syndrome episodes.

An analysis of 107 incidents of emetic syndrome food poisoning in the United Kingdom in which diagnostic laboratories had carried out quantitative microbiology on samples of the incriminated foods (usually cooked rice) produced a range of *B. cereus* counts from 1.0×10^3 to 5.0×10^{10} cfu/g, with a median of 1.0×10^7 cfu/g (Kramer and Gilbert, 1989). Moreover, a study of 18 outbreaks from which clinical material was available for examination established that *B. cereus* was readily detectable in 32 of 40 (80%) fecal specimens at levels up to 3×10^9 cfu/g (Gilbert, 1979). The eight cases from whom the organism could not be isolated submitted specimens several days after cessation of symptoms.

Thus, several epidemiological features of *B. cereus* emetic syndrome food poisoning can be identified: (1) the food vehicles responsible are almost invariably farinaceous, containing either cereal (mainly rice) or cereal-derived ingredients such as flour; (2) in the vast majority of episodes, that food vehicle will have been held for too long at unsatisfactory storage temperatures; (3) as a result of (2), the incriminated food will be found to contain substantial levels of *B. cereus*; and (4) acute-phase fecal specimens from those affected by this form of gastroenteritis will carry significant numbers of *B. cereus*.

Epidemiologically similar outbreaks are increasingly being recognized and reported from many countries around the world (Kramer and Gilbert, 1989), including Canada (Lefebvre et al., 1973; Mathias et al., 1976; Todd, 1982, 1985a,b, 1987), Finland (Raevuori et al., 1977; Hirn and Aho, 1986), India (Jauhari and Kulshrestha, 1986), Japan (Itoh et al., 1982), the Netherlands (Beckers, 1976, 1982, 1985), Norway (Iverson et al., 1982), Singapore (Tay et al., 1982), and the United States (Holmes et al., 1981; Thompson et al., 1985).

C. Ecology of *B. cereus*

Both spore and vegetative forms of *B. cereus* are frequent inhabitants of a wide range of environments, including soils and clays (particularly those associated with the rhizosphere), sediments, dust, natural waters, vegetation, and many food types, notably cereals and cereal derivatives, milk and dairy products, dried foods, spices, meat products, and vegetables (Goepfert et al., 1972; Norris et al., 1981; Johnson, 1984).

1. *Prevalence in Foods*

A comprehensive study of the incidence of *B. cereus* in food materials has been carried out by Nygren (1962), whose examination of 3888 samples revealed a contamination rate of 51.6% among 1546 food ingredients, 43.8% of 1911 cream and dessert dishes, and 52.2% of 431 meat and vegetable products.

Given the significant association of the emetic syndrome with cooked rice, it is not surprising that *B. cereus* is frequently found in this commodity. Schiemann (1978), for example, in an investigation of the bacteriological quality of Chinese take-away foods, reported direct isolation of the organism from 33% of fried rice samples. From a similar survey, Shinagawa et al. (1979) found 66% of cooked rice samples to be contaminated.

Bacillus species comprise approximately 90% of rice paddy soil bacteria (Asanuma et al., 1979), and *B. cereus* in particular remains closely associated with the rice plant throughout its development. Raw rice, even in the refined polished form, is a reliable source of *B. cereus* strains, and reported isolation rates have ranged from 46 to 100% (Gilbert and Parry, 1977; Shinagawa et al., 1979; Blakey and Priest, 1980; Bryan et al., 1981; Vijayalakshmi et al., 1981).

Apart from the various rice dishes, a typical Oriental menu may include several other food items known to harbor *B. cereus*, including tofu, noodles, sushi, egg roll, fried meat, and vegetable dishes (Schiemann, 1978; Shinagawa et al., 1979; Ushioda et al., 1980; Sly and Ross, 1982). As with cooked rice, these items may also become hazardous through mishandling, and consequently should not be overlooked as a possible cause of *B. cereus* food poisoning where this is attributed to an Oriental meal.

Before its potential pathogenicity was appreciated, *B. cereus* was recognized as a frequent contaminant of milk and cream (Donovan, 1959). The organism is responsible for a common spoilage defect in milk variously referred to as "broken" or "bitty" cream (Stone and Rowlands, 1952; Billing and Cuthbert, 1958) or "sweet curdling" (Overcast and Atmaram, 1974). Both raw and pasteurized milk are susceptible, especially during warmer weather (15°C or higher), and the condition is believed to arise from the activities of *B. cereus* lecithinase on the fat globules present in milk.

The source of the milk contamination has been traced to the storage of hay in milking sheds (Billing and Cuthbert, 1958), to cans of milk allowed to stand after emptying (Donovan, 1959), and more recently, to mastitic cows (Raevuori and Koiranen, 1978).

Several investigators have studied the incidence of *B. cereus* in milk and milk products. Ionescu and colleagues (1966) recovered the organism at counts of up to 10^4 cfu/ml from 12.4% of fresh raw milk samples and 86.7% of bottled pasteurized milk. Similarly, Ahmed et al. (1983) isolated *B. cereus* from samples of raw milk (9%), pasteurized milk (35%), cheddar cheese (14%), and ice cream (48%). Some concern has been raised over the survival of *Bacillus* spores in UHT processed milk (Mostert et al., 1979; Shinagawa et al., 1984), and the fate of *B. cereus* during the cheese-making process (Mikolajcik et al., 1973). The rabbit ligated ileal loop test was used by Chopra and co-workers (1980) to determine that 6 out of 25 milk isolates were potentially pathogenic. Powdered milk, used in the preparation of vanilla slices (Pinegar and Buxton, 1977), a milk-gelatin dessert (Anon., 1977), and macaroni and cheese (Holmes et al., 1981), was thought to be the source of *B. cereus* contamination contributing to outbreaks involving these foods.

2. *Fecal Carriage of* B. cereus

References to *B. cereus* in the feces of individuals other than in the context of food poisoning, though rare, date back to 1919 (Batchelor, 1919), when it was recorded that *B. cereus* was isolated from approximately two thirds of over 50 Baltimore children.

The ingestion of *B. cereus* may be regarded as an inevitable consequence of the widespread contamination of our food supply with this organism. In healthy individuals, the low levels of *B. cereus* normally associated with food do not pose any risk of illness, and spores surviving passage through the upper alimentary tract eventually become part of the transitory intestinal flora. Observations in one individual taking a proprietary pharmaceutical product whose active ingredient was a mutant atoxigenic strain of *B. cereus* have shown that the organism could be detected in the feces by direct aerobic culture just 4 days after ingestion of a dose of 8×10^9 spores (Turnbull, 1981).

Ghosh (1978), in a survey aimed at determining the prevalence of *B. cereus* in the feces of healthy persons, isolated the bacterium from 14% of single fecal specimens from 711 adults in the general population using an enrichment technique. *B. cereus* was also found in 15% of 400 fecal specimens from healthy individuals in Japan (Itoh et al., 1982). Turnbull and Kramer (1985) compared the fecal carriage of *B. cereus* among three unrelated groups of individuals: two from South Africa, one from the United Kingdom. Isolation rates from the first South African group (120 children of ages 6–11 years) ranged from 24.3% during the autumn season to 43% during the summer months: the seasonal variation was regarded as significant. Within the U.K. group, isolation rates varied from 0 to 40% over a 3-week period. These authors concluded that *Bacillus* species in general are commonly present in normal feces, and that their presence, particularly that of *B. cereus* solely reflects dietary intake. Small numbers of *B. cereus* are unable to persist or colonize the intestine following dietary ingestion in the normal healthy individual.

V. ANTIGENIC CONSTITUTION AND SEROLOGY

The serology of the genus *Bacillus*—and *B. cereus* in particular—has formed the subject of several review papers (Norris, 1962; Baba, 1969; Goepfert et al., 1972; Gilbert, 1979; Berkeley et al., 1984). Although antigenic relationships within the genus remain to be comprehensively defined, attempts to develop serological procedures as diagnostic aids have been notably successful in a number of areas.

A. Spore Antigens

The ability to form endospores is a key characteristic of the genus, and many investigations have been undertaken into the nature of spore antigens and their potential use in species and strain discrimination. Norris (1962) reviewed the earliest studies on *Bacillus* spore antigens and the technical problems encountered in their use for serological analysis. In general, the problems stemmed from three sources: (1) contamination of spore antigen preparations with vegetative cell debris, (2) germination of spores in vivo during the course of serum production (resulting, as with (1), in the formation of anti-vegetative cell immunoglobulins), and (3) in vitro spore germination occurring during the immunoassay.

Bacillus endospores possess hydrophobic surface properties (Lamanna and Eisler, 1960) and thus an intrinsic tendency to autoagglutinate. Noble (1919), however, devised a technique for producing homogeneous spore suspensions of *B. anthracis* using actively growing, serially cultured vegetative cells to seed the sporulation medium. This method was adapted by Norris and Wolf (1961) for studying the spore antigens of other *Bacillus* species, although these authors encountered strains whose spores still remained prone to autoagglutination, which could not, therefore, be examined by direct agglutination tests.

Lamanna (1940) attempted to classify the large-celled Group 1 bacilli on the basis of their spore agglutinins. Although differentiation from *B. megaterium* was possible, *B. cereus* strains could not be distinguished from those of *B. mycoides*—an observation consistent with the present classification of *B. mycoides* as a variant of *B. cereus*. The multiplicity of spore surface antigens in a single strain of *B. cereus* was later demonstrated by Doak and Lamanna

(1948), who also showed that spore preparations of certain *B. brevis* and *B. sphaericus* strains could cross-react with *B. cereus* antisera.

Further evidence of the close taxonomic relationship of *B. cereus*, *B. anthracis*, and *B. thuringiensis* was indirectly obtained from the results of two studies (Lamanna and Eisler, 1960; Lamanna and Jones, 1961), which revealed extensive cross-agglutination between the spores of the three species.

In a detailed study of *Bacillus* species antigens, Norris and Wolf (1961) determined the higher species specificity of the spore antigens, and showed that these presented as heat-resistant agglutinogens and precipitinogens which were absent in the corresponding vegetative cell structures. No single heat-stable agglutinogen could be found in all strains of *B. cereus*. However, a spore precipitinogen common to all strains of *B. cereus* was found, antibodies to which also gave cross-precipitin reactions with *B. thuringiensis* spore extracts.

Further work with *B. cereus* spore antigens was carried out by Kim and Goepfert (1972) using a fluorescent-labeled antibody technique. This approach was adopted to overcome the problem of spore aggregation frequently encountered in direct agglutination tests.

B. Somatic Antigens

The specificity of vegetative cell somatic (O) antigens of *B. cereus* was first investigated in detail by Sievers and Zetterberg (1940), who observed cross-reactions between strains of a number of *Bacillus* species, including *B. subtilis* and *B. cereus* O-antisera. Ivanovics and Foldes (1958) evaluated a gel diffusion precipitation test using antigenic polysaccharides extracted from vegetative cells of *B. cereus* and concluded that two broad groups of *B. cereus* strains could be distinguished according to their reaction with antisera raised against somatic *B. anthracis* polysaccharide antigens. Tomcsik and Baumann-Grace (1959) were able to recognize 13 O-antigenic types within a group of 23 *B. cereus* strains. However, extracted polysaccharides from vegetative cells reacted with *B. anthracis* O-antisera (Baumann-Grace et al., 1959). Norris and Wolf (1961) failed to demonstrate the presence of a species-common vegetative cell precipitinogen among strains of *B. cereus*. Walker et al. (1966) reported the presence of vegetative cell somatic antigens in spores. These antigens were, however, located along the cortical membrane and were not therefore available to directly stimulate antibody formation.

C. Flagellar Antigens

Flagellar (H) antigens have found extensive application in serological studies of *Bacillus* species. This can most probably be attributed to the higher strain specificity conferred by the flagellar (as opposed to the spore and somatic) antigens (Norris and Wolf, 1961). In addition, H-antigens have proved less problematic to handle than spore antigens.

One successful application of H-antigens has been the development of a serological typing scheme for *B. cereus* strains by Taylor and Gilbert (1975) and

Gilbert and Parry (1977). The scheme is used routinely by the Food Hygiene Laboratory, both in the laboratory investigation of food poisoning outbreaks and other *B. cereus*–associated problems, and also for serotyping strains from nongastrointestinal infections in man and animals.

The work of Taylor and Gilbert (1975) followed that of LeMille and colleagues (1969), who demonstrated 17 H-serotypes among a group of 33 *B. cereus* strains isolated mainly from insects. In further tests using other *Bacillus* species, two strains of *B. megaterium* were found to cross-react with the *B. cereus* antisera. Conversely, some of the original *B. cereus* strains cross-reacted with a *B. subtilis* H-antiserum.

Taylor and Gilbert (1975) based their provisional typing scheme on 17 prototype strains isolated from foods and clinical specimens associated with outbreaks of food poisoning in the United Kingdom, Canada, the Netherlands and the United States and one strain from a neonatal brain abscess. The scheme has subsequently been enlarged to increase the number of H-antigenic types that can be recognized (Gilbert and Parry, 1977; Gilbert, 1979; Gilbert et al., 1981; Kramer et al., 1982; Gilbert and Kramer, 1986; Kramer and Gilbert, 1989).

Currently the scheme comprises 42 H-antisera raised against prototype strains of diverse origin: foods and clinical specimens related to both emetic- and diarrheal-type food-poisoning episodes, foods not associated with illness, non–food related clinical infections, and environmental sources.

Details of antisera production and the serological typing procedure are given by Taylor and Gilbert (1975) and Kramer et al. (1982). *B. cereus* H-specific antisera are not available commercially, but laboratories both in the United Kingdom and abroad, isolating *B. cereus* from well-documented incidents of foodborne gastroenteritis, may refer such strains to the Food Hygiene Laboratory at Colindale for serological typing. A similar serotyping facility is also provided by the Tokyo Metropolitan Research Laboratory of Public Health in Japan, based on the UK types H.1 to H.18 and supplemented with an additional 12 antisera to Japanese isolates. Reported applications have included the investigation of food-poisoning outbreaks and the study of serotype distributions among various food groups (Terayama et al., 1978; Itoh et al., 1982).

B. cereus prototype strains H.1 (from an emetic syndrome outbreak) and H.2 (from a diarrheal syndrome outbreak) have been lodged with the National Collection of Type Cultures (Central Public Health Laboratory, Colindale Avenue, London NW9 5HT, United Kingdom, from whom they can be obtained as NCTC 11143 and 11145, respectively.

Cao et al. (1984) recently published data relating to the performance of an H-serotyping scheme for *B. cereus* developed at the Lanzhou Institute of Biological Products in China. This comprises a set of 11 H-specific antisera raised against "epidemic" isolates, having agglutination titers of 1:3200–1:12,800 after absorption. Sixty-seven percent of isolates (of undisclosed source, but believed to be of food-poisoning origin) were typable with the scheme, 30 (32%) of the 94 strains examined being of a single antigenic type 5/V.

The epidemiological application of the U.K. serotyping scheme in the investigation of *B. cereus* gastroenteritis is well documented. Table 4 shows the distribution of serotypes of *B. cereus* from 200 outbreaks of emetic syndrome food poisoning originating from 11 countries between 1971 and 1986. Overall, 91% of isolates from separate incidents proved typable, and 15 H-antigen types were represented. The majority of strains (63.5%), however, were of one type, H.1, followed by H.8 and H.3 accounting for 8.0% and 4.0% of strains, respectively. From some 18% of outbreaks a combination of (usually two or three) serotypes was recovered (e.g., H.1, H.4, and H.14). In these circumstances, the causative association is attributed equally to all the strains represented, as practicable methods for determining emetic toxin production capability (believed to be the main criterion of pathogenicity for this syndrome) are not yet available.

Despite the reported prevalence of *B. cereus* diarrheal syndrome food poisoning, particularly among northern and eastern European countries, relatively few isolates have been available for serological examination. Table 5 lists the serotypes associated with 20 such outbreaks, the types of food involved, and the countries in which the episodes occurred. As with isolates from emetic syndrome outbreaks, the high proportion of strains of serotype H.1 associated

Table 4 *B. cereus* Emetic Syndrome Food Poisoning: Distribution of Serotypes from 200 Outbreaks

Country (no. outbreaks)	Source of strains	H-serotypes isolated	No. (%) outbreaks by serotype
United Kingdom (144)			
		1[b]	127 (63.5)
Netherlands (19)		3	8
		4[b]	5
Japan (15)		5	5
		8[b]	16 (8.0)
India (6)		10	1
	Implicated food[a]	11/(15)	1
China (5)	and/or vomitus	12[b]	5
	and/or feces	14[b]	3
Australia (3)		19	1
		20[b]	2
Eire (3)		24	1
		iii/iv[b]	3
United States (2)		v	2
		G[†]	2
Bulgaria, Finland, Spain (1 each)		Not typable	18 (9.0)

[a]Implicated foods (no. outbreaks): Fried/boiled rice (167); other rice dishes (5); fried/boiled pasta (12); cakes/sweets/desserts (7); infant feeds (3); cooked vegetables (2); miscellaneous (3).
[b]Either as the sole serotype isolated, or in combination with other serotypes (iii, iv, v, and G are provisional serotype designations).
Source: Kramer and Gilbert, 1989.

Table 5 *B. cereus* Diarrheal Syndrome Food Poisoning: Distribution of Serotypes from 20 Outbreaks

Food incriminated[a]	H-serotypes isolated	Country
Vanilla sauce (2 outbreaks)	1	Norway
Boiled sausage	1	Eire
Vegetable stew	1	Denmark
Meat sausage	1 + 3	China
Meat loaf	2	United States
Barbecued chicken	6	Canada
Wheat flour dessert	8	Bulgaria
Indonesian rice dish	8	Netherlands
Vanilla pudding	9	Netherlands
Indonesian rice dish	10	Netherlands
Forcemeat	11/(15)	China
Tongue and ragout rolls	12 + NT	Netherlands
Turkey loaf	19 + NT	United States
Beef stew	26	United States
Boiled cod	C[b]	Spain
Pea soup	NT	Netherlands
Veal broth	NT	Bulgaria
Lobster paté	NT	United Kingdom
Cooked turkey	NT	United Kingdom

[a]Reported levels of *B. cereus*, 10^5–10^9 cfu/g.
[b]Provisional serotype designation.
NT = not typable.
Source: Gilbert and Kramer, 1986.

with the diarrheal syndrome illness is noteworthy. Spores produced by food-poisoning strains of this type have been shown to possess markedly greater heat resistance than those of other serotypes isolated from samples of uncooked rice (Parry and Gilbert, 1980) (see also Sec. II.B), and these would tend to selectively survive cooking procedures.

The evidence for selection of serotypes is further substantiated by the results of serotype distribution surveys which have been undertaken on different groups of *B. cereus* isolates from foods, fecal specimens, and environmental sources not associated with food poisoning (Gilbert and Parry, 1977; Ghosh, 1978; Gilbert et al., 1981; Itoh et al., 1982; Turnbull and Kramer, 1985; Gilbert and Kramer, 1986). These data are summarized in Table 6. The preponderance of *B. cereus* type H.1 strains—and to a lesser degree, other serotypes more commonly associated with food poisoning, such as H.5 and H.8—in cooked rice is not matched by the serotype distribution patterns characteristic of raw rice (in which types H.17, H.20, H.15, and H.12 predominate) and environmental sources in general (types H.C, H.20, and H.17 predominant). The selection of type H.1 strains in other heat-treated products is also suggested by the serotype distribution data for pasteurized milk and cream and cooked meat and poultry, although equivalent data for the raw commodities have yet to be obtained in order to confirm this supposition.

Table 6 Predominant Serotypes of *B. cereus* Isolated from Food, Feces, and Environmental Sources Not Associated with Food Poisoning

Source	Number of isolates examined	Predominant H-serotypes detected (frequency >4%)	Not typable (%)
Environment[a]	200	C[d] (8%), 20 (7%), 17 (5%), 11/(15) (4%)	49
Human feces[b]	336	1 (10%), 18 (6%), 17 (5%), 20 (4%)	49
Raw rice	100	17 (15%), 20 (7%), 15 (6%), 12 (6%), 18 (4%)	46
Cooked rice	100	1 (23%), 5 (6%), 8 (6%), 19 (6%), 20 (5%)	40
Pulses and cereals[c]	100	8 (17%), 12 (7%), 4 (6%), 17 (4%)	48
Pasteurized milk and cream	100	1 (11%), 22 (8%), 21 (6%), 8 (5%)	54
Cooked meat and poultry	100	1 (15%), 11 (6%), 19(6%), 3 (5%), 20 (5%), 12 (4%)	51

[a]Including mud, soil, gravel, dust, surface water, vegetation, natural fibers.
[b]From healthy adult and child population in the United Kingdom, Japan, and South Africa.
[c]Excluding rice.
[d]Provisional serotype designation.
Source: Kramer and Gilbert, 1989.

The serotyping results from fecal carriage surveys reveal the ubiquitous nature of *B. cereus* and indicate that the presence of the organism in normal feces is solely a reflection of dietary intake. Where selection does occur during passage through the intestinal tract, this is most likely to favor the survival of spores rather than vegetative cell forms of the organism.

In a survey of *B. cereus* carriage in the feces of 711 healthy adults in the United Kingdom, Ghosh (1978) obtained an isolation rate of 14% with 15 serotypes represented. Fifty-two of the 100 strains isolated proved nontypable. Turnbull and Kramer (1985) reported the results of a similar study of 120 healthy African schoolchildren. The fecal carriage rate ranged from 24.3 to 43%, and 24 serotypes were recovered, 9 of which were also found in food samples representative of the daily diet.

Other applications of the U.K. serotyping scheme have included studies on the distribution of *B. cereus* strains in various foods and food additives (Gilbert and Parry, 1977; Blakey and Priest, 1980; Roberts et al., 1982), in imported contaminated wound dressings (Marples, 1983), from nongastrointestinal infections in humans (Turnbull et al., 1977b; Turnbull and Kramer, 1983; Dryden and Kramer, 1987), bovine mastitis (Johnston, 1986; Jones and Turnbull, 1981), and hospital cross-infection outbreaks involving neonates (Gostling et al., 1980; Birch et al., 1981; Youngs et al., 1985).

B. thuringiensis strains have also been successfully classified on the basis of their flagella antigens (Barjac and Bonnefoi, 1962, 1968), and a serological typing scheme for this species has been developed. Fourteen serotypes can be recognized (Barjac, 1981), some of which can be further characterized according to the presence of H-antigenic subfactors.

There is evidence that certain strains of *B. cereus* and *B. thuringiensis* share common H-antigens. Taylor and Gilbert (1975) reported that agglutinating antibodies to *B. cereus* type H.18 were completely absorbed by suspensions of *B. thuringiensis* type 4a,b. An isolate of *B. thuringiensis* type 5a,b has also been observed to agglutinate with antisera to *B. cereus* type H.20 (Gilbert et al., 1981).

VI. PATHOGENICITY

A. Exotoxins Associated with Food Poisoning

Most strains of *B. cereus* are capable of elaborating an unusually wide range of extracellular metabolites, mainly during the exponential growth phase, and including a number of toxins or virulence factors identified on the basis of their behavior in in vivo models and their epidemiological association with disease. Table 7 attempts to present in some order the rather confused nomenclature applied to the various toxic moieties associated with *B. cereus* and to summarize from the literature their respective biochemical and pathological characteristics. However, the precise relationship of the toxin described by Ezepchuk and Fluer (1973) and Ezepchuk et al. (1979) to others studied remains uncertain. The principal toxic metabolites of *B. cereus* are the subject of an extensive and detailed review by Turnbull (1986).

1. *Diarrheal Enterotoxin*

The results of human volunteer feeding studies carried out by Hauge (1955) supported the concept of *B. cereus*–induced diarrhea. Nikodemusz (1965, 1966a,b, 1967) also established that cats and dogs fed experimental diets containing $>10^5$ *B. cereus*/g developed severe diarrhea and dehydration. More recently, the feeding of whole-cell cultures of strains isolated from food-poisoning incidents to rhesus monkeys (Melling et al., 1976; Goepfert, 1978; Logan et al., 1979; Gilbert and Kramer, 1986) and similarly, cell-free culture filtrates and ammonium sulfate–precipitated preparations (Goepfert, 1973, 1978) have been shown to induce diarrhea in these animals.

Goepfert et al. (1972) and Spira and Goepfert (1972a,b) indicated the possible existence of an enterotoxin, following experiments involving the injection of whole-cell *B. cereus* cultures into ligated rabbit intestinal loops. Positive fluid accumulation responses were obtained with 19 of 22 *B. cereus* and 4 of 6 *B. thuringiensis* cultures. From these studies, a number of significant observations followed (Spira and Goepfert, 1972a), to be later substantiated by other workers (Turnbull, 1976; Turnbull et al., 1977): (1) that, under optimal growth and test conditions, different strains produced different degrees of fluid accumulation; (2) that Brain Heart Infusion (BHI) medium consistently engendered the greatest loop response, while nutrient broth cultures were weakly reactive or loop-negative, irrespective of the bacterial growth levels obtained; (3) that loop response did not differentiate *B. cereus* strains associated with food poisoning from those of other sources; (4) that young rabbits (<1200 g) were a more sensitive and reproducible model than were their adult

Table 7 Principal Exotoxins of *B. cereus*

Exotoxin (synonyms)	Properties	Ref.
Diarrheal enterotoxin (diarrheagenic factor, LRIL fluid accumulation factor, intestinonecrotic toxin, vascular permeability factor, dermonecrotic toxin, mouse lethal factor #1)	Thermolabile antigenic protein. MW ca. 38,000–57,000; pI 4.9–5.6. "Multicomponent" or subunit structure. Inactivated by proteolytic enzymes. Necrotic, lethal. Pathogenic role in foodborne illness and extraintestinal infection.	Kramer et al., 1978; Kramer, 1984; Spira and Goepfert, 1975; Shinagawa et al., 1985b; Turnbull, 1976; Thompson et al., 1984; Turnbull et al., 1977, 1979a
Emetic toxin/factor Vomiting toxin/factor	Highly stable. Probably a peptide. MW < 10,000. Not formed above 40°C. Resistant to proteolytic enzymes. Thermostable at 126°C for 90 min. Sporulation associated?	Melling et al., 1976; Melling and Capel, 1978; Turnbull et al., 1979a; Turnbull, 1986
Primary hemolysin (cereolysin, hemolysin I, mouse lethal factor #2)	Thermolabile antigenic protein. MW ca. 49,000–59,000; pI 6.3–6.7. Thiol-activated cytolysin. Neutralized by cholesterol and antistreptolysin O. Necrotic, lethal. Pathogenic role in extraintestinal infection.	Bernheimer and Grushoff, 1967a,b; Burnheimer et al., 1968; Cowell et al., 1976; Turnbull et al., 1979a; Turnbull and Kramer, 1983
Secondary hemolysin (hemolysin II)	Thermolabile antigenic protein. MW ca. 29,000–34,000; pI 4.9–5.3. Protease susceptible. In vitro activity unaffected by thiols, cholesterol and antistreptolysin O. In vivo toxicity not yet established.	Fossum, 1964; Coolbaugh and Williams, 1978; Kramer et al., 1978; Parker and Goepfert, 1978
Phospholipases C (lecithinase, egg yolk turbidity factor)	Relatively stable enzyme complex: (a) phosphatidylcholine hydrolase: MW 23,000, pI ca. 6.5–8.5. (b) phosphatidylinositol hydrolase: MW 29,000, pI 5.4 (phosphatasemia factor). (c) Sphingomyelinase: MW 24,000, pI 5.6. Hemolytic.	Ikezawa et al., 1976, 1977, 1978, 1980; Slein and Logan, 1963, 1965; Mollby, 1978; Zwaal et al., 1971
Exoenterotoxin described by Ezepchuk and Fluer	Thermolabile antigenic protein. MW 57,000. Inactivated by 60°C for 20 min. Lethal to rodents. IV administration to cats induces emesis. Possibly related to diarrheal enterotoxin.	Ezepchuk and Fluer, 1973; Gorina et al., 1975, 1976
Toxin isolated by Ezepchuk et al.	Protein. MW 100,000. Activity unaffected by trypsin. Lethal. IV administration to cats induces fever. LRIL fluid accumulation negative. VPR test positive. Relationship to exoenterotoxin not known.	Ezepchuk et al., 1979

counterparts, and (5) that if one or more loops was strongly positive, the animals were likely to die within 10 h.

These same authors also observed that cultures introduced directly into unligated ilea or by stomach catheter failed to elicit diarrhea and that positive fluid accumulation was significantly associated with an increase in bacterial numbers within the respective loops, whereas strains that were negative in this model showed a reduction in numbers. In contrast, in vivo growth of established loop-positive strains following resuspension in fresh BHI medium prior to injection failed to elicit a response. From these data, the authors concluded that an increase in cell numbers was a consequence of, rather than a cause of, fluid accumulation, that intraluminal multiplication was not involved in fluid accumulation, and that by inference, *B. cereus*–induced diarrhea was likely to be the result of intoxication rather than infection.

This important study was the first of a series by Goepfert and co-workers in which a hitherto undefined activity of *B. cereus* was elucidated. On the basis of its ability to stimulate fluid accumulation in the ligated rabbit ileal loop (LRIL) test, the toxic factor was classified as an enterotoxin. Evidence was presented (Spira and Goepfert, 1972a,b) of nonidentity between the enterotoxin and both the hemolysin and lecithinase activities of the organism.

For a number of enteric pathogens, a direct correlation has been established between fluid accumulation in the LRIL test and the responses of guinea pigs and rabbits to intradermal injection of culture filtrates. Glatz and co-workers (Glatz and Goepfert, 1973; Glatz et al., 1974) confirmed that the correlation also held true for *B. cereus* between fluid-inducing capability in the LRIL test and the extent of reaction in the guinea pig skin and vascular permeability reaction (VPR) in rabbit skin. Moreover, with both dermal assays, the formation of a zone of necrosis accompanied the activities of more potent enterotoxic culture filtrates. These same authors further established the likely identities of the LRIL fluid–inducing and VPR factors by demonstrating a highly significant linear regression for the two activities, although it was also found that the necrotic component of the reaction did not fit the line of regression (Glatz et al., 1974).

Spira (1974) and Spira and Goepfert (1972a) studied in greater detail the properties of the enterotoxin in both crude and partially purified (by Sephadex G-75 gel filtration) preparations. Evidence was obtained, using the LRIL test, that the effect of the enterotoxin on intestinal permeability was transient and that the molecule bound weakly to receptor sites in the ileum. In contrast to the enterotoxins of *V. cholerae* and *V. perfringens*, *B. cereus* enterotoxin activity was inhibited by injection of antiserum 10 min after injection of an enterotoxic culture filtrate into a test loop. Also, LRIL activity was not affected by antisera raised against choleragen, *C. perfringens* enterotoxin, or the *B. cereus* lethal factor (Johnson and Bonventre, 1967). On Sephadex G-75 gel filtration, LRIL fluid–inducing, VPR, and lethal activities eluted coincidentally, distinct from phospholipase C but incompletely resolved from hemolysin.

The original groundwork in *B. cereus* toxinology laid down by the FRI research group at Wisconsin (Spira and Goepfert, 1972a,b; 1975; Glatz and Goepfert, 1973; Goepfert, 1973, 1974; Spira, 1974; Glatz et al., 1974, 1976,

1977) has been developed and expanded by workers in other countries. In particular it has been shown that the majority of strains of *B. cereus* exhibit characteristic toxigenicity, and that food-poisoning isolates cannot be distinguished from strains from other sources solely on this basis (Turnbull, 1976; Turnbull et al., 1979a,b; Turnbull and Kramer, 1983; Shinagawa et al., 1984). The correlation between LRIL-fluid accumulation, the guinea-pig skin reaction, and the rabbit skin vascular permeability reaction has also been reported by Turnbull and colleagues (1977, 1979a,b), who observed that strongly toxigenic strains gave rise to varying degrees of dermonecrosis in the skin tests and mucosal necrosis in the LRIL test. The necrotic activity is believed to be a significant contributory factor in the pathogenesis of nongastrointestinal *B. cereus* infection (Turnbull et al., 1979b; Turnbull and Kramer, 1983).

With the ultimate objective of preparative-scale purification, Carpenter and co-workers (1975), Glatz and Goepfert (1976, 1977), and Spira and Silverman (1979) investigated growth conditions necessary to achieve optimum yields of the diarrheal enterotoxin in fermenter systems using semi-defined media. From their collective findings a number of salient criteria emerged: (1) an inoculum of between 0.1 and 1% v/v of either stationary or exponential growth phase culture of the producer strain gave significantly higher yields than did the same inoculum at 10% v/v or greater; (2) addition of 0.5–1.0% w/v glucose to the growth medium stimulated enterotoxin production; (3) pH control within the range 7.0–8.0 dramatically improved yields, compared to no pH control or control within other ranges; (4) enterotoxin production occurred within the temperature range 18–43°C, with an optimum of 32°C; (5) the maximum agitation rate achievable without foaming generated the highest yields; and (6) the optimum incubation period prior to harvest under such conditions was 5 h. By applying these conditions, enterotoxin yields up to 50-fold greater than those produced by conventional shake-flask techniques could be achieved.

There is some disagreement in the literature as to appropriate dissolved oxygen (DO) levels: Spira and Silverman (1979) and Carpenter et al. (1975) both found very low levels to be preferable, whereas Glatz and Goepfert (1976, 1977) recorded maximal yields at DO levels around 80% saturation. These workers agreed, however, that significant enterotoxin levels could also be obtained during anaerobic growth.

Given that the conditions necessary to obtain optimum yields in closed culture systems had been well defined, nonetheless, attempts to isolate and purify the enterotoxin were repeatedly hampered by a combination of factors associated with *B. cereus* toxigenesis. These included: (1) the labile nature of the molecule; (2) its susceptibility to proteolytic enzymes; (3) the attenuation of toxigenicity that occurred in producer strains on repeated subculture; and (4) separation methodology problems posed by the co-production of other metabolites sharing similar molecular properties. However, experiments with various novel biochemical approaches to these problems eventually led to several research groups independently reporting on the purification and characterization of the enterotoxin, and the development of immunoassay techniques (Ezepchuk and Fluer, 1973; Gorina et al., 1975, 1976; Kramer et al.,

1978; Ezepchuk et al., 1979; Kramer, 1984; Thompson et al., 1984; Shinagawa et al., 1985b).

Preparative gel isoelectric focusing was used by Kramer and colleagues (Kramer et al., 1978; Turnbull et al., 1979a) to isolate a protein of MW 50,000 and pI 4.9 from the culture filtrate of a *B. cereus* strain (F4433/73) implicated in diarrheal syndrome food poisoning. This molecule was considered to be a diarrheal enterotoxin on the basis of its in vivo behavior: positive LRIL fluid accumulation, VPR, dermonecrotic, and mouse lethal activities were exhibited. Although completely resolved from cereolysin (the primary hemolysin) and phospholipase C components, the enterotoxin preparations were found to possess low-level hemolytic activity derived from the close proximity in the isoelectric profile of a secondary hemolysin. A PAG electrophoretic separation of the purified enterotoxin revealed three distinct bands (Turnbull, 1986). Under high resolution analytical isoelectric focusing, two moieties associated with the enterotoxin were observed (Kramer, 1984), having pIs of 5.1 and 5.6, respectively. Both components possessed VPR, dermonecrotic, and cytotoxic activities. LRIL activities, however, were not determined.

Further experimental evidence of a probable multicomponent or subunit enterotoxin structure was also provided by Thompson and co-workers (Thompson et al., 1984). Chromatography on Amberlite CG-400, QAE-Sephadex, Sephadex G-75, and hydroxylapatite was used to separate extracellular proteins produced by *B. cereus* strain B-4ac, a fraction containing three detectable antigens of MW 38,000, 39,500, and 43,000 was obtained, having positive LRIL, VPR, dermonecrotic, mouse lethal, and cytotoxic properties. Two other fractions showed no toxic activity when tested individually, although each was shown to contain two of the three antigens detectable in the toxic fraction. When the nontoxic fractions were combined, activity in all the biological assays was restored. Furthermore, antisera against either of the nontoxic fractions was found to neutralize the dermonecrotic activity of the combined material. The isoelectric points of two of the antigens were found to be around 5.3.

A similar protein exotoxin has been described by Ezepchuck and Fluer (1973) and Gorina and colleagues (1975, 1976) the purification of which was monitored using mouse lethality and the emetic response in cats as bioassays. On the basis of its reported molecular weight (57,000 daltons), this toxin would appear to be either related to or identical with the enterotoxin isolated by Spira and Goepfert (1975), Kramer et al. (1978), Turnbull et al. (1979a), Thompson et al. (1984), and Shinagawa et al. (1985b). However, the relationship of the more recently described 100,000 dalton MW/VPR-positive/LRIL-negative/lethal toxin of Ezepchuck et al. (1979) to the toxins of *B. cereus* that have now been characterized is not at present clear.

2. *Emetic Toxin*

The epidemiological features of the emetic syndrome type of *B. cereus* food poisoning were detailed in Sec. IV.B. Since the majority of incidents have been associated with rice dishes, Melling and colleagues (1976) devised a rice slurry medium for studies on the pathogenic mechanisms involved in this syndrome.

Isolates cultured in rice medium were subsequently fed to rhesus monkeys by intragastric intubation. Of the three strains selected for initial tests, one (F4810/72) associated with an emetic syndrome episode, produced emesis in approximately half the feedings. On the other hand, a strain causative of a diarrheal syndrome outbreak (F4433/73) and an isolate from raw rice both failed to induce emesis, although F4433/73 did cause diarrhea in more than half the feeding trials. The specificity of rice as a vehicle and growth medium was demonstrated when cultures of F4810/72 in protein hydrolysate media, with or without a starch supplement, failed to induce emesis. This observation supported the finding of Goepfert (1978) that BHIG cultures of isolates from emetic syndrome incidents failed to induce a vomiting response in rhesus monkeys.

Following the observation that approximately 50% of monkeys were unresponsive towards the emetic toxin, Melling and Capel (1978) subsequently selected for further feeding studies only those animals identified through screening as positive responders. From experimental evidence obtained using *B. cereus* strain F4810/72, a number of significant features of this toxin emerged: (1) cell-free rice culture supernatant preparations possessed emetic activity—the first definite evidence of the involvement of an extracellular toxin in the syndrome; (2) attempts to concentrate the emetic toxin revealed that is passed through a 10,000 MW cutoff molecular exclusion filter and was not retained by dialysis tubing—indicative of a relatively small molecular size; (3) the toxin proved to be highly stable, surviving autoclaving at 121°C for 90 min, pH extremes of 2 to 11, and exposure to the proteolytic enzymes trypsin and pepsin; and (4) no apparent resistance developed in monkeys fed up to 16 times during an 8-month period, indicating the low antigenicity of the molecule. The authors concluded that, in contrast to the nature of the diarrheal enterotoxin, the emetic toxin was an entirely distinct molecule of low molecular weight, poor antigenicity, and unusual stability.

Given the obvious restrictions of using a toxin assay based on the feeding of monkeys, Melling and Capel (see Turnbull, 1986) sought to investigate whether the relationship between the emetic syndrome and cooked rice might be linked to sporulation of the organism in this medium. Two growth and toxin-production studies were carried out using strain F4810/72, in which spore counts were also determined. In the first, emetic activity appeared in the late exponential growth phase before spore levels had become detectable. In the second study, emetic activity was not apparent until several hours into the stationary phase, when the spore count had reached a maximum. Thus, on the basis of data obtained so far, a relationship between sporulation and production of emetic toxin has neither been confirmed nor refuted. However, if such a link does exist, it is not a direct correlation, as cultures of F4810/72 in artificial sporulation media have failed to induce emesis in monkeys at 98% sporulation (Melling et al., 1976; Turnbull, 1986). The emetic syndrome outbreaks associated with foods other than cooked rice (see Table 4) indicate that production of the emetic toxin is not exclusive to rice. However, it is likely that in many types of food the level of bacterial multiplication necessary to produce hazardous amounts of preformed toxin also results in noticeable spoilage, and that these foods would consequently be discarded.

Table 8 Comparative Properties of *B. cereus* Diarrheal and Emetic Toxins

Property	Diarrheal enterotoxin	Emetic toxin
Nature/MW	Protein/38,000–46,000 (SDS PAGE) 50,000–57,000 (G. 100)	Peptide (?)/<10,000
Isoelectric point (pI)	4.9–5.6	ND[a]
Stabilities		
Heat	Inactivated at 56°C for 5 min	Stable at 126°C for 90 min
pH	Unstable <4 and >11	Stable 2 to 11
Proteases	Pronase, trypsin, and pepsin sensitive	Trypsin and pepsin resistant
Other enzymes, etc.	EDTA, β-glucuronidase, and alkylation resistant	ND[a]
Production		
In foods	Preformed (?)	Preformed
Optimum laboratory media	BHIG, CAM[b]	Rice culture slurry
Optimum temperature	32–37°C	25–30°C
Growth phase	Late exponential	Late exponential-stationary (? sporulation related)
Biological activities		
Monkey challenge	Diarrhea 0.5–3.5 h	Emesis 1.0–5.0 h
Rabbit ileal loop	Positive (150–300 μg). Necrotic	Negative
Mouse ileal loop	Positive (12 μg)	ND[a]
Rabbit VPR[c]	Positive (0.05–1.25 μg). Necrotic	Negative
Mouse VPR[c]	Positive (0.2 μg)	ND[a]
Suckling mouse FAT[d]	Positive (ND)[a]	ND[a]
Mouse lethality (i.v.)	Positive (12–30 μg)	ND[a]
Cytotoxicity (HFS, CHO, INT-407)[e]	Positive (0.1–0.5 μg)	ND[a]
Antigenicity	Positive.[f] May be “multicomponent”	Low or negative antigenicity

Action	Fluid (and Na^+, Cl^-) absorption reversed Strongly necrotic; mucosal damage; other tissues affected Glucose and amino acid malabsorption May stimulate adenylate cyclase-cAMP system, or reduce cell energy through microvilli damage Capillary permeability altered	Not known
Laboratory detection		
In vivo assays	Ligated ileal loop test Vascular permeability reaction Suckling mouse test	Monkey challenge
In vitro assays	Tissue culture (Vero, CHO, INT-407)[e] Immunodiffusion Immunoelectrophoresis Reverse passive hemagglutination Reverse passive latex agglutination	Vacuolation of HEp-2 cells (Hughs et al., 1988)

[a]ND, no data.
[b]BHIG, brain heart infusion with glucose; CAM, casamino acids medium.
[c]VPR, vascular permeability reaction.
[d]FAT, fluid accumulation test.
[e]CHO, Chinese hamster ovary; INT-407, human embryonic intestinal epithelium.
[f]No cross-reactivities with *Shigella dysenteriae, Vibrio cholerae, Clostridium perfringens*, or *Escherichia coli* LT enterotoxins.

The optimal temperature range for emetic toxin production in rice culture was found to be 25–30°C (Melling and Capel, 1978). At temperatures of between 35 and 45°C, despite equivalent or higher vegetative cell and spore counts being obtained, the emetic activity was lower than that obtained with 30°C cultures.

The limitations of the monkey feeding assay (i.e., low sensitivity, reproducibility, and practicality) have hampered research into the nature and properties of the emetic toxin. It is not yet known, for example, whether different strains produce this toxin to different degrees. The variation in response between animals is too great to enable this to be accurately determined.

On the basis of current evidence, however, there appears to be no consistent relationship between diarrheal and emetic toxin production by any given strain of *B. cereus*. In VPR tests on isolates from emetic syndrome incidents which have been cultured in BHI medium, but which in rice cultures have also induced emesis in monkeys, toxin production categories 1–4 have all been represented (Turnbull, 1979a). One implication of these findings is that certain strains could give rise to either (or both) vomiting or diarrheal symptoms according to the nature of the food in which they have been allowed to multiply. Later-onset diarrhea is occasionally reported as a secondary feature of emetic syndrome episodes, and this could be construed to arise through the activities of both toxins. In contrast, out of four strains associated with diarrheal syndrome episodes that were fed to monkeys as rice cultures, only one induced emesis in just one out of eight feedings—evidence that not all *B. cereus* strains are able to produce both these toxins.

Table 8 is a summary of the comparative properties of *B. cereus* diarrheal enterotoxin and emetic toxin as they are currently understood and is based on data pooled from research groups in the United Kingdom (Melling et al., 1976; Turnbull, 1976, 1979a; Kramer et al., 1978; Melling and Capel, 1978; Gilbert and Kramer, 1984; Kramer, 1984; Hughes et al., 1988), the United States (Spira and Goepfert, 1972a,b, 1975; Spira and Silverman, 1979; Thompson et al., 1984), Japan (Shinagawa et al., 1985a,b), and the USSR (Ezepchuk and Fluer, 1973; Gorina et al., 1975, 1976; Ezepchuk et al., 1979).

REFERENCES

Ahmed, A. A.-H., Moustafa, M. K., and Marth, E. H. (1983). Incidence of *Bacillus cereus* in milk and some milk products. *J. Food Prot. 46*: 126–128.

Anon. (1977). An outbreak of food poisoning in three schools. Public Health Laboratory Service, London. Communicable Disease Report No. 44.

Asanuma, S., Tanaka, H., and Yatazawa, M. (1979). Rhizoplane microorganisms of rice seedlings as examined by scanning electron microscopy. *Soil Sci. Plant Nutr. 25*: 539–551.

Baba, T. (1969). Analytical serology of *Bacillaceae*. In *Analytical Serology of Microorganisms*, Vol. 2, J. B. G. Kwapinski, ed. Wiley & Sons, Inc., New York, pp. 609–642.

Batchelor, M. D. (1919). Aerobic spore-bearing bacteria in the intestinal tract of children. *J. Bacteriol. 4*: 23–34.

Baumann-Grace, J. B., Kovics, H., and Tomcsik, J. (1959). Extraktion von Polysaccharid-hapatenen aus der Zellwand des *B. anthracis* und des *B. cereus*. *Schweiz. Z. Pathol. Bakteriol.* *22*: 158–176.

Beckers, H. J. (1976). The bacteriological quality of boiled and fried rice from Chinese restaurants in relation to *Bacillus cereus* food poisoning. *Arch. Lebensmittelhyg.* *27*: 66–68.

Beckers, H. J. (1982). Incidence of foodborne disease in the Netherlands: Annual summary, 1979. *J. Food Prot.* *45*: 1338–1341.

Beckers, H. J. (1985). Incidence of foodborne disease in the Netherlands: Annual summary, 1980. *J. Food Prot.* *48*: 181–187.

Berkeley, R. C. W., Logan, N. A., Shute, L. A., and Capey, A. G. (1984). Identification of *Bacillus* species. In *Methods in Microbiology*, Vol. 16, T. Bergan, ed. Academic Press, London, pp. 291–328.

Bernheimer, A. W., and Grushoff, P. (1967a). Cereolysin: Production, purification, and partial characterization. *J. Gen. Microbiol.* *46*: 143–150.

Bernheimer, A. W., and Grushoff, P. (1967b). Extracellular hemolysin of aerobic sporogenic bacilli. *J. Bacteriol.* *93*: 1541–1543.

Bernheimer, A. W., Grushoff, P., and Avigad, L. S. (1968). Isoelectric analysis of cytolytic bacterial proteins. *J. Bacteriol.* *95*: 2439–2441.

Beuchat, L. R., Ma-Lin, C. F. A., and Carpenter, J. A. (1980). Growth of *Bacillus cereus* in media containing plant seed materials and ingredients used in Chinese cookery. *J. Appl. Bacteriol.* *48*: 397–407.

Billing, E., and Cuthbert, W. A. (1958). "Bitty" cream: The occurrence and significance of *Bacillus cereus* spores in raw milk supplies. *J. Appl. Bacteriol.* *21*: 65–78.

Birch, B. R., Perera, B. S., Hyde, W. A., Ruehorn, V., Ganguli, L. A., Kramer, J. M., and Turnbull, P. C. B. (1981). *Bacillus cereus* cross-infection in a maternity unit. *J. Hosp. Infect.* *2*: 349–354.

Blakey, L. J., and Priest, F. G. (1980). The occurrence of *Bacillus cereus* in some dried foods including pulses and cereals. *J. Appl. Bacteriol.* *48*: 297–302.

Bradshaw, J. G., Peeler, J. T., and Twedt, R. M. (1975). Heat resistance of ileal loop reactive *Bacillus cereus* strains isolated from commercially canned food. *Appl. Microbiol.* *30*: 943–945.

Brekenfeld, H. (1926). Lebensmittelbakterien und Vergiftungen. *Zentralbl. Bakteriol.* I Orig. *99*: 353–385.

Brekenfeld, H. (1929). Eine Presskopfvergiftungen und ihre Lehren. *Zentralbl. Bakteriol.* I Orig. *110*: 139–147.

Bryan, F. L., Bartleson, C. A., and Christopherson, N. (1981). Hazard analyses, in references to *Bacillus cereus*, of boiled and fried rice in Cantonese-style restaurants. *J. Food Prot.* *44*: 500–512.

Cao, R., Liu, G., Chang, S., Fen, D., and Dong, S. (1984). Studies on the biological characters and serotypes of 94 cultures of *Bacillus cereus*. *Chinese J. Microbiol. Immunol.* *4*: 298–301.

Carpenter, D. F., Spira, W. M., and Silverman, G. J. (1975). Effects of dissolved oxygen tension on bacterial enterotoxin production. *Developments in Industrial Microbiology* (Soc. Industrial Microbiol.) *17*: 363–374.

Chopra, P., Singh, A., and Kalra, M. S. (1980). Occurrence of *Bacillus cereus* in milk and milk products. *Indian J. Dairy Sci.* *33*: 248–252.

Coolbaugh, J. C., and Williams, R. P. (1978). Production and characterization of two hemolysins of *Bacillus cereus*. *Can. J. Microbiol.* *24*: 1289–1295.

Cowell, J. L., Grushoff-Kosyk, P. S., and Bernheimer, A. W. (1976). Purification of cereolysin and the electrophoretic separation of active (reduced) and inactive (oxidized) forms of the purified toxin. *Infect. Immun.* *14*: 144–154.

de Barjac, H. (1981). Insect pathogens in the genus *Bacillus*. In *The Aerobic Endospore-forming Bacteria: Classification and Identification*, R. C. W. Berkeley and M. Goodfellow, eds. Academic Press, London, pp. 241–250.

de Barjac, H., and Bonnefoi, A. (1962). Essai de classification biochimique et serologique de 24 souches de *Bacillus* du type *B. thuringiensis*. *Entomophaga 7*: 5–31.

de Barjac, H., and Bonnefoi, A. (1968). A classification of strains of *Bacillus thuringiensis* Berliner with a key to their differentiation. *J. Invert. Pathol. 11*: 335–347.

DeBuono, B. A., Brondum, J., Kramer, J. M., Gilbert, R. J., and Opal, S. M. (1988). Plasmid, serotypic, and enterotoxin analysis of *Bacillus cereus* in an outbreak setting. *J. Clin. Microbiol. 26*: 1571–1574.

Doak, B. W., and Lamanna, C. (1948). On the antigenic structure of the bacterial spore. *J. Bacteriol. 55*: 373–380.

Donovan, K. O. (1959). The occurrence of *Bacillus cereus* in milk and on dairy equipment. *J. Appl. Bacteriol. 22*: 131–137.

Dryden, M. S., and Kramer, J. M. (1987). Toxigenic *Bacillus cereus* as a cause of wound infections in the tropics: Results of an Operation Raleigh survey. *J. Infect. 15*: 207–212.

Ezepchuk, Y. V., and Fluer, F. S. (1973). The enterotoxic effect. *Moderne Medizin 3*: 20–25.

Ezepchuk, Y. V., Bondarenko, V. M., Yakovleva, E. A., and Koryagina, I. P. (1979). The *Bacillus cereus* toxin: Isolation of permeability factor. *Zentralbl. Bakteriol. Hyg.*, I Abt. Orig. A. *244*: 275–284.

Fluer, F. S., and Ezpechuk, Y. Z. (1970). Formation of lecithinase by *Bacillus cereus* (English translation). *Mikrobiologya* (Moscow) *39*: 396–401.

Foegeding, P. M., and Busta, F. F. (1981). Bacterial spore injury—an update. *J. Food Prot. 44*: 776–786.

Fossum, K. (1964). The heat sensitivity of *Bacillus cereus* hemolysin. *Acta Path. Microbiol. Scand. 60*: 523–527.

Franklin, J. G. (1970). Spores in milk: Problems associated with UHT processing. *J. Appl. Bacteriol. 33*: 180–191.

Ghosh, A. C. (1978). Prevalence of *Bacillus cereus* in the faeces of healthy adults. *J. Hyg.*, Camb. *80*: 233–236.

Gibson, T., and Gordon, R. E. (1974). Genus I *Bacillus*. In *Bergey's Manual of Determinative Bacteriology*, 8th ed., R. E. Buchanan and N. E. Gibbons, eds. Williams and Wilkins, Baltimore, pp. 529–550.

Gilbert, R. J. (1979). *Bacillus cereus* gastroenteritis. In *Food-borne Infections and Intoxications*, 2nd ed., H. Riemann and F. L. Bryan, eds. Academic Press, New York, pp. 495–518.

Gilbert, R. J., and Kramer, J. M. (1984). *Bacillus cereus* enterotoxins: Present status. *Biochem. Soc. Trans. 12*: 198–200.

Gilbert, R. J., and Kramer, J. M. (1986). *Bacillus cereus* food poisoning. In *Progress in Food Safety*, D. O. Cliver and B. A. Cochrane, eds. Food Research Institute, University of Wisconsin—Madison, pp. 85–93.

Gilbert, R. J., and Parry, J. M. (1977). Serotypes of *Bacillus cereus* from outbreaks of food poisoning and from routine foods. *J. Hyg.*, Camb. *78*: 69–74.

Gilbert, R. J., and Taylor, A. J. (1976). *Bacillus cereus* food poisoning. In *Microbiology in Agriculture, Fisheries and Food*, F. A. Skinner and J. G. Carr, eds. Society for Applied Bacteriology Symposium Series, No. 4. Academic Press, London, pp. 197–213.

Gilbert, R. J., Stringer, M. F., and Peace, T. C. (1974). The survival and growth of *Bacillus cereus* in boiled and fried rice in relation to outbreaks of food poisoning. *J. Hyg.*, Camb. *73*: 433–444.

Gilbert, R. J., Turnbull, P. C. B., Parry, J. M., and Kramer, J. M. (1981). *Bacillus cereus* and other *Bacillus* species: Their part in food poisoning and other clinical infections. In *The Aerobic Endospore-forming Bacteria: Classification and Identification*, R. C. W. Berkeley and M. Goodfellow, eds. Academic Press, London, pp. 297–314.

Glatz, B. A., and Goepfert, J. M. (1973). Extracellular factor synthesized by *Bacillus cereus* which evokes a dermal reaction in guinea pigs. *Infect. Immun. 8*: 25–29.

Glatz, B. A., and Goepfert, J. M. (1976). Defined conditions for synthesis of *Bacillus cereus* enterotoxin by fermenter-grown cultures. *Appl. Environ. Microbiol. 32*: 400–404.

Glatz, B. A., and Goepfert, J. M. (1977). Production of *Bacillus cereus* enterotoxin in defined media in fermenter-grown cultures. *J. Food Prot. 40*: 472–474.

Glatz, B. A., Spira, W. M., and Goepfert, J. M. (1974). Alteration of vascular permeability in rabbits by culture filtrates of *Bacillus cereus* and related species. *Infect. Immun. 10*: 299–303.

Goepfert, J. M. (1973). Pathogenicity patterns in *Bacillus cereus* foodborne disease. In *Proc. First International Congress of Food Science and Technology*, Jerusalem, Vol. 1, pp. 140–141.

Goepfert, J. M. (1978). Monkey feeding trials in the investigation of the nature of *Bacillus cereus* food poisoning. Fourth International Congress of Food Science and Technology, Madrid, Vol. 3, pp. 178–181.

Goepfert, J. M., Spira, W. M., and Kim, H. U. (1972). *Bacillus cereus*: Food poisoning organism. A review. *J. Milk Food Technol. 35*: 213–227.

Gordon, R. E. (1977). The genus *Bacillus*. In *CRC Handbook of Microbiology*, 2nd ed., Vol. I: *Bacteria*, A. I. Laskin and H. A. Lechevalier, eds. CRC Press, Inc., Cleveland, OH, pp. 319–336.

Gordon, R. E., Haynes, W. C., and Pang, C. H.-N. (1973). The genus *Bacillus*. Handbook No. 427. USDA, Washington, DC.

Gorina, L. G., Fluer, F. S., Olovnikov, A. M., and Ezepchuk, Y. V. (1975). Use of the aggregate-hemagglutination technique for determining exo-enterotoxin of *Bacillus cereus. Appl. Microbiol. 29*: 201–204.

Gorina, L. G., Fluer, F. S., Olovnikov, A. M., and Ezepchuk, Y. V. (1976). Highly sensitive determination of *Bacillus cereus* exo-enterotoxin using the method of aggregate haemagglutination. *J. Hyg. Epidem. Microbiol. Immunol. 20*: 361–367.

Gostling, J. V. T., Richold, J. C., Turnbull, P. C. B., and Kramer, J. M. (1980). *Bacillus cereus* in a maternity unit. Public Health Laboratory Service, London, Communicable Disease Report No. 36.

Gutkin, B. J. (1975). *Bacillus cereus* intoxication followed by periorbital oedema. *Brit. Med. J. 4*: 24.

Hauge, S. (1950). *Bacillus cereus* as a cause of food poisoning. *Nord. Hyg. Tigskr. 31*: 189–206.

Hauge, S. (1955). Food poisoning caused by aerobic spore-forming bacilli. *J. Appl. Bacteriol. 18*: 591–595.

Hirn, J., and Aho, M. (1986). Foodborne disease outbreaks in Finland 1975–1984. In *Proc. Second World Congress on Foodborne Infections and Intoxications*, Berlin, Vol. 1, Institute of Veterinary Medicine—Robert von Ostertag Institute, West Berlin.

Holmes, J. R., Plunkett, T., Pate, P., Roper, W. L., and Alexander, W. J. (1981). Emetic food poisoning caused by *Bacillus cereus. Arch. Intern. Med. 141*: 766–767.

Hughes, S., Bartholomew, B. A., Hardy, J. C., and Kramer, J. M. (1988). Potential application of a HEp-2 cell assay in the investigation of *Bacillus cereus* emetic-syndrome food poisoning. *FEMS Microbiol. Lett. 52*: 7–12.

Ikezawa, H., Yamanegi, M., Taguchi, R., Miyashita, T., and Ohyabu, T. (1976). Studies on phosphatidylinositol phosphodiesterase (phospholipase C type) of *Bacillus cereus*.

1. Purification, properties and phospatase-releasing activity. *Biochim. Biophys. Acta 450*: 154–164.

Ikezawa, H., Yamanegi, M., Taguchi, R., Miyashita, T., and Ohyabu, T. (1977). A phosphatidylinositol phospholipase C (phosphatasemia factor) of *Bacillus cereus*. *Jap. J. Med. Sci. Biol. 30*: 81–82.

Ikezawa, H., Mori, M., Ohyabu, T., and Taguchi, R. (1978). Studies on sphingomyelinase of *Bacillus cereus*. 1. Purification and properties. *Biochim. Biophys. Acta 528*: 247–256.

Ikezawa, H., Mori, M., and Taguchi, R. (1980). Studies on sphingomyelinase of *Bacillus cereus*; hydrolytic and hemolytic actions on erythrocyte membranes. *Arch. Biochem. Biophys. 199*: 572–578.

Ingram, M. (1969). Sporeformers as food spoilage organisms. In *The Bacterial Spore*, G. W. Gould and A. Hurst, eds. Academic Press, London, pp. 549–610.

Ionescu, G., Ienistea, C., and Ionescu, C. (1966). Freeventa *B. cereus* in laptele crud si in laptele pasteurizat. *Microbiol. Parazitol. Epidemiol. 11*: 423–430.

Itoh, T., Kai, A., Saito, K., Yanagawa, Y., Inaba, M., Takahashi, M., Takano, I., Shingaki, M., Sakai, S., Shinohara, T., Kato, K., Tamura, N., Tsuchiya, N., and Komai, Y. (1982). Epidemiological and bacteriological examination of fifteen vomiting-type outbreaks of food poisoning due to *Bacillus cereus* in Tokyo. *Ann. Rep. Tokyo Metr. Res. Lab. Publ. Hlth. 33*: 9–18.

Ivanovics, G., and Foldes, J. (1958). Problems concerning the phylogenesis of *B. anthracis*. *Acta Microbiol. Hung. 5*: 89–109.

Iverson, H., Rosef, O., and Selas, P. (1982). Outbreak of food poisoning caused by *Bacillus cereus* at a geriatric and health care centre. *Norsk. Veterinaertidsskrift. 94*: 337–340.

Jauhari, J. S., and Kulshrestha, S. B. (1986). Food poisoning episode in a family due to *B. cereus*. In *Proc. Second World Congress on Foodborne Infections and Intoxications*, Berlin, Vol. I. Institute of Veterinary Medicine—Robert von Ostertag Institute, West Berlin.

Johnson, C. E., and Bonventre, P. F. (1967). Lethal toxin of *Bacillus cereus*. I. Relationships and nature of toxin, hemolysin, and phospholipase. *J. Bacteriol. 94*: 306–316.

Johnson, K. M. (1984). *Bacillus cereus* foodborne illness—an update. *J. Food Prot. 47*: 145–153.

Johnson, K. M ., Nelson, C. L., and Busta, F. F. (1982). Germination and heat resistance of *Bacillus cereus* spores from strains associated with diarrheal and emetic food-borne illnesses. *J. Food Sci. 47*: 1268–1271.

Johnson, K. M., Nelson, C. L., and Busta, F. F. (1983). Influence of temperature on germination and growth of spores of emetic and diarrheal strains of *Bacillus cereus* in a broth medium and in rice. *J. Food Sci. 48*: 286–287.

Johnston, K. G. (1986). *Bacilus cereus* mastitis in lactating cows. *Proc. XIV International Congress on Diseases of Cattle*, Dublin, 1986.

Jones, T. O., and Turnbull, P. C. B. (1981). Bovine mastitis caused by *Bacillus cereus*. *Vet. Rec. 108*: 272–274.

Kim, H. U., and Goepfert, J. M. (1971). Enumeration and identification of *Bacillus cereus* in foods. I. 24-hour presumptive test medium. *Appl. Microbiol. 22*: 581–587.

Kim, H. U., and Goepfert, J. M. (1972). Efficacy of a fluorescent-antibody procedure for identifying *Bacillus cereus* in foods. *Appl. Microbiol. 24*: 708–713.

Knaysi, G. (1964). Effect of temperature on the rate of germination in *Bacillus cereus*. *J. Bacteriol. 87*: 619–622.

Kramer, J. M. (1984). *Bacillus cereus* exotoxins: Production, isolation, detection and properties. In *Bacterial Protein Toxins*, J. E. Alouf, J. H. Freer, F. J. Fehrenbach, and J. Jeljaszewicz, eds. Academic Press, London, pp. 385–386.

Kramer, J. M., and Gilbert, R. J. (1989). *Bacillus cereus* and other *Bacillus* species. In *Foodborne Bacterial Pathogens*, M. P. Doyle, ed. Marcel Dekker, New York, pp. 21–70.

Kramer, J. M., Turnbull, P. C. B., Jorgensen, K., Parry, J., and Gilbert, R. J. (1978). Separation of exponential growth exotoxins of *Bacillus cereus* and their preliminary characterization. *J. Appl. Bacteriol.* *45*: xix.

Kramer, J. M., Turnbull, P. C. B., Munshi, G., and Gilbert, R. J . (1982). Identification and characterization of *Bacillus cereus* and other *Bacillus* species associated with foods and food poisoning. In *Isolation and Identification Methods for Food Poisoning Organisms*, J. E. L. Corry, D. Roberts, and F. A. Skinner, eds. Academic Press, London, pp. 261–286.

Lamanna, C. (1940). The taxonomy of the genus *Bacillus*. III. Differentiation of the large-celled species by means of spore antigens. *J. Infect. Dis.* *67*: 205–212.

Lamanna, C., and Eisler, D. (1960). Comparative study of the agglutinogens of the endospores of *B. anthracis* and *B. cereus*. *J. Bacteriol.* *79*: 435–441.

Lamanna, C., and Jones, L. (1961). Antigenic relationship of the endospores of *B. cereus*-like insect pathogens to *B. cereus* and *B. anthracis*. *J. Bacteriol.* *81*: 622–625.

Larkin, J. M., and Stokes, J. L. (1966). Isolation of psychrophilic species of *Bacillus*. *J. Bacteriol.* *91*: 1667–1671.

Lee, M. S., and Chang, D. S. (1980). Distribution and physiological characteristics of *Bacillus cereus* in rice and rice products. *Bull. Korean Fish. Soc.* *13*: 163–171.

Lefebvre, A., Gregoire, C. A., Brabant, W., and Todd, E. (1973). Suspected *Bacillus cereus* food poisoning. *Epidemiol. Bull. Ottawa* *17*: 108–110.

LeMille, F., de Barjac, H., and Bonnefoi, A. (1969). Etude serologique de *Bacillus*. Mise en evidence de divers serotypes bases sur les antigenes flagellaires. *Annales Inst. Pasteur* *117*: 31–38.

Logan, N. A., Capel, B. J., Melling, J., and Berkeley, R. C. W. (1979). Distinction between emetic and other strains of *Bacillus cereus* using the API system and numerical methods. *FEMS Microbiol. Lett.* *5*: 373–375.

Lubenau, C. (1906). *Bacillus peptonificans* als Erreger einer Gastroenteritis-Epidemie. *Zentralbl. Bakteriol.*, I Orig. *40*: 433–437.

Marples, R. R. (1983). Contaminated first-aid dressings: Report of a working party of the PHLS. *J. Hyg.*, Camb. *90*: 241–252.

Mathias, R. G., Todd, E., Szabo, R., and Martin, D. (1976). Illness from fried rice—St. John's, Newfoundland. *Can. Dis. Week. Rep.* *2*: 78–79.

Melling, J., and Capel, B. J. (1978). Characteristics of *Bacillus cereus* emetic toxin. *FEMS Microbiol. Lett.* *4*: 133–135.

Melling, J., Capel, B. J., Turnbull, P. C. B., and Gilbert, R. J. (1976). Identification of a novel enterotoxigenic activity associated with *Bacillus cereus*. *J. Clin. Pathol.* *29*: 938–940.

Midura, T., Gerber, M., Wood, R., and Leonard, A. R. (1970). Outbreak of food poisoning caused by *Bacillus cereus*. *Publ. Hlth. Rep.* *85*: 45–48.

Mikolajcik, E. M. (1970). Thermodestruction of *Bacillus* spores in milk. *J. Milk Food Technol.* *33*: 61–63.

Mikolajcik, E. M., Kearney, J. W., Kristofferson, T. (1973). Fate of *Bacillus cereus* in cultured and direct acidified skim milk and cheddar cheese. *J. Milk Food Technol.* *36*: 317–320.

Mol, J. H. H. (1957). The temperature characteristics of spore germination and growth of *Bacillus cereus*. *J. Appl. Bacteriol.* *20*: 454–459.

Molin, N., and Snygg, B. G. (1967). Effect of lipid materials on heat resistance of bacterial spores. *Appl. Microbiol.* *15*: 1422–1426.

Mollby, R. (1978). Bacterial phospholipases. In *Bacterial Toxins and Cell Membranes*, J. Jeljaszewicz and T. Wadstrom, eds. Academic Press, London, pp. 367–424.

Morita, T. N., and Woodburn, M. J. (1977). Stimulation of *Bacillus cereus* growth by protein in cooked rice combinations. *J. Food Sci. 42*: 1232–1235.

Mortimer, P. R., and McCann, G. (1974). Food-poisoning episodes associated with *Bacillus cereus* in fried rice. *Lancet i*: 1043–1045.

Mostert, J. F., Luck, H., and Husmann, R. A. (1979). Isolation, identification, and practical properties of *Bacillus* species from UHT and sterilized milk. *S. Afr. J. Dairy Technol. 11*: 125–132.

Nikodemusz, I. (1964). Die Reproduzierbarkeit der von *Bacillus cereus* verursachteten Lebensmittelvergiftungen bei Katzen. *Zentralbl. Bakteriol.*, I Orig. *196*: 81–87.

Nikodemusz, I. (1986a). Comparison du pouvoir pathogene experimental de *Bacillus cereus* et de *Bacillus laterosporus* administeres par voie orale. *Annales Inst. Pasteur 17*: 229–232.

Nikodemusz, I. (1966b). Die Wirkung langfristigen Verabreichung von *Bacillus cereus* verunreinigten Lebensmitteln bei Katzen. *Zentralbl. Bakteriol.*, I Orig. *199*: 64–67.

Nikodemusz, I. (1967). Die enteropathogene Wirkung von *Bacillus cereus* bei Hunden. *Zentralbl. Bakteriol.*, I Orig. *202*: 533–538.

Noble, A. (1919). A method for the production of a homogeneous suspension of *Bacillus anthracis* to be used in agglutination reactions. *J. Immunol. 4*: 105–109.

Norris, J. R. (1962). Bacterial spore antigens: A review. *J. Gen. Microbiol. 28*: 393–408.

Norris, J. R., and Wolf, J. (1961). A study of the antigens of the aerobic spore-forming bacteria. *J. Appl. Bacteriol. 24*: 42–56.

Norris, J. R., Berkeley, R. C. W., Logan, N. A., and O'Donnell, A. G. (1981). The genera *Bacillus* and *Sporolactobacillus*. In *The Prokaryotes—A handbook on Habitats, Isolation and Identification of Bacteria*, Vol. II, M. P. Starr, H. Stolp, H. G. Truper, A. Balows, and H. G. Schlegel, eds. Springer-Verlag, Berlin, pp. 1711–1742.

Nygren, B. (1962). Phospholipase C-producing bacteria and food poisoning. *Acta Pathol. Microbiol. Scand. Suppl. 160*: 1–89.

Overcast, W. W., and Atmaram, K. (1974). The role of *Bacillus cereus* in sweet curdling of fluid milk. *J. Milk Food Technol. 37*: 233–236.

Parker, D. A., and Goepfert, J. M. (1978). Enhancement of synthesis of *Bacillus cereus* enterotoxin using a sac-culture technique. *J. Food Prot. 41*: 116–117.

Parry, J. M., and Gilbert, R. J. (1980). Studies of the heat resistance of *Bacillus cereus* spores and growth of the organism in boiled rice. *J. Hyg.*, Camb. *84*: 77–82.

Pinegar, J. A., and Buxton, J. D. (1977). An investigation of the bacteriological quality of retail vanilla slices. *J. Hyg.*, Camb. *78*: 387–394.

Priest, F. G. (1981). DNA homology in the genus *Bacillus*. In *The Aerobic Endospore-Forming Bacteria: Classification and Identification*, R. C. W. Berkeley and M. Goodfellow, eds. Academic Press, London, pp. 33–57.

Public Health Laboratory Service (1972). Food poisoning associated with *Bacillus cereus*. *Brit. Med. J. i*: 189.

Raevuori, M. (1976). Effect of sorbic acid and potassium sorbate on growth of *Bacillus cereus* and *Bacillus subtilis* in rice filling of Karelian pastry. *Eur. J. Appl. Microbiol. 2*: 202–213.

Raevuori, M., and Genigeorgis, C. (1975). Effect of pH and sodium chloride on growth of *Bacillus cereus* in laboratory media and certain foods. *Appl. Microbiol. 29*: 68–73.

Raevuori, M., and Koiranen, L. (1978). *Bacillus cereus* as a cause of mastitis, and its occurrence in milk and milk products. *Suomen Elainlaakarilehti 84*: 5–10.

Raevuori, M., Kiutamo, T., and Niskanen, A. (1977). Comparative studies of *Bacillus cereus* strains isolated from various foods and food poisoning outbreaks. *Acta Vet. Scand. 18*: 397–407.

Rapport, H., and Goepfert, J. M. (1978). Thermal injury and recovery of *Bacillus cereus*. *J. Food Prot. 41*: 533–537.

Roberts, D., Watson, G. N., and Gilbert, R. J. (1982). Contamination of food plants and plant products with bacteria of public health significance. In *Bacteria and Plants*, Society for Applied Bacteriology Symposium Series No. 10, M. E. Rhodes-Roberts and F. A. Skinner, eds. Academic Press, London, pp. 169–195.

Saleem, Z. M., and Al-Delaimy, K. S. (1982). Inhibition of *Bacillus cereus* by garlic extracts. *J. Food Prot. 45*: 1007–1009.

Schiemann, D. A. (1978). Occurrence of *Bacillus cereus* and the bacteriological quality of Chinese "take-out" foods. *J. Food Prot. 41*: 450–454.

Seitz, M. (1913). Pathogener *Bacillus subtilis. Zentralbl. Bakteriol.*, I Orig. *70*: 113–114.

Shehata, T. E., and Collins, E. B. (1971). Isolation and identification of psychophilic species of *Bacillus* from milk. *Appl. Microbiol. 21*: 466–469.

Shehata, T. E., and Collins, E. B. (1972). Sporulation and heat resistance of psychrophilic strains of *Bacillus. J. Dairy Sci. 55*: 1405–1409.

Shinagawa, K., Kunita, N., Sasaki, Y., and Okamoto, A. (1979). Biochemical characteristics and heat tolerance of strains of *Bacillus cereus* isolated from uncooked and cooked rice after food poisoning outbreaks. [In Japanese, English summary.] *J. Food Hyg. Soc. Japan 20*: 431–436.

Shinagawa, K., Konuma, H., Kurata, H ., Tanabayashi, K., and Matsusaka, M. (1984). Surveillance of raw meat, meat products and meat-product additives for contamination with *Bacillus cereus* and enterotoxigenicity of the isolated strains. *J. Faculty of Agriculture of Iwate Univ., Japan 17*: 175–182.

Shinagawa, K., Matsusaka, N., Konuma, H., and Kurata, H. (1985a). Purification and characterization of *Bacillus cereus* diarrheal toxin. *Proceedings Ninth International Symposium of the World Association of Veterinary Food Hygienists*, Budapest, Hungary.

Shinagawa, K., Matsusaka, N., Konuma, H., and Kurata, H. (1985b). The relation between the diarrheal and other biological activities of *Bacillus cereus* involved in food poisoning outbreaks. *Japan J. Vet. Sci. 47*: 557–565.

Sievers, O., and Zetterberg, B. (1940). A preliminary investigation into the antigenic character of spore-forming aerobic bacteria. *J. Bacteriol. 40*: 45–56.

Slein, M. W., and Logan, G. F., Jr. (1963). Partial purification and properties of two phospholipases of *Bacillus cereus. J. Bacteriol. 85*: 369–381.

Slein, M. W., and Logan, G. F., Jr. (1965). Characterization of the phospholipases of *Bacillus cereus* and their effects on erythrocytes, bone cells, and kidney cells. *J. Bacteriol. 90*: 69–81.

Sly, T., and Ross, E. (1982). Chinese foods: Relationship between hygiene and bacterial flora. *J. Food Prot. 45*: 115–118.

Smith, N. R., Gordon, R. E., and Clark, F. E. (1946). Aerobic mesophilic spore-forming bacteria. USDA Misc. Publ. No. 559.

Smith, N. R., Gordon, R. E., and Clark, F. E. (1952). Aerobic spore-forming bacteria. USDA Monograph No. 16.

Spira, W. M. (1974). Animal assay systems for the qualitative and quantitative determination of *Bacillus cereus* enterotoxin. Ph.D. thesis, University of Wisconsin–Madison, WI.

Spira, W. M., and Goepfert, J. M. (1972a). *Bacillus cereus*-induced fluid accumulation in rabbit ileal loops. *Appl. Microbiol. 24*: 341–348.

Spira, W. M., and Goepfert, J. M. (1972b). An enterotoxic factor produced by *Bacillus cereus* and assayed in the ligated ileal loop of rabbits. Abstr. Annu. Meet. Amer. Soc. Microbiol., p. 33.

Spira, W. M., and Goepfert, J. M. (1975). Biological characteristics of an enterotoxin produced by *Bacillus cereus*. *Can. J. Microbiol. 21*: 1236–1246.

Spira, W. M., and Silverman, G. J. (1979). Effects of glucose, pH, and dissolved-oxygen tension on *Bacillus cereus* growth and permeability factor production in batch culture. *Appl. Environ. Microbiol. 37*: 109–116.

Stadhouders, J., Hup, G., and Langeveld, L. P. M. (1980). Some observations on the germination, heat resistance and outgrowth of fast-germinating and slow-germinating spores of *Bacillus cereus* in pasteurized milk. *Neth. Milk Dairy J. 34*: 215–228.

Stone, M. J., and Rowlands, A. (1952). 'Broken' or 'bitty' cream in raw and pasteurized milk. *J. Dairy Res. 19*: 51–62.

Tay, L., Goh, K. T., and Tan, S. E. (1982). An outbreak of *Bacillus cereus* food poisoning. *Singapore Med. J. 23*: 214–217.

Taylor, A. J., and Gilbert, R. J. (1975). *Bacillus cereus* food poisoning: A provisional serotyping scheme. *J. Med. Microbiol. 8*: 543–550.

Terayama, T., Shingaki, M., Yamada, S., Ushioda, H., Igarashi, H., Sakai, S., and Zen-Yoji, H. (1978). Incidence of *Bacillus cereus* in commercial foods and serological typing of isolates. *J. Food Hyg. Soc.*, Japan *19*: 98–104.

Thompson, N. E., Ketterhagen, M. J., Bergdoll, M. S., and Schantz, E. J. (1984). Isolation and some properties of an enterotoxin produced by *Bacillus cereus*. *Infect. Immun. 43*: 887–894.

Thompson, N. E., Aschenbach, J. M., Schantz, E. J., and Bergdoll, M. S. (1985). *Bacillus cereus* food poisoning. In *Food Research Institute 1985 Annual Report*. University of Wisconsin–Madison, WI, pp. 452–453.

Todd, E. C. D. (1982). Foodborne and waterborne disease in Canada—1977 Annual Summary. *J. Food Prot. 45*: 865–873.

Todd, E. C. D. (1985a). Foodborne and waterborne disease in Canada—1978 Annual Summary. *J. Food Prot. 48*: 990–996.

Todd, E. C. D. (1985b). Foodborne and waterborne disease in Canada—1979 Annual Summary. *J. Food Prot. 48*: 1071–1078.

Todd, E. C. D. (1987). Foodborne and waterborne disease in Canada—1980 Annual Summary. *J. Food Prot. 50*: 420–428.

Tomcsik, J., and Baumann-Grace, J. B. (1959). Serologische Typen von *Bacillus cereus* und ihre Verwandtschaft mit *Bacillus anthracis*. *Schweiz Zeit. Pathol. Bakteriol. 22*: 144–157.

Turnbull, P. C. B. (1976). Studies on the production of enterotoxins by *Bacillus cereus*. *J. Clin. Pathol. 29*: 941–948.

Turnbull, P. C. B. (1981). *Bacillus cereus* toxins: *Pharmacol. Ther. 13*: 453–505.

Turnbull, P. C. B. (1986). *Bacillus cereus* toxins. In *Pharmacology of Bacterial Toxins*, F. Dorner and J. Drews, eds. Pergamon Press, Oxford, pp. 397–448.

Turnbull, P. C. B., Nottingham, J. F., and Ghosh, A. C. (1977). A severe necrotic enterotoxin produced by certain food, food poisoning and other clinical isolates of *Bacillus cereus*. *Brit. J. Exp. Pathol. 58*: 273–280.

Turnbull, P. C. B., and Kramer, J. M. (1983). Non-gastrointestinal *Bacillus cereus* infections: An analysis of exotoxin production by strains isolated over a two-year period. *J. Clin. Pathol. 36*: 1091–1096.

Turnbull, P. C. B., and Kramer, J. M. (1985). Intestinal carriage of *Bacillus cereus*: Faecal isolation studies in three population groups. *J. Hyg.*, Camb. *95*: 629–638.

Turnbull, P. C. B., Kramer, J. M., Jørgensen, K., Gilbert, R. J., and Melling, J. (1979a). Properties and production characteristics of vomiting, diarrheal, and necrotizing toxins of *Bacillus cereus*. *Amer. J. Clin. Nutr. 32*: 219–228.

Turnbull, P. C. B., Jørgensen, K., Kramer, J. M., Gilbert, R. J., and Parry, J. M. (1979b). Severe clinical conditions associated with *Bacillus cereus* and the apparent involvement of exotoxins. *J. Clin. Pathol. 32*: 289–293.

Ushioda, H., Igarashi, H., Takahashi, M., Shigaki, M., Terayama, T., and Sakai, S. (1980). Survey on contamination of commercial foods with *Bacillus cereus*-biotypes and serotypes of the isolates. *Ann. Rep. Tokyo Metr. Res. Lab. Publ. Hlth. 31*: 109–114.

Vas, K., and Proszt, G. (1957). Observation on heat destruction of spores of *Bacillus cereus. J. Appl. Bacteriol. 20*: 431–441.

Vijayalakshmi, G., Dwarakanath, C. T., and Murthy, V. S. (1981). Studies on *Bacillus cereus* contamination of rice and rice preparations. *J. Food Sci. Technol. 18*: 231–234.

Walker, P. D., Baillie, A., Thomson, R. O., and Batty, I. (1966). The use of ferritin-labeled antibodies in the location of spore and vegetative antigens of *B. cereus. J. Appl. Bacteriol. 29*: 512–518.

Youngs, E. R., Roberts, C., Kramer, J. M., and Gilbert, R. J. (1985). Dissemination of *Bacillus cereus* in a maternity unit. *J. Infect. 10*: 228–232.

Yrios, J. W., Goepfert, J. M., Skinner, H. G., and Belinky, S. (1975). *Bacillus cereus* food poisoning—Wisconsin. *Morbid. Mortal. Week. Rep. 24*: 306.

Zwaal, R. F. A., Roelofsen, B., Comfurius, P., and van Deenen, L. L. M. (1971). Complete purification and some properties of phospholipase C from *Bacillus cereus. Biochim. Biophys. Acta 233*: 474–479.

7

Cholera Infection and Poisoning

Charles A. Kaysner

United States Food and Drug Administration, Bothell, Washington

I. INTRODUCTION

Cholera, the "scourge of Asia," is a gastrointestinal disease caused by a bacterium, *Vibrio cholerae* serogroup 0:1, that is endemic to parts of the Asian continent, primarily India and the Ganges basin. In past centuries, this catastrophic disease has caused thousands of deaths. Cholera has usually infected impoverished people who live in unsanitary conditions. In these areas, drinking water is often taken from sources that are also used for sewage disposal and other human activities. The original description of the etiological agent of cholera is attributed to Pacini in 1854, but many bacteriologists remained skeptical of his findings because similar but harmless vibrios could be isolated from diverse environments.

Cholera is considered by some to be an ancient human affliction (Pollitzer, 1959; De, 1961). The distinct symptoms and explosive epidemic onslaught of the disease are believed to be depicted in early Arabian, Chinese, Hindu, Greek, and Roman writings (McNicol and Doetsch, 1983). For 2500 years the word cholera was used to describe diarrhea and vomiting from any cause, not only bacterial. Whatever the origin of the word or the disease, cholera still afflicts a large number of people in the world yearly. Recently, in a report to the World Health Organization, more than 48,000 cases of cholera were recorded from 39 countries in 1989 (Anonymous, 1990). Approximately 75% of the cases were in African countries.

The pandemic cholera that is clinically recognized today emerged in India around 1817 (Longmate, 1966). Since this time, seven pandemics have been recorded, the latest spreading from Indonesia in 1959 to Asia, Africa, and Eastern Europe by the early 1970s, with a total of 41 countries reporting cases. Interestingly, the seventh was caused by the El Tor biotype, the hemolytic biotype, of *V. cholerae* 0:1, while previous pandemics were caused by the classical biotype. The El Tor biotype essentially replaced the classical biotype in Asia. For more than 10 years beginning in 1973, the isolation of the classical biotype was rare in cases investigated by the International Centre for Diarrhoeal Disease Research in Dacca (Cook et al., 1983). Since September 1982, there has been a gradual reemergence in Asia of the classical strain, which eventually accounted for over 90% of the cholera cases occurring in January 1983. It is interesting that the El Tor biotype surfaced in the United States in the early 1970s, and as yet the classical biotype has not been identified as being responsible for illness in this country. One wonders if the El Tor biotype is more transient in nature or more adaptable to new environments than its 0:1 cousin.

II. EPIDEMIOLOGY

A. *V. cholerae* 0:1 in the United States

Prior to 1970 in the United States, cholera was not well known—a few cases occurred at the turn of the century and the last identified outbreak was recorded in 1911. These illnesses were primarily thought to occur in individuals who had traveled to Asia and the Orient and had returned to the United States with the infection. It was not until 1973 that an apparent cholera problem surfaced in the United States when a man from Port Lavaca, Texas, was diagnosed with the disease (Weissman et al., 1974). Although the source of the infection was not identified, the patient had consumed raw oysters. Shortly thereafter, a woman in Massachusetts was found to be ill with what was eventually identified as a noncholera *Vibrio* (Harrington et al., 1974). In the past, bacterial strains that were biochemically similar to *V. cholerae* but did not agglutinate in the O group antisera were called noncholera vibrios. The source of the infection was not identified, but the patient had traveled to Mexico prior to the onset of severe diarrhea. Also in 1974, a second illness caused by a noncholera vibrio was reported (DeGermane and Smith, 1974). In Alabama in 1977, another illness caused by *V. cholerae* 0:1 Inaba was reported by Cameron et al. (1977), in which the patient had been known to consume large numbers of raw oysters and had done so for many years.

In 1978, the state of Louisiana became the focal point for cholera incidence after a man from Abbeville was diagnosed with the disease. Persistent investigation by a medical technician of a bacterial isolate from the patient led to a later identification of it by the Centers for Disease Control (CDC) in Atlanta as toxigenic *V. cholerae* serogroup 0:1 Inaba (Bradford, 1984). This diagnosis led to an intensive investigation by state and federal health officials of a potential cholera problem in Louisiana. During a 2-month investigation, 11 cases of cholera were identified. Eight of these cases were symptomatic, and all 11 cases were associated with the consumption of either boiled or steamed home-cooked crabs. The contaminated crabs were caught in a variety of places, miles apart, suggesting no single point of contamination. A large number of environmental samples were analyzed including estuarine water, shellfish, and crustaceans. Less than 0.5% of these samples were found to contain *V. cholerae* 0:1, which suggested that this pathogen was endemic to Louisiana, but in very low numbers. Of interest during this time was the fact that the strain of *V. cholerae* 0:1 isolated in Texas in 1973 and the strains isolated from the 11 patients in Louisiana were identical to each other by phage type. This would suggest that this particular strain had become endemic in both states and had persisted for some time environmentally. It was concluded by Kaper et al. (1982) that a single strain of *V. cholerae* 0:1 is a resident in the U.S. Gulf Coast, based on genetic sequences, and that a second reservoir of cholera toxin genes exists in non-0:1 *V. cholerae* strains in Louisiana.

In subsequent years, isolation of *V. cholerae* 0:1 were made in various locales in Louisiana. Again the incidence level was quite low for the amount of sampling that was done. Several of the isolates, however, were nontoxigenic strains of the 0:1 Inaba serogroup. In 1979, an unusual observation was made in New Orleans when a nontoxigenic *V. cholerae* 0:1 was isolated from a sewage system. An investigation of a patient with a broken leg from an automobile accident revealed a lesion on the lower leg after convalescence. A nontoxigenic strain was isolated from a culture of this lesion. The patient while redressing the lesion was discarding the bandages into his toilet, which was subsequently discharged into the sewage system of New Orleans.

In 1981, *V. cholerae* 0:1 Ogawa was isolated from the Lake Charles, Louisiana, sewage system. This was one of the first reports of this serovar in the country. Most 0:1 serovars causing human illness and found environmentally have been from the 0:1 Inaba *V. cholerae* strain. Another isolation of 0:1 Ogawa was reported by Motes et al. (1983) from Apalachicola Bay, Florida, which again was unrelated to human illness. This serovar remains rare in the United States, even to this date, as there are still no reports in the literature of the isolation of toxigenic strains.

An excellent piece of epidemiological work was published in 1983 (Johnston et al.)—the findings of a cholera outbreak onboard a floating oil rig off the coast of Texas in 1981. This proved to be the largest outbreak of cholera in the United

States in over a century and was caused by toxigenic *V. cholerae* 0:1 El Tor Inaba. One individual, ill prior to reporting to work on the oil rig, was the cause of 15 other individuals becoming infected. It was found that a cross-connection occurred between the drinking water system and sewage disposal piping. The contamination of the sewage system by the infected individual (index case) allowed the drinking water to become contaminated. Cooked rice for a meal on the day the cross-connection was found was rinsed with the contaminated water and was held for most of the day at a temperature that permitted the pathogen to grow. It was concluded that this interesting outbreak occurred due to a combination of factors: the occurrence of sporadic toxigenic *V. cholerae* 0:1 infections along the Gulf Coast, the failure to adequately treat sewage, the presence of a cross-connection, the failure to chlorinate the drinking water, and the failure to maintain cooked food at a temperature that prevents bacterial growth. In other words, all the lessons a student of public health learns for preventing human foodborne disease were ignored.

In areas where there are only sporadic cases of cholera, there may be environmental reservoirs that need to be monitored. If a reservoir exists, the risk that it poses will be decreased by thorough cooking of food and chlorination of water from that source. Health authorities should conduct an epidemiological investigation to determine the vehicle and should search for additional cases or asymptomatic carriers. Since infected individuals can discharge tremendous numbers of the pathogen in their stools, there can be a continual contamination of an area.

B. Incidence Studies

One interesting fact regarding the previous reported human illnesses is the food histories of these patients. Consumption of raw shellfish or cooked crustaceans was reported by several individuals. In addition, numerous reports have also incriminated seafoods as the vehicle of transmission, for example, raw oysters from Florida (Lewis et al., 1979; Picardi et al., 1980; Morris et al., 1984) and Louisiana acquired in Colorado (Doran et al., 1989), raw clams in New Hampshire (MacRae et al., 1982) and crab cakes in Maryland, although the crab originated from Texas (Lin et al., 1986). Even though the incriminated foods were primarily from Gulf Coast estuarine environments, investigations were conducted into the incidence of *V. cholerae* in other estuarine environments of the United States. Seafoods have been actively promoted for human diets; therefore environmental investigations were prudent to assess potential health risks due to the presence of *V. cholerae* in these seafoods. It has been shown that non-0:1 *V. cholerae* is an inhabitant of virtually all estuaries in the United States, while the 0:1 serogroup has been isolated from several. Chronologically, these incidence reports appeared shortly after the 1978 outbreak with a report from the Chesapeake Bay (Kaper et al., 1979). Thereafter various researchers published research on, for example, the incidence in Chesapeake Bay and Louisiana of serogroup 0:1 (Colwell et al., 1981), Maryland (Hoge et al., 1989), non-0:1 in Florida and Louisiana (Madden et al., 1982), 0:1 and non-0:1 in the Louisiana Gulf Coast (Roberts et al., 1982), non-0:1 from Texas to Florida (DePaola et al., 1983), 0:1 and non-0:1 in two Florida estuaries (Hood et al., 1983), non-0:1 in Monterey Bay, California (Kenyon et al., 1983), and Oregon estuaries (Tison et al., 1986), and from three West Coast states with nontoxigenic 0:1 being isolated from Morro Bay, California (Kaysner et al., 1987a). The El Tor 0:1 strains isolated were of the Inaba serogroup, which again shows the rarity of the Ogawa serogroup in the United States. Similarly, the low isolation rate of toxigenic strains in both the 0:1 and non-0:1 groups in these reports leads one to believe that the contraction of the illness called cholera would remain rare in this country. Indeed, during the 5-year period 1983–1987 only one outbreak of foodborne illness caused by *V. cholerae* was reported to CDC (Bean et al., 1990). This figure may be misleading, in that an outbreak is defined as an incident involving two or more persons and, in addition, in 62% of the outbreaks the etiological agent was not identified even though bacterial pathogens caused the largest number of outbreaks (66%) and cases (92%). A most recent report from FDA (Glatzer, 1990) compiled a total of eight shellfish-related illnesses due to *V. cholerae*: two from the 0:1 serogroup and six from non-0:1 *V. cholerae*. The majority of the cases were associated with the consumption of raw oysters harvested primarily from Louisiana and Florida. One death was reported from a non-0:1 infection. All cases involved only one individual and thus would not be included in a report from CDC. Most recently (Lee and Hanek, 1990), the first case of non-0:1 gastroenteritis was reported in the state of Alaska. The patient, who previously had heart surgery, had consumed oysters harvested from Puget Sound in the state of Washington. The oysters were the implicated vehicle, although other circumstances were known to exist in the patient history. If the Washington state oysters were truly the vehicle, it would be the first such case reported. Thus, it seems that neither coastline of the United States is free of potential illness from non-0:1 *V. cholerae*. However, the presence of *V. cholerae* in U.S. coastal estuaries has brought about an increased awareness by public health officials and has focused investigations into the food history of a patient to see if seafood was involved.

C. *V. mimicus*

Another *Vibrio* species closely resembles *V. cholerae* in both phenotype and disease-producing ability. This species, *V. mimicus*, was recently identified (although biochemically atypical but closely related) because of its distinct genetic difference from *V. cholerae* (Davis et al., 1981). Strains of this species have caused illnesses similar to those caused by non-0:1 *V. cholerae*, having been isolated from wounds and also from stools of patients with gastroenteritis, many of whom had consumed raw oysters prior to onset of diarrhea. Several strains at CDC had been shown to produce either a heat-labile or a heat-stable enterotoxin or, in some cases, both. Strains of this species did agglutinate with the antisera of the type scheme of Smith (1979) for *V. cholerae* (Shandera et al., 1983). The one noticeable difference between the two species is that *V. mimicus* does not ferment sucrose. Enterotoxins produced by *V. mimicus* have been purified and appear to be identical to cholera toxin (Spira and Fedorka-Cray,

1984). There is reactivity in the Y-1 adrenal cell assay, the rabbit intestinal loop, and other assays used for cholera toxin determination. One of these strains, used as a control strain in our laboratory, even hybridizes with the enterotoxin gene of *V. cholerae* (Lockman et al., 1984) that we use as a gene probe for our *V. cholerae* isolates. In the most recent report by Glatzer (1990), five cases of gastroenteritis caused by *V. mimicus* were reported in the total of shellfishborne illnesses. The food history of four of five patients pointed to raw oysters harvested from the Gulf Coast as the vehicle of the infections. Thus physicians treating patients with acute gastroenteritis after ingestion of seafood should consider *V. mimicus* in the differential diagnosis along with *V. cholerae*. It has been suggested that appropriate media for *Vibrio* isolation, such as thiosulfate citrate bile salts agar (TCBS), be used in conjunction with those used for isolation of other enteric pathogens.

Most illnesses after consumption of raw oysters involves the oyster being served "on the half shell" and eaten without a previous heat treatment. This means that the oyster is harvested, shipped to a location as "shellstock" (in the shell), and freshly shucked and served. The oyster will stay alive in the shell after harvest for days if handled properly (cool, damp storage). Once the oyster is shucked, cut open with a knife—a technique that requires considerable practice—both to retain the esthetics of the product and to prevent cuts and punctures of the shucker, the oyster dies quite rapidly. It is after death of the animal that decomposition, both microbial and chemical, occurs, which, at least from experience in our lab, has a deleterious effect on the survival of *Vibrio* species. During decomposition, glycolysis occurs, which lowers the pH of the oyster. This drop in pH can rapidly destroy viability of *V. cholerae* and other species as well. Shucked oysters seem to offer a built-in safety factor in prevention of gastroenteritis caused by *Vibrio* species.

III. MEDICAL ASPECTS

A. Human Infection

As mentioned earlier, humans usually contract cholera from water or food that has been contaminated by feces of a cholera victim. The pathogen is ingested and must then survive the first nonspecific defense mechanism of the host, the gastric acid. One known predisposition to a severe infection is hypochlorhydria (Nalin et al., 1978). If *V. cholerae* survive this perilous transit, they pass beyond the pylorus and establish in the proximal small intestine, the duodenum, and jejunum. The bacteria multiply and after 2–5 days cause the sudden onset of nausea, vomiting, abdominal cramping, and acute diarrhea. This occurs only if they survive and overcome several defenses of a healthy individual against enteric pathogens. These barriers include peristalsis, which serves to continually move the bacteria on to the colon; the intestinal mucosa layer that separates the bacteria from mucosal erythrocytes; and the presence of normal intestinal flora, particularly lactobacilli, which are inhibitory to enteric pathogens (Levine et al., 1984).

Mucinase and other proteolytic enzymes, motility, and chemotaxis are some of the multiple virulence properties of *V. cholerae* that allow the organism to overcome the protective mucus barrier. Once penetration of the mucus layer occurs and *V. cholerae* reaches the erythrocytes of the intestinal mucosa, they adhere to mucosal cells, particularly on the villus crypts. Several adhesion mechanisms have been reported in the form of hemagglutins (Jones et al., 1976; Finkelstein et al., 1978; Finkelstein and Hanne, 1982). The findings by Jones and coworkers (1976) that *V. cholerae* hemagglutinated to human blood group O but not chicken erythrocytes brings out an interesting point. Studies in endemic areas and in volunteers have shown that severe cholera occurs more commonly in humans of blood group O than in those with the other blood groups (Levine et al., 1979). Furthermore, in Bengal, called the ancestral endemic home of cholera, the population has the lowest prevalence of blood group O in the world (Bodmer and Cavalii-Sforza, 1976). One would speculate then that in that geographical area chronic or asymptomatic carriers must be in abundance to help continue the presence of *V. cholerae* in the environment.

Once *V. cholerae* has established itself and adheres to the mucosal erythrocytes, enterotoxin is produced (cholera toxin) as the organism multiplies. Generally, after 2–5 days there is a sudden onset of nausea and vomiting and painless diarrhea. In severe cases, the loss of fluid from the gut, in the form of liquid feces, is referred to quite descriptively as "rice-water stools." The fluid loss may be as great as 20 L/day, which leads to extreme dehydration. Symptoms progress to suppressed renal function, thirst, leg and abdominal cramps, and progressive weakness and collapse due to marked dehydration and electrolyte loss (Sakazaki and Balows, 1981). Without adequate therapy the mortality rate can reach 60% of cases, but can be reduced to less than 1% by intravenous replacement of fluid and electrolytes. Symptoms of the disease rarely last more than a few days if adequate treatment is obtained (Stephen and Pietrowski, 1983).

Ingestion of as few as 10^3 viable *V. cholerae* 0:1 initiated diarrheal infection in 60% of challenged individuals if the gastric barrier was overcome. The resulting illness was mild. Inocula of 10^5–10^6 administered with food or $NaHCO_3$, to buffer the gastric acid, caused diarrhea in 80–100% of volunteers. Rice-water purging occurred in some of those individuals (Cash et al., 1974; Levine et al., 1984). Volunteer studies clearly demonstrated an inverse relationship between basal levels of gastric acid and severity of diarrhea (Nalin et al., 1978).

B. Non-0:1 *V. cholerae*

Gastroenteritis due to non-0:1 *V. cholerae* predominates over enteric infections caused by *V. cholerae* 0:1 in the United States (Morris et al., 1981). There is some indication of "noncholera vibrios" causing diarrheal illness as early as 1954 (McIntyre and Feeley, 1965). Diarrheal illness due to non-0:1 strains is sporadic and rarely associated with defined outbreaks. Symptoms range from a milder gastroenteritis to a more fulminant diarrhea which resembles cholera, from toxigenic O group 1 strains, although most cases are of less severity than the true cholera. However, a surfer from Santa Cruz, California, contracted a non-0:1 *V. cholerae* infection, suffered extreme dehydration, and was close to expiration from the disease (Kenyon et al., 1983; Kumar et al., 1984).

There is a strong epidemiological association between non-0:1 *V. cholerae* infection and the consumption of raw oysters. Geographically, the oysters involved were primarily harvested from growing areas of the Gulf Coast states (Wilson et al., 1981; Morris et al., 1981). Recent reports seem to follow the same trend for reported cases in 1989 and 1990 (Glatzer, 1990). Six of eight reported cases in 1989 and six of six in 1990 involved raw oysters predominantly harvested from Gulf Coast waters, if the harvesting point was determined. It was also reported by Janda et al. (1988) that during an 8-year span (1980–1987) 44% of all *Vibrio* cases reported in the state of California were caused by non-0:1 *V. cholerae*.

Of interest is the fact that the predominant number of non-0:1 *V. cholerae* isolates from confirmed cases of gastroenteritis were nontoxigenic (Morris et al., 1981; Janda et al., 1988) reacting neither in tissue cell lines nor in biological assays, i.e., ligated-adult rabbit ileal loop. However, whole-cell preparations yielded positive results in animal bioassays (Madden et al., 1982). It appears then that non-0:1 infections are probably related to other virulence mechanisms. The average duration of symptoms reported was approximately 6 days, longer than for true cholera. Also noted in approximately 30% of the cases is the presence of bloody diarrhea, which is not found with the 0:1 serogroup infections (Morris et al., 1981).

It was reported early that some non-0:1 *V. cholerae* strains produced an enterotoxin similar to CT (Ohashi et al., 1972; Zinnaka and Carpenter, 1972; Craig et al., 1981; Yamamoto et al., 1983) or identical to CT (Yamamoto et al., 1982). One of these non-0:1 toxins (Yamamoto et al., 1982) was indistinguishable from CT biologically, immunologically, and in molecular structure, while the others report physicochemical differences between their non-0:1 enterotoxins and CT. Whether CT or CT-like enterotoxins are always necessary to cause diarrheal illness is unlikely in that other non-0:1 strains isolated from patients were nontoxigenic. Thus, other factors must also be involved. The production of a cytolysin by non-0:1 *V. cholerae* may be one of the pathogenic mechanisms present in nontoxigenic strains (McCardell et al., 1985). This heat-labile cytolysin produced by a number of environmental isolates was cytotoxic to Y-1 mouse adrenal cells and Chinese hamster ovary cells, lysed rabbit red blood cells, produced a hemorrhagic zone in rabbit skin, was lethal to adult mice when injected intravenously and caused fluid accumulation in rabbit ileal loops. At present good markers of pathogenicity for non-0:1 *V. cholerae* are lacking. Animal assays and biochemical markers exist, but they have not been completely evaluated as to their role in human illness.

C. Extraintestinal Infections

Of no less importance medically, particularly to patients involved, are extraintestinal infections caused by *V. cholerae* non-0:1, summarized nicely by Janda et al. (1988). This organism has been isolated from a number of sites including blood, ears, cerebrospinal and peritoneal fluids, wounds, respiratory and biliary tracts, and the gall bladder and appendix. Unlike *V. cholerae* 0:1, which is rarely associated with extraintestinal infection (Morris and Black, 1985), non-0:1 infections are increasingly reported. The most common extraintestinal infection appears to be bacteremia sometimes accompanied by central nervous system involvement. Septicemia has been described in two newborn infants caused by non-0:1 *V. cholerae* (Rubin et al., 1981; Morgan et al., 1985), both of whom had meningitis. One was culturally confirmed by isolation of *V. cholerae* from the cerebrospinal fluid.

In most of these reported cases, except for wound infections and the infants, patients were much more likely to have underlying diseases. Some of the more common predisposing conditions were cirrhosis, diabetes, malignancy, peripheral vascular disease (Hughes et al., 1978; Safrin et al., 1988), and abnormalities of the gastrointestinal tract, for example, gastrectomy (Toeg et al., 1990). The mortality rate associated with infections by this organism, which has a tendency for bloodstream invasion, is above 60%. Antibiotic therapy with tetracycline and chloramphenicol has been reported (Safrin et al., 1988), although non-0:1 strains have shown susceptibility to other antibiotics.

It would appear then that non-0:1 *V. cholerae* is an opportunistic pathogen, and individuals who have underlying diseases have a lowered resistance to infection by the strains. It would be prudent for those individuals to refrain from consumption of raw seafoods, particularly shellfish. With the awareness in the medical community over the past decade regarding *V. cholerae*, it would not be surprising to see more reports in the literature of these types of infections.

In the late summer of 1988, a patient presented to a county hospital in Shelton, Washington, and died within 5 hours. Non-0:1 *V. cholerae* was isolated from the patient's blood, spinal fluid, and a bullae on the lower extremity. The patient had been feverish for 2 days prior to admission and was a recovering alcoholic. There was no history of ingestion of raw seafoods and the attending physician found no wounds on the patient. The isolate from the patient was found to be nontoxigenic in our laboratory in tissue cell assay and also did not hybridize with the radiolabeled CT gene probe used by FDA (Lockman et al., 1984). The isolate was quite lethal to adult mice supplemented with iron dextran to increase the serum iron level (FDA, 1984). The estimated 50% lethal dose of intraperitoneally injected cells was 2 cfu compared to 3.6×10^5 cfu for non–iron-treated mice with the same isolate. These values compare to 3.7×10^4 and 2.1×10^4 cfu for *V. cholerae* 0:1 El Tor Inaba and 0:1 Classical (569B) for iron-supplemented mice and 4.2×10^7 and 3×10^9 cfu for non–iron-treated mice, respectively. It appears then that non-0:1 strains have enhanced virulence in individuals with increased serum iron. The lethality results for the non-0:1 patient strain are similar to those obtained for virulent strains of *V. vulnificus* in our laboratory (Kaysner et al., 1987b). Even though the point of entry to the patient was not identified, this was the first case of a lethal *V. cholerae* non-0:1 infection in the state of Washington.

It was shown several years ago (Robins-Browne et al., 1977) that a strain of non-0:1 *V. cholerae* was capable of invading rabbit ileal mucosal cells. This, coupled with the production of a siderophore (Payne and Finkelstein, 1978; Griffiths et al., 1984), may give the non-0:1 strains an advantage of infectivity of patients with high serum iron levels or other liver ailments.

IV. TOXICOLOGICAL

A. Cholera Toxin

Enterotoxins refer to bacterial products that act on the mucosal epithelium of the small intestine. This action causes fluid secretion, related to the enzymatic effect of the enterotoxin on the intestinal cells, often through specific receptors and increased cyclic nucleotide concentrations, resulting in profuse diarrhea. Enterotoxin action does not damage the intestinal mucosa (Ashkenazi and Pickering, 1989). Cholera toxin is perhaps the most studied of any of the bacterial toxins; indeed, it was the prototype for the research done on enterotoxins. Several excellent review articles describe cholera toxin (Finkelstein, 1988; Moss and Vaughan, 1988).

Cholera toxin (CT or choleragen) was initially described in 1959 by two laboratories working quite independently (De, 1959; Dutta et al., 1959). It was another 10 years before Finkelstein and LoSpalluto (1969) reported the purification of the toxin, which enabled the pathogenesis of the disease to be studied at the molecular level. Since that time knowledge of CT and other enterotoxins has increased tremendously. The search for an appropriate animal model, one that would manifest diarrhea in response to the toxin, was one drawback slowing the study of CT. Demonstration of CT production can be shown in tissue cells lines, Y-1 adrenal cell or Chinese hamster ovary cells, or ligated intestinal segments in rabbits. FDA presently uses the tissue cell lines.

In the late 1960s, the mode of action of CT was "discovered" when sterile filtrates of toxigenic *V. cholerae* mimicked the effects of cyclic AMP, which reverses the direction of chloride ion transport, allowing active secretion of chloride from the mucosal surface of the ileum. Absorption of sodium ions was also reduced. The changes in ion balance caused a passive efflux of water from the mucosal surface, bringing about diarrhea (Field, 1971; Holmgren, 1981). It was also demonstrated that the amount of cholera toxin produced in vitro is not by itself a predictor of virulence of a toxigenic strain (Levine et al., 1981). Miller and Mekalanos (1984) cloned the regulatory gene (toxR) that controls CT transcription. They found that even nontoxigenic strains possessed the regulator but lacked the structural genes (ctx) for CT production.

Cholera toxin is an oligomeric protein first purified in 1969 (Finkelstein and LoSpalluto, 1969) having a molecular weight of approximately 83,000 daltons and composed of subunits A_1 (21,000 d) and A_2 (7,000 d), and five B subunits (11,000 d each). The orientation of subunits of the CT molecule has also been proposed (Gill, 1976). Separately, neither the A nor B subunits had significant biological activity (Finkelstein et al., 1974). The initial CT action is the binding of the B subunit to the receptor, ganglioside G_{m1}, on the cell membrane. The A_1 subunit is required for stimulation of adenylate cyclase, causing increased levels of cyclic AMP and hypersecretion of salt and water (Gill and Meren,

1978). The A subunit is synthesized as a single polypeptide which undergoes subsequent proteolytic cleavage (nicking) to the A_1 and A_2 subunits outside the cell. This heat-labile enterotoxin has been well characterized at the molecular and genetic level (Moseley and Falkow, 1980). Recently, the role of a specific pilus structure in colonization of the human intestine by *V. cholerae* 0:1 was shown by Herrington et al. (1988).

There are still questions that need to be answered in the study of CT. For example, what is the actual mechanism by which the A_1 subunit stimulates adenylate cyclase activity, and how does the A_1 subunit penetrate the cell membrane or enter the cytoplasm to reach its target?

B. Noncholera Vibrio Toxins

It was mentioned previously that certain strains of non-0:1 *V. cholerae* produce CT or CT-like proteins. Toxigenic non-0:1 strains may produce severe, watery diarrhea indistinguishable from classical cholera (Kelly et al., 1982). It would appear then that the mode of action of the enterotoxins of non-0:1 strains is similar to CT. In fact, as was discussed previously, Yamamoto et al. (1983) found similar subunits A and B in a toxin produced by the non-0:1 strain that was physicochemically different than CT. Further study of non-0:1 *V. cholerae* is necessary to elaborate the mechanism(s) necessary for both toxigenic and nontoxigenic strains to cause diarrheal illness. Non-0:1 *V. cholerae* isolated from cases of diarrhea appears to produce disease through some mechanism other than cholera-like toxin, yet it is unclear how other toxins and hemolysins affect pathogenicity (Spira et al., 1983).

Cytotoxins are a distinct group of diarrhea-related toxins (O'Brien and Holmes, 1987). They are defined by their ability to kill mammalian cells, usually by inhibition of protein synthesis. In vitro, cytotoxic activity can be demonstrated on several tissue culture cell lines. In vivo, they cause damage to epithelial cells of the intestine and interfere with normal absorptive mechanisms. The loss of fluids is possibly related to this impaired absorption. Cytotoxins apparently do not cause active fluid secretion by the gut, unlike enterotoxins, nor do they leave the gut undamaged. Shiga toxin is the prototype of the cytotoxin group (Ashkenazi and Pickering, 1989). It appears that *V. cholerae* produces at least one cytolysin, as do some strains of *V. mimicus* (McCardell et al., 1985). This cytolysin may be a pathogenic mechanism present in non-CT or non–CT-like strains of *V. cholerae*; however, further studies need to be done to determine pathogenesis.

REFERENCES

Anonymous. (1990). Cholera-Worldwide, 1989. *Morbid Mortal. Week. Rep. 39*: 365–367.

Askenazi, S., and Pickering, L. K. (1989). Pathogenesis and diagnosis of bacterial diarrhea. *Eur. J. Clin. Microbiol. Infect. Dis. 8*: 203–206.

Bean, N. H., Griffin, P. M., Goulding, J. S., and Ivey, C. B. (1990). Foodborne disease outbreaks, 5-year summary, 1983-1987. *J. Food Prot. 53*: 711–728.

Bodmer, W. F., and Cavalii-Sforza, L. L. (1976). Evolution, human welfare and society. In *Genetics, Evolution and Man*. W. H. Freeman, New York, pp. 562–604.

Bradford, H. B., Jr. (1984). An epidemiological study of *V. cholerae* in Louisiana. In *Vibrios in the Environment*, R. R. Colwell, ed. John Wiley & Sons, New York, pp. 59–72.

Cameron, J. M., Hester, K., Smith, W. L., Caviness, E., Hosty, T., and Wolf, F. S. (1977). *Vibrio cholerae*-Alabama. *Morbid. Mortal. Week. Rep. 26*: 159.

Cash, R. A., Music, S. I., Libonatti, J. P., Snyder, M. J., Wenzel, R. P., and Hornick, R. B. (1974). Response of man to infection with *Vibrio cholerae*. I. Clinical, serologic and bacteriologic responses to a known inoculum. *J. Infect. Dis. 129*: 45–52.

Colwell, R. R., Seidler, R. J., Kaper, J., Joseph, S. W., Garges, S., Lockman, H., Maneval, D., Bradford, H., Roberts, N., Remmers, E., Huq, I., and Huq, A. (1981). Occurrence of *Vibrio cholerae* serotype 0:1 in Maryland and Louisiana estuaries. *Appl. Environ. Microbiol. 41*: 555–558.

Cook, W. L., Wachsmuth, K., Feeley, J., and Huq, I. (1983). The question of classical cholera. *Lancet*, Apr. 16, 879–880.

Craig, J. P., Yamamoto, K., Takeda, Y., and Miwatani, T. (1981). Production of cholera-like enterotoxin by a strain of *Vibrio cholerae* Non-0:1, isolated from the environment. *Infect. Immun. 34*: 90–97.

Davis, B. R., Fanning, G. R., Madden, J. M., Steigerwalt, A. G., Bradford, H. B., Jr., Smith, H. L., Jr., and Brenner, D. J. (1981). Characterization of biochemically atypical *Vibrio cholerae* strains and designation of a new pathogenic species, *Vibrio mimicus*. *J. Clin. Microbiol. 14*: 631–639.

De, S. N. (1959). Enterotoxicity of bacteria-free culture filtrate of *Vibrio cholerae*. *Nature 183*: 2533–2534.

De, S. N. (1961). *Cholera. Its Pathology and Pathogenesis*. Oliver and Boyd, Edinburgh, Scotland.

DeGermane, J. H ., and Smith, M. T. (1974). Non cholera vibrio enteritis contracted in the United States by an American. *J. Infect. Dis. 129*: 587–589.

DePaola, A., Presnell, M. W., Motes, M. L., Jr., McPhearson, R. M., Twedt, R. M., Becker, R. E., and Zywmo, S. (1983). Non 0:1 *Vibrio cholerae* in shellfish, sediment and waters of the U.S. Gulf Coast. *J. Food Prot. 46*: 802–806.

Doran, M., Shillam, P., Hoffman, R. E., and McFarland, L. M. (1989). Toxigenic *Vibrio cholerae* 0:1 infection acquired in Colorado. CDC *Morbid. Mortal. Week. Rep. 38*: 19–20.

Dutta, M. K., Panse, M. W., and Kulkarni, D. R. (1959). Role of cholera toxin in experimental cholera. *J. Bacteriol. 78*: 594–595.

Field, M. (1971). Intestinal secretion: Effect of cyclic AMP and its role in cholera. *N. Engl. J. Med. 284*: 1137–1144.

Finkelstein, R. A. (1988). Structure of cholera enterotoxin (choleragen) and the immunologically related ADP-ribosylating heat-labile enterotoxins. In *Handbook of Natural Toxins*, Vol. 4, *Bacterial Toxins*, Hardegree, M. C., and Tu, A. T., eds. Marcel Dekker, Inc., New York, pp. 1–38.

Finkelstein, R. A., and LoSpalluto, J. J. (1969). Pathogenesis of experimental cholera: Preparation and isolation of choleragen and choleragenoid. *J. Exper. Med. 130*: 185–202.

Finkelstein, R. A., and Hanne, L. F. (1982). Hemagglutinins (colonization factors?) produced by *Vibrio cholerae*. In *Proc. 17th Joint Conference on Cholera*. U.S.-Japan Cooperative Medical Science Program, Baltimore, MD.

Finkelstein, R. A., Boesman, M., Neoh, S. H., LaRue, M. K., and Delaney, R. (1974). Dissociation and recombination of the subunits of the cholera enterotoxin (choleragen). *J. Immunol. 113*: 145–150.

Finkelstein, R. A., Arita, M., Clements, J. D., and Nelson, E. T. (1978). Isolation and purification of an adhesive factor ("Cholera Lectin") from *Vibrio cholerae*. In *Proc.*

12th Joint Conference on Cholera. U.S.-Japan Cooperative Medical Science Program, Atlanta, GA (DHEW Publ. No. 79-1590), pp. 137–151.

Food and Drug Administration. (1984). *Bacteriological Analytical Manual*, 6th ed. Association of Official Analytical Chemists, Arlington, VA.

Gill, D. M. (1976). The arrangement of subunits in cholera toxin. *Biochem. 15*: 1242–1248.

Gill, D. M., and Meren, R. (1978). ADP-ribosylation of membrane proteins catalyzed by cholera toxin: Basis of the action of adenylate cyclase. *Proc. Natl. Acad. Sci. 75*: 3050–3054.

Glatzer, M. B. (1990). Shellfish-related illnesses for fiscal year 1990. Department of Health and Human Services, Food and Drug Administration, Atlanta, GA, Aug. 15.

Griffiths, G. L., Sigel, S. P., Payne, S. M., and Neilands, J. B. (1984). Vibriobactin, a siderophore from *Vibrio cholerae. J. Biol. Chem. 259*: 383–385.

Harrington, D., McKenna, R. F., Waterman, G. P., and M. Holmes. (1974). Non-cholera vibrio diarrhea-Massachusetts. *Morbid. Mortal. Week. Rep. 23*: 415.

Herrington, D. E., Hall, R. H., Losonsky, G., Mekalanos, J. J., Taylor, R. K., and Levine, M. M. (1988). Toxin, toxin-coregulated pili, and the toxR regulon are essential for *Vibrio cholerae* pathogenesis in humans. *J. Exper. Med. 168*: 1487–1492.

Hoge, C. W., Watsky, D., Peeler, R. N., Libonati, J. P., Israel, E., and Morris, J. G., Jr. (1989). Epidemiology and spectrum of vibrio infections in a Chesapeake Bay community. *J. Infect. Dis. 160*: 985–993.

Holmgren, J. (1981). Actions of cholera toxin and the prevention and treatment of cholera. *Nature 292*: 413–417.

Hood, M. A., Ness, G. E., Rodrick, G. E., and Blake, N. J. (1983). Distribution of *Vibrio cholerae* in two Florida estuaries. *Microbiol. Ecol. 9*: 65–75.

Hughes, J. M., Hollis, D. G., Gangarosa, E. J., and Weaver, R. E. (1978). Non-cholera *Vibrio* infections in the United States: Clinical, epidemiological and laboratory features. *Ann. Intern. Med. 88*: 602–606.

Janda, J. M., Powers, C., Bryant, R. G., and Abbott, S. L. (1988). Current perspectives on the epidemiology and pathogenesis of clinically significant *Vibrio* spp. *Clin. Microbiol. Rev. 1*: 245–267.

Johnston, J. M., Martin, D. L., Perdue, J., McFarland, L. M., Caraway, C. T., Lippy, E. C., and Blake, P. A. (1983). Cholera on a Gulf Coast oil rig. *N. Engl. J. Med. 309*: 523–526.

Jones, G. W., Abrams, G. D., and Freter, R. (1976). Adhesive properties of *Vibrio cholerae*: Adhesion to isolated rabbit brush border membranes and hemagglutinating activity. *Infect. Immun. 14*: 232–239.

Kaper, J. B., Lockman, H., Colwell, R. R., and Joseph, S. W. (1979). Ecology, serology and enterotoxin production of *Vibrio cholerae* in Chesapeake Bay. *Appl. Environ. Microbiol. 37*: 91–102.

Kaper, J. B., Bradford, H. B., Jr., Roberts, N. C., and Falkow, S. (1982). Molecular epidemiology of *Vibrio cholerae* in the U.S. Gulf Coast. *J. Clin. Microbiol. 16*: 129–134.

Kaysner, C. A., Abeyta, C., Jr., Wekell, M. M., DePaola, A., Jr., Stott, R. F., and Leitch, J. M. (1987a). Incidence of *Vibrio cholerae* from estuaries of the United States West Coast. *Appl. Environ. Microbiol. 53*: 1344–1348.

Kaysner, C. A., Abeyta, C., Jr., Wekell, M. M., DePaola, A., Jr., Stott, R. F., and Leitch, J. M. (1987b). Virulent strains of *Vibrio vulnificus* isolated from estuaries of the United States West Coast. *Appl. Environ. Microbiol. 53*: 1349–1351.

Kelly, M. T., Peterson, J. W., Sarles, H. B., Jr., Romanko, M., Martin, D., and Hafkin, B. (1982). Cholera on the Texas Gulf Coast. *JAMA 247*: 1598–1599.

Kenyon, J. E., Gillies, D. C., Piexoto, D. R., and Austin, B. (1983). *Vibrio cholerae* (non-0:1) isolated from California coastal waters. *Appl. Environ. Microbiol. 46*: 1232–1233.

Kumar, S., Shorenstein, M. L., Niven, N., and Stroe, M. (1984). Non-0:1 *Vibrio cholerae* gastroenteritis in northern California. *West J. Med. 140*: 783–784.

Lee, L., and Hanek, R. (1990). Non-01 *Vibrio cholerae* infection from raw oysters, Alaska's first case. *State of Alaska Epidemiol. Bull.*, No. 20. (10/5/90). Dept. Health and Human Services, Anchorage, AK.

Levine, M. M., Nalin, D. R., Rennels, M. B., Nornick, R. B., Sotman, S., VanBlerk, G., Hughes, T. P., and O'Donnell, S. (1979). Genetic susceptibility to cholera. *Ann. Human. Biol. 6*: 369–374.

Levine, M. M., Black, R. E., Clements, M. L., Cisneros, L., Nalin, D. R., and Young, C. R. (1981). Duration of infection-derived immunity to cholera. *J. Infect. Dis. 143*: 818–820.

Levine, M. M., Black, R., and Clements, M. L. (1984). Pathogenesis of enteric infections caused by *Vibrio*. In *Vibrios in the Environment*, R. R. Colwell, ed. John Wiley & Sons, New York, pp. 109–122.

Lewis, C., Harris, J., Hausfeld, K., Prather, E. C., Roberts, A. E., Gunn, R. A., Janowoski, H., Lieb, S., and Gissendanner, E. (1979). Non-0:1 *Vibrio cholera* infections—Florida. *Morbid. Mortal. Week. Rep. 28*: 571–577.

Lin, F. Y., Morris, J. G., Jr., Kaper, J. B., Gross, T., Michalski, J., Morrison, C., Libonati, J. P., and Israel, E. (1986). Persistence of cholera in the United States: Isolation of *Vibrio cholerae* 0:1 from a patient with diarrhea in Maryland. *J. Clin. Microbiol. 23*: 624–626.

Lockman, H. A., Galen, J. E., and Kaper, J. B. (1984). *Vibrio cholerae* enterotoxin genes: nucleotide sequence analysis of DNA encoding ADP-ribosyltransferase. *J. Bacteriol. 159*: 1086–1089.

Longmate, N. (1966). *King Cholera, the Biology of a Disease*. Hamish Hamilton, London, England.

MacRae, S., Clements, T., and Cournoyer, J. (1982). Non-0:1 *Vibrio cholerae* gastroenteritis-New Hampshire. CDC. *Morbid. Mortal. Weekly Rep. 31*: 538.

Madden, J. M., McCardell, B. A., and Read, R. B., Jr. (1982). *Vibrio cholerae* in shellfish from U.S. coastal waters. *Food Technol. 36*: 93–96.

McCardell, B. A., Madden, J. M., and Shah, D. B. (1985). Isolation and characterization of a cytolysin produced by *Vibrio cholerae* serogroup non-0:1. *Can. J. Microbiol. 31*: 711–720.

McIntyre, O. R., and Feeley, J. C. (1965). Characteristics of non-cholera vibrios isolated from cases of human diarrhoea. *Bull. WHO 32*: 627–632.

McNicol, L. A., and Doetsch, R. M. (1983). A hypothesis accounting for the origin of pandemic cholera: A retrograde analysis. *Perspect. Biol. Med. 26*: 547–552.

Miller, V. L., and Mekalanos, J. J. (1984). Synthesis of cholera toxin is positively regulated at the transcriptional level by toxR. *Proc. Natl. Acad. Sci. 81*: 3471–3475.

Morgan, D. R., Moore, D. G., Ball, B. D., and Kohl, S. (1985). Severe *Vibrio cholerae* sepsis and meningitis in a young infant. *Tex. Med. 81*: 37–38.

Morris, J. G., Jr., and Black, R. E. (1985). Cholera and other vibrios in the United States. *N. Engl. J. Med. 312*: 343–350.

Morris, J. G., Jr., Wilson, R., Davis, B. R., Wachsmuth, I. K., Riddle, C. F., Wathen, H. G., Pollard, R. A., and Blake, P. A. (1981). Non 0 group 1 *Vibrio cholerae* gastroenteritis in the United States. *Ann. Intern. Med. 94*: 656–658.

Morris, J. G., Jr., Picardi, J. L., Lieb, S., Lee, J. V., Roberts, A., Hood, M., Gunn, R. A., and Blake, P. A. (1984). Isolation of nontoxigenic *Vibrio cholerae* 0 Group 1 from a patient with severe gastrointestinal disease. *J. Clin. Microbiol. 19*: 296–297.

Moseley, S. L., and Falkow, S. (1980). Nucleotide sequence homology between the heat-labile enterotoxin gene of *Escherichia coli* and *Vibrio cholerae* deoxyribonucleic acid. *J. Bacteriol. 144*: 444–446.

Moss, J., and Vaughan, M. (1988). Cholera toxin and *E. coli* enterotoxins and their mechanisms of action. In *Handbook of Natural Toxins*, Vol. 4, *Bacterial Toxins*, Hardegree, M. C., and Tu, A. T., eds. Marcel Dekker, Inc., New York, pp. 39–87.

Motes, M. L., Jr., Zywno, S. R., DePaola, A., Becker, R. E., and Presnell, M. W. (1983). Isolation of *Vibrio cholerae* serotype Ogawa from a Florida estuary. *Appl. Environ. Microbiol. 45*: 321–322.

Nalin, D. R., Levine, R. J., Levine, M. M., Hoover, D., Bergquist, E., McLaughlin, J., Libonati, J., Alam, J., and Hornick, R. B. (1978). Cholera, non-vibrio cholera and stomach acid. *Lancet 2*: 856–859.

O'Brien, A. D., and Holmes, R. K. (1987). Shiga and shiga-like toxin. *Microbiol. Rev. 21*: 206–220.

Ohashi, M., Shimada, T., and Fukumi, H. (1972). In vitro production of enterotoxin and hemorrhagic principle by *Vibrio cholerae*, NAG. *Jpn. J. Med. Sci. Biol. 25*: 179–194.

Payne, S. M., and Finkelstein, R. A. (1978). Siderophore production of *Vibrio cholerae*. *Infect. Immun. 20*: 310–311.

Picardi, J. L., Field, C. R., Grant, E., Grimsley, W. E., Tousignant, H., Wells, F. B., Gunn, R. A., Lieb, S., Roberts, A., Schnieder, N., Lunsford, W., and Steidinger, K. (1980). Cholera-Florida. *Morbid. Mortal. Week. Rep. 29*: 601.

Pollitzer, R. (1959). *Cholera*. Monograph No. 43. World Health Organization, Geneva, Switzerland.

Roberts, N. C., Siebeling, R. J., Kaper, J. B., and Bradford, H. B., Jr. (1982). Vibrios in the Louisiana Gulf Coast environment. *Microb. Ecol. 8*: 299–312.

Robins-Browne, R. M., Still, C. S., Isaäcson, M., Koornhof, H. J., Appelbaum, P. C., and Scragg, J. N. (1977). Pathogenic mechanisms of a non-agglutinable *Vibrio cholerae* strain: Demonstration of invasive and enterotoxigenic properties. *Infect. Immun. 18*: 542–545.

Rubin, L. G., Altman, J., Epple, L. K., and Yolken, R. H. (1981). *Vibrio cholerae* meningitis in a neonate. *J. Pediatr. 98*: 940–942.

Safrin, S., Morris, J. G., Jr., Adams, M., Pons, V., Jacobs, R., and Conte, J. E., Jr. (1988). Non-0:1 *Vibrio cholerae* bacteremia: Case report and review. *Rev. Infect. Dis. 10*: 1012–1017.

Sakazaki, R., and Balows, A. (1981). The genera *Vibrio, Plesiomonas*, and *Aeromonas*. In *The Prokaryotes. A Handbook on Habitats, Isolation, and Identification of Bacteria*, Starr, M. P., Stolp, H., Trüper, H. G., Balows, A., and Schlegel, H. G., eds. Springer-Verlag, New York, pp. 1272–1301.

Shandera, W. X., Johnston, J. M., Davis, B. R., and Blake, P. A. (1983). Disease from infection with *Vibrio mimicus*, a newly recognized *Vibrio* species. *Ann. Intern. Med. 99*: 169–171.

Smith, H. L., Jr. (1979). Serotyping of non-cholera Vibrios. *J. Clin. Microbiol. 10*: 85–90.

Spira, W. M., and Fedorka-Cray, P. J. (1984). Purification of enterotoxins from *Vibrio mimicus* that appear to be identical to cholera toxin. *Infect. Immun. 45*: 679–684.

Spira, W. M., Fedorka-Cray, P. J., and Pettebone, P. (1983). Colonization of the rabbit small intestine by clinical and environmental isolates of non-0:1 *Vibrio cholerae* and *Vibrio mimicus*. *Infect. Immun. 41*: 1175–1183.

Stephen, J., and Pietrowski, R. A. (1983). *Bacterial Toxins*. Aspects of Microbiology 2. American Society for Microbiology, Washington, DC, pp. 16–25.

Tison, D. L., Nishibuchi, M., Seidler, R. J., and Siebeling, R. J. (1986). Isolation of non-0:1 *Vibrio cholerae* serovars from Oregon coastal environments. *Appl. Environ. Microbiol. 51*: 444–445.

Toeg, A., Berger, S. A., Battat, A., Hoffman, M., and Yust, I. (1990). *Vibrio cholerae* bacteremia associated with gastrectomy. *J. Clin. Microbiol. 28*: 603–604.

Weissman, J. B., Dewitt, W. E., Thompson, J., Muchnick, C. N., Portnoy, B. L., Feeley, J. C., and Gangarosa, E. J. (1974). A case of cholera in Texas. *Amer. J. Epidemiol.* *100*: 487–490.

Wilson, R., Lieb, S., Roberts, A., Stryker, S., Janowski, H., Gunn, R., Davis, B., Riddle, C. F., Barrett, T., Morris, J. G., Jr., and Blake, P. A. (1981). Non-0:1 group *Vibrio cholerae* gastroenteritis associated with eating raw oysters. *Amer. J. Epidemiol. 114*: 293–298.

Yamamoto, K., Takeda, Y., Miwatani, T., and Craig, J. P. (1982). Purification and some properties of a non-0:1 *Vibrio cholerae* enterotoxin that is identical to cholera enterotoxin. *Infect. Immun. 39*: 1128–1135.

Yamamoto, K., Takeda, Y., Miwatani, T., and Craig, J. P. (1983). Evidence that a non-0:1 *Vibrio cholerae* produces enterotoxin that is similar but not identical to cholera enterotoxin. *Infect. Immun. 41*: 896–901.

Zinnaka, Y., and Carpenter, C. C. J. (1972). An enterotoxin produced by non-cholera vibrios. *Johns Hopkins Med. J. 131*: 403–411.

8

Botulism in Home-Processed Foods

John N. Sofos

Colorado State University, Fort Collins, Colorado

I. GENERAL

The disease of botulism is defined as an acute descending flaccid paralysis that occurs when the neurotoxin of the bacterium *Clostridium botulinum* blocks neuromuscular transmission (Arnon, 1989). Botulism is a relatively rare type of poisoning, but *C. botulinum* is widely distributed in the soil and in waters throughout the world, contaminating agricultural commodities and food products.

Foodborne botulism occurs when a food is contaminated with *C. botulinum* spores or vegetative cells; processing and preparation of the food is not adequate to inactivate *C. botulinum* or its toxins, or the food is contaminated after processing; the food composition and handling conditions are such that they support growth of *C. botulinum* and toxin production; or the food appears acceptable to the consumer and is consumed without cooking or after insufficient heating to inactivate the toxin (Eklund, 1982). In general, foodborne botulism is caused by eating improperly preserved food in which *C. botulinum* has grown and produced toxin (Wallen, 1983).

The toxins of *C. botulinum* are some of the most potent biological poisons known. There are reports of deaths from eating a single string bean or a few kernels of home-canned corn. One individual was reported to die after only tasting and then spitting out a mouthful of home-preserved peppers. Some outbreaks have been notable, as the one in Albany, Oregon, in 1924 which resulted in the death of an entire family of 12 after eating contaminated home-canned green beans (Wallen, 1983).

Low-acid, commercially canned foods in the United States are consumed to an extent of more than 10 billion cans per year, but the extent of botulism outbreaks from these products has been extremely low (Schaffner, 1982). The number of botulism outbreaks from home-processed foods, however, is approximately 10 times larger than that from commercially canned products (Table 1). Thus, the title of this chapter signifies the great involvement of home-processed foods in outbreaks of botulism.

Before 1926, botulism outbreaks from commercially canned foods were nearly as prevalent as they are now from consumption of home-processed foods (Denny, 1982). The safety record of commercially canned products was improved through research and education of its member companies by the National Canners Association (now National Food Processors Association), which was founded in 1907, and through government regulatory actions. In general the lower incidence of botulism from consumption of commercial compared to home-processed products reflects the greater awareness and controls

Table 1 Foodborne Outbreaks of Botulism in the United States, 1899–1981

Foods	Number of outbreaks	
	Home-processed	Commercially processed
Low acid products		
Vegetables	432	40
Meat and fish	50	14
Acid products	40	1

Source: Schaffner, 1982.

applied by the industry, which result in better avoidance of *C. botulinum* growth and toxic production. Home processors and consumers, however, must be aware that control measures, such as proper heating and cold storage, must be maintained before product consumption. If mishandled, even a commercial product may lead to a botulism outbreak. Foods canned at home should also be processed under proper conditions for the type of food. Problems develop only when improper canning, salting, or pickling procedures for vegetables, meat, fish, and other foods are employed (Sperber, 1982). In recent years, botulism has been caused by consumption of locally prepared foods in some areas of the world in which its existence was not fully realized. Examples of such outbreaks include those in Kenyan natives consuming a traditional food of white ants and sour milk, and those caused by fermented fish products in Iran (Sugiyama and Sofos, 1988).

II. HISTORICAL

Botulism has probably been associated with humans since they first attempted to preserve foods (Eklund, 1982), and its history has been reviewed by Dolman (1964), Smith and Sugiyama (1988), and Hauschild (1989). The association of the disease with sausages, especially smoked blood sausage in Germany, led to introduction of the term "botulism," which is derived from the Latin word *botulus*, meaning sausage (Dolman, 1964). The common German term for botulism was *Wurstvergiftung* which also means sausage poisoning (Hauschild, 1989). In recent years, sausages, and in many countries meats in general, are involved in only a small fraction of the recorded botulism outbreaks, while consumption of vegetables or fish has become the primary cause of the disease.

The etiologic agent of botulism was first isolated in 1896 by Emile Pierre Marie van Ermengem (1897), a professor of bacteriology at the University of Ghent in Belgium. Van Ermengem investigated an outbreak from consumption of improperly salted ham in the Belgian village of Ellezelles in the province of Hainot. The outbreak involved 34 cases and three deaths. Van Ermengem isolated an anaerobic organism from the home-cured ham and from the spleen of one of the victims, and named it *Bacillus botulinus*, later renamed *Clostridium botulinum*. His studies indicated that the organism was destroyed after 1 hour of heating at 80°C and characterized it as a motile, gram-positive, anaerobic sporeformer with optimum growth at 25–30°C. He also suggested that "ichthyism" or "ichthyosismus," a well-documented illness resulting from consumption of preserved fish, was another manifestation of botulism (Hauschild, 1989).

Based on the excellent description of van Ermengem, the isolate from the salted ham would now be classified as nonproteolytic type B strain. Additional types of *C. botulinum* strains, A through G, were identified in later years. Based on the heat resistance of van Ermengem's culture, however, a farmer's bulletin was published in the United States in 1909, which outlined procedures for home canning of foods. Due to lack of knowledge of existence of more heat-resistance *C. botulinum* strains, the heat treatments recommended were inadequate, and may have led to a number of botulism outbreaks in the early 1900s from consumption of underprocessed home-canned foods (Eklund, 1982).

Botulism as a disease was first recognized in the United States in 1899, and since then records of reported outbreaks have been maintained. In the period 1899–1978 there were 778 outbreaks of botulism in the United States, involving 2019 individual cases, of whom 1002 died. This is equivalent to a 50% mortality rate, which has declined in recent years to less than 10%. This decline is due to improved detection methods, availability of antitoxins, and treatment of victims with appropriate mechanized ventilation. In the period 1983–1987 in the United States (Table 2) there were 74 reported outbreaks with 256 cases and 10 fatalities (Bean et al., 1990). In the same period, 56 of the outbreaks involved foods eaten at home, 2 in restaurants or delicatessens, and 16 were of unknown origin.

From 1973 to 1987 in the United States (Table 3), 99 outbreaks were due to consumption of fruits and vegetables, 35 due to fish, 5 due to meat and poultry products, and 5 due to mushrooms (Bean and Griffin, 1990). The number of reported deaths was 47 in the United States, or 3.13 per year. Major contributing factors and number of outbreaks were inadequate cooking (91) and improper holding temperature (34). The types of foods associated with botulism outbreaks are limitless. In recent years, the disease has been associated with consumption of unusual food items such as sautéed onions, garlic in oil, and foil-wrapped baked potatoes (Sugiyama and Sofos, 1988).

Table 2 Reported Foodborne Botulism Outbreaks in the United States, 1983–1987

	Number			Food consumed at		
Year	Outbreaks	Cases	Deaths	Home	Food service	Unknown
1983	13	162	3	11	1	1
1984	11	16	0	10	1	0
1985	17	33	2	17	0	0
1986	22	27	3	15	0	7
1987	11	18	2	3	0	8
Total	74	256	10	56	2	16

Source: Bean et al., 1990.

Table 3 Food Products Involved in Botulism Outbreaks in the United States, 1973–1987

Food product	Number of outbreaks
Beef	2
Pork	1
Turkey	1
Chicken	1
Fish	35
Dairy	1
Fruits and vegetables	99
Mushrooms	5
Nondairy beverages	5
Mexican-style food	3
Other	40
Unknown	38
Total	231

Source: Bean and Griffin, 1990.

III. DISEASE

A. Forms of Botulism

Botulism as a disease is divided into three or four categories based on the introduction of toxin to its victims (Sugiyama and Sofos, 1988). These categories include:

1. Foodborne botulism, which is the classical intoxication caused by consumption of food contaminated with preformed toxin of *C. botulinum*, which has proliferated in the food.
2. Wound botulism, which is rare and is the result of infection of a wound, growth of *C. botulinum*, and in vivo elaboration of toxin.
3. Infant botulism, which is an infection that involves infants of less than 1 year of age, and is caused by ingestion of spores of *C. botulinum*, colonization of the intestinal tract, and elaboration of toxin in the lumen of the intestine.
4. An "undetermined" classification in which scientists include the rare occasions of botulism caused by intestinal infection and in vivo toxin production in humans older than 1 year of age. This unclassified form appears to be associated with abnormalities in the gastrointestinal system and its microflora.

B. Infant Botulism

This syndrome of infants, characterized by hypotonia, was first identified in 1976, and now is reported as the most common form of botulism in the United States, with 68 cases reported in California in 1988–89 (Midura and Arnon, 1976; Arnon, 1989). The illness appears as isolated cases with no evidence of toxin-containing food being ingested, but toxin and the organism (*C. botulinum*) are found in the feces of the patient (Sugiyama and Sofos, 1988).

The average length of hospital stay in 1988–89 in California was 4.9 weeks at a cost of $62,670 (Anonymous, 1990). The fatality rate in hospitalized infants was approximately 2% (Arnon, 1989).

In infant botulism, spores of *C. botulinum* are ingested; they colonize the intestine, germinate, and form botulinal toxin in the intestinal lumen. The toxin is absorbed and causes the disease, which is thus characterized as an intestinal toxemia of infancy (Arnon, 1989). The toxico-infection then results in excretion of *C. botulinum* organisms and toxin for several weeks in the feces of the infant. The minimum infective dose of *C. botulinum* spores for infants is estimated to be 10–100 spores, but during the acute stages of the illness levels of 10^8 cfu of the pathogen and 10^5 mouse LD_{50} doses of toxin are found in the feces of the patients (Foster, 1986; Sugiyama and Sofos, 1988; Arnon, 1989).

The disease afflicts only infants, with 94% of the over 700 U.S. cases (as of 1988) involving patients of less than 6 months of age at onset, while 50% of the patients were 1–3 months of age at onset. The youngest and oldest patients reported were 2 and 52 weeks of age, respectively. Although the disease was first described in California, it has now been identified in many states, countries, and most continents. The affected infants show signs of neurological distress, including inability to cry, suckle, and hold the head up properly, which explain the syndrome being called "limp baby disease" in some cases (Foster, 1986). More details on the clinical aspects of the disease are presented by Arnon (1989).

The cultures involved in infant botulism, with the exception of four reported cases, have been types A and B of Group I. The exceptions were caused by a Bf subtype; a strain of *Clostridium barati* producing type F neurotoxin; and two cases in Italy were attributed to a strain of *Clostridium butyricum* producing type E botulinal toxin (Arnon, 1989). The lack of reports for infant botulism cases caused by strains of Group II may be due to the fact that these strains grow better at below body temperatures (Sugiyama and Sofos, 1988).

Conventional adult mice have been found resistant to enteric botulinal infection even when challenged with 10^6 or more spores. In germ-free mice or when the intestinal microflora had been distributed by feeding antibiotics, the animals were infected if fed only 10 spores of *C. botulinum* (Sugiyama, 1982). In addition, it was reported that certain organisms of the normal intestinal microflora of healthy infants may inhibit growth of *C. botulinum* in vitro, while their absence in patients may contribute to infant botulism susceptibility (Arnon, 1989).

Although the source of spores for most reported cases of infant botulism has remained undetected, about 20% of the patients in California were fed honey before the illness developed (Arnon, 1989). In addition, *C. botulinum* spores were isolated regularly from honey samples ingested by patients and from retail samples of honey. Arnon (1989) concluded that the evidence was sufficient to recommend that infants under the age of 12 months not be fed honey. Spores of *C. botulinum* were found at low levels in some corn syrup samples (Kautter et al., 1982), but epidemiological and laboratory studies indicated that this product was not a risk factor for infants. Spores of the pathogens have also been isolated from yard soil samples and vacuum cleaner dust of patients and healthy infants. Breast feeding appears to be associated with slower onset of infant botulism and with protection against sudden death (Arnon, 1989).

C. Foodborne Botulism

Conventional botulism food poisoning, or botulism, results from consumption of food that has supported growth of *C. botulinum* and elaboration of its deadly neurotoxin. The toxin interferes with transmission of nerve stimuli, causing paralysis and resulting in death due to asphyxiation (Foster, 1986; Pierson and Reddy, 1988; Smith and Sugiyama, 1988). The incubation period varies from a few hours to several days, but in most cases the first symptoms are noticed within 12–48 hours after consumption in food contaminated with the neurotoxin. The first symptoms (Hughes et al., 1981) include nausea and vomiting and are followed by neurological symptoms and signs, which include blurred or double vision and related impairments, difficulty in swallowing and speaking, muscle weakness and lack of coordination, and respiratory impairment which leads to death. Other gastrointestinal but nonspecific symptoms may include diarrhea, abdominal pain, and, at the later stages of the disease, constipation.

The epidemiology of the disease has been reviewed by Hauschild (1989). Strains of type A are the main cause of foodborne botulism in the United States, Argentina, and China, while type B is involved in most outbreaks of continental Europe, with type E predominating in the cooler regions of the Northern Hemisphere. Foods associated with type A outbreaks are mostly vegetables, while meat and marine products are mostly associated with types B and E, respectively. Countries with sporadic or no reported outbreaks of foodborne botulism include Great Britain, Sweden, Finland, The Netherlands, Switzerland, Austria, Greece, Australia, and New Zealand (Hauschild, 1989).

Outbreaks in the mainland of the United States are most commonly associated with home-processed vegetable products and type A, while most outbreaks in Alaska involve seafood contaminated with type E *C. botulinum*. Similarly, over 90% of the Japanese and Canadian outbreaks are caused by type E and consumption of marine products. In addition to common seafood, raw, fermented, or parboiled meats from sea mammals and salmon eggs are associated with the high number of outbreaks affecting native people of Alaska and Canada. The most common foods associated with botulism in the Soviet Union are mushrooms, vegetables, and cured fish. In China, there were nearly 1000 outbreaks reported in the period 1958–1989, and most involved type A from consumption of vegetables, especially bean products (Hauschild, 1989). As indicated in Table 4, 60–100% of the outbreaks in various countries are associated with home-processed foods.

The duration of the illness is 1–10 days or more, depending on the type and amount of toxin and food ingested and the resistance of the victim. Full recovery may take several weeks or months, but the fatality rate has decreased from over 50% in the past to less than 10% in recent years. This decrease is due to better diagnosis of the disease, availability and treatment with antisera, and facilitation of respiratory function with modern equipment. Treatment of the disease includes removal or inactivation of unbound botulinal toxin and

Table 4 Food Products Involved in Botulism Outbreaks Worldwide

Country or state	Food products (%)				Processing (%)	
	Meat	Fish	Plant	Other	Home	Commercial
Alaska	45[a]	55	0	0	100	0
Argentina	3	10	73	13	77	23
Belgium	60	20	20	0	60	40
Canada	70[a]	22	8	0	97	3
Czechoslovakia	72	7	14	7	100	0
China	10	0	86	4	—	—
France	86	5	7	2	88	12
Hungary	67	0	3	29	100	0
Iran	3	97	0	0	—	—
Japan	0	99	1	0	98	2
Poland	87	11	2	0	68	32
Spain	42	0	58	0	92	8
Sweden	17	83	0	0	83	17
United States	14	17	60	9	90	10
U.S.S.R.	17	67	16	0	97	3

[a]Includes sea mammals.
Source: Hauschild, 1989.

respiratory support. Free toxin in the gastrointestinal tract is removed by administration of cathartics, enema, or emetics, or is neutralized with administration of antiserum (Hatheway et al., 1984; Hauschild, 1989).

The economic losses involved in botulism outbreaks can be major (Todd, 1985a,b). The following examples give an estimate of the range and extent in costs. An outbreak of type E botulism from Alaskan canned salmon consumed in Great Britain in 1978 resulted in direct and indirect costs of approximately $6 million. Two cases of type E botulism from the same product in Belgium in 1982 cost an estimated $148 million. The estimated total cost of an outbreak from consumption of contaminated potato salad eaten at a restaurant was $8,400,000 (Sugiyama and Sofos, 1988).

IV. ORGANISM

A. Characteristics

The species *C. botulinum* includes a group of organisms of the family Bacillaceae which are distinguished by their ability to produce toxins of similar pharmacological neurotoxic action (Sugiyama and Sofos, 1988). The toxins are 150,000 dalton dichain proteins which bind irreversibly to peripheral cholinergic synapses (Arnon, 1989). The organisms are gram-positive, obligate anaerobic, rod-shaped, sporeforming soil bacteria with a worldwide distribution. From the soil they contaminate water and many foods, from which they can be isolated (Hauschild, 1989; Conner et al., 1989).

The various strains of *C. botulinum* are classified into four groups based on their proteolytic activity and other properties such as resistance to heat and type of toxin being produced (Smith and Sugiyama, 1988; Sugiyama and Sofos, 1988; Hauschild, 1989). Group I strains include all known cultures producing toxin type A, which are proteolytic, and the proteolytic cultures which produce toxin types B and F. Nonproteolytic, but saccharolytic, cultures producing toxin types B, E, or F are Group II strains. Mildly proteolytic or nonproteolytic cultures producing toxin types C_1, C_2, and D are classified as Group III strains. Finally, weakly proteolytic and nonsaccharolytic cultures producing toxin type G are Group IV strains (Solomon et al., 1985). This chapter deals mostly with Group I and II strains, because they are the ones involved in documented human outbreaks of botulism. Group II cultures have been associated with botulism outbreaks in aquatic birds, chickens, turkeys, cattle, sheep, and captive lions (Sugiyama and Sofos, 1988). Group IV includes only a few known strains and has not been implicated in documented botulism outbreaks. The strains included in type G of Group IV include the original isolates from a soil sample in Argentina (Gimenez and Ciccarelli, 1970), and those isolated in Switzerland from postmortem examination of humans in a hospital (Sonnabend et al., 1981).

The classification of *C. botulinum* strains into groups is practical because it includes in one species all cultures that produce neurotoxins of similar pharmacological action. The validity of subdividing the species into toxin types, however, is being questioned, since the toxin type of some cultures is variable, and species other than *C. botulinum* were found to produce toxins of the pathogen (Sugiyama and Sofos, 1988; Hauschild, 1989). There is a known interchange of dominant toxin in C and D organisms. In addition, there is transfer of C_1 toxigenicity to *Clostridium novyi*; two toxigenic cultures of *C. butyricum* produced type E toxin, which was involved in two separate cases of infant botulism in Italy; and a culture of *C. barati* produced type F toxin, which was involved in a case of infant botulism (Hall et al., 1985; McCroskey et al., 1986; Aureli et al., 1986).

In addition to differences expected among groups, types, and strains, spores of the same strain but of different origin, or produced under different conditions, can behave differently in the same environment (Blocher et al., 1982; Sofos et al., 1986). In addition, there may be major differences between laboratory and naturally occurring spores (Sugiyama and Sofos, 1988). Spores prepared from cultures freshly isolated from a botulism outbreak produced toxin more readily in the implicated food than spores of laboratory stock cultures (Solomon and Kautter, 1986). Furthermore, conditions, such as pH, under which cultures are produced may influence their behavior and resistance (Hobbs, 1976).

B. Habitat and Incidence

The natural habitat of *C. botulinum* is the soil, from where its spores contaminate dust, water, and agricultural commodities, including human foods (Arnon, 1989). In general, the species is found worldwide, but it has been more commonly reported in the Northern Hemisphere, where it occurs as far north as Alaska. It should be noted, however, that more studies on *C. botulinum* incidence have examined environmental samples from the Northern than the Southern Hemisphere (Sugiyama and Sofos, 1988).

Clostridium botulinum does not appear to have a living host, although it has been found in some infant mammals and in small numbers in healthy vertebrate and invertebrate animals. The strains of Group I are the main soil inhabitants, while strains of Group II, with type E being the most prevalent, are found in moist environments, including sediments of salt and fresh waters and commercial fish ponds (Cann et al., 1975). Relative incidences of Group I types vary with geographic location (Hauschild, 1989). The region of the United States west of the Rocky Mountains is mostly contaminated with type A spores, while type B is more prevalent in soil samples east of the Mississippi River.

Hauschild (1989) summarized a number of quantitative surveys for *C. botulinum* spores in the environment and in foods. Most of the soil surveys were conducted in North America and Europe. In general, there was an agreement among types and numbers of spores found in the environment, and the botulism outbreaks documented in each region. In addition to the western United States, type A appears to predominate in soils of Argentina and Brazil, while type B is a major type not only in soil samples from the eastern United States but also in Great Britain, Denmark, the Netherlands and other European countries, where most reported outbreaks are attributed to this type of *C. botulinum*. In addition to aquatic environments, type E is also prevalent in the interior of countries like Sweden and Japan (Hauschild, 1989).

The environmental and food concentration of *C. botulinum* contamination appears to be low, because the organism is found in only a few samples and in low numbers. If the organism multiplies, however, even in localized areas, large numbers can occur in pockets, without being present in adjacent areas. In addition, even a single spore has the ability to outgrow and produce enough toxin to result in a fatal outbreak of botulism (Sugiyama and Sofos, 1988).

Concentrations of organisms in terrestrial and aquatic samples reported in most probable numbers (MPN) range from less than 1 to 2500 per kg. Surveys for the incidence of *C. botulinum* in foods have focused on meats, fish, and honey with MPN values of 0.1–7, 1–170, and 1–10 per kg, respectively (Hauschild, 1989). A variety of infant foods were analyzed for presence of *C. botulinum*, and spores were found only in 13 of 1001 25-g samples of corn syrup analyzed, at a level of approximately 1 spore per kg (Kautter et al., 1982).

V. NEUROTOXINS

A. General

The neurotoxins produced by *C. botulinum* are classified by antigenic specificities as types A, B, C_1, C_2, D, E, F, and G (Sugiyama and Sofos, 1988; Hauschild, 1989), and the same classification is used for cultures, since most strains produce only one type of toxin. Known exceptions to this classification are cultures producing C_1, C_2, and D toxins, and those producing toxin types in pairs, or other clostridia producing *C. botulinum* toxins. Cultures producing C_1, C_2, and D toxins usually form toxin mixtures and are typed based on the toxin with the highest concentration. When C_1 toxin is dominant, the cultures are classified as C_a, C_s when C_2 toxin is dominant, and D when D type toxin is dominant in the mixture (Eklund and Poysky, 1972). The culture fluid of a soil isolate was completely neutralized only with a mixture of type A and F antitoxins, designated as subtype Af, since 90–95% of the total toxicity was neutralized by type A antitoxin (Sugiyama and Sofos, 1988). A mixture of A and B antitoxins at a ratio of 10:1 was needed to neutralize the culture fluid of an isolate from a home-made meat pie involved in an outbreak, and the culture was designated as subtype Ab. In another situation, however, the 1:4 toxicity ratio of A:B, resulted in the isolate from an infant botulism case being classified as subtype Ba (Hatheway et al., 1981). As mentioned before, a different aspect of botulinal toxigenesis was observed with cultures of *C. barati* and *C. butyricum* producing *C. botulinum* toxins (Sugiyama and Sofos, 1988).

Formation of toxin types C_1 and D was shown to be mediated by bacteriophages, but control of toxigenesis by bacteriophages has not been established for other types of *C. botulinum* (Hauschild, 1989). Also, there has been no association reported between ability for toxin formation and botulinal plasmids (Scott and Duncan, 1978; Strom et al., 1984; Weickert et al., 1986). Botulinal toxins are formed within the clostridial cell during growth and accumulate in the culture fluid towards the end of the growth phase, mostly through cell lysis. Toxin is also released by the cell during the logarithmic growth phase and before cell lysis (Hauschild, 1989).

B. Structure

Although there is variation, the molecular weight of toxins ranges from 128,000 for type F to 170,000 for type B. All toxin types are similar proteins, and an average molecular weight of 150,000 is used when they are considered as a single class of toxins (Sugiyama, 1980; Simpson, 1981). The toxic part of all types consists of a smaller (L; 50,000 molecular weight) and a larger (H; 100,000 molecular weight) subunit (Sugiyama and Sofos, 1988; Hauschild, 1989). These subunits are linked by a covalent disulfide bond(s), but noncovalent attractions may also be important in holding them together. Toxin type C_2 is the exception because its subunits are separate molecules.

The toxins may exist in culture fluids or foods as molecular complexes of approximate molecular weights of 150,000–900,000 daltons (Sugiyama, 1980; Hauschild, 1989). This happens because in the natural state they may occur as noncovalently associated complexes with at least one nontoxic, antigenically distinct botulinal protein (Sugiyama and Sofos, 1988). Bimolecular complexes of type A and B toxins may become trimolecular through association with a second, different nontoxic protein that has hemagglutinating activity. The individual molecules of a complex, however, are similar in size, and thus, the molecular weight is doubled or tripled in bimolecular or trimolecular complexes compared to that of the toxin itself. The toxicity of the bimolecular and trimolecular complexes is only one-half or one-third, respectively, that of the purified toxin (Sugiyama and Sofos, 1988). The toxin and its complexes are called "derivative" and "progenitor" toxins, respectively, because the toxins are isolated as complexes and then purified to derive the toxic molecule. The bi- and trimolecular toxin forms are also known as medium (M) or 12S (Svenberg units) and large (L) or 16S progenitor toxins, respectively (Sugiyama and Sofos, 1988; Hauschild, 1989).

C. Activation

The intracellularly formed toxins are released as intact proteins of relatively low toxicity. In the culture fluid, however, toxins of proteolytic (Group I) strains are exposed to protease enzymes, which activate them and increase their toxicity to the maximum potential level. Possibly a different enzyme converts the molecule into the two subunit form, mentioned earlier, by cleaving (nicking) a peptide bond(s). This peptide bond is located about one-third the distance from the amino terminal group of the protein (Sugiyama and Sofos, 1988; Hauschild, 1989). Group II toxins of types B, E, and F and other nonproteolytic cultures of types C_2 and G are especially susceptible to activation, and their lethality may increase by several $\log_{10}$ units in the presence of proteolytic enzymes such as trypsin (Solomon and Kautter, 1979; Solomon et al., 1985).

Activation is accompanied by nicking of the toxin, but they seem to be unrelated (Sugiyama and Sofos, 1988; Hauschild, 1989). The two components of a nicked toxin are the light (L) and the heavy (H) chains of 50,000 and 100,000 molecular weight, respectively. Individually the two chains are nontoxic, but their toxicity is restored by reestablishing their disulfide bond(s) through oxidation (Sakaguchi, 1983; Hauschild, 1989). The two individual chains are antigenically distinct, and their individual antibodies can neutralize the complete toxin, with anti-H serum being generally more effective than anti-L serum (Sugiyama, 1980).

The activation mechanism may involve breakage of a lysyl or arginyl peptide bond at a site near a chain end or under an interchain disulfide bridge. An alternative mechanism of activation may involve hydrolysis of a lysine ester, while nicking probably involves the carboxyl group of arginine (Hauschild, 1989).

D. Action

The neurotoxins become attached at the neuromuscular junction causing blockage of transmitter release, which leads to general paralysis. In other words, the toxin poisons the endings of cholinergic nerves so that the amounts of acetylcholine released by incoming nerve stimuli progressively decrease (Sugiyama and Sofos, 1988; Hauschild, 1989). This neurotoxic action is the result of the complementary action of the two toxin subunits, with the H subunit binding to membrane receptors at the nerve endings, enabling the L subunit to translocate and interfere with release of acetylcholine (Sugiyama, 1980; Smith and Sugiyama, 1988).

The action of the C_2 toxin is different than the above for the other toxin types. The C_2 toxin causes respiratory difficulty through hypotension, which follows extravasation of fluids, especially in the lungs. In general, the effects of C_2 toxin are cytotoxic and not neurogenic, indicating that it may have become cytotoxic as it evolved into a binary toxin of separated subunits (Hauschild, 1989).

E. Lethality

The oral lethal doses for humans are estimated as the most likely amount ingested in untreated cases of fatal or near fatal botulism (Hauschild, 1989). These doses range from 5×10^3 to 1×10^5 intraperitoneal (i.p.) mouse LD_{50} for type A and Group I type B toxins, and from 1×10^5 to 5×10^5 i.p. mouse LD_{50} for Group II type B and E toxins. In general, toxins of *C. botulinum* are considered as the most potent biological poison known to humans.

Intraperitoneal toxicities of type A toxin for mice are 2.4×10^8, 3.0×10^8, and 5.0×10^8 LD_{50}/mg for monomolecular (S), bimolecular (M), and trimolecular (L) toxins. This indicates that on a molar basis, derivative and progenitor toxins of the same type are of similar toxicities when administered by the parenteral route. Apparently the atoxic fraction of the toxin only functions to protect the toxin from inactivation in the digestive tract. This action ends when the toxin enters into the lymph, which occurs mostly in the duodenum and the jejunum. The toxin then transverses the intestinal wall and enters as derivative toxin (S) into the lymph and bloodstream (Sugiyama, 1980; Sakaguchi, 1983; Hauschild, 1989).

F. Inactivation

The most effective inactivation of botulinal toxins in foods is through heat treatment. Inactivation curves for toxin, however, are nonlinear and appear as diphasic with an initial major decline which levels off as heating time increases (Woolford et al., 1978; Woodburn et al., 1979). The shape of these inactivation curves may be due to differences in the size of toxic complexes and to variations in the degree of hydrogen bonding or aggregation during heating (Hauschild, 1989).

Since toxin inactivation by heat is nonlinear, it is impossible to express their heat resistance with the traditional D-values used for microorganisms. F-values have been determined, however, and expressed as the time needed for a known toxin concentration to be reduced to a single LD_{50} dose. When the initial toxin concentration was 10^4 mouse LD_{50}/g, the F-values of type A, B, F, and G toxins in beef and mushroom patties were determined to be 1–2 minutes at 70–80°C (Bradshaw et al., 1979; 1981). The z-values were calculated to be 3–5, 4–6, and 7–8°C for types A and B, F and G, and E toxins, respectively (Hauschild, 1989).

In general, toxin destruction by heat is more difficult in foods than in buffer systems. Times which have been recommended for thermal inactivation of up to 10^5 LD_{50}/g of all types of toxins in foods were 20 and 5 minutes at 79 and

85°C, respectively (Woodburn et al., 1979). A general recommendation for the public is to heat food at boiling temperatures for 10 minutes, provided that the food has not been tasted before heating and that no contamination of other unheated foods or utensils has occurred.

Other effective means of toxin destruction involve chlorine and ozone treatments, while freezing is relatively ineffective (Woolford et al., 1978). The toxin in water may be inactivated by chlorine treatments or removed in purification plants using an alum treatment and filtration, or by active charcoal treatment (Hauschild, 1989).

VI. METHODOLOGY

A. General

For confirmation of a botulism outbreak, in addition to the signs and symptoms, botulinal neurotoxin or viable cells or spores of *C. botulinum* should be detected in suspect foods or clinical specimens. Methodologies for detection of the pathogen and its toxins have been reviewed by Sugiyama and Sofos (1988) and Hauschild (1989). When laboratory confirmation is difficult, confirmation of clinical diagnosis of botulism can be supported by electromyography (Arnon et al., 1977; Hauschild, 1989). It should be mentioned, however, that it is not imperative to isolate a pure culture of *C. botulinum*, if the toxin is formed in an enrichment culture fluid of a sample. In general, there is a more frequent need for detection of the neurotoxins than isolation of the organism.

Samples to be analyzed for the organism and its toxins include suspect food products and clinical specimens such as feces, stomach contents, enema fluids, and autopsy sections of the intestines or the liver. Serum is analyzed only for toxin, while in infant botulism cases the stools are the most likely specimen to contain viable *C. botulinum* and toxin (Hauschild, 1989).

B. Detection of Neurotoxin

The traditional and standard method for detection of botulinal neurotoxins is the mouse bioassay. This method is based on demonstrating presence of a mouse lethal agent that can be neutralized by one or more of the botulinal antitoxins (Sugiyama and Sofos, 1988). The method is the only one officially accepted by regulatory authorities in the United States (Kautter and Lynt, 1984a,b) and has remained basically unchanged for many years (Hauschild, 1989). The bioassay and its slight variations are described in several publications (Anonymous, 1979; Hobbs et al., 1982; Kautter and Lynt, 1984a,b).

The method involves intraperitoneal injection of mice with a liquid sample or an extract of solid samples in the presence or absence of antitoxins. The antiserum is usually mixed with the sample before injection, rather than injecting it in the mice before injection of the suspect sample. Extracts of the samples are prepared by blending, homogenizing, or macerating in a slightly acidic (pH 6.2) gelatin-phosphate buffer. Gastric contents may also need adjustment of pH to about 6.0 to maintain toxicity and viability of spores (Hauschild, 1989). Extraction of toxin may be improved by inclusion of 1–2 M urea in the buffer (Wang and Sugiyama, 1983).

The preparations are clarified by centrifugation and, when feasible, sterilized by filtration to prevent mouse deaths from infection. Infection can also be avoided with addition of tetracycline or other antibiotics in the sample extract (Sugiyama and Sofos, 1988; Hauschild, 1989). Boiling of the sample inactivates the toxin, and the mice should survive. Using only the presence of a heat-stable, lethal agent as evidence for the absence of botulinal toxin ignores the possibility of both being present (Sugiyama and Sofos, 1988).

When presence of toxin of nonproteolytic strains is suspected, or when low levels of toxins form proteolytic strains are present, treatment of the sample extracts with trypsin improves detection of toxin (Kautter and Lynt, 1984a,b). Sometimes trypsinization may result in death of mice in the absence of toxin (Tanaka et al., 1986).

Endotoxins of gram-negative *Escherichia* and other bacteria that may be present in samples and interfere with defection of botulinal neurotoxins may be neutralized with bovine serum (Solberg et al., 1985). Actually, several modifications can be used to detect botulinal toxin in cases of interference by nonspecific agents (Sugiyama and Sofos, 1988). Inorganic salts can be removed by dialysis, while freezing and subsequent thawing before testing can also eliminate interfering toxicity. Dilution of the sample can also reduce nonspecific agents to levels below lethality, while the dose of botulinal toxin may still be lethal (Kautter and Lynt, 1984a,b). If nonspecific deaths of mice cannot be eliminated, there may at least be presumptive evidence of botulism from the signs and symptoms of the disease and their prevention by presence of antitoxin.

Mice injected with toxic samples show signs of ruffled fur, pinching of the waist, labored breathing, limp paralysis, and finally general paralysis which leads to death (Hauschild, 1989). Time of death is enhanced with increased concentration of toxin, but if death occurs within 2 hours of injection, presence of nonspecific lethal agents is very likely. The mice are observed for 4 days, but most deaths occur within 24 hours. When toxin concentration is very low the mice may show signs of botulism but eventually survive. Confirmation of toxin in these cases may require injection of new mice with 0.8–1.0 ml instead of 0.4–0.5 ml of sample extract.

Several in vitro tests for detection of botulinal toxin have been developed (Hobbs et al., 1982), but their major drawback has been lack of sensitivity and, in many cases, specificity and reliability (Sugiyama and Sofos, 1988). The extremely high lethality of botulinal toxins per unit weight makes the sensitivity of the mouse bioassay difficult to surpass. The most sensitive of the in vitro methods can detect approximately 1 ng of neurotoxin per ml, which is equivalent to 100 mouse LD_{50} doses. The more sensitive procedures are electroimmunodiffusion, reverse passive hemagglutination radioimmunoassay, countercurrent immunoelectrophoresis, enzyme-linked immunoabsorbent assays (ELISA), and a reversed passive latex agglutination test (Hauschild, 1989).

Another problem of in vitro methods such as ELISA is the potential for cross-reactions among toxins. In one situation, the test for B type toxin reacted slightly with type A toxin, and the type E system cross-reacted with type A and B toxins. Tubes coated with a mixture of types A, B, and E antitoxins, however, could be used to screen for presence of any one of the three toxins, but sensitivity would still be lower than the bioassay. These methods, however, may be useful when the sensitivity of the mouse biotest is not necessary (Sugiyama and Sofos, 1988).

C. Detection and Isolation of the Organism

The first step in detection of *C. botulinum* usually involves enrichment of a sample from the suspect food in a broth. The most commonly used enrichment media are cooked meat medium with or without glucose, chopped meat-glucose-starch medium, and tryptone-peptone-glucose-yeast extract broth (Kautter and Lynt, 1984a,b). Trypsin may be added to inactivate inhibitory bacteriocins and activate toxin of nonproteolytic strains. Inoculated tubes of broth are incubated with and without prior heat treatment (60–80°C) for 10–20 minutes, depending on suspected type, to detect spores and cells of *C. botulinum*, respectively. Alcohol (50%) treatment of the sample for 1 hour prior to inoculation may also be used to inactivate vegetative cells (Kautter and Lynt, 1984a,b). Addition of lysozyme to the broth may help in reversing heat injury of spores of nonproteolytic strains (Sofos, 1989b).

After incubation of inoculated enrichment broths, presence of *C. botulinum* is detected by mouse bioassay toxin analysis of the supernatant culture fluids. Immunofluorescent assays have also been evaluated for detection of toxin (Glasby and Hatheway, 1984), but they have disadvantages such as occasional false-positive reactions and cross-reactions among types of *C. botulinum*. The fluorescent antibody tests, however, could be useful as rapid screening tests for suspect foods and fecal samples in suspected outbreaks of botulism (Hauschild, 1989).

Traditional culture media for isolation of pure cultures of *C. botulinum* use blood or egg yolk as differential ingredients (Sugiyama and Sofos, 1988; Hauschild, 1989). Blood demonstrates hemolysis, whereas in presence of egg yolk, colonies likely to be *C. botulinum* develop a lipase-induced surface iridescence. Presence of lysozyme in the recovery agar medium may improve isolation of nonproteolytic Group II cultures (Scott and Bernard, 1985). Egg yolk also provides lysozyme in the medium. Proteolytic *C. botulinum* have been isolated from feces samples of infant botulism cases with culture media containing D-cycloserine, sulfamethoxazole, and trimethoprine or thymidine phosphorylase (Glasby and Hatheway, 1985; Mills et al., 1985; Sugiyama and Sofos, 1988). Heat or alcohol treatment before plating should improve isolation of spores by reducing the numbers of vegetative cells in the enrichment broth.

Colonies of *C. botulinum* can be identified directly by ELISA (Dezfulian and Bartlett, 1985), because individual colonies of types A and B contain

10^2–10^4 mouse LD_{50} doses (Sugiyama and Sofos, 1988). In recent years, there have also been developed differential media containing botulinal antitoxins instead of blood or egg yolk. The antitoxins are included either in the plating medium or as an overlay agar (Lilly et al., 1984). The antitoxin then reacts with the toxin in the colony and forms an immune precipitate that can be seen after staining. This may fail, however, if the toxin level is very low or very high. Thus, the amounts of antitoxins included in the formulation of these media are critical for the development of detectable precipitation zones (Hauschild, 1989).

Use of gas-liquid chromatography for detection of fatty acid patterns may only be useful for detection of different groups (proteolytic vs. nonproteolytic) of *C. botulinum*, which have their own characteristic fatty acid profiles (Hauschild, 1989).

VII. CONTROL

A. General

Growth and toxin production of *C. botulinum* in foods are enhanced by high-moisture (water activity > 0.94) low salt (<5–10%), low acid (pH > 4.6), reduced oxygen, and increased temperature (> 3.3°C) conditions (Pierson and Reddy, 1988). Since many foods meet most of these conditions, the food industry has developed a variety of methods for control of *C. botulinum* either through destruction or inhibition of its growth with physical and chemical treatments.

B. Destruction

Use of appropriate heat treatments is the most practical method of destroying *C. botulinum* spores in foods. Low acid (pH > 4.6), high water activity foods need to be heated to a minimum process equivalent to 2–4 minutes at 121°C. This is known as 12D, "botulinum cook," or commercial sterilization process, which results in the destruction of 10^{12} viable spores of *C. botulinum* to a single surviving spore (Hauschild, 1989). Foods of pH lower than 4.6 can be preserved with milder (pasteurization) heat treatments, which are not lethal to spores, but they are heat damaged and inhibited by the reduced pH (Blocher and Busta, 1983).

Spores of Group I strains are more heat resistant than those of Group II strains (Lynt et al., 1982a,b; Sperber, 1982; Hauschild, 1989). Differences in heat resistance also exist among types of strains within the same group. Type B spores of nonproteolytic strains were up to 30% more heat resistant than type E spores, which are classified in the same group (II) (Scott and Bernard, 1982; Simunovic et al., 1985).

Resistance of spores to destruction by gamma irradiation and chemical sanitizers is discussed by Hauschild (1989), Foegeding (1983), and Cook and Pierson (1983). These agents, however, are not permitted in foods at levels able to destroy *C. botulinum* spores.

C. Inhibition

1. *General*

Control of *C. botulinum* in most foods that permit its growth is through inhibition rather than destruction. Inhibition of cell proliferation and elaboration of toxin is generally achieved by manipulation of one or more of the factors that affect growth (Sperber, 1982). Important to inhibition and the potential for toxin production is also the number of spores of *C. botulinum* present in a food. In general, the inhibitory activity of various factors is inversely related to the level of inoculum (Hauschild, 1982; Robinson et al., 1982; Baker and Genigeorgis, 1990).

2. *Temperature*

The minimum growth temperature for strains of Groups I and II are 10 and 3.3°C, respectively (Hobbs, 1976; Smith and Sugiyama, 1988). These minimum temperatures, however, apply only to certain strains, while most others are inhibited at somewhat higher temperatures (Hauschild, 1989). Maximum growth is obtained at temperatures of 35–37, 30–35, and 40–42°C for strains of Groups I, II, and III, respectively, while maximum temperatures allowing growth are in the range of 45–50°C.

Since Group II strains are psychrotrophic, refrigeration above 3.3°C may be inadequate for inhibition of *C. botulinum*. Temperatures below 10°C, however, should be adequate for control of proteolytic strains (Sperber, 1982). Group II strains have produced toxin in ≥ 31 days at 3.3°C, when all other conditions were favorable, and in ≤ 10 days at 10°C (Ohye and Christian, 1967; Simunovic et al., 1985).

Although home refrigeration at <10°C may not be adequate for complete inhibition, acidity, salt, and other factors enhance inhibition and are more effective at lower temperatures. In general, use of refrigeration in combination with other inhibitory parameters permits formulation of products with more acceptable sensory characteristics (Sugiyama and Sofos, 1988).

3. *Acidity*

The pH range allowing growth of *C. botulinum* is between 4.7 and 8.5, with Group I cultures inhibited in foods of pH values ≤ 4.6, while a pH ≤ 5.0 is sufficient to inhibit Group II organisms (Odlaug and Pflug, 1978; Sugiyama and Sofos, 1988). This led to development of the government regulation that moist foods of pH values 4.6 or lower may be preserved and be safe from botulism with heat-processing treatments less severe than sterilization (Sperber, 1982).

Most fruits and some vegetable products are acidic enough to inhibit development of toxin by *C. botulinum* (Sugiyama and Sofos, 1988; Hauschild, 1989). Other foods, with insufficiently low pH, are acidified artificially (pickled) or fermented biologically during processing to achieve pH values below 4.6 and be preserved. Addition of various acids may achieve inhibition of *C. botulinum* at different pH values. One study reported that the most to the least inhibitory sequence of acidulants was acetic, lactic, citric, and hydrochloric (Smelt et al., 1982).

Although lowering the pH to <4.7 is adequate for inhibition of *C. botulinum* and is used in some foods, many more products are preserved with less severe acidification when pH is one in a series of factors that, when combined, inhibit the pathogen. In addition, at pH values less than optimum, other inhibitors, such as storage temperature, water activity, and chemical preservatives, are more effective than at pH values optimal for growth of *C. botulinum*.

As indicated above, foods have traditionally been divided as high or low acid products when their pH values are <4.6 or ≥4.7, respectively, based on inhibition of growth of *C. botulinum* at pH values < 4.7. Moist, high acid foods are made shelf-stable and free of botulism only with pasteurization heat (<100°C) treatments, which inactivate vegetative cells. The pH then should inhibit development of the surviving spores. For low acid, moist foods to become shelf-stable, they need either fermentation and acidification combined with mild heating or commercial sterilization (canning) heat (>100°C) treatments.

Occasional cases of botulism, however, have been associated with consumption of foods classified as high acid (Sperber, 1982). Of the 722 foodborne botulism outbreaks reported in the United States in the period 1899–1975, 35 were attributed to high acid or acidified foods (pH < 4.6), of which 34 were home-processed products (Odlaug and Pflug, 1978). Fourteen of these outbreaks were due to consumption of fruits or fruit juices, three from consumption of pickles, and 18 involved tomato products. For example, two deaths were associated with consumption of home-canned pears, which have average pH values < 4.0. Microbiological analyses indicated presence of yeasts in the product, which raised the pH to >6.0 (Meyer and Gunnison, 1929), which permitted toxin production by *C. botulinum*. Several of the above implicated foods were found contaminated with yeasts, molds, diplococci, and other microorganisms able to grow at low pH values (Sperber, 1982).

Sugiyama and Sofos (1988) presented four situations that may permit formation of toxin by *C. botulinum* at pH values below 4.6.

1. Since complete acidification and pH equilibration of certain particulate foods may require several days, depending on type and particle size of food, as well as type of acidulant, such foods may become toxic before complete acidification if storage temperatures and other factors permit development of *C. botulinum*.
2. The natural pH of certain high acid foods may vary considerably around 4.6. For example, certain tomato cultivars grown in certain soils or overripened and bruised may yield products with pH values > 4.6.
3. This situation involves the metabiotic effect indicated earlier, where organisms such as yeasts, mold and species of bacteria, such as *Bacillus licheniformis*, are able to grow at pH values below 4.6. As they develop, these organisms increase product pH, at least in their microenvironment, to levels that permit growth of *C. botulinum* spores if present in their vicinity. Acidity gradients associated with fungal mats have been demonstrated in tomato products (Huhtanen et al., 1976; Odlaug and Pflug, 1978; 1979).
4. Spore inocula of types A, B, and E have been able to develop and produce toxin after incubation of several weeks in certain high acid (pH as low as

4.0) substrates under specified conditions. These conditions involved culture media containing high amounts of precipitated protein and strictly anaerobic conditions (Raatjes and Smelt, 1979; Smelt et al., 1982; Tanaka, 1982; Tsang et al., 1985; Young-Perkins and Merson, 1987; Wong et al., 1988). It is very likely that under these conditions the pathogen is able to develop in microenvironments of pH >4.6 within the protein precipitate, while average pH of the substrate remains <4.6 (Tanaka, 1982). The above conditions, however, are unlikely to be present in foods. Thus, the existing regulations concerning processing of high acid foods have not been changed.

4. Water Activity

The amount of water in a food which is unbound and available to support microbial growth is defined as water activity (a_w). Water activity of foods is reduced by removal of water through drying and by addition of humectants which bind water and reduce its availability for chemical reactions and microbial growth. In addition, water activity is reduced in frozen food where a large portion of the water exists in the crystallized form. Different species of microorganisms cease their growth at different minimum levels of water activity (Sperber, 1982, 1983; Beuchat, 1987). Minimum water activities reported as permitting growth of Group I *C. botulinum* strains are in the range of 0.94–0.96, while nonproteolytic strains cease growth at water activities of 0.97 and lower. These water activity minima (<0.94 and <0.97) are applicable when common salt (sodium chloride) is the humectant used to control the water activity. The actual salt (or brine) levels (in the water phase) needed to yield water activity values of 0.97 and 0.94 are 5 and 10%, respectively (Sugiyama and Sofos, 1988).

In general, the minimum water activity allowing growth varies, not only with types and strains, but also with the nature of the solute used to control the amount of free water in the substrate. Some solutes protect instead of inhibiting enzymatic reactions, or are "compatible" solutes causing less osmotic stress (Sperber, 1983; Bell and DeLacy, 1985). These ingredients are less effective inhibitors of growth than others (Sugiyama and Sofos, 1988). When glycerol replaces salt in control of water activity, the minimum value permitting growth of type E becomes 0.94 instead of 0.97 (Troller, 1973). Thus, salt is an important factor in the control of *C. botulinum* (Hauschild, 1989). When the level of salt, however, is undesirable organoleptically, then less salt may be used in combination with other factors inhibitory to growth, such as pH and refrigeration. Combinations of such inhibitors allow the development of low salt and sodium products, which are preferred by certain consumers suffering from high blood pressure (Sofos,1984).

5. Gas Atmosphere

Growth and toxin production by *C. botulinum* are influenced by the oxidation-reduction or redox potential (Eh) of the substrate. Although difficult to measure, redox potential depends on the interrelationships of partial pressure of oxygen, pH, and concentration of reducing compounds, such as those containing thiol groups (Sugiyama and Sofos, 1988).

As an anaerobe, *C. botulinum* initiates growth at an electronegative Eh, but, in some instances, it has grown even at +250 mV (Sperber, 1982). As *C. botulinum* germinates or other organisms grow, the Eh of the substrate is reduced to values even below –200 mV (Lund and Wyatt, 1984). Maximum growth occurs at –350 mV (Smoot and Pierson, 1979). Oxygen raises the redox potential and should inhibit *C. botulinum*, but the limiting Eh depends on several conditions, including pH, type of substrate, and presence of inhibitors. Food packaged in metal cans demonstrated lower redox potential than when in glass containers (Montville and Conway, 1982). Upper values of Eh reported as allowing growth of *C. botulinum* are on the order of +200 mV (Hauschild, 1989), but stress factors, such as acidity and presence of salt, lower these levels (Smoot and Pierson, 1979).

It is commonly assumed that exposing food to air will prevent growth of *C. botulinum*. This, however, is incorrect, since microenvironments of suitable Eh can exist in nonhomogeneous foods exposed to air which are suitable for growth of the pathogen (Sperber, 1982; Lund and Wyatt, 1984).

The extension of shelf life of refrigerated foods by changing the composition of the air surrounding them, either to complete vacuum or increased carbon dioxide and nitrogen and reduced oxygen levels, is called modified atmosphere packaging (MAP), and its usefulness has been established (Eklund, 1982; Genigeorgis, 1985). The modified atmosphere inhibits growth of gram-negative bacteria, such as pseudomonads, and other spoilage psychrotrophs. These aerobic organisms, when uninhibited, grow more rapidly than others and develop off-odors and flavors in foods, which are perceived by consumers as product spoilage. The modified atmospheres usually allow growth of gram-positive lactic acid–producing bacteria, which grow slower and produce less objectionable changes in the organoleptic qualities of the foods. There is thus a need to evaluate various products, MAP conditions, and storage temperatures to determine whether the anaerobic *C. botulinum*, especially the psychrotrophic nonproteolytic strains, are able to grow and form toxin before product spoilage is evident. This applies especially to fish products, which are often contaminated with type E spores, and there is a need to extend their refrigerated shelf life with methods such as MAP.

In general, for fish stored in MAP, the extent of time needed for development of detectable spoilage and toxin production becomes shorter as the storage temperature is increased from 0 to 10°C (Genigeorgis, 1985; Post et al., 1985; Lindroth and Genigeorgis, 1986). The situation is reversed at temperatures around 10°C and above (Sugiyama and Sofos, 1988). Overall, it has been stated that a potential health hazard may exist if the seafood packaged in modified atmosphere is stored above 5°C (Eklund, 1982).

It should be mentioned, however, that most seafood is usually cooked before consumption, which should inactivate toxin if no cross-contamination has occurred before cooking. A recently published study examined 1074 samples of commercial, vacuum-packaged fresh fish for development of toxin during 12 days of storage at 12°C (Lilly and Kautter, 1990). Even when the seafood was marginally acceptable (after 12 days at 12°C), none of the 1074 samples were found positive for toxin of *C. botulinum*. This is reassuring, and it indicates that the fish either contained no spores of *C. botulinum*, or the spores were unable to grow and produce toxin in the fish within 12 days at 12°C. The high incidence of type E botulism outbreaks among native people in Alaska and Canada, however, may be attributed to the practice of fermenting their products while wrapped in plastic bags (Sugiyama and Sofos, 1988; Hauschild, 1989).

6. *Chemical Additives*

Several chemical additives are approved and used in food processing with the objective of extending the shelf life or maintaining product safety by inhibiting microorganisms (Branen and Davidson, 1983). A common preservative that inhibits *C. botulinum* and maintains safety during temperature abuse of cured meat products is sodium or potassium nitrite (Sofos et al., 1979; Sofos and Busta, 1980; Benedict, 1980; Anonymous, 1981, 1982; Roberts and Gibson, 1986). In addition to its antimicrobial activity, nitrite is involved in curing, color fixation, flavor development, and antioxidant activity of meat products. Sorbic acid was proposed as an alternative to nitrite because it is an effective inhibitor of botulinal spore germination, growth, and toxin production (Sofos and Busta, 1981, 1983; Robach and Sofos, 1982; Sofos, 1989a).

A variety of phenolic compounds, including parabens and antioxidants, have demonstrated inhibitory activity against *C. botulinum* (Davidson, 1983). Certain phosphate salts, which are used in foods for pH control, emulsifying, water-holding, binding, and flavoring objectives, may also inhibit *C. botulinum* (Kautter et al., 1979; Tompkin, 1984; Sofos, 1986; 1989c; Wagner, 1986). In pasteurized process cheese spreads, the antibotulinal activity is increased with phosphate compared to citrate use as emulsifying agents (Tanaka et al., 1979).

Other agents reported as inhibiting *C. botulinum* include sulfur dioxide, sodium hypophosphite, liquid smoke flavorings, sodium lactate, spices, seasonings, and their extracts (Sofos and Busta, 1980; Sperber, 1982; Sugiyama and Sofos, 1988; Maas et al., 1989; Rhodehamel et al., 1990).

7. *Biological Inhibitors*

Interest in using biological agents (Daeschel, 1989) to preserve foods has increased in recent years, even though lactic acid–producing bacteria have been used to ferment and preserve foods for centuries. Also, competitive microorganisms are important in products such as semipreserved meats, where, if the product is temperature abused, they develop and inhibit *C. botulinum* or warn the consumer by causing product spoilage (Hauschild, 1982; 1989). Inoculation with lactic acid bacteria and addition of a fermentable carbohydrate allows curing of bacon with reduced nitrite levels because the lactics produce acid and inhibit *C. botulinum* in case of product abuse (Tanaka et al., 1980, 1985). In addition to acid, lactic acid bacteria produce bacteriocins, which may be involved in extension of product shelf life (Daeschel, 1989).

8. *Interactions of Factors*

The major factors controlling growth of *C. botulinum* in foods are storage temperature, product pH and water activity, added chemical preservatives, and competitive microflora. Preservation of certain foods is based exclusively on any one of these factors. This applies to canned products, frozen or dried foods, and fermented or acidified items. Many foods, however, combine the inhibitory activity of several preservative factors to ensure their stability and safety. The botulism safety record of commercially produced cured meat products in the United States is an excellent example of product preservation through interaction of various inhibitory parameters. This concept in food preservation has been compared to various hurdles or barriers ("hurdles concept") that the microorganism has to surmount before it spoils or renders the food toxic (Leistner, 1977). Thus, it is possible to maintain the botulinal safety of a product by reducing the amount of one inhibitor (e.g., sodium chloride or nitrite) while increasing the activity of another (e.g., pH). This principle has allowed the safe marketing of the various semipreserved foods which add convenience and variety to our diet.

A few studies have provided experimental data on the contribution of various hurdles to inhibition of *C. botulinum* in meat and cheese products (Roberts et al., 1981a,b,c; Tanaka et al., 1986), while predictive modeling is gaining interest as a procedure for quantifying the risk of toxin formation in variable food formulations of refrigerated products (Baker and Genigeorgis, 1990). These models should be able to predict quantitatively the time to toxin development in products of variable formulations stored under different conditions (Conner et al., 1989).

VIII. FOODS

A. General

Growth of *C. botulinum* is favored by complex substrates containing readily available amino acids, vitamins, and inorganic salts (Smith and Sugiyama, 1988). Most foods, however, are nutritionally adequate for *C. botulinum* growth and toxin production, as demonstrated by outbreaks that have involved products such as garlic in oil and sautéed onions (Sugiyama and Sofos, 1988). In general, both plant and animal food products provide the nutrients needed for *C. botulinum* growth and toxin production.

Numerous foods have been implicated in foodborne outbreaks of botulism. Between 1899 and 1976 in the United States, about 53% of the outbreaks were associated with vegetable products. Home-processed foods caused 72% of the outbreaks, while commercially processed products were involved in 8.6%, and undetermined foods in 19.8%. Improperly canned, low acid vegetable products provide excellent growth environments for *C. botulinum* spores (Wallen, 1983). While cured meats were commonly associated with botulism outbreaks in the United States in the past, this is no longer the case. They continue, however, to cause problems in European countries (Tompkin, 1980).

Several recent outbreaks have been associated with foods prepared and served in food-service establishments. They resulted from product mishandling, which demonstrates that many products may have the ability to support toxin production if environmental conditions permit development of *C. botulinum*.

B. Foods of Recent Concern

Changes in consumer lifestyles and activities have resulted in increased demand for fresh, high quality, convenient food products or meals, which require minimal preparation effort and time (Anonymous, 1988a,b; Scott, 1989; Conner et al., 1989). This need has resulted in the development and availability of large numbers of partially processed ready-to-eat and heat-and-serve products that are of longer than usual shelf life but need refrigeration or freezing. Although these products, such as soups, sauces, salads, and complete meals, appear to be successful in the marketplace, there is concern involving potential abuse and development of foodborne health hazards such as *C. botulinum* (Conner et al., 1989).

The heat treatment received by these products extends their refrigerated shelf life, but is usually inadequate to inactivate *C. botulinum* spores, thus, nonproteolytic spores, which can grow at refrigeration temperatures, may have adequate time to do so when the shelf life is extended. In addition, potential temperature abuse not only will enhance growth of nonproteolytic types, but it may also allow growth of proteolytic strains (Solomon et al., 1982). Furthermore, the mild heat treatment received by these products and packaging under vacuum or other modified atmospheres may eliminate or reduce growth of competitive spoilage microorganisms, and may allow toxin development while the product appears to be still organoleptically acceptable. Thus, consumers should be aware of these potential dangers and keep the products under recommended storage conditions, while processors may need to introduce multiple barriers for inhibition of *C. botulinum* and other pathogens in case of temperature abuse. The manufacturers and processors of these extended shelf life, modern refrigerated foods must presume that *C. botulinum* spores are present in the raw ingredients; that the heat treatment is inadequate to destroy these spores, but reduces competitive, inhibitory, spoilage microflora; and that proper refrigeration will not be maintained at some point during product handling. Thus, they need to assure their safety by other means in case these conditions are met and *C. botulinum* develops before product consumption.

Involvement of refrigerated foods in botulism outbreaks is very low, but certain outbreaks have attracted attention in recent years. Furthermore, some research challenge studies have illustrated the potential for botulism hazards with some of these products (Sugiyama and Sofos, 1988; Hauschild, 1989; Conner et al., 1989).

When garlic in oil was kept unrefrigerated for unspecified amounts of time, it caused two outbreaks of type B botulism (Solomon and Kautter, 1988). It should be noted that the product was labeled "keep refrigerated." A study with inoculated chopped garlic in oil stored at room temperature indicated that 5 spores per bulb of garlic produced toxin, while the product still appeared organoleptically acceptable. The spores of the pathogen were also found to be naturally present in garlic bulbs (Solomon and Kautter, 1988).

Restaurant-served potato salads have been involved in as many as three reported outbreaks of botulism. In two of the outbreaks the potato salad was prepared with aluminum foil–wrapped baked potatoes, which after baking, had been kept for several days at room temperature. It is logical to assume that the soil contaminated the potatoes with *C. botulinum*, the spores survived baking, and then developed and formed toxin during storage of the potatoes or the potato salad (Sugiyama and Sofos, 1988). Thus, baked potatoes should be stored at temperatures ≤7°C or ≥60°C (Hauschild, 1989). A study with artificially inoculated potatoes which were wrapped in aluminum foil and baked demonstrated survival of *C. botulinum* spores and production of toxin during storage at room temperature (Sugiyama et al., 1981).

Commercially cooked, vacuum-packaged potatoes are available as a convenience item in Europe with a refrigerated shelf life of approximately 6 weeks. It was demonstrated, however, that these products can become toxic, when spores of *C. botulinum* are present, if temperature abused, even before spoilage is noticeable (Notermans et al., 1981). Proteolytic as well as nonproteolytic spores survived cooking at 95°C for 40 min (the typical process) and formed toxin within 6 weeks at 10°C. No toxin was detected when the vacuum-packaged potatoes were stored at 4°C. A subsequent study demonstrated that a hurdle in addition to refrigeration was adequate to extend the period of safety of the product (Notermans et al., 1985). The treatment involved dipping of the potatoes before cooking in a solution of ascorbic and citric acids.

When kept warm for several hours and then served on a meat patty sandwich, sautéed onions were involved in 28 cases of type A botulism (MacDonald et al., 1985; Solomon and Kautter, 1986). The raw onions in the restaurant were found to be contaminated with botulinal spores. When onions were inoculated with spores and treated under the same conditions, they became toxic in 2 days at 35°C (Solomon and Kautter, 1986). It appears that immersion in fat or oil creates an anaerobic environment, which allows toxin formation when stored at the appropriate temperature for the needed length of time (Sugiyama and Sofos, 1988; Hauschild, 1989).

It was shown that packaging fresh mushrooms in semipermeable, polyvinylchloride film allowed toxin production within 3–4 days at 20°C, when an inoculum of 5×10^4C *C. botulinum* spores was introduced in the product (Sugiyama and Yang, 1975). This potential problem can be avoided, however, by opening one or two holes (3 mm in diameter) in the packaging film, which supply enough oxygen in the package to inhibit the pathogen (Sugiyama and Rutledge, 1978; Kautter et al., 1978; Sugiyama, 1982).

Although marketed frozen, meat pies have been involved in at least three incidents of botulism due to abuse at home (Sugiyama and Sofos, 1988; Hauschild, 1989). This, of course, demonstrates a situation of extreme abuse or mishandling after heating. Recently, cabbage was also suspected as a possible vehicle of botulism (Solomon et al., 1990).

Smoking of fish from the Great Lakes did not inactivate type E spores of *C. botulinum* and resulted in three outbreaks of human botulism in the 1960s. The products were toxic with no evident signs of spoilage (Eklund, 1982). Three outbreaks of botulism have involved consumption of "kapchunka." This is a ready-to-eat ethnic food prepared with uneviscerated fish which is salt-cured and air-dried with or without smoking (Conner et al., 1989).

Tofu is a soybean curd food of the Orient, which has gained popularity in the United States. A study indicated that type A and B spore inocula produced toxin in tofu in 1 and 3 weeks at 25 and 15°C, respectively. No toxin was detected in tofu stored for 6 weeks at 5 or 10°C (Kovats et al., 1984).

Hard-boiled eggs cooled in water contaminated with 100 spores of Group I/ml and then stored at 30°C allowed formation of toxin within 2–7 days (Lubin et al., 1985). This resembles the outbreak of staphylococcal food poisoning in which approximately 300 children were afflicted after consumption of hard-boiled eggs (Merrill et al., 1984). Boiling damages the egg cuticle and shell membranes allowing absorption of contaminated water by the heated eggs. Thus, water-cooled, hard-boiled eggs should be refrigerated at ≤7°C. Commercially hard-boiled resin-coated eggs, which are air-cooled, were found free of botulinal toxin and may be marketed without refrigeration (Hauschild, 1989).

Hamburger sandwiches inoculated with type E spores and stored under nitrogen were toxic within 30 days at 12°C, while still organoleptically acceptable (Kautter et al., 1981). At room temperature, hamburger and sausage sandwiches inoculated with type A and B spores were toxic within 7 days.

Foods having discrete particles of variable composition, which are individually unsuitable for toxin production, may become toxic when they are combined to formulate a new product (Sugiyama and Sofos, 1988). An example of this possibility occurred in Japan and resulted in an outbreak of type A botulism (Hayaishi et al., 1986). Mustard-miso was used as stuffing to fill holes of raw lotus roots. During heating and storage the two components equilibrated so that the original pH of 5.0 and water activity of 0.92 became pH 5.3 and water activity 0.98, which permitted formation of botulinal toxin.

IX. CONCLUSIONS

Clostridium botulinum is a soil organism that can grow and produce toxin in a variety of food products, which may still appear acceptable to consumers. As a human pathogen it is of great concern because its neurotoxins are extremely potent poisons. Even at certain refrigeration temperatures (>3.3°C) given sufficient time nonproteolytic *C. botulinum* strains may grow and form toxin. Extensive heating (canning), reduced pH (<4.6), drying (water activity < 0.94), or constant refrigeration or freezing (<3.3°C) can prevent botulism hazards. A variety of foods, however, are preserved by combining various parameters which collectively provide an environment unfavorable for growth of the pathogen. In general, as a pathogen causing infectious infant botulism or foodborne botulism poisoning, *C. botulinum* should be of concern to food processors and handlers as well as consumers.

REFERENCES

Anonymous (1979). Handbook for epidemiologists, clinicians, and laboratory workers. U.S. Department of Health, Education and Welfare, CDC, Atlanta, GA.

Anonymous (1981). *The Health Effects of Nitrate, Nitrite and N-nitroso Compounds*, National Research Council, National Academy Press, Washington, DC.

Anonymous (1982). *Alternatives to the Current Use of Nitrite in Foods*, National Research Council, National Academy Press, Washington, DC.

Anonymous (1988a). Refrigerated Foods and Microbiological Criteria Committee. Safety considerations for new generation refrigerated foods. *Dairy Food Sanit. 8*: 5–7.

Anonymous (1988b). Refrigerated Foods and Microbiological Criteria Committee. Factors to be considered in establishing good manufacturing practices for the production of refrigerated foods. *Dairy Food Sanit. 8*: 288–291.

Anonymous (1990). Infant botulism in California, 1988–89. Department of Health Services, State of California—Health and Welfare Agency, February 23.

Arnon, S. S. (1989). Infant botulism. In *Anaerobic Infections in Humans*. Academic Press, San Diego, CA, pp. 601–609.

Arnon, S. S., Midura, T. F., Clay, S. A., Wood, R. M., and Chin, J. (1977). Infant botulism: Epidemiological, clinical, and laboratory aspects. *JAMA 237*: 1946–1951.

Aureli, P., Fenicia, L., Pasolini, B., Gianfranceschi, M., McCroskey, L. M., and Hatheway, C. L. (1986). Two cases of type E infant botulism caused by neurotoxigenic *Clostridium butyricum* in Italy. *J. Infect. Dis. 154*: 207–211.

Baker, D. A., and Genigeorgis, C. (1990). Predicting the safe storage of fresh fish under modified atmospheres with respect to *Clostridium botulinum* toxigenesis by modeling length of the lag phase of growth. *J. Food Prot. 53*: 131–140.

Bean, N. H., and Griffin, P. M. (1990). Foodborne disease outbreaks in the United States, 1983–1987: Pathogens, vehicles, and trends. *J. Food Prot. 53*: 804–817.

Bean, N. H., Griffin, P. M., Goulding, J. S., and Ivey, C. B. (1990). Foodborne disease outbreaks, 5-year summary, 1983–1987. *J. Food Prot. 53*: 711–728.

Bell, R. G., and DeLacy, K. M. (1985). The effect of nisin-sodium chloride interactions on the outgrowth of *Bacillus licheniformis* spores. *J. Appl. Bacteriol. 59*: 127–132.

Benedict, R. C. (1980). Biochemical basis for nitrite-inhibition of *Clostridium botulinum* in cured meat. *J. Food Prot. 43*: 877–891.

Beuchat, L. R. (1987). Influence of water activity on sporulation, germination, outgrowth, and toxin production. In *Water Activity: Theory and Applications to Food*, L. B. Rockland and L. R. Beuchat, eds. Marcel Dekker, New York, pp. 137–152.

Blocher, J. C., and Busta, F. F. (1983). Bacterial spore resistance to acid. *Food Technol. 37*(11): 87–99.

Blocher, J. C., Busta, F. F., and Sofos, N. J. (1982). Influence of potassium sorbate and pH on ten strains of type A and B *Clostridium botulinum*. *J. Food Sci. 47*: 2028–2032.

Bradshaw, J. G., Peeler, J. T., and Twedt, R. M. (1979). Thermal inactivation of *Clostridium botulinum* toxin types A and B in buffer, and beef and mushroom patties. *J. Food Sci. 44*: 1653–1657.

Bradshaw, J. G., Peeler, J. T., and Twedt, R. M. (1981). Thermal inactivation of *Clostridium botulinum* toxin types F and G in buffer and in beef and mushroom patties. *J. Food Sci. 46*: 688–690, 696.

Branen, A. L., and Davidson, P. M. (1983). *Antimicrobials in Foods*. Marcel Dekker, New York.

Cann, D. C., Taylor, L. Y., and Hobbs, G. (1975). The incidence of *Clostridium botulinum* in farmed trout raised in Great Britain. *J. Appl. Bacteriol. 39*: 331–336.

Conner, D. E., Scott, V. N., and Bernard, D. T. (1989). Potential *Clostridium botulinum* hazards associated with extended shelf-life refrigerated foods: A review. *J. Food Safety 10*: 131–153.

Cook, F. K., and Pierson, M. D. (1983). Inhibition of bacterial spores by antimicrobials. *Food Technol. 37*(11): 115–125.

Daeschel, M. A. (1989). Antimicrobial substances from lactic acid bacteria for use as food preservatives. *Food Technol. 43*(1): 164–167.

Davidson, P. M. (1983). Phenolic compounds. In *Antimicrobials in Foods*, A. L. Branen and P. M. Davidson, eds. Marcel Dekker, New York, pp. 37–74.

Denny, C. B. (1982). Industry's response to problem solving in botulism prevention. *Food Technol. 36*(12): 116–118.

Dezfulian, M., and Bartlett, J. G. (1985). Selective isolation and rapid identification of *Clostridium botulinum* types A and B by toxin detection. *J. Clin. Microbiol. 21*: 231–233.

Dolman, C. E. (1964). Botulism as a world health problem. In *Botulism. Proceedings of a Symposium*, K. H. Lewis, and K. Cassel, eds. Public Health Service Publ. No. 999-FP-1, Cincinnati, OH, pp. 5–32.

Eklund, M. W. (1982). Significance of *Clostridium botulinum* in fishery products preserved short of sterilization. *Food Technol. 36*(12): 107–112, 115.

Eklund, M. W., and Poysky, F. T. (1972). Activation of a toxic component of *Clostridium botulinum* types C and D by trypsin. *Appl. Microbiol. 24*: 108–113.

Foegeding, P. M. (1983). Bacterial spore resistance to chlorine compounds. *Food Technol. 37*(11): 100–104, 110.

Foster, E. M. (1986). *Clostridium botulinum. Food Technol. 40*(8): 18–19.

Genigeorgis, C. (1985). Microbial safety implications of the use of modified atmospheres to extent the storage life of fresh meat and fish. A review. *Int. J. Food Microbiol. 1*: 237–251.

Gimenez, D. F., and Ciccarelli, A. S. (1970). Another type of *Clostridium botulinum. Zentralbl. Bakteriol. Parasitenkd. Infektionskr. Hyg. Abt. I Orig. 215*: 221–224.

Glasby, C., and Hatheway, C. L. (1984). Fluorescent-antibody reagents for the identification of *Clostridium botulinum. J. Clin. Microbiol. 18*: 1378–1383.

Glasby, C., and Hatheway, C. L. (1985). Isolation and enumeration of *Clostridium botulinum* by direct inoculation of infant fecal specimens on egg yolk agar and *Clostridium botulinum* isolation media. *J. Clin. Microbiol. 21*: 264–266.

Hall, J. D., McCroskey, L. M., Pincomb, B. J., and Hatheway, C. L. (1985). Isolation of an organism resembling *Clostridium barati* which produces type F botulinal toxin from an infant with botulism. *J. Clin. Microbiol. 21*: 654–655.

Hatheway, C. L., McCroskey, L. M., Lombard, G. L., and Dowell, V. R. (1981). A typical toxin variant of *Clostridium botulinum* type B associated with infant botulism. *J. Clin. Microbiol. 14*: 607–611.

Hatheway, C. L., Snyder, J. D., Seals, J. E., Edell, T. A., and Lewis, G. E. (1984). Antitoxin levels in botulism patients treated with trivalent equine botulism antitoxin of toxin types A, B, and E. *J. Infect. Dis. 150*: 407–412.

Hauschild, A. H. W. (1982). Assessment of botulism hazards from cured meat products. *Food Technol. 36*(12): 95–104.

Hauschild, A. H. W. (1989). *Clostridium botulinum*. In *Foodborne Bacterial Pathogens*, M. P. Doyle, ed. Marcel Dekker, New York, pp. 111–189.

Hayaishi, K., Sakaguchi, S., and Sakaguchi, G. (1986). Primary multiplication of *Clostridium botulinum* type A in a mustard-miso stuffing of "karashi-renkon" (deep-fried mustard-stuffed lotus root). *Int. J. Food Microbiol. 3*: 311–320.

Hobbs, G. (1976). *Clostridium botulinum* and its importance in fishery products. *Adv. Food Res. 22*: 135–185.

Hobbs, G., Crowther, J. S., Neaves, P., Gibbs, P. A., and Jarvis, B. (1982). Detection and Isolation of *Clostridium botulinum*. In *Isolation and Identification Methods for Food Poisoning Organisms*, J. E. L. Corry, D. Roberts, and F. A. Skinner, eds. Soc. Appl. Bacteriol. Symp. Ser. 17, pp. 151–164.

Hughes, J. M., Blumenthal, J. R., Merson, M. H., Lombard, G. L., Dowell, V. R., Jr., and Gangarosa, E. J. (1981). Clinical features of types A and B food-borne botulism. *Ann. Inter. Med. 95*: 442–445.

Huhtanen, C. N., Naghski, J., Custer, C. S., and Russell, R. W. (1976). Growth and toxin production by *Clostridium botulinum* in moldy tomato juice. *Appl. Environ. Microbiol. 32*: 711–715.

Kautter, D. A., and Lynt, R. K. (1984a). *Clostridium botulinum.* In *Bacteriological Analytical Manual of Food and Drug Administration*, 6th ed. Association of Official Analytical Chemists, Arlington, VA, pp. XIV-1 to XIV-16.

Kautter, D. A., and Lynt, R. K. (1984b). *Clostridium botulinum.* In *Compendium of Methods for the Microbiological Examination of Foods*, 2nd ed., M. L. Speck, ed. American Public Health Association, Washington, D.C., pp. 468–482.

Kautter, D. A., Lilly, T., Jr., and Lynt, R. (1978). Evaluation of the botulism hazard in fresh mushrooms wrapped in commercial polyvinylchloride film. *J. Food Prot. 41*: 120–121.

Kautter, D. A., Lilly, T., Jr., Lynt, R. K., and Solomon, H. M. (1979). Toxin production by *Clostridium botulinum* in shelf-stable pasteurized process cheese spreads. *J. Food Prot. 42*: 784–786.

Kautter, D. A., Lynt, R. K., Lilly, T. Jr., and Solomon, H. M. (1981). Evaluation of the botulism hazard from nitrogen-packed sandwiches. *J. Food Prot. 44*: 59–61.

Kautter, D. A., Lilly, T., Solomon, H. M., and Lynt, R. K. (1982). *Clostridium botulinum* in infant foods: A survey. *J. Food Prot. 45*: 1028–1029.

Kovats, S. K., Doyle, M. P., and Tanaka, M. (1984). Evaluation of the microbiological safety of tofu. *J. Food Prot. 47*: 618–622.

Leistner, L. (1977). Hurdle effect and energy saving. In *Food Quality and Nutrition*, W. K. Downey, ed. Applied Science Publ., London, pp. 553–557.

Lilly, T., Jr., and Kautter, D. A. (1990). Outgrowth of naturally occurring *Clostridium botulinum* in vacuum-packaged fresh fish. *J. Assoc. Offic. Anal. Chem. 73*: 211–212.

Lilly, T., Kautter, D. A., Lynt, R. K., and Solomon, H. M. (1984). Immunodiffusion detection of *Clostridium botulinum* colonies. *J. Food Prot. 47*: 868–870.

Lindroth, S. E., and Genigeorgis, C. A. (1986). Probability of growth and toxin production by nonproteolytic *Clostridium botulinum* in rockfish stored under modified atmospheres. *Int. J. Food Microbiol. 3*: 169–181.

Lubin, L. B., Morton, R. D., and Bernard, D. T. (1985). Toxin production in hard-cooked eggs experimentally inoculated with *Clostridium botulinum. J. Food Sci. 50*: 969–970, 984.

Lund, B. M., and Wyatt, G. M. (1984). The effect of redox potential, and its interaction with sodium chloride concentration, on the probability of growth of *Clostridium botulinum* type E from spore inocula. *Food Microbiol. 1*: 49–65.

Lynt, R. K., Kautter, D. A., and Solomon, H. M. (1982a). Differences and similarities among proteolytic and nonproteolytic strains of *Clostridium botulinum* types A, B, E and F: A review. *J. Food Prot. 45*: 466–474.

Lynt, R. K., Kautter, D. A., and Solomon, H. M. (1982b). Heat resistance of proteolytic *Clostridium botulinum* type F in phosphate buffer and crabmeat. *J. Food Sci. 47*: 204–206, 230.

Maas, M. R., Glass, K. A., and Doyle, M. P. (1989). Sodium lactate delays toxin production by *Clostridium botulinum* in cook-in-bag turkey products. *Appl. Environ. Microbiol. 55*: 2226–2229.

MacDonald, K. L., Spengler, R. F., Hatheway, C. L., Hargrett, N. T., and Cohen, M. L. (1985). Type A botulism from sautéed onions: Clinical and epidemiologic observations. *JAMA 253*: 1275–1278.

McCroskey, L. M., Hatheway, C. L., Fenicia, L., Pasolini, B., and Aureli, P. (1986). Characterization of an organism that produces type E botulinal toxin but which resembles *Clostridium butyricum* from the feces of an infant with type E botulism. *J. Clin. Microbiol. 23*: 201–202.

Merrill, G. A., Werner, S. B., Bryant, R. G., Fredson, D., and Kelly, K. (1984). Staphylococcal food poisoning associated with Easter egg hunt. *JAMA 252*: 1019–1022.

Meyer, K. F., and Gunnison, J. B. (1929). Botulism due to home canned Bartlett pears. *J. Infect. Dis. 45*: 134–141.

Midura, T. F., and Arnon, S. S. (1976). Infant botulism: Identification of *Clostridium botulinum* and its toxins in feces. *Lancet 2*: 934–936.

Mills, D. C., Midura, T. F., and Arnon, S. S. (1985). Improved selective medium for the isolation of lipase-positive *Clostridium botulinum* from feces of human infants. *J. Clin. Microbiol. 21*: 947–950.

Montville, T. J., and Conway, L. K. (1982). Oxidation-reduction potentials of canned foods and their ability to support *Clostridium botulinum* toxigenes. *J. Food Sci. 47*: 1879–1882.

Notermans, S., Dufrenne, J., and Keybets, M. J. H. (1981). Vacuum-packed cooked potatoes: Toxin production by *Clostridium botulinum* and shelf-life. *J. Food Prot. 44*: 572–575.

Notermans, S., Dufrenne, J., and Keybets, M. J. H. (1985). Use of preservatives to delay toxin formation by *Clostridium botulinum* (type B, strain okra) in vacuum-packed, cooked potatoes. *J. Food Prot. 48*: 851–855.

Odlaug, T. E., and Pflug, I. J. (1978). *Clostridium botulinum* and acid foods. *J. Food Prot. 41*: 566–573.

Odlaug, T. E., and Pflug, I. J. (1979). *Clostridium botulinum* growth and toxin production in tomato juice containing *Aspergillus gracilis*. *Appl. Environ. Microbiol. 37*: 496–504.

Ohye, D. F., and Christian, J. H. B. (1967). Combined effects of temperature, pH and water activity on growth and toxin production by *Clostridium botulinum* types A, B, and E. In *Botulinum 1966*, M. Ingram, and T. A. Roberts, eds. Chapman & Hall, London, pp. 217–223.

Pierson, M. D., and Reddy, N. R. (1988). *Clostridium botulinum*. *Food Technol. 42*(4): 196–198.

Post, L. S., Lee, D. A., Solberg, M., Furgang, D., Specchio, J., and Graham, C. (1985). Development of botulinal toxin and sensory deterioration during storage of vacuum and modified atmosphere packaged fish fillets. *J. Food Sci. 50*: 990–996.

Raatjes, G. J. M., and Smelt, J. P. P. M. (1979). *Clostridium botulinum* can grow and form toxins at pH values lower than 4.5. *Nature 281*: 398–399.

Rhodehamel, E. J., Pierson, M. D., and Leifer, A. M. (1990). Hypophosphite: A review. *J. Food Prot. 53*: 513–518.

Robach, M. C., and Sofos, J. N. (1982). Use of sorbates in meat products, fresh poultry and poultry products. *J. Food Prot. 44*: 614–622.

Roberts, T. A., and Gibson, A. M. (1986). Chemical methods for controlling *Clostridium botulinum* in processed meats. *Food Technol. 40*(40): 163–171.

Roberts, T. A., Gibson, A. M., and Robinson, A. (1981a). Prediction of toxin production by *Clostridium botulinum* in pasteurized pork slurry. *J. Food Technol. 16*: 337–355.

Roberts, T. A., Gibson, A. M., and Robinson, A. (1981b). Factors controlling the growth of *Clostridium botulinum* types A and B in pasteurized, cured meats. I. Growth in pork slurries prepared from 'low' pH meat (pH range 5.5–6.3). *J. Food Technol. 16*: 239–266.

Roberts, T. A., Gibson, A. M., and Robinson, A. (1981c). Factors controlling the growth of *Clostridium botulinum* types A and B in pasteurized, cured meats. II. Growth in pork slurries prepared from 'high' pH meat (range 6.3–6.8). *J. Food Technol. 16*: 267–281.

Robinson, A., Gibson, A. M., and Roberts, T. A. (1982). Factors controlling the growth of *Clostridium botulinum* types A and B in pasteurized, cured meats. V. Prediction of toxin production: Non-linear effects of storage temperature and salt concentration. *J. Food Technol.* *17*: 727–744.

Sakaguchi, G. (1983). *Clostridium botulinum* toxins. *Pharmac. Ther.* *19*: 165–194.

Schaffner, R. M. (1982). Government's role in preventing foodborne botulism. *Food Technol.* *36*(12): 87–88, 115.

Scott, V. N. (1989). Interactions of factors to control microbial spoilage of refrigerated foods. *J. Food Prot.* *52*: 431–435.

Scott, V. N., and Bernard, D. T. (1982). Heat resistance of spores of nonproteolytic type B *Clostridium botulinum*. *J. Food Prot.* *45*: 909–912.

Scott, V. N., and Bernard, D. T. (1985). The effect of lysozyme on the apparent heat resistance of nonproteolytic type G *Clostridium botulinum*. *J. Food Safety* *7*: 145–154.

Scott, V. N., and Duncan, D. L. (1978). Cryptic plasmids in *Clostridium botulinum* and *Clostridium botulinum*-like organisms. *FEMS Microbiol. Lett.* *4*: 55–58.

Simpson, L. L. (1981). The origin, structure, and pharmacological activity of botulinum toxin. *Pharmacol. Rev.* *33*(3): 155–188.

Simunovic, J., Oblinger, J. L., and Adams, J. P. (1985). Potential for growth of non-proteolytic types of *Clostridium botulinum* in pasteurized restructured meat products: A review. *J. Food Prot.* *48*: 265–276.

Smelt, J. P. P. M., Raatjes, G. J. M., Crowther, J. S., and Verrips, C. T. (1982). Growth and toxin formation by *Clostridium botulinum* at low pH values. *J. Appl. Bacteriol.* *52*: 75–82.

Smith, L. DS., and Sugiyama, H. (1988). *Botulism: The Organism, Its Toxins, the Disease*, 2nd ed. Charles C. Thomas, Springfield, IL.

Smoot, L. A., and Pierson, M. D. (1979). Effect of oxidation-reduction potential on the outgrowth and chemical inhibition of *Clostridium botulinum* 10755 A spores. *J. Food Sci.* *44*: 700–704.

Sofos, J. N. (1984). Antimicrobial effects of sodium and other ions in foods: A review. *J. Food Safety* *6*: 45–78.

Sofos, N. J. (1986). Use of phosphates in low-sodium meat products. *Food Technol.* *40*(9): 52–69.

Sofos, J. N. (1989a). *Sorbate Food Preservatives*. CRC Press, Boca Raton, FL.

Sofos, J. N. (1989b). Detection of injured spore-forming bacteria from foods. In *Injured Index and Pathogenic Bacteria: Occurrence and Detection in Foods, Water and Feeds*, B. Ray, ed. CRC Press, Boca Raton, FL, pp. 147–177.

Sofos, J. N. (1989c). Phosphates in meat products. In *Developments in Food Preservation-5*, S. Thorne, ed. Elsevier Science Publishing Co., Amsterdam, pp. 207–252.

Sofos, J. N., and Busta, F. F. (1980). Alternatives to the use of nitrite as an antibotulinal agent. *Food Technol.* *34*(5): 244–251.

Sofos, J. N., and Busta, F. F. (1981). Antimicrobial activity of sorbate. *J. Food Prot.* *44*: 614–622.

Sofos, J. N., and Busta, F. F. (1983). Sorbates. In *Antimicrobials in Foods*, A. L. Branen and P. M. Davidson, eds. Marcel Dekker, New York, pp. 141–175.

Sofos, J. N., Busta, F. F., and Allen, C. E. (1979). Botulism control by nitrite and sorbate in cured meats: A review. *J. Food Prot.* *42*: 739–770.

Sofos, J. N., Pierson, M. D., Blocher, J. C., and Busta, F. F. (1986). Mode of action of sorbic acid on bacterial cells and spores. *Int. J. Food Microbiol.* *3*: 1–17.

Solberg, M., Post, L. S., Furgang, D., and Graham, C. (1985). Bovine serum eliminates rapid nonspecific toxic reactions during bioassay of stored fish for *Clostridium botulinum* toxin. *Appl. Environ. Microbiol.* *49*: 644–649.

Solomon, H. M., and Kautter, D. A. (1979). Sporulation and toxin production by *Clostridium botulinum* type G. *J. Food Prot.* *42*: 965–967.

Solomon, H. M., and Kautter, D. A. (1986). Growth and toxin production by *Clostridium botulinum* in sautéed onions. *J. Food Prot. 49*: 618–620.

Solomon, H. M., and Kautter, D. A. (1988). Outgrowth and toxin production by *Clostridium botulinum* in bottled chopped garlic. *J. Food Prot. 51*: 862–865.

Solomon, H. M., Kautter, D. A., and Lynt, R. K. (1982). Effect of low temperature on growth of nonproteolytic *Clostridium botulinum* types B and F and proteolytic type G in crabmeat and broth. *J. Food Prot. 45*: 516–518.

Solomon, H. M., Kautter, D. A., and Lynt, R. K. (1985). Common characteristics of the Swiss and Argentine strains of *Clostridium botulinum* type G. *J. Food Prot. 48*: 7–10.

Solomon, H. M., Kautter, D. A., Lilly, T., and Rhodehamel, E. J. (1990). Outgrowth of *Clostridium botulinum* in shredded cabbage at room temperature under a modified atmosphere. *J. Food Prot. 53*: 831–833.

Sonnabend, O., Sonnabend, W., Heinzle, R., Sigrist, T., Dirnhofer, R., and Krech, U. (1981). Isolation of *Clostridium botulinum* type G and identification of type G botulinal toxin in humans: Report of five sudden unexpected deaths. *J. Infect. Dis. 143*: 22–27.

Sperber, W. H. (1982). Requirements of *Clostridium botulinum* for growth and toxin production. *Food Technol. 36*(12): 89–94.

Sperber, W. H. (1983). Influence of water activity on foodborne bacteria—A review. *J. Food Prot. 46*: 142–150.

Strom, M. S., Eklund, M. W., and Poysky, F. T. (1984). Plasmids in *Clostridium botulinum* and related *Clostridium* species. *Appl. Environ. Microbiol. 48*: 956–963.

Sugiyama, H. (1980). *Clostridium botulinum* neurotoxin. *Microbiol. Rev. 44*: 419–448.

Sugiyama, H. (1982). Botulism hazards from nonprocessed foods. *Food Technol. 36*: 113–115.

Sugiyama, H., and Sofos, J. N. (1988). Botulism. In *Developments in Food Microbiology—4*, R. K. Robinson, ed. Elsevier Applied Science, London, pp. 77–120.

Sugiyama, H., and Rutledge, K. S. (1978). Failure of *Clostridium botulinum* to grow in fresh mushrooms packaged in plastic film overwraps with holes. *J. Food Prot. 41*: 348–350.

Sugiyama, H., and Yang, K. H. (1975). Growth potential of *Clostridium botulinum* in fresh mushrooms packaged in semi-permeable plastic film. *Appl. Microbiol. 30*: 964–969.

Sugiyama, H., Woodburn, M., Yang, K. H., and Movroydis, C. (1981). Production of botulinum toxin in inoculated pack studies of foil-wrapped baked potatoes. *J. Food Prot. 44*: 896–898, 902.

Tanaka, N. (1982). Toxin production by *Clostridium botulinum* in media at pH lower than 4.6. *J. Food Prot. 45*: 234–237.

Tanaka, N., Goepfert, J. M., Traisman, E., and Hoffbeck, W. M. (1979). A challenge of pasteurized process cheese spread with *Clostridium botulinum* spores. *J. Food Prot. 42*: 787–789.

Tanaka, N., Traisman, E., Lee, M. H., Cassens, R. G., and Foster, E. M. (1980). Inhibition of botulinum toxin formation in bacon by acid development. *J. Food Prot. 43*: 450–457.

Tanaka, N., Meske, L., Doyle, M. P., Traisman, E., Thayer, D. W., and Johnston, R. W. (1985). Plant trials of bacon made with lactic acid bacteria, sucrose and lowered sodium nitrite. *J. Food Prot. 48*: 679–686.

Tanaka, N., Traisman, E., Plantinga, P., Finn, L., Flom, W., Meske, L., and Guggisberg, J. (1986). Evaluation of factors involved in antibotulinal properties of pasteurized processed cheese spreads. *J. Food Prot. 49*: 526–531.

Todd, E. C. D. (1985a). Economic loss from foodborne disease and non-illness related recalls because of mishandling by food processors. *J. Food Prot. 48*: 621–633.

Todd, E. C. D. (1985b). Economic loss from foodborne disease outbreaks associated with foodservice establishments. *J. Food Prot. 48*: 169–180.

Tompkin, R. B. (1980). Botulism from meat and poultry products—a historical perspective. *Food Technol. 34*(5): 229–236, 259.

Tompkin, R. B. (1984). Indirect antimicrobial effects in foods: Phosphates. *J. Food Safety 6*: 13–27.

Troller, J. A. (1973). The water relations of food-borne bacterial pathogens. *J. Milk Food Technol. 36*: 276–288.

Tsang, N., Post, L. S., and Solberg, M. (1985). Growth and toxin production by *Clostridium botulinum* in model acidified systems. *J. Food Sci. 50*: 961–965.

Van Ermengem, E. P. M. (1897). Über einen neuen anaeroben Bacillus und seine Beziehungen zum Botulismus. *Z. Hyg. Infedtionskr. 26*: 1–56. Translated by S. Desch in *Rev. Infect. Dis. 1*: 701–719, 1979.

Wagner, M. K. (1986). Phosphates as antibotulinal agents in cured meats: A review. *J. Food Prot. 49*: 482–487.

Wallen, S. E. (1983). Understanding botulism. *Dairy Food Sanit. 3*: 4–8.

Wang, Y., and Sugiyama, H. (1983). Extraction of botulinum toxin with urea buffer. *J. Food Prot. 46*: 861–863.

Weickert, M. J., Chambliss, G. H., and Sugiyama, H. (1986). Production of toxin by *Clostridium botulinum* type A strains cured of plasmids. *Appl. Environ. Microbiol. 51*: 52–56.

Wong, D. M., Young-Perkins, K. E., and Merson, R. L. (1988). Factors influencing *Clostridium botulinum* spore germination, outgrowth and toxin formation in acidified media. *Appl. Environ. Microbiol. 54*: 1446–1450.

Woodburn, M. J., Somers, E., Rodriguez, J., and Schantz, E. J. (1979). Heat inactivation rates of botulinum toxins A, B, E and F in some foods and buffers. *J. Food Sci. 44*: 1658–1661.

Wooldord, A., Schantz, E. J., and Woodburn, M. J. (1978). Heat inactivation of botulinal toxin type A in some convenience foods after frozen storage. *J. Food Sci. 43*: 622–624.

Young-Perkins, K. E., and Merson, R. L. (1987). *Clostridium botulinum* spore germination, outgrowth and toxin production below 4.6; interactions between pH, total acidity and buffering capacity. *J. Food Sci. 52*: 1084–1088, 1096.

III

PLANT AND FUNGAL ORIGIN

9

Mushroom Poisons

Heinz Faulstich and Theodor Wieland

Max-Planck-Institut für Medizinische Forschung, Heidelberg, Germany

I. INTRODUCTION

This chapter is intended to summarize our present knowledge of toxic components occurring in mushrooms. While the toxicity of most of the poisonous mushroom species has long been known, that of others has been recognized only in recent decades. Each of the sections dealing with the various toxic components will first cite the mushroom species most frequently involved and then describe the symptoms and the chemistry of the toxic compounds. Included is the concentration of the toxin in the mushroom tissue and methods of detection. Whenever possible, toxicology and the mechanism of action are discussed. No information is given on the treatment of the various intoxications.

Most of this chapter deals with the syndromes produced by amatoxins and orrellanine, which cause by far the greatest number of fatalities. These two sections include the most up-to-date data available in this field at present. Other kinds of mushroom poisoning are discussed in a less detailed manner, but references for further information are given. For further general studies the following are recommended: Rumack and Salzman, 1978; Faulstich et al., 1980; Flammer and Horak, 1983; Bresinsky and Besl, 1985; and Flammer, 1985a,b.

II. AMATOXINS

A. Amatoxin-Accumulating Species

By far the largest number of cases of severe mushroom poisoning are produced by the green death cap *Amanita phalloides*. Given its high content of amatoxins and its abundance all over Europe, it is easy to understand that this species accounts for more than 90% of all fatal cases on the continent. Estimates of amatoxin poisonings in Europe vary between 50 and 500 cases per year.

Considering that 64 children were treated for amatoxin poisoning in 1988 at the Children's Health Center in Warsaw alone and that 16 of these died (Socha, personal communication, 1990), the higher number is probably realistic. Increasingly, cases of *A. phalloides* poisoning are reported in North America (Frank and Cummins, 1987).

Among the white *Amanitas*, the white subspecies *A. phalloides* var. *verna* is very rare and only occasionally causes poisoning (Hazani et al., 1983). In contrast, the destroying angel, *A. virosa* is frequent on the East Coast of the United States as well as in some places in Europe, for example southern Sweden or central France. While its content of amatoxins may be somewhat lower than that of the green species, it still represents one of the most dangerous mushroom species (Piering and Bratanow, 1990). Although visually not very attractive for mushroom hunters, some amatoxin-containing species of the genera *Lepiota* and *Galerina* appear to be increasingly involved in casualties. For example, *L. helveola* and *L. fulvella* (Piqueras, 1984; Sanz et al., 1989), *L. josserandi* (Bon and Boif) (Haines et al., 1985), and *L. brunneoincarnata* (Schulz-Weddingen, 1986; Langer et al., 1990) have been identified as the cause of severe mushroom poisonings.

Other species of the genera *Amanita, Galerina,* and *Lepiota* such as *A. bisporigera, A. tenuifolia, A. ocreata, A. suballiacea, G. autumnalis,* and *L. brunneolilacea* must be regarded as potentially deadly following the identification of amatoxins in their tissues.

B. Symptoms, Diagnosis, and Prognosis

First symptoms of *Amanita* poisoning occur after a latency period of 6–24 h (usually 8–12 h, rarely up to 48 h), sometimes referred to as phase I. Such a long symptomless period is one of the most important indications of amatoxin poisoning. In meals of mixed mushrooms containing toxic *Amanita* spp. as well as species causing gastrointestinal disorders within a short latency period, the presence of amatoxins may, however, be masked. In the second phase, defined as the gastrointestinal phase, heavy vomiting, severe abdominal cramps, and nausea occur, accompanied by water diarrhea causing severe dehydration and oliguria, together with loss of electrolytes and acid-base disorders. Persistence of diarrhea during this period is a strong indication for amatoxin poisoning (Zilker, 1987). During phase II, which lasts for 24–36 h, disturbances of blood coagulation begin, in particular a decrease of prothrombin time. Phase III, lasting 12–24 h, is characterized by an improvement of clinical symptoms, while elevated values of transaminases AST and ALT (SGOT, SGPT) reveal the beginning of liver necrosis. The last phase (IV) is determined by hepatic failure, encephalopathy, and very often acute renal failure. In addition, internal bleeding is observed and may cause complications or even death. Patients usually die within days 5–8, but deaths may occur as late as 20 days (Marugg and Reutter, 1985) or even 25 days (Hruby et al., 1979) after the mushroom meal.

In order to decide whether or not a patient is to be submitted to intensive care treatment, it is of great importance to know the existence and severity of amatoxin poisoning. Physical, chemical, and immunological methods for the identification of amatoxins in body fluids have been proposed (see below), but there is considerable evidence today that no correlation exists between the amatoxin concentration in urine or peripheral blood and the severity of an amatoxin poisoning (Jankowska et al., personal communication, 1990). Besides anamnesis and the identification of the offending mushroom, the latency period is one of the most reliable tools for diagnosis as well as for prognosis. Experimental studies with laboratory animals, as well as clinical experience, have shown that a short latency period (6–9 h) is indicative for the ingestion of large amounts of amatoxins and, correspondingly, a severe course of intoxication (Marugg and Reutter, 1985; Piqueras, personal communication, 1990). Another important tool for prognosis is the prothrombin time, particularly the rate at which this parameter decreases. There is general agreement today that a steep decline of this laboratory value (<10% after 48 h) suggests a poor prognosis. Similarly, an early and steep increase of transaminase values (AST, ALT > 2000 U/L) or bilirubin (>50 μmol/L) is indicative of a poor prognosis, more so than the maximum values reached (Marugg and Reutter, 1985; Socha, personal communication, 1990). Early prognostic parameters are desirable with respect to liver transplantation, because by the time the indications for this life-saving surgery are clear, the patient's overall state of health may have deteriorated too much.

C. Chemistry

Amatoxins are cyclic peptides built from eight amino acids. While all the amino acids are in the L-configuration, three of them differ from amino acids in proteins in the hydroxylation of their side chains: OH-proline, $(OH)_2$-isoleucine, (6′-OH)-tryptophan. Another unusual feature of the toxins is an R-configurated sulfoxide bridge between the side chains of cysteine and (6′-OH)-tryptophan, resulting in a rigid, pretzel-like shape of the molecules (Wieland and Faulstich, 1978). The family of amatoxins comprises nine members; most of them, however, are found in very small amounts or even traces, so that they will not contribute to poisoning. In *A. phalloides* mushrooms amatoxins are made up of nearly equal amounts of α-amanitin, the acidic β-amanitin and some γ-amanitin (<10%) (Fig. 1). On average, *A. phalloides* mushrooms contain amatoxins in amounts of ca 3.5 mg/g dry weight. Recent toxicity studies in the mouse show that the LD_{50} of all three main amatoxins are nearly equal (ca. 0.5–0.75 mg/kg bwt, depending on the strain).

In *A. virosa* mushrooms the acidic amatoxin component can be absent, while α-amanitin is found in amounts of 2.0 mg/g dry weight. Interestingly, some *A. virosa* mushroom samples collected in Virginia were found to contain no α-amanitin but amaninamide (Fig. 1) instead, which is α-amanitin without the 6′ hydroxy group at the tryptophan moiety (Buku et al., 1980). Since Yocum and Simons (1977) also reported on an American *A. virosa* sample in which α-amanitin was absent and only amanin (probably amaninamide) was detected, the possibility exists that *A. virosa* mushrooms growing at some locations in North America lack the ability to hydroxylate the aromatic

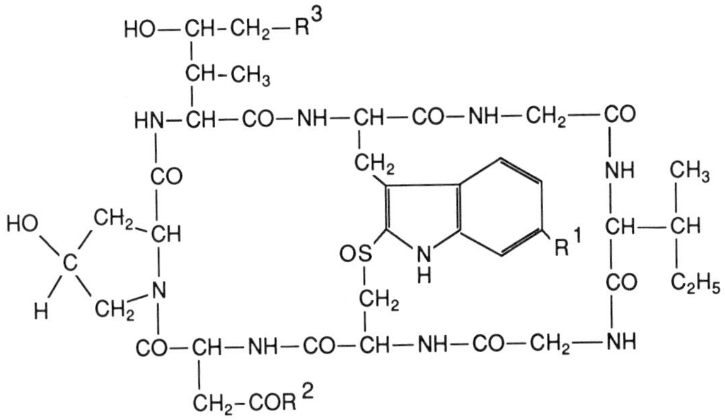

Figure 1 Structures of α-amanitin (R^1 = OH, R^2 = NH_2, R^3 = OH), β-amanitin (R^1 = OH, R^2 = OH, R^3 = OH), γ-amanitin (R^1 = OH, R^2 = NH_2, R^3 = H), and amaninamide (R^1 = H, R^2 = NH_2, R^3 = OH).

side chain. Some samples of toxic *Galerina* and *Lepiota* spp. analyzed previously contained α-amanitin in amounts of ca 1.0 mg/g dry weight, while acidic or minor components of the amatoxins were absent. More recent work, however, shows that *Galerina* mushrooms exist that also contain β- and γ-amanitin (Enjalbert, pers. comm.), and that the amatoxin content of small Lepiotas may be distinctly higher (3.2–3.5 mg/g dry weight) (Haines et al., 1985; Piqueras, personal communication, 1990) than known so far.

Most of the *Amanita* species (*A. phalloides, A. phalloides* var. *verna, A. virosa, A. bisporigera*) contain a second family of toxic peptides, the phallotoxins. These toxic peptides do not contribute to amatoxin poisoning, as is obvious from the fact that toxic *Lepiota* or *Galerina* spp. cause the same amatoxin syndrome but completely lack phallotoxins. In addition, it was shown that all symptoms described as typical for human amatoxin poisoning, including gastrointestinal disease, could be produced in dogs by sole administration of pure amatoxins. The failure of phallotoxins to contribute may be understood by their lower toxicity (LD_{50} in the mouse is ca 2.0 mg/kg bwt) and/or by an insufficient absorption of these toxins in the gastrointestinal tract. *A. virosa* mushrooms contain, beside the phallotoxins, a third family of toxic peptides, the virotoxins (Faulstich et al., 1980). They exhibit biological activities very similar to phallotoxins and are therefore likewise thought not to contribute to poisonings of *A. virosa*.

D. Methods of Detection

For the detection of amatoxins in mushroom tissue, a simple assay, the Newspaper Test by Wieland (1949), has been reported. A drop of mushroom juice is applied on lignine-containing paper, dried, and treated with concentrated (10 N) hydrochloric acid. After a couple of minutes a blue or—if the mushroom juice was colored—greenish-blue stain develops if amatoxins are present. The limit of detection is 20 μg amatoxin/ml. It is important to note that with this assay amanin and amaninamide, which can represent the whole amatoxin content of *A. virosa* mushrooms, remain undetected. A screening assay by Seeger (1984) showed that of 335 gill-bearing mushroom species submitted to the Newspaper Test, 19% were found to be positive but did not contain amatoxins. On the other hand, none of the esteemed edible mushroom species were among the 63 excluded by this study. On paper and thin layer chromatograms, small amounts of amatoxins are detected as purple spots by spraying with cinnamaldehyde and exposing to vapors of hydrochloric acid (Wieland et al., 1949).

For the detection of amatoxins in biological fluids (urine, serum, gastric or duodenal juice) immunological methods have been developed. A radioimmunoassay established in our own laboratory (Faulstich et al., 1982) is based on the replacement of a tritiated amatoxin from nylon-supported antibodies. With a limit of detection of ca 3 ng amatoxin/ml, it has been used for several years for the detection of amatoxins in patients' urine. No cross-reaction of the antibodies used is known, so the presence of amatoxins in urine samples unambiguously indicates the ingestion of amanitin- or amaninamide-containing mushrooms. However, cases of severe amanitin intoxication were recently reported where urine values of amatoxins were <20 ng/ml. A careful evaluation of clinical parameters and RIA-determined amatoxin concentrations of urine of more than 100 patients at the Children's Health Center in Warsaw revealed that a significant correlation does not exist (Jankowska et al., personal communication, 1990). A sensitivity approximately 10 times greater than for the tritium assay is reached by a radioimmunoassay established recently by a Swiss group (Andres et al., 1986; Andres and Frei, 1987). This assay measures the amount of a ^{125}I-labeled amatoxin bound—in competition to the native toxin to be determined—to an amatoxin-specific antibody and thus avoids the quench problems of tritium. It seems particularly suited for amatoxin determination in patients' serum, where the concentration is usually distinctly lower than that in urine. However, many experts today also question the existence of a correlation between the severity of amatoxin poisoning and the concentration of amatoxins in peripheral blood.

Physical determinations of amatoxins use high performance liquid chromatography (HPLC), mass spectrometry, or fluorometry. HPLC, as introduced by Beutler and Der-Marderosian (1981) and further developed by others (Jehl et al., 1985; Caccialanza et al., 1985; Donner et al., 1987; Rieck and Platt, 1988), has been claimed to possess a limit of detection of 10 ng amatoxin/ml. A limitation of this method is, however, that at the typical R_F values substances different from amatoxins may show up. Furthermore, some of the assays do not include β-amanitin. This is a considerable deficit, because in some *A. phalloides* samples analyzed in our laboratory β-amanitin accounted for more than 60% of the whole amatoxin content. Fast-atom-bombardment mass spectrometry (Pudill, 1989) and fluorescence spectroscopy of amatoxins (Little and Preston, 1984) have so far only been explored with solutions containing pure toxins.

E. Toxicokinetics

The toxicokinetics of the amatoxins are largely determined by their low molecular weight (ca. 900) and amphilic nature, i.e., solubility in water as well as in polar organic solvents. Absorption of the toxins from the intestinal tract must occur quickly, because in one case of amatoxin poisoning the amatoxins could be detected in urine only ca. 2 h after ingestion (Homann et al., 1986). In dogs it was shown that after i.v. administration of a radioactively labeled amanitin the toxin was distributed into the extracellular space (Faulstich et al., 1985). Excretion by urine was high and accounted for more than 80% of the whole dose (Faulstich, 1980). Uptake of amatoxins from the portal blood is achieved by a multispecific transporting system present on the sinusoidal side of hepatocytes (Kröncke et al., 1986). With amatoxins this transporting system works at a relatively low rate, accounting for only 5% of the phallotoxin transporting rate. However, it seems to be efficient enough to achieve an intracellular concentration of amatoxins that is able to block the transcription enzyme RNA polymerase II.

Considering that the concentration of RNA polymerase II in hepatocytes is ca. 5×10^{-8} M (Cochet-Meilhac et al., 1974) and that the K_D value of the amatoxin–RNA polymerase II complex is ca. 1×10^{-8} M (Cochet-Meilhac and Chambon, 1974), a considerable part of the toxin complex must be present in the dissociated state. This may explain the high elimination rate of amatoxins into bile. We determined that after a 30-min perfusion of rat liver, approximately two-thirds of the amount of the radioactive amatoxin taken up could be recovered in the bile fluid (Jahn et al., 1980). By such efficient self-purification, an amatoxin-poisoned liver may be free from amatoxins within a few hours—provided the uptake is completely interrupted. This, however, is not easily achieved. Even in cases where by extensive cleaning of the bowel the primary absorption of the toxins is stopped, the liver would be exposed to amatoxins excreted into bile and reabsorbed by the gastrointestinal tract. Proof of the importance of the enterohepatic circulation of amatoxins was given in 1973, when we showed that dogs poisoned with otherwise lethal doses of amanitin could be saved by means of a choledochus drainage (Fauser and Faulstich, 1973). Piqueras (personal communication, 1990) and Frank and Cummins (1987) have shown that biliary endoscopic diversion in humans removed amatoxins and may therefore represent an effective therapy. Interruption of the enterohepatic circulation is also possible using drugs. Among several drugs examined in our laboratory in the perfused rat liver, silibindihemisuccinate (silibinin) was the most efficient in suppressing the uptake of a radioactive-labeled amatoxin (Jahn et al., 1980).

F. Toxicology

Amatoxins primarily affect three types of cells: mucosal cells of the gastrointestinal tract, hepatocytes, and probably renal tubular cells. Specificity for these three kinds of cells may be understood by the fact that permeation of the toxins through the membranes of these cells is facilitated. In hepatocytes the transporting system responsible for the uptake of amatoxins has been identified (Kröncke et al., 1986), and a similar transporting system probably exists in mucosal cells. Absorption of amatoxins by mucosal cells may explain most of the symptoms observed during the gastrointestinal phase, such as vomiting and diarrhea. Renal cells are thought to be affected because the kidney excretes large amounts of amatoxins. Reabsorption of the toxins in the proximal tubules, however, seems unlikely. Interestingly, vomiting and diarrhea were also observed in dogs administered a lethal dose of amanitin parenterally (Faulstich and Fauser, 1980). Here, however, it cannot be excluded that the toxin had taken a route from liver to intestine. The gastrointestinal symptoms cause serious losses of water and salt that have to be balanced.

Among the first liver symptoms is hypoglycemia. The spontaneous drop of blood glucose may result from impaired glycogenolysis and/or gluconeogenesis and thus reflect the beginning of liver failure (Bivins et al., 1985), but it may also be due to a rise of insulin as stated recently by Kelner and Alexander (1987). In the experiments with dogs, hypoglycemia was found to be the cause of death of many animals if blood glucose was not substituted. Since balance of glucose together with substitution of water and electrolytes is a must in all protocols of amatoxin treatment, hypoglycemia is usually not a problem in human *Amanita* poisoning.

A serious symptom is disorder of blood coagulation. Disseminated intravasal coagulation (DIC) has been diagnosed in many cases and was seen as the cause of necrotic areas in the kidney (Wagner-Thiessen, 1983). From the second day, prothrombin activity is found decreased in all severe cases and may become lower than 10% of the normal value. As a consequence extended gastrointestinal bleeding may occur. Another sign of severe liver necrosis is the increase of serum concentrations of transaminases, AST, and ALT, which are taken as parameters of diagnosis as well as prognosis. Only after the third day were bilirubin elevated and the patients jaundiced. In severe cases a hepatic encephalopathy develops, which may reach the stage of coma.

Acute kidney failure as reported to occur frequently in the late phase of *Amanita* poisoning represents in most cases a hepato-renal symptom. (During the gastrointestinal phase a functional renal failure due to hypovolemia is observed.) A direct impact of amatoxins on kidney cells is still a matter of controversy (Marugg and Reutter, 1985; Zilker, 1987; Homann, 1989). For patients (Zilker, 1987) as well as for laboratory animals (Faulstich and Fauser, 1980) it was reported that individuals can die after a long delay showing all symptoms of renal failure while hepatic functions are fully recovered. Typical signs of kidney failure are the increase of blood creatinine and a significant loss of serum phosphate (Marugg and Reutter, 1985; Ryzko et al., 1987).

According to Socha (personal communication, 1990) the following symptoms developed in the course of poisoning in patients that subsequently died: coma (100%); oliguria/anuria (70%); a PT index < 30% (96%); transaminase > 2000 U/ml (92%). Today, mortality following amatoxin poisoning is commonly reported to be 10–20%. A more precise estimate is not available because any ratio reported will depend on whether less severe cases of mushroom poisoning have been identified correctly as *Amanita* poisoning.

G. Mechanism of Action

Tracing back nuclear lesions in livers of mice poisoned with α-amanitin such as condensation of chromatin and fragmentation of nucleoli to the biochemical event, Stirpe and Fiume (1967) detected that amanitin inhibits one of the transcription enzymes, RNA polymerase II. Independent of their origin, all mammalian enzymes of this type show similar susceptibility to α-amanitin, with K_i values around 10^{-8} M. Other transcription enzymes of mammalian origin are much less susceptible (RNA polymerase III, $K_i = 10^{-5}$ M) or not at all (RNA polymerase I, $K_i > 10^{-3}$ M).

Since in mammalian cells no other proteins are known that bind to α-amanitin as strongly as does RNA polymerase II, all toxic effects caused by amanitin are likely due to the inhibition of this enzyme. RNA polymerase II transcribes hn RNA, which after processing yields mRNA, the template for protein synthesis. If amanitin penetrates into cells, the inhibition of transcription must result in a lack of RNA copies and, consequently, of the corresponding proteins necessary to maintain the functions of life. The crucial parameter in this process seems to be the period of time a cell is exposed to amatoxins. Although no damage becomes visible during this stage, the stock of RNA molecules kept by the cell is continuously decreasing by natural degradation. This process is silent and may last for hours or even days. However, at the moment, when the information for an essential protein is lacking, leading to a deficit that can no longer be balanced, the point of no return is reached, and the cell turns necrotic.

RNA polymerases II of eukaryotic cells are complex enzymes consisting of numerous subunits, the largest being 180–220 kd, the smallest ca. 20 kd (see, for example, Kedinger and Chambon, 1972). Through affinity labeling experiments, Brodner and Wieland (1976) pinpointed the second largest subunit (140 kd) as the binding site of amatoxins. Vaisius and Wieland (1982) reported that RNA polymerase II, in the presence of α-amanitin, can still form a dinucleotide, but not oligomers composed of three or more nucleotides. It was concluded that elongation, but not initiation, is inhibited by amatoxins.

Because the formation of a trinucleotide, unlike the formation of a dinucleotide, requires movement of the enzyme on the single-stranded DNA, it can be concluded that amatoxins actually block the ability of the enzyme to move on the template. If amatoxins indeed act as a brake shoe in the moving of a mechanical system, an antidote cannot easily be envisaged. Classical antidotes like atropin against muscarine poisoning act on complex systems where binding and toxic activity may represent two different events. In amatoxin poisoning, reactivation of the enzyme could only occur by removal of the toxin. One possibility for this might be the administration of amatoxin-binding proteins able to sequester free toxin in the cardiovascular system. It was proved, however, that such amatoxin-binding proteins cannot be immunoglobulins. In a study aiming at the neutralization of amatoxins—in analogy to snake bites—by injection of monoclonal antibodies or Fab fragments into mice, we detected that due to glomerular filtration and reabsorption of the toxin complexes in proximal tubular cells of kidney, toxicity of α-amanitin was increased tremendously, up to 50-fold (Faulstich et al., 1988).

III. GYROMITRIN; OTHER HEPATOTOXINS

A. *Gyromitra esculenta*

Gyromitra esculenta (Pers. ex Fr.), the false morel, a short-stalked mushroom with a brainlike folded cap of red to dark brown color was considered a delicious edible mushroom for centuries until it turned out to contain, in the raw state, toxic substances that can cause death. Franke et al. (1967) presented a compilation of 513 cases of poisoning including 14.5% fatalities. The severe cases occurred after ingestion of raw or insufficiently cooked false morels, while after extensive cooking and discarding the water, or after drying the mushrooms, poisoning occurred only rarely.

B. Symptoms

The symptoms of intoxication are similar to those of poisoning by *Amanita phalloides*. After a latency period of 6–20 h a gastrointestinal phase develops including symptoms like vomiting, abdominal pain, nausea, and headache, and in some patients also diarrhea. In most cases this phase ends with recovery within 2–6 days. However, after ingestion of large amounts of weakly cooked false morels, a hepatorenal phase can follow with symptoms of liver injury, haemoglobinuria, or anuria. Predominant symptoms of this phase are nervous disturbances like difficulties in moving, cramps, deliria, and even unconsciousness. Death can occur through collapse of circulation.

Besides acute liver illness, the toxic components of *G. esculenta* can cause cancer. This was shown for pentanalmethylformylhydrazone, which induced tumors in lungs, liver, and preputial glands in Swiss mice (Toth and Raha, 1987).

C. Chemistry and Detection

The main component of *Gyromitra esculenta*, gyromitrin, is a volatile compound, the formylmethylhydrazone of acetaldehyde (Fig. 2a) (List and Luft, 1968). By gas chromatographic analysis of *Gyromitra* mushrooms, small amounts of formylmethylhydrazones of eight higher alphatic aldehydes were detected by Pyysalo (1975). Gyromitrin is an unstable substance, prone to hydrolysis and oxidation. By hydrolysis, which occurs also in the intestinal tract, gyromitrin is cleaved into methylformylhydrazine (Fig. 2b), which after loss of the formyl residue yields *N*-methylhydrazine (Fig. 2c), the real poison. The instability of gyromitrin suggests that in the mushroom it will exist not in the free state but bound to high molecular components, possibly as a glycoside (Stijve, 1978). Indeed, for determining the poison in mushroom material it cannot simply be extracted from dry mushroom powder with water-free solvents (List and Luft, 1969) but has to be heated with water to 120°C in a closed tube for several hours and extracted as *N*-methylhydrazine from the water phase by chloroform in an atmosphere of nitrogen.

By gas chromatography, according to Pyysalo and Niskanen (1977) or Stijve (1978), several micrograms of gyromitrin can be detected. More sensitive is a thin-layer chromatographic method using Kieselgel 60 F 254 (nanoDC) described by Stijve (1978) by which, after development in chloroform:methanol (9:1) as few as 0.02 μg of gyromitrin can be identified. For visualization, the plate is sprayed with cinnamaldehyde/HCl and heated to 80°C for several minutes, until the substance appears as bright yellow spots. One kilogram of fresh mushroom contains from 1.0 to 1.5 g of the poison. The lethal dose for children is assumed to be about 10–30 mg/kg body weight, for adults 20–50 mg/kg. One can estimate that for children a few mushrooms must be sufficient to cause illness.

D. *Amanita abrupta*

Recently hepatotoxic agents have been reported to occur in a rare *Amanita* species from Japan, *A. abrupta* (Yamaura et al., 1986). Although distinctly less toxic than *A. phalloides* or *A. virosa, A. abrupta* causes symptoms similar to *A. phalloides*, such as decrease of serum glucose, depletion of liver glycogen, and a transient and moderate rise of serum transaminases (AST, ALT). While amatoxins were shown to be absent, an unsaturated amino acid, L-2-amino-4-pentynoic acid, has been proposed as the hepatotoxic agent of this mushroom (Yamaura et al., 1986). Besides this amino acid, L-2-amino-4,5-hexadienoic acid and a chlorohydrin, (2S,4Z)-2-amino-5-chloro-6-hydroxy-4-hexenoic acid (Ohta et al., 1987), were isolated from *A. abrupta*.

IV. ORELLANINE

A. Toxic *Cortinarius* Species

Cortinarius is the largest genus of fungi in Europe, and at least two species are severely toxic. The toxicity of *Cortinarius orellanus* (*Fries*), a medium sized, fox-colored mushroom, became first apparent in 1952 when 102 inhabitants of Bydgosz (Poland) fell ill after ingestion of this mushroom (Grzymala, 1957, 1962). Eleven of them died 4–16 days after the mushroom meal with acute renal failure. Similarly, the closely related, rust-brown species *Cortinarius*

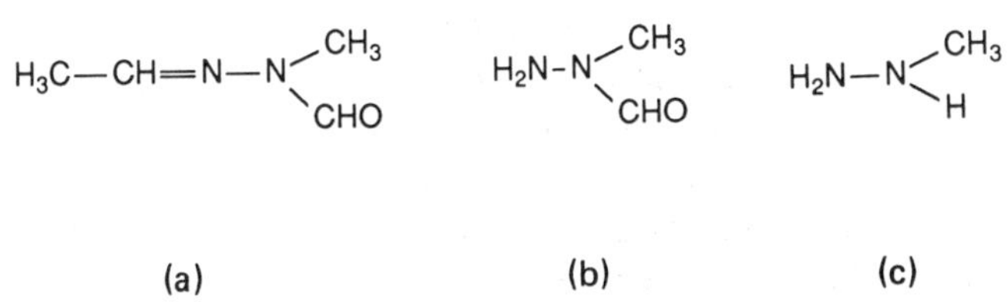

Figure 2 Structures of (a) gyromitrine, (b) *N,N*-formylmethylhydrazine, and (c) *N*-methylhydrazine.

speciosissimus (*Kühn et Romagn*), which is found more frequently in northern Europe, was proved toxic (Hulmi et al., 1974; Möttönen et al., 1975), presumably by the same principle. More recently, intoxications by *Cortinarius splendens* have been reported from France (Gérault, 1981), again with symptoms similar to those indicated above. Poisoning by *Cortinarius* species must certainly have occurred in earlier times, too; however, the connection between the ingestion of these mushrooms and the symptoms had not been realized, owing to a very long latency period which may amount to more than 2 weeks. Several cases of *Cortinarius* poisoning reported from various countries in the past decades have been extensively described in a review by Schumacher and Høiland (1983).

B. Symptoms

Flammer (1982) describes the symptoms as tiredness, excessive thirst, dryness and burning pain in the mouth, gastric and abdominal pain, nausea, emesis, chills and pains in the loins, diarrhea, and pains of muscles and joints. In a later phase, oliguria or even anuria may appear as a consequence of kidney damage, apparent even in the early stages from increasing blood concentrations of urea and creatinine. In severe cases irreversible renal failure may develop, which today, however, can be managed by timely hemoperfusion or renal transplantation.

C. Chemistry

In 1962, Grzymala prepared from *Cortinarius* mushrooms an almost pure toxin fraction for which he coined the name orellanine. Antkowiak and Gessner (1975) identified two homogeneous toxic substances and proposed their structures. According to these authors orellanine, the main component is 3,3′-, 4,4′-tetrahydroxy-2,2′-bipyridyl-*N,N*′-dioxide (Fig. 3a), while the second component orellinine was suggested to be the monodeoxo derivative (Fig. 3b) (Antkowiak and Gessner, 1979). The structures have been confirmed by chemical synthesis (Dehmlow and Schulz, 1985, 1987; Tiecco et al., 1986; Hasseberg and Gerlach, 1988). Due to sterically hindered rotation, orellanine and orellinine may exist in two atropisomeric forms. In addition, both orellanine and orellinine can adopt tautomeric chinonelike structures. In crystals of the trichloroacetic acid complex of orellanine, the two rings were found in a position virtually perpendicular to each other (Cohen-Addad et al., 1987). Chemically, the pyridine-*N*-oxide structures of orellanine are unstable. On heating, or on UV irradiation on cellulose thin layer plates, orellanine is decomposed into its bisdeoxo form (Fig. 3c), orelline, a yellow and blue fluorescent compound that is nontoxic for animals (Antkowiak and Gessner, 1985). Other substances isolated or claimed to have been isolated from *Orellanus* species play no role in mushroom poisoning. Evidence for the existence of a neurotoxin has been given by Kürnsteiner and Moser (1981) and confirmed by Prast et al. (1985). However, paralytic effects in mice were observed only after intraperitoneal injection of extremely high doses, but not after peroral administration. The existence of

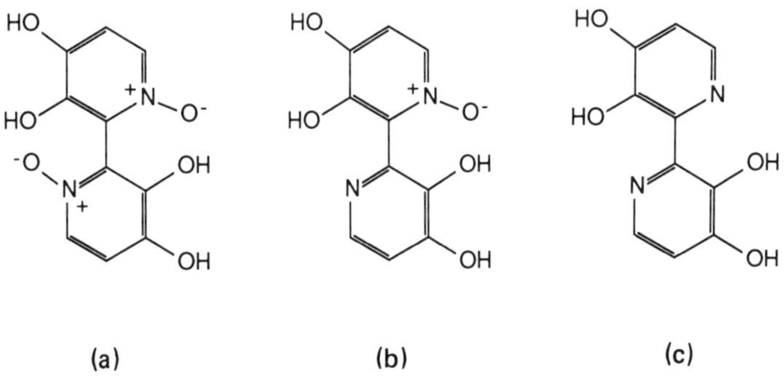

Figure 3 Structures of (a) orellanine, (b) orellinine, and (c) orelline.

cyclic kidney-toxic peptides called cortinarin A, B, and C (Tebbett and Caddy, 1984) has so far not been confirmed by others (Laatsch and Matthies, 1991).

D. Methods of Detection

A simple method for detecting orellanine in an aqueous extract of fresh or dried mushroom was described by Schumacher and Høiland (1983). It makes use of the grey-blue color generated by orellanine with $FeCl_3$ in acidic solution. This reaction can also be applied to thin layers after chromatography in *n*-butanol:acetic acid:water (3:1:1) where the compound either appears as a streak of R_F = 0.0–0.5 (on silica) or R_F = 0.68 (on cellulose) (Prast and Pfaller, 1988). In their photodecomposition experiments on cellulose thin-layer plates, Antkowiak and Gessner (1985) used isopropanol:conc. HCl:water (85:22:18) as solvent and detected the single components by their typical hues of blue fluorescence under UV light: navy blue for orellanine (R_F = 0.78), dark blue for orellinine (R_F = 0.66), and light blue for the nontoxic orelline (R_F = 0.48). Due to composition in daylight or during inspection of the plates under UV light, the color of orellanine may change. Thin-layer chromatography (TLC) on cellulose plates with a complex solvent system consisting of *n*-butanol:HCl:chloroform:water (40:20:15:3.8) was employed for detecting the decomposition products of orellanine in biological fluids and renal biopsies by Rapior et al. (1989). Besides TLC, HPLC has been reported as a method for the analysis of mushroom extracts (Holmdahl et al., 1987). The concentration of 1.5% orellanine in dried mushrooms as determined by Antkowiak and Gessner (1975) was roughly confirmed by Prast et al. (1985) who by TLC found 1.4% in dried *C. orellanus* and 0.9% in *C. speciosissimus*. Cantin et al. (1989) using reversed-phase HPLC on two different silica phases under relatively strong acidic conditions found 1.2%. These authors also reinvestigated several thin-layer systems described by former authors.

E. Toxicology

As mentioned above, the mushroom poisoning reported in 1952 differed from others by two remarkable features: the mushroom predominantly caused nephrotoxic effects, and it produced its first symptoms after 2–6 days, in one case as late as 17 days. The unusually prolonged incubation time represents a typical symptom of *C. orellanus* poisoning as already shown by S. Grzymala. He reported that various animals poisoned either orally or intraperitoneally with his purified mushroom extract died after a long lag period of 5–12 days. The histopathological findings of the kidneys of these animals were similar to those found in humans. In the following years evaluation of clinical data was intensified, and investigations were started with small laboratory animals using whole dried *Cortinarius* mushrooms as well as pure orellanine. Recent toxicity data reported LD_{50} values of 12.5–20 mg orellanine/kg mouse (Prast et al., 1985; Holmdahl et al., 1987; Richard et al., 1988) if the toxin was administered intraperitoneally. For peroral administration the doses were 2–3 times higher (33–90 mg/kg mouse). According to Prast et al. (1985) 31 mg of orellanine correspond to 2.2 g of dried *C. orellanus* mushrooms. The data indicate that resorption of orellanine from the gastrointestinal tract must be slow.

The clinical expression of *orellanus* toxicosis is oliguria or anuria and acute renal failure. Occasionally, vomiting after 4–24 h was reported. Kidney damage was verified by biopsy, e.g., by Marichal et al. (1977) and Short et al. (1980). The main target of the toxin is the tubular system where the primary urine is concentrated and where xenobiotic substances are accumulated. This may explain why tissues such as glomeruli or liver, when perfused with toxin concentrations as low as in blood, show no signs of injury. On the other hand, free orellanine disappears rapidly from urine as indicated by the observation that, in male rats fed with *C. orellanus*, orellanine was detectable in urine only during the first 24 h (Prast and Pfaller, 1988).

The histopathological alterations in kidneys of experimental animals were examined by several groups using light microscopy (Nieminen et al., 1975; Holmdahl et al., 1987; Richard et al., 1988) or electron microscopy (Lahtiperä et al., 1986; Prast and Pfaller, 1988). There is general agreement today that even conspicuous effects such as those occurring in epithelial cells after administration of high doses of orellanine cannot be observed until 2 days after administration, while tubular necrosis is fully developed only after 5 days. In accordance with this, cultures of epithelial cells of proximal tubules of pig kidney showed disruption of confluent monolayers after 48 h incubation with orellanine (Heufler et al., 1987). Biochemically, the activities of membrane-bound alkaline phosphatase and cytosolic lactate dehydrogenase were found decreased. Since cell membranes were not affected (exclusion of trypan-blue), an intracellular mode of action was suggested.

F. Mechanism of Action

The structure of orellanine, a bisquaternary 2,2′-dipyridinium compound (Fig. 3) prompted experiments comparing it with diquat (Fig. 4a) and paraquat (Fig. 4b) (methylviologen), which are widely used toxic herbicides causing renal failure in animals and man. Studying the toxic effects of these herbicides on rat kidney, Lock and Ishmael (1979) found that 24 h after subcutaneous

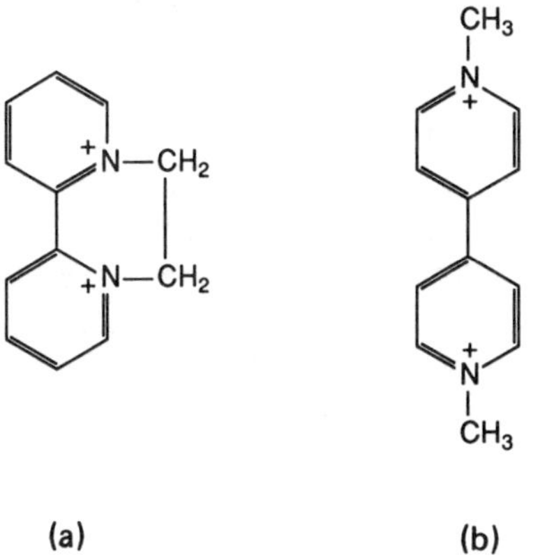

Figure 4 Structures of (a) diquat and (b) paraquat.

administration of about 20 mg/kg in rats, both compounds caused focal hydropic degeneration in proximal tubules. The effect, however, was mild as compared with that caused by orellanine or $HgCl_2$. This is in line with studies of Gstraunthaler and Prast (1983), who found that the dipyridylium herbicides are less toxic than orellanine for rats as well as for cultures of tubular epithelial cells. When assayed by the inhibition of monolayer formation, the cytotoxicity of orellanine on growing cells was 12 times higher than that of diquat and 20 times higher than that of paraquat.

The herbicides and the extracts of *Cortinarius* were also studied for their toxic effects on the photosynthetic apparatus of a green plant, *Lemna minor* (duckweed) (Høiland, 1983). These studies gave rise to the assumption that the mechanism of inhibition for orellanine and the herbicides may be the same (Schumacher and Høiland, 1983). The generally accepted theory is that the bis-quaternary herbicides are easily transformed into radicals by transmitting one electron to dioxygen, O_2, thus generating O_2 radicals ($O_2^{\circ-}$), which might damage phospholipids in membrane systems or interfere with the electron transfer in chloroplasts. On reinvestigation, however, Richard et al. (1987) found that orellanine (0.4 mM) efficiently inhibited the photosynthetic activity of *Lemna minor* but did not interfere with the chloroplastic electron transfer chain in thylakoids. A comparison of the electrochemical behavior of orellanine and paraquat revealed that voltametric reduction of orellanine is irreversible, whereas paraquat is reduced in two steps, the first being a reversible one-electron process. Hence, the modes of action of the two kinds of inhibitors seem to be different. As mentioned above, epithelial kidney cells damaged by orellanine retained intact cytoplasmic membranes (trypan-blue test) but exhibited decreased rates of nucleic acid and protein synthesis. This and the long latency period could point to an inhibition of other fundamental processes, since alterations of nuclei have been detected by electron microscopy (Lahtiperä et al., 1986).

The target structures of orellanine and orellinine, as well as their modes of action, have not yet been identified. Studies on structure-toxicity relationships by Richard et al. (1985) led to the conclusion that orellanine and orellinine are the most active components of a series of 22 molecules containing either pyridine or bipyridine structures with one or two hydroxyl groups and with the pyridine-nitrogen either in the oxidized or reduced form. Syntheses of analogs closer to the structures of the toxins have to our knowledge not been carried out. From the three naturally occurring mushroom components it can be concluded that at least one of the two *N*-oxide moieties is necessary for activity. Considering the long-term effect of orellanine, it seems possible that the toxin does not act by itself but after conversion into the proper toxic agent by unknown metabolic processes.

V. MUSCARINE

A. Mushrooms Producing Muscarine

Muscarine certainly represents the most famous mushroom poison. Moreover, muscarine was long considered to be the toxin produced by all poisonous mushrooms (Schmiedeberg and Koppe, 1869). Correspondingly, the search for this toxic ingredient played a prominent role in the history of mycotoxin research. The name was derived from the beautiful red-capped and white-spotted fly agaric, *Amanita muscaria* (*musca* = fly), which was reputed to be dangerous to man and toxic for flies when sliced and soaked in milk. *Amanita muscaria*, however, contains muscarin in only traces, while it is found in large amounts in mushrooms of the genera *Clitocybe* and *Inocybe*. It is instructive how this enduring misconception arose.

When extracts of *A. muscaria* were applied to the classical object of early pharmacologists, the frog heart, a decrease in beat amplitude and finally standstill was observed. Guided by this test, Schmiedeberg and Koppe, as early as in 1869, were able to obtain a crude preparation of muscarine. Since the drug exerts a distinct effect when only a few micrograms are applied to the frog heart in situ—a fact not envisaged by the researchers at that time—the concentration of muscarine in *A. muscaria* was overestimated for a long time. Kögl et al. (1931), who were the first to isolate muscarine as a crystalline Reineckatsalt, expected to obtain ca. 17 g of the alkaloid from 1250 kg of fly agaric but obtained only a few hundred milligrams. These workers attributed the loss to the destruction of muscarine, due to the time elapsed between the crop of the mushrooms and the preparation of the methanolic extract. Later on, however, Eugster and Waser (1951) showed that the concentration of muscarine in fly agarics is indeed only about 0.0003% of fresh weight. These authors obtained muscarine hydrochoride in a crystalline state and elucidated its structure (Eugster, 1969).

Concentrations of muscarine approximately 100-fold higher than in *A. muscaria* are present in *Inocybe* and *Clitocybe* species. Of the numerous *Inocybe* species the red staining *I. patouillardi* (Bres.) should be mentioned, which in the fresh state contains about 0.04% of the toxic substance (Eugster,

1957). A large number of similar-looking *Inocybe* species also exist that contain varying amounts of muscarine, among them *I. fastigiata* (*Schiff. ex. Fr.*), the straw-colored fiber head, *I. fibrosa*, the white *Inocybe*, and *I. geophylla*. An enumeration of all muscarine-containing *Inocybe* species is found in the work of Bresinksi and Besl (1985). *Clitocybe* species are known in Germany as *Trichterlinge*, the name being derived from the funnel-shaped hat. Among these small- to medium-sized, pale-colored mushroom species, about a dozen have been found to contain muscarine in amounts again much higher than in *A. muscaria*. Of these, only *Clitocybe dealbata*, the ivory *Clitocybe*, may be mentioned, which grows on meadows or lawns.

B. Symptoms and Toxicity

In mice, muscarine has an LD_{50} of ca. 0.25 mg/kg bwt when administered intraperitoneally, and higher if administered orally. Even if humans were several times more sensitive to muscarine than mice, a severe intoxication of man would require a large amount of *A. muscaria*. So it is unlikely that any human has ever died from muscarine after the ingestion of fly agarics.

Symptoms of poisoning caused by muscarine include salivation, lacrimation, perspiration, nausea, vomiting, headache, visual disturbances, abdominal colic, diarrhea bradycardia, and hypotension. The symptoms appear 30 min to 2 h following the ingestion of muscarine-rich carpophores. All these symptoms are understood as consequences of the parasympaticomimetic effect of muscarine. Among the psychoneurotic alterations are dizziness, disturbances of movement, excitement, and the feeling of drunkenness.

C. Chemistry and Detection

In 1931 Kögl et al., though possessing only a small amount of muscarine, recognized the trimethylammonium moiety and the presence of a hydroxyl group in the molecule, whose gross composition could be analyzed nearly correctly. Only 25 years later Eugster (1956a,b) and simultaneously Kögl et al. (1957) revealed the complete structure of 2-methyl-3-hydroxy-5-trimethylammonium-methyl-tetrahydrofuran and confirmed it by X-ray analysis. The compound has three chirality centers and hence exists in eight diastereometric forms. Among them only one, the isomer shown in Fig. 5a, exhibits the strong muscarinic effect. Other isomers were detected in traces in various mushrooms but possess only weak muscarinic activity. All isomers have been obtained by chemical synthesis (see Waser, 1961).

For a long time detection and quantitation of muscarine was a difficult task, because no sensitive color reactions or other specific chemical reactions of muscarine were known. Accordingly, mainly biological test methods have been used (Malone et al., 1969). These, however, can give erroneous results because of the existence of cholinesterlike substances that exert muscarinelike effects. Today, thin-layer methods, HPLC, and mass spectrometric methods are used, for example, high performance TLC (Stijve, 1981), by which 0.1 μg muscarine can be detected. This method uses so-called cellulose-nanoplates (Merck), which are run with a mixture of 2-butanol:95% ethanol:acetic acid:water

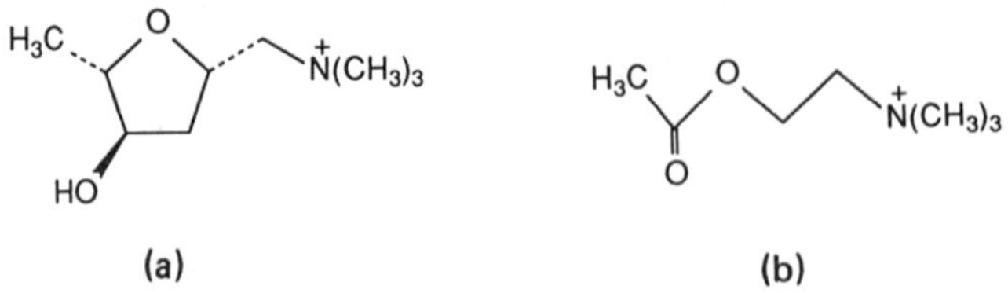

Figure 5 Structures of (a) muscarine and (b) acetylcholine.

(80:20:10:30). Muscarine is visualized by Dragendorff's reagent (a bismuth–iodide complex) and appears as an orange-colored spot of $R_F = 0.55$.

D. Mechanism of Action

Through its structural similarity to acetylcholine (Fig. 5b), muscarine binds to the acetylcholine receptor on synapses of the nerve endings of smooth muscles and endocrine glands, causing the well-known parasympaticomimetic effects. Because muscarine is not an ester like acetylcholine and hence resists esterase activity, it is not degraded but can cause continuous stimulation of the affected neurons. Incidentally, *A. muscaria* mushrooms also contain acetylcholine. A detailed survey of the pharmacology of muscarine and other muscarinelike compounds on animals as well as on isolated organs has been compiled by Waser (1961). A natural antidote is atropine, which in competition to muscarine will bind to the receptor, but not evoke a signal.

VI. MUSCIMOL, IBOTENIC ACID

A. Mushrooms Producing Muscimol

Symptoms of illness as occurring after ingestion of the fly agaric *A. muscaria* cannot be attributed to muscarine, which is present in this mushroom in only tiny amounts. The same is true for the panther cap, *A. pantheria*, and for *A. strobiliformis* which occasionally causes cases of poisoning in Japan. This inconsistency prompted Takemoto et al. (1964) in Japan and Bowden et al. (1965) in England to start a closer investigation of the active components produced by these mushrooms. At the same time Eugster et al. (1965) investigated *A. muscaria* in order to detect in these mushrooms the principle that acts on the central nervous system.

B. Chemistry and Detection

The three laboratories isolated from the mushrooms two isoxazoles, ibotenic acid (from *ibotengutake*, Japanese for *A. strobiliformis*) and muscimol, which were shown to be responsible for the insecticidal property of the mushrooms. In addition, an oxazolone, muscazone, was isolated. As shown in Figure 6a, ibotenic acid is α-amino-(4-hydroxy-isoxazole-2)-yl-acetic acid, a structure related to and possibly derived from β-oxo-L-glutamine. Muscimol (Fig. 6b) is

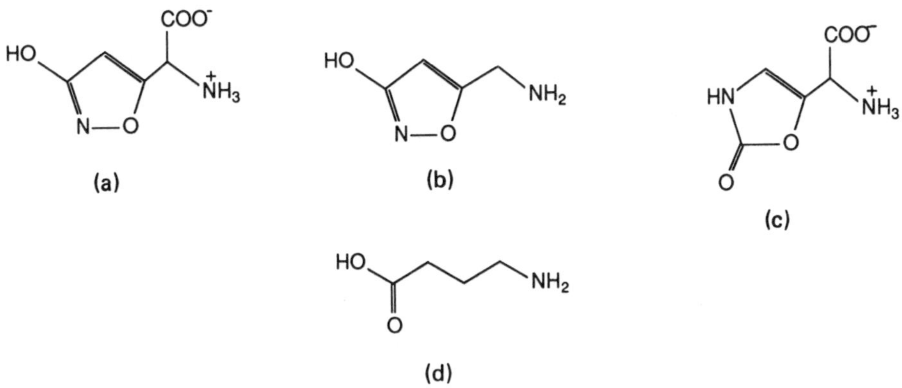

Figure 6 Structures of (a) ibotenic acid, (b) muscimol, (c) muscazone, and (d) γ-aminobutyric acid (GABA).

the decarboxylation product of ibotenic acid. It was suggested that muscazone (Fig. 6c) is formed from ibotenic acid by a photoinduced rearrangement (Göth et al., 1967). For qualitative analysis, paper chromatography or electrophoresis can be used. TLC on cellulose plates with 2-butanol:95% ethanol:acetic acid:water (75:25:5:7.5) shows, after spraying with ninhydrin and heating, muscimol as a yellow spot at $R_F = 0.35$ (Stijve, 1981). Column chromatography (Gore and Jordan, 1982) or HPLC (Lund, 1979) were also recommended for the separation and quantitation of the components of *A. muscaria* and related mushrooms. For a more recent determination of ibotenic acid and muscimol in *A. muscaria, A. pantherina*, and *A. gemmata* by two-dimensional TLC, see Beutler and DerMarderosian (1981). The amounts of the isoxazoles present in mushrooms were estimated by several authors, who reported average values of 0.2% for dried *A. muscaria* and 0.4% for *A. pantherina*. In rats the LD_{50} of muscimol was determined to be 45 mg/kg bwt by oral and about 4.5 mg/kg by i.v. administration; the corresponding values for ibotenic acid are 129 and 42 mg/kg, respectively. Perhaps ibotenic acid exerts its effect only as a source of muscimol that is generated in the body by decarboxylation (Theobald et al., 1968).

C. Symptoms and Toxicity

When eaten in larger amounts, the three mushroom species cause, beside gastrointestinal irritation, dizziness and erratic, sometimes manic, behavior, which may last for several hours. In the past these mushrooms were eaten deliberately in several places in Europe in order to produce these hallucinogenic effects. More recently, a few alarming incidents of poisoning have been reported in the United States, Europe, and South Africa, especially in children (see, e.g., Gosselin et al., 1984).

According to Theobald et al. (1968) muscimol, and to a lesser extent ibotenic acid, mainly affect psychomotor functions, while vegetative functions are left intact. Since the structure of muscimol resembles that of γ-aminobutyric acid (Fig. 6d), it was suggested by Brehm et al. (1972) that the GABA receptor of the central nervous system is the primary target of the drug. It is interesting to note that the symptoms produced by the two isoxazol components are not completely congruent with those produced by the mushrooms themselves. Therefore it cannot be excluded that other active components not yet identified may contribute to the syndrome.

VII. HALLUCINOGENIC INDOLE DERIVATIVES

A. Psilocybin, Psilocin

Mushrooms containing hallucinogenic indole derivatives are found in the genera *Psylocybe, Panaeolus, Pholiotina* (*Conocybe*), *Gymnopilus*, and, possibly, *Panaeolina*. Most widely spread in Europe and North America is *Psylocybe semilanceata*. Particularly in England and the United States, mushrooms of this and related species are used as a drug and sometimes sold, in dried form, on the black market. For reviews of this field see Francis and Murray, (1983) and Schwartz and Smith (1988). In one case the toxin was administered intravenously (Curry and Rose, 1985). Poisoning was also reported for *Panaeolus cyanescens* (Heim et al., 1966). Hallucinogenic compounds were further detected in *Pholiotina cyanopus* and *Gymnopilus spectabilis* (Hatfield et al., 1978).

According to Stamets (1978) the history of hallucinogenic mushrooms started with the use of teonanacatl in shamanic rites by certain Mexican and Central American tribes. An excursion to the American mushroom eaters and experiments performed on themselves by the Wassons (1957) resulted in cultivation of the Mexican mushrooms, probably *Psilocybe cubensis*, in the greenhouse by Heim (1978), followed by chemical investigation of the active substances by Hofmann and coworkers (1958, 1959). Psilocybin is a derivative of tryptamine, 4-phosphoryloxy-dimethyltryptamine, or 4-phosphoryloxy-3-[2-(dimethyamino)-ethyl]-indole (Fig. 7a). It was obtained by chemical synthesis in the laboratory of Hofmann et al. (1958). The dephosphorylated compound, psilocin, is not hallucinogenic and, unlike the phosphoric ester, easily decomposed by oxidation. Dried mushrooms contain approximately 0.2–0.7% of psilocybin. Baeocystine and norbaeocystine are the monomethylated and nonmethylated derivatives of psilocybin, respectively, detected in *Psilocybe baeocystis* by Leung and Paul (1968).

TLC is the method of choice for identifying indole compounds in mushrooms. Hydroxyindoles readily couple with Pauly's reagent (diazotated sulfanilic acid) to yield spots of different colors. Alternatively, detection by dimethylaminocinnamaldehyde has been recommended (Stijve et al., 1976).

Symptoms after ingestion of about 20 g of fresh mushrooms, or 4–8 mg psilocybin, start within the first half hour. Reactions to the drug vary between individuals from a feeling of relaxation to one of tension, anxiety, or dizziness. Sometimes nausea and abdominal discomfort including vomiting and diarrhea may occur. During the second half hour the occurrence of visual effects is

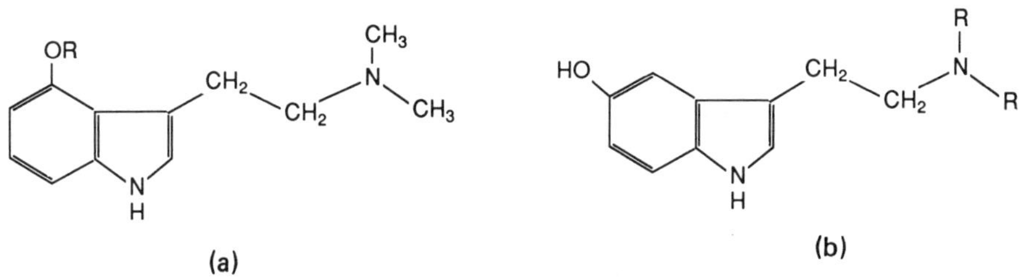

Figure 7 Structures of (a) psilocybin (R = PO_3H_2) and psilocin (R = H) and (b) bufotenine (R = CH_3). (Serotonin is structure b with R = H.)

reported, including the perception of brilliant colors and objects with closed eyes. Panic reactions have been reported, such as fear of death or insanity. During the following hours the visual effects increase and then disappear. Systemic effects are mostly due to the stimulation of the central or sympathetic nervous system, and may comprise pupillary dilation, rapid heart beat, and high blood pressure combined with low blood sugar and decreased body temperature. More details are found in a review by Vergeer (1983).

B. Bufotenin

The 5-hydroxy isomer of psilocin, bufotenine (Fig. 7b), previously isolated from toad skin (Wieland et al., 1934), has been extracted from the harmless yellow mushroom *Amanita citrina* (Wieland et al., 1953). Besides this base, precursors like 5-hydroxytryptophan and 5-hydroxytryptamine (serotonin) have been detected in various mushrooms, e.g., by Tyler (1961) and Tyler and Gröger (1964). The concentrations of the psychoactive amines, however, are too small to cause any toxicity of these mushroom species.

VIII. COPRINE

On roadsides or in grassland, mushrooms with egg-shaped grey-white fruiting bodies show up, deliquescing into ink-colored liquid when older. In the young state the inky cap, *Coprinus atramentarius*, is edible, but will cause gastrointestinal and cardiovascular disturbances when consumed together with alcoholic beverages. The reaction is similar to that of disulfiram (Antabuse) employed in the treatment of alcoholism.

Typical symptoms include flushes, mydriasis, paresthesia, tachycardia, sweating, hypertension, and nausea. The effects normally disappear after 3–4 h, but occasionally may last up to 50 h (Flammer, 1985a). The agent causing these symptoms was identified simultaneously in the United States (Hatfield and Schaumberg, 1975) and in Sweden (Lindberg et al., 1975). It was named coprine and is the amidohemiketal of cyclopropanone and L-glutamine (Fig. 8). According to Wisemann and Abeles (1979), its mode of action is understood as blocking of an essential SH-group of the liver enzyme aldehyde dehydrogenase

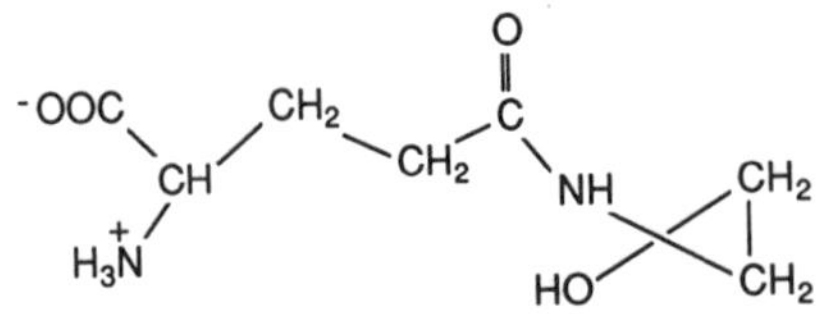

Figure 8 Structure of coprine.

under formation of a hemithioketal of cyclopropanone, released from coprine in liver. Inhibition of this enzyme leads to an elevated concentration of acetaldehyde, causing the symptoms described above.

IX. OTHERS

A. Mushrooms Causing Gastrointestinal Disorders

Although poisonings with gastrointestinal symptoms have been estimated to amount to up to 40% of all cases of mushroom poisoning (Alder, 1960), reports on them are not numerous because fatalities are very rare, and patients normally recover within a few days. In the few casualties reported so far, only children were involved (Chapuis, 1984).

Among the species most frequently involved are *Entoloma sinuatum* and *Agaricus xanthoderma*. The latter may be confused with edible *Agaricus* species, but can be easily distinguished from them by its bad odor. The odor is caused by phenols to which the gastrointestinal symptoms are also attributed. Very violent courses of gastrointestinal disorders are reported from *Tricholoma pardinum*. *Omphalotus olearius*, a mushroom that occasionally causes poisonings in southern Europe, and the related North American Jack O'Lantern are rare (French and Garretson, 1988). The gastrointestinal disorders following ingestion of these mushrooms are at least in part due to the presence of the sesquiterpene illudin S. Occasionally, poisonings caused by the genera *Lactarius* (e.g., *L. helvus*) or *Ramaria* (e.g., *R. pallida*) became known. More details are found in Bresinsky and Besl (1985).

A mushroom that since the end of the last century has been reported to sporadically cause cases of human poisoning is *Chlorophyllum molybditis*. Most of the cases occurred in the central south and southeast of the United States. *C. molybdatis*, the "green parasol," is a tall, attractive mushroom that favors grassy areas and may be mistaken for *Lepiotas*. It typically causes nausea, vomiting, and cramps, but most cases recover with supportive care within 48 h. For a review of this poisoning, see Whitaker and Box (1985).

B. Mushrooms Causing Allergic Reactions

Two mushroom species have been identified that can cause hemolytic anemia by immunoreaction: *Paxillus involutus* and *Suillus luteus* (for review see Flammer, 1985b). Both are abundant and sometimes consumed in large amounts. The severe allergic reaction must not be confused with the gastrointestinal disorders that occasionally can occur with *P. involutus* when the mushrooms are insufficiently cooked. The immune reaction can be distinguished from the gastrointestinal symptoms by a hemagglutination test described by Lefèvre (1982). The antibody produced—typically only after consumption of the mushrooms for several years—is of the IgG class. In the absence of antigen it has no effect on erythrocytes. Only when the extract of cooked mushroom, containing the still unknown antigenic component, is added, agglutination of red cells occurs ending with hemolysis. Disposition towards this immunoreaction is of course individual, and thus may lead to one participant of a mushroom meal being affected, but not others. One case has been reported where death by shock occurred $3^1/_2$ days after ingestion (Winkelmann et al., 1982).

Recently, irritations caused by an unknown toxic or allergenic compound of the shiitake mushroom, *Lentinus edodes*, were reported. This mushroom is a highly esteemed ingredient of Japanese and Chinese cuisine; however, Nakamura nd Kobayashi (1985) describe the occurrence of pruritus caused by pinhead-sized papules in 30 patients, recorded over a period of 9 years. The toxicodermia mostly developed 1 day after the ingestion of shiitake and disappeared within 8–10 days with treatment with antihistamines or glucocorticosteroids.

REFERENCES

Alder, A. E. (1960). Die Pilzvergiftungen in der Schweiz während 40 Jahren. *Schweiz. Zeitschrift Pilzkunde 38*: 65–73.

Andres, R. Y., and Frei, W. (1987). ^{125}I-Amatoxin and antiamatoxin for radioimmunoassay prepared by a novel approach of chemical and structural consideration. *Toxicon 25*: 915–922.

Andres, R. Y., Frei, W., Gautschi, K., and Vonderschmitt, D. J. (1986). Radioimmunoassay for amatoxin by a rapid ^{125}I tracerbased system. *Clin. Chem. 32*: 1751–1755.

Antkowiak, W. Z., and Gessner, W. P. (1975). Isolation and characteristics of toxic components of *Cortinarius orellanus Fries. Bull. Acad. Po. Sci. Chim. 23*: 729–733.

Antkowiak, W. Z., and Gessner, W. P. (1979). The structures of orellanine and orelline. *Tetrahedron Lett. 21*: 1931–1934.

Antkowiak, W. Z., and Gessner, W. P. (1985). Photodecomposition of orellanine and orellinine, the fungal toxins of *Cortinarius orellanus Fries* and *C. speciosissimus. Experientia 41*: 769–771.

Beutler, J. A., and DerMarderosian, A. H. (1981). Chemical variation in *Amanita. J. Nat. Prod.* (Lloydia) *44*: 422–431.

Bivins, H. G., Knopp, R., Lammers, R., McMicken, D. B., and Wolowodik, O. (1985). Mushroom ingestion. *Ann. Emergency Med. 14*: 101–106.

Bowden, K., Drysdale, A. C., and Mogey, G. A. (1965). Constituents of *Amanita muscaria. Nature 206*: 1359–1360.

Brehm, L., Hjeds, H., and Krogsgaard-Larsen (1972). The structure of muscimol, a GABA analogue of restricted conformation. *Arch. Chem. Scand. 26*: 1298–1299.

Bresinsky, A., and Besl, H. (1985). *Giftpilze*. Wissenschaftl. Verlagsges, Stuttgart.

Brodner, O. G., and Wieland, Th. (1976). Identification of the amatoxin-binding subunit of RNA polymerase B by affinity labeling experiments. Subunit B3—the true amatoxin receptor protein of multiple RNA polymerase B. *Biochemistry 15*: 3480–3484.

Buku, A., Wieland, Th., Bodenmüller, H., and Faulstich, H. (1980). Amaninamide, a new toxin of *Amanita virosa* mushrooms. *Experientia* (Basel) *36*: 33–34.

Caccialanza, G., Gandini, C., and Ponci, R. (1985). Direct, simultaneous determination of α-amanitin, β-amanitin and phalloidin by high performance liquid chromatography. *J. Pharmaceut. Biomed. Anal. 3*: 179–185.

Cantin, D., Richard, J.-M., and Alary, J. (1989). Chromatographic behaviour and determination of orellanine, a toxin from the mushroom *Cortinarius orellanus. J. Chromatogr. 478*: 231–237.

Chapuis, J.-R. (1984). Jahresbericht der Verbandstoxikologen für das Jahr 1983. *Schweiz. Zeitschr. Pilzkunde 62*: 196–197.

Cochet-Meilhac, M., and Chambon, P. (1974). Animal DNA-dependent RNApolymerases. 11. Mechanism of inhibition of RNA polymerases B by amatoxins. *Biochem. Biophys. Acta 353*: 160–184.

Cochet-Meilhac, M., Nuret, P., Courvalin, J. C., and Chambon, P. (1974). Animal DNA-dependent RNA-polymerases. 12. Determination of the cellular number of RNA polymerase B molecules. *Biochim. Biophys. Acta 353*: 185–192.

Cohen-Addad, C., Richard, J.-M., Giutel, J.-C., (1987). Structure of an orellanine-trifluoroacetic acid complex: Evidence of a very short O-hydrogen bond. *Acta Cryst. C43*: 504–507.

Curry, S. C., and Rose, M. C. (1985). Intravenous mushroom poisoning. *Ann. Emergency Med. 14*: 900–902.

Dehmlow, W. V., and Schulz, H.-J. (1985). Synthesis of orellanine, the lethal poison of a toadstool. *Tetrahedron Lett. 26*: 4903–4906.

Dehmlow, W. V., and Schulz, H.-J. (1987). Das Pilztoxin Orellanin. *Liebigs Ann. Chem. 1987*: 857–861.

Donner, A., Mascher, H., and Hruby, K. (1987). Quantitative Bestimmung von Amanitin im Serum mit HPLC. *J. Clin. Chem. Clin. Biochem. 25*: 605–606.

Eugster, C. H. (1956a). Über Muscarin aus Fliegenpilzen. *Helv. Chim. Acta. 39*: 1002–1023.

Eugster, C. H. (1956b). Zur Konstitution des Muscarins. 3. *Mitt. Helv. Chim. Acta 39*: 1023–1037.

Eugster, C. H. (1957). Isolierung von Muscarin aus *Inocybe patouillardi* (Bres.). *Helv. Chim. Acta 40*: 884–887.

Eugster, C. H. (1969). Chemie der Wirkstoffe aus dem Fliegenpilz, *Amanita muscaria. Fortschr. Chem. Org. Naturstoffe 27*: 231–261.

Eugster, C. H., Müller, G. F. R., and Good, R. (1965). Wirkstoffe aus *Amanita muscaria*: Ibotensäure und Muscazon. *Tetrahedron Lett.* 1813–1815.

Eugster, C. H., and Waser, P. G. (1951). Zur Kenntnis des Muscarins. *Experientia 10*: 298–300.

Faulstich, H. (1980). Pharmacokinetics of amatoxins in the dog. In *Amanita Toxins and Poisoning*, H. Faulstich, B. Kommerell, and T. Wieland, eds. Witzstrock, New York, pp. 88–89.

Faulstich, H., and Fauser, U. (1980). The course of *Amanita* intoxication in beagle dogs. In *Amanita Toxins and Poisoning*, H. Faulstich, B. Kommerell, and T. Wieland, eds. Witzstrock, New York, pp. 115–120.

Faulstich, H., Buku, A., Bodenmüller, H., and Wieland, Th. (1980). Virotoxins: Actin-binding cyclic peptides of *Amanita virosa* mushrooms. *Biochemistry 19*: 3334–3343.

Faulstich, H., Zobeley, S., and Trischmann, H. (1982). A rapid radioimmunoassay using a nylon support for amatoxins from *Amanita* mushrooms. *Toxicon 20*: 913–924.

Faulstich, H., Talas, A., and Wellhöner, H. H. (1985). Toxicokinetics of labeled amatoxins in the dog. *Arch. Toxicol. 56*: 190–194.

Faulstich, H., Kirchner, K., and Derenzini, M. (1988). Strongly enhanced toxicity of the mushroom toxin α-amanitin by an amatoxin-specific Fab or monoclonal antibody. *Toxicon 26*: 491–499.

Fauser, U., and Faulstich, H. (1973). Beobachtungen zur Therapie der Knollenblätterpilzvergiftung. Besserung der Prognose durch Unterbrechung des enterohepatischen Kreislaufs (Choledochusdrainage). *Dtsche Med Wschr. 98*: 2259–2259.

Flammer, R. (1982). Das Orellanus Syndrom: Pilzvergiftung mit Niereninsuffizienz. *Schweiz. Med. Wschr. 112*: 1181–1184.

Flammer, R. (1985a). Brechdurchfälle als Leitsymptom—Pilze und Alkohol. *Schweiz. Rundschau Med. (Praxis) 74*: 992–996.

Flammer, R. (1985a). Das Paxillussyndrom: Immunhämolyse nach wiederholtem Pilzgenuβ. *Schweiz. Rundschau Med. (Praxis) 74*: 997–999.

Flammer, R., and Horak, E. (1983). Giftpilze-Pilzgifte. Kosmos, Stuttgart.

Francis, J., and Murray, V. S. G. (1983). Review of enquiries made to the NPIS concerning Psilocybe mushroom ingestion 1978-1981. *Human Toxicol. 3*: 349–352.

Frank, I. C., and Cummins, L. (1987). Amanita poisoning treated with endoscopic biliary diversion. *J. Emerg. Nurs. 13*: 132–136.

Franke, S., Freimuth, U., and List, P. H. (1967). Über die Giftigkeit der Frühjahrslorchel *Gyromitra (Helvella) esculenta. Arch. Toxikol. 22*: 293–332.

French, A. L., and Garretson, L. K. (1988). Poisoning with the North American Jack O'Lantern, *Omphalotus illudens. Clin. Toxicol. 26*: 81–88.

Gérault, A. (1981). Intoxication collective de type orellanien provoquée par *Cortinarius splendens. R. Hry. Bull. Soc. Myc. Fr. 97*: 67–72.

Gore, M. C., and Jordan, P. M. (1982). Microbore single column analysis of pharmacologically active alkaloids from the fly agaric mushroom *Amanita muscaria. J. Chromatogr. 243*: 323–328.

Gosselin, R. E., Smith, R. P., and Hodge, H. C. (1984). Mushroom toxins. In *Clinical Toxicology of Commercial Products: Acute Poisoning*, 5th ed., R. E. Gosselin, ed. Williams and Wilkins, Baltimore, pp. 289–309.

Göth, H. A. R., Gagneux, C., Eugster, C. H., and Schmid, H. (1967). 2(3H)-Oxazolone durch Photoumlagerung von 3-Hydroxyoxazolen. Synthese von Muscazon. *Helv. Chim. Acta 50*: 137–142.

Gryzmala, S. (1957). Massenvergiftung durch den orangefuchsigen Hautkopf. *Z. Pilzkd. 23*: 139–142.

Gryzmala, S. (1962). L'isolement d'orellanine poison du *Cortinarius orellanus Fries* et l'étude des ses effects anato-pathologiques. *Bull. Trimest. Soc. Mycol. Fr. 78*: 394–404.

Gstraunthaler, G., and Prast, H. (1983). Studies on the nephrotoxicity of *Cortinarius orellanus (Fr)*: The effect of dipyridyles on renal epithelial cell cultures. *Sydowia 34*: 53–58.

Haines, J. H., Lichstein, E., and Glickerman, D. (1985). A fatal poisoning from an amatoxin-containing *Lepiota. Mycopathologica 93*: 15–17.

Hasseberg, H.-A., and Gerlach, H. (1988). Synthese von Orellin. *Helv. Chim. Acta 71*: 957–962.

Hatfield, G. M., and Schaumberg, J. P. (1975). Isolation and structural studies of coprin, the disulfiram-like constituent of *Coprinus attramentarius. Lloydia 38*: 489–496.

Hatfield, G. M., Waldes, L. J., and Smith, A. H. (1978). The occurrence of psilocybin in *Gymnopilus* species. *Lloydia 41*: 140–144.

Hazani, E., Taitelman, U., and Shasha, S. M. (1983). *Amanita verna* poisoning in Israel—Report of a rare case and of time and place. *Arch. Toxicol.*, Suppl. *6*: 186–189.

Heim, R. (1978). *Les Champignons Toxique et Hallucinogènes*. 2nd ed. Boubée, Paris.

Heim, R., Hofmann, A., and Tscherter (1966). Sur une intoxication collective, une syndrome psilocybien causée en France par un Copelandia. *C. R. Acad. Sci. 262*: 519–523.

Heufler, C., Feldmayer, G., and Prast, H. (1987). Investigations on the mode of action of the fungus toxin orellanine on renal cell cultures. *Agents and Actions 21*: 203–208.

Hofmann, A., Frey, A., Ott, H., Petrzilka, T., and Troxler, F. (1958). Konstitutionsaufklärung und Synthese von Psilocybin. *Experientia 14*: 397–399.

Hofmann, A., Heim, R., Brack, A., Kobel, A., Frey, H., Ott, H., Petrzilka, T., and Troxler, F. (1959). Psilocybin und Psilocin, zwei psychotrope Wirkstoffe aus mexikanischen Rauschpilzen (*Psilocybe*). *Helv. Chim. Acta 42*: 1557–1572.

Holmdahl, J., Ahlmen, J., Berge, S., Lundberg, S., and Persson, S.-A. (1987). Isolation and nephrotoxic studies of orellanine from the mushroom *Cortinarius speciosissimus. Toxicon. 25*: 195–199.

Høiland, K. (1983). Extracts of *Cortinarius speciosissimus* affecting the photosynthetic apparatus of *Lemna minor. Trans. Br. Mycol. Soc. 81*: 633–639.

Homann, J. (1980). Knollenblätterpilzvergiftung. *Die med. Welt 40*: 1171–1178.

Homann, J., Rawer, P., Bleyl, H., Matthes, K.-J., and Heinrich, D. (1986). Early detection of amatoxins in human mushroom poisoning. *Arch. Toxicol. 59*: 190–191.

Hulmi, S. P., Sipponen, P., Forsström, J., and Vilska, J. (1974). Seitikkisienen aiheuttama vakava munuaisvaurio (Mushroom poisoning caused by *Orellanus speciosissimus*). *Duodecim* (Helsinki) *90*: 1044–1050.

Hruby, K., Lenz, K., Moser, C. D., Bachner, J., and Korninger, C. (1979). Knollenblätterpilzvergiftungen in Österreich. *Wiener Klin. Wschr. 91*: 509–513.

Jahn, W., Faulstich, H., and Wieland, Th. (1980). Pharmacokinetics of ^{3}H-methyl-dehydroxymethyl-α-amanitin in the isolated perfused rat liver, and the influence of several drugs. In *Amanita Toxins and Poisoning*, H. Faulstich, B. Kommerell, and Th. Wieland, eds. Witzstrock, New York, pp. 79–85.

Jehl, F., Gallion, C., Birkel, P., Jaeger, A., Flesh, F., and Minck, R. (1985). Determination of α-amanitin and β-amanitin in human biological fluids by high-performance liquid chromatography. *Anal. Biochem. 149*: 35–42.

Kedinger, C., and Chambon, P. (1972). Animal DNA-dependent RNApolymerases. 3. Purification of calf thymus BI and BII enzymes. *Europ. J. Biochem. 28*: 283–290.

Kelner, M. J., and Alexander, N. M. (1987). Endocrine hormone abnormalities in *Amanita* poisoning. *Clin. Toxicol. 25*: 21–37.

Kögl, F., Duisberg, H., and Erxleben, H. (1931). Über Muscarin I. *Liebig's Ann. Chem. 489*: 156–192.

Kögl, F., Salemink, C. A., Schoúten, H., and Jellinek, F. (1957). Über Muscarin III. *Rec. Trav. Chim. Pays-Bas 76*: 109-127.

Kröncke, K. D., Fricker, G., Meier, P. J., Gerok, W., Wieland, T., and Kurz, G. (1986). Alpha-amanitin uptake into hepatocytes. *J. Biol. Chem. 27*: 2562–2567.

Kürnsteiner, H., and Moser, M. (1981). Isolation of a lethal toxin from *Cortinarius orellanus. Mycopathologica 74*: 65–72.

Laatsch, H., and Matthies, L. (1991). Fluorescent compounds in Cortinarius speciosissimus: Investigation for the presence of cortinarins. *Mycologia 83*: 492-500.

Lahtiperä, S., Naukkarinen, A., and Collan, Y. (1986). Mushroom poisoning due to *Cortinarius speciosissimus*: Electron microscope studies in rats. *Arch. Toxicol. Suppl. 9*: 315–319.

Langer, M., Vesconi, S., and Costantino, D. (1990). In *Update in Intensive Care and Emergency Medicine*, Vol. 10, J. L. Vincent, ed. Springer, Berlin, pp. 483–493.

Lefévre, H. (1982). Immunhämolytische Anämie nach Genuβ des Kahlen Krempling (*Paxillus involutus*). *Dtsch. Med. Wschr. 107*: 1374–1374.

Leung, A. Y., and Paul, A. G. (1968). Baeocystin, a monomethyl analog of psilocybin from *Psilocybe baeocystis* saprophytic culture. *J. Pharm. Sci. 57*: 1667–1671.

Lindberg, P., Bergman, R., and Wickberg, B. (1975). Isolation and structure of coprine, a novel physiologically active cyclopropane derivative from *Coprinus atramentarius* and its synthesis via 1-aminocyclopropanol. *J. Chem. Soc. Chem. Commun. 1975*: 946–947.

List, P. H., and Luft, P. (1968). Gyromitrin, das Gift der Frühjahrslorchel. *Arch. Pharm. 301*: 294–305.

List, P. H., and Luft, P. (1969). Nachweis und Gehaltbestimmung von Gyromitrin in frischen Lorcheln. *Arch. Pharm. 302*: 143–146.

Little, M. C., and Preston, J. F. (1984). The fluorimetric detection of amatoxins, phallotoxins and other peptides in *Amanita suballiacea. J. Natural Products 47*: 93–97.

Lock, E. A., and Ishmael, J. (1979). The acute toxic effects of paraquat and diquat on the rat kidney. *Toxicol. Appl. Pharmacol. 50*: 67–76.

Lund, W. (1979). Estimation of muscimol and ibotenic acid in *Amanita muscaria* using high performance liquid chromatography. *Arch. Pharm. Chem. Sci. Ed. 7*: 115–118.

Malone, M. H., Robichaud, R. C., Tyler, V. E., and Brady, L. R. (1969). A bioassay for muscarine activity and its detection in certain *Inocybe. Lloydia 24*: 204–210.

Marichal, J. F., Triby, F., Wiederkehr, J. L., and Carbiener, R. (1977). Insufficance rénale chronique après intoxication par champignon de type *Cortinarius orellanus Fries. Nouv. Presse Med.* (France) *6*: 2973–2975.

Marugg, D., and Reutter, F. W. (1985). Die Amanita-phalloides-Intoxikation—Moderne therapeutische Maβnahmen und klinischer Verlauf. *Schweiz. Rdsch. Med. (Praxis) 74*: 972–982.

Möttönen, M., Nieminen, L., and Heikkilae, H. (1975). Damage caused by two finnish mushrooms *Cortinarius speciosissimus* and *C. gentiles* on the rat kidney. *Z. Naturforsch. 30c*: 668–679.

Nakamura, T., and Kobayashi, A. (1985). Toxikodermie durch den Speisepilz Shiitake (*Lentinus edodes*). *Der Hautarzt 36*: 591–593.

Niemimen, L., Möttönen, M., Tirri, R., and Ikonen, S. (1975). Nephrotoxicity of *Cortinarius speciocissimus*: A histological and enzyme histochemical study. *Exp. Pathol. 11*: 239–246.

Ohta, T., Nakajima, S., Hasanaka, S.-I., Yamamoto, M., Shinmen, Y., Nishimura, C., Yamaizumi, Z., and Nozoe, S. (1987). A chlorohydrin amino acid from *Amanita abrupta. Phytochemistry 26*: 565–566.

Piering, W. F., and Bratanow, N. (1990). Role of the clinical laboratory in guiding treatment of *Amanita virosa* mushroom poisoning: Report of two cases. *Clin. Chem. 36*: 571–574.

Piqueras, J. (1984). Intoxicacion de tipo ciclopeptidico (Faloidina) producida por pequenas Lepiotas. *Bull. Soc. Catalana Micol. 8*: 33–37.

Prast, H., Pfaller, W. E. R., and Moser, M. (1985). Toxic properties of the mushroom *Cortinarius orellanus* I. Chemical characterization of the main toxin of *Cortinarius orellanus (Fries)*, and *C. speciosissimus (Kühn & Romagn)* and acute toxicity in mice. *Arch. Toxicol. 62*: 81–88.

Prast, H., and Pfaller, W. (1988). Toxic properties of the mushroom *Cortinarius orellanus (Fries)* II. Impairment of renal functions in rats. *Arch. Toxicol. 62*: 89–96.

Pudill, R. (1989). Die Bestimmung von Amatoxinen und Phallotoxinen mit Fast Atom Bombardement-Massenspektrometrie (FAB-MS) Diagnostik und Klinik der Knollenblätterpilz-Vergiftung. *GIT Labor Med. 1989*: 320–327.

Pyysalo, H. (1975). Some new toxic compounds in false morels *Gyromitra esculenta. Naturwissenschaften 62*: 395–395.

Pyysalo, H., and Niskanen, A. (1977). Occurrence of N-methyl-N-formylhydrazones in fresh and processed false morel. *J. Agric. Food Chem. 25*: 644–647.

Rapior, S., Delpech, N., Andary, C., and Huchard, G. (1989). Intoxication by *Cortinarius orellanus*: Detection and assay of orellanine in biological fluids and renal biopsies. *Mycopathologia 108*: 155–161.

Richard, J.-M., Taillandier, G., and Benoit-Guyod (1985). A quantitative structure-activity relationship study on substituted pyridines as a contribution to the knowledge of the toxic effects of orellanine, a toxin from the mushroom *Cortinarius orellanus. Toxicon 23*: 815–824.

Richard, J.-M., Ravanel, P., and Cantin, D. (1987). Phytotoxicity of orellanine, a mushroom toxin. *Toxicon 25*: 350–354.

Richard, J.-M., Louis, J., and Cantin, D. (1988). Nephrotoxicity of orellanine, a toxin from the mushroom *Cortinarius orellanus. Arch. Toxicol. 62*: 242–245.

Rieck, W., and Platt, D. (1988). High-performance liquid chromatographic method for the determination of α-amanitin and phalloidin in human plasma using column-switching technique and its application in suspected cases of poisoning by the green species of Amanita mushroom (*A. phalloides*). *J. Chromatogr. 425*: 121–134.

Rumack, B. H., and Salzman, E. (1978). *Mushroom Poisoning and Treatment*. CRC-Press, West Palm Beach, FL, U.S.A.

Ryzko, J., Socha, J., and Jankowska, I. (1987). Estimation of calcium and phosphorous metabolism in children with acute hepatic failure due to *Amanita phalloides* poisoning, presented at Falk Symposium 48, Calcium dependent processes in the liver, Titisee, June 1987.

Sanz, P., Reig, R., Piqúeras, J., Marti, G., and Corbella, J. (1989). Fatal mushroom poisoning in Barcelona, 1986–1988. *Mycopathologia 108*: 207–209.

Schmiedeberg, O., and Koppe, R. (1869). In *Das Muscarin, das Giftige Alkaloid des Fliegenpilzes*, F. C. W. Vogel, ed. Leipzig.

Schulz-Weddingen, I. (1986). Beiträge zur Kenntnis der Gattung Lepiota. I. Eine Intoxikation mit *Lepiota brunneo-incarnata* in Nordwestdeutschland. *Zschr. f. Mykol. 52*: 91–110.

Schumacher, T., and Høiland, K. (1983). Mushroom poisoning caused by species of the genus *Cortinarius Fries. Arch. Toxicol. 53*: 87–106.

Schwartz, R.-H., and Smith, D. E. (1988). Hallucinogenic mushrooms. *Clin. Pediatr. 27*: 70–73.

Seeger, R. (1984). Zeitungspapiertest für Amanitine—falsch positive Ergebnisse. *Zschr. f. Mykol. 50*: 353–359.

Short, A. I. K., Watling, R., McDonald, M. K., and Robson, J. S. (1980). Poisoning by *Cortinarius speciosissimus. Lancet 1980*: 942–944.

Stamets, P. (1978). *Psilocybe Mushrooms and Their Allies*. Homstead Book Company, Seattle.

Stijve, T. (1978). Ethylen gyromitrin and N-methyl-N-formyl-hydrazine in commercially available dried false morels. *Mitt. Geb. Lebensmittelunters. Hyg. 69*: 492–504.

Stijve, T. (1981). High performance thin layer chromatographic determination of the toxic principles of some poisonous mushrooms. *Mitt. Geb. Lebensm. Unters. Hyg. 72*: 44–54.

Stijve, T., Hischenhuber, C., and Ashley, D. (1976). Occurrence of 5-hydroxylated indole derivatives in *Panaeolina foenisecii (Fries)* Küchner from various origin. *Z. Mykol. 50*: 361–368.

Stirpe, F., and Fiume, L. (1967). Studies on the pathogenesis of liver necrosis by α-amanitin. Effect of α-amanitin on ribonucleic acid polymerase in mouse liver nuclei. *Biochem. J. 105*: 779–782.

Takemoto, T., Nakajima, T., and Sakuma, P. (1964). Isolation of an flycidal constituent "ibotenic acid" from *Amanita muscaria* and *A. pantherina. Yakugaku Zasshi 84*: 1232–1233.

Tebbett, I. R., and Caddy, B. (1984). Mushroom toxins of the genus *Cortinarius. Experientia 40*: 441–446.

Theobald, W., Büch, O., Kunz, H. A., Krupp, P., Stenger, E. G., and Heimann, H. Z. (1968). Pharmakologische und experimental-psychologische Untersuchungen mit 2 Inhaltsstoffen des Fliegenpilzes (*Amanita muscaria*). *Arzneim. Forsch. (Drug. Res.) 18*:311–315.

Tiecco, M., Tingoli, L., Testaferri, L., Chianelli, D., and Wenkert, E. (1986). Total synthesis of orellanine, the lethal toxin of *Cortinarius orellanus Fries* mushroom. *Tetrahedron 42*: 1475–1485.

Toth, B., and Raha, C. R. (1987). Carcinogenesis by pentanal methylformylhydrazone of *Gyromitra esculenta* in mice. *Mycopathologia 98*: 83–89.

Tyler, V. E., Jr. (1961). Indole derivatives in certain North American mushrooms. *Lloydia 24*: 71–74.

Tyler, V. E., Jr., and Gröger, D. (1964). Amanita alkaloids II. *Amanita citrina* and *Amanita porphyria*. *Planta Med. 12*: 397–402.

Vaisius, A. C., and Wieland, Th. (1982). Formation of a single phosphodiester bond by RNA polymerase B from calf thymus is not inhibited by α-amanitin. *Biochemistry 21*: 3097–3101.

Vergeer, P. P. (1983). Poisonous fungi: Mushrooms. In *Fungi Pathogenic for Humans and Animals*, Part B, H. D. H. Howard and L. F. Howard, eds. Marcel Dekker, New York, pp. 374–412.

Wagner-Thiessen, E. (1983). Gastrointestinale Blutung nach Knollenblätterpilzvergiftung. *Die med. Welt. 34*: 895–899.

Waser, P. G. (1961). Chemistry and pharmacology of muscarine, muscarone and some related compounds. *Pharmacol. Rev. 13*: 465–506.

Wasson, V. P., and Wasson, R. G. (1957). *Mushrooms, Russia and History*, Vols. 1 and 2. Pantheon Books, New York.

Wieland, H., Konz, W., and Mittasch, H. (1934). Die Konstitution von Bufotenin und Bufotenidin. Über Krötengiftstoffe VII. *Liebigs Ann. Chem. 513*: 1–25.

Wieland, Th. (1986). *Peptides of Poisonous Amanita Mushrooms*, Rich, A., ed. Springer-Verlag.

Wieland, Th., and Faulstich, H. (1978). Amatoxins, phallotoxins, phallolysin, and antamanide: The biologically active components of poisonous *Amanita* mushrooms. *Crit. Rev. Biochem. 5*: 185–260.

Wieland, Th., Wirth, L., and Fischer, E. (1949). β-Amanitin, eine dritte Komponente des Knollenblätterpilzgiftes. *Liebig's Ann. Chem. 564*: 152–160.

Wieland, Th., Motzel, W., and Merz, H. (1953). Über das Vorkommen von Bufotenin im gelben Knollenblätterpilz. *Liebigs Ann. Chem. 577*: 10–16.

Whitaker, G. R., and Box, J. F. (1985). *Chlorophyllum molybditis* mushroom poisoning: A case report and review of the syndrome. *J. Arkansas Med. Soc. 82*: 220–222.

Winkelmann, M., Borchard, F., Stangel, W., and Grabensee, B. (1982). Tödlich verlaufene immunhämolytische Anämie nach Genuβ des Kahlen Kremplings (*Paxillus involutus*). *Dtsche. Med. Wschr. 107*: 1190–1194.

Wisemann, J. S., and Abeles, R. H. (1979). Mechanism of inhibition of aldehyde dehydrogenase by cyclopropanone hydrate and the mushroom toxin coprine. *Biochemistry 18*: 427–435.

Yamaura, Y., Fukuhara, M., Takabatake, E., Ito, N., and Hashimoto, T. (1986). Hepatotoxic action of a poisonous mushroom *Amanita abrupta* in mice and its toxic component. *Toxicology 38*: 161–173.

Yocum, R. R., and Simons, D. M. (1977). Amatoxins and phallotoxins in *Amanita* species of the northeastern United States. *Lloydia 40*: 178–190.

Zilker, T. (1987). Diagnose und Therapie der Pilzvergiftungen (Teil II). *Leber, Magen, Darm 1987*: 173–197.

10

The Toxicology of Alkaloids in Foods and Herbs

Ryan J. Huxtable

University of Arizona, Tucson, Arizona

I. INTRODUCTION

Alkaloids are nitrogenous secondary metabolites found in plants. Typically, they are formed from amino acids by decarboxylation plus other modifications or derived, in part, from acetate or mevalonate. In many cases, they form part of the chemical defense system of the species elaborating them. Alkaloids show great structural variation, particularly among the angiosperms, or flowering plants. There are estimated to be around 500,000 flowering plant species. This is a highly successful group, having evolved in the presence of grazing and browsing animals, insect pests, parasites, and bacteria, that owes its success largely to its chemical ingenuity. Unsurprisingly, many of the alkaloids elaborated by angiosperms and other plants have marked pharmacological actions on humans. Alkaloids of therapeutic importance include morphine, vincristine, vinblastine, quinine, atropine, cocaine, pilocarpine, reserpine, colchicine, and a host of others.

About 40% of plant families contain alkaloid-bearing plants, although alkaloids are present in only around 9% of genera. In a given species, alkaloid content can vary widely, depending on the part of the plant, its maturity, the time of year, geographic location, and type of soil. Even plants examined from the same location at the same time of the year can show wide variations in alkaloid content from one year to the next. Thus, *Senecio longilobus* leaves show an 80-fold variation in alkaloid content, and *S. riddellii* a 100-fold variation (Johnston et al., 1985). Storage conditions can also markedly affect alkaloid content. With potatoes, for example, a 50-fold increase in alkaloid level can occur on inappropriate storage (Sharma and Salunkhe, 1989), while conversely alkaloid levels in certain *Crotalaria* species can decrease on storage (Heath et al., 1975).

When alkaloids are taken by mouth, toxicity can be expressed in the gastrointestinal tract. In certain cases, however, bioactivation in the liver is required for toxicity. In such cases, gastrointestinal toxicity is minimized, toxicity, instead, being expressed in the liver, the lungs (which receives the brunt of substances leaving the liver), and the kidneys, in which alkaloids and metabolites may be concentrated and excreted. Fetuses and neonates lack bioactivating enzymes such as the mixed function oxidases, and therefore tend to accumulate alkaloids, such as caffeine (see Fig. 6), which depend on metabolism for excretion. Hence, while the half-life of caffeine in adults is 4.9 ± 1.8 h, in full-term babies it is 80 ± 26 h, and in premature babies 102.9 ± 17.9 h (Aldridge et al., 1979; Dews, 1984). Neonates may also show less susceptibility to the toxicity of alkaloids requiring bioactivation. However, other factors also affect the response of the developing organism to alkaloids, so generalization is dangerous.

Depending on their lipid solubility, alkaloids can exhibit central nervous system toxicity. Lipid solubility is also a function of the basicity of an alkaloid. The higher the pK_a, the higher the fraction of alkaloid that is ionized at physiological pH, and the lower the partition coefficient into lipid compartments, such as the brain (Fig. 1). The central nervous system effects are often the primary reason alkaloids are intentionally taken, other than for medical

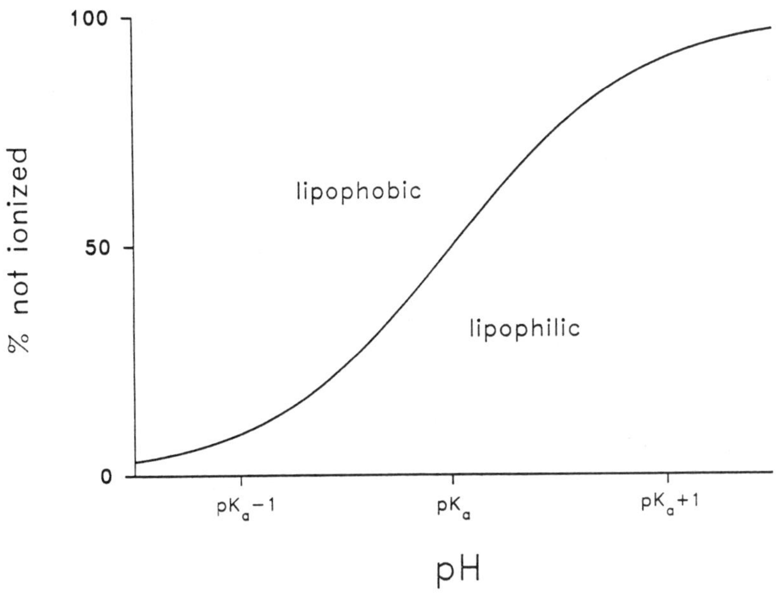

Figure 1 Pharmacokinetic relationship between the pK_a of an alkaloid and its ability to penetrate the brain. The more basic the alkaloid, the higher the value of the pK_a relative to physiological pH, and the greater the fraction of the alkaloid in the body in the ionized, conjugate acid, form, and the lower the fraction in the lipophilic form.

reasons. The use of caffeine in the form of coffee or tea, nicotine (see Fig. 6) in the form of tobacco, or, in various forms, of cocaine (see Fig. 6), morphine, and a host of other alkaloids is predicated on their central actions.

Hepatic metabolism typically consists of hydroxylation and conjugation. In general, hepatic metabolites have increased aqueous solubility and lower lipid partition coefficients than the parent alkaloid, and thus are likely to have less effect on the central nervous system. These characteristics also hasten excretion from the body.

Many alkaloids, such as coniine (see Fig. 6), nicotine, cocaine or tropane alkaloids such as scopolamine or atropine (see Fig. 6) are readily absorbed across mucous membranes or through the skin. Hamlet's father was fraternally murdered by means of a plant extract being poured into his ear as he slept. The plant has been tentatively identified as *Conium maculatum*, a source of coniine (Max, 1988). Such alkaloids can be absorbed directly from the oral cavity or by the lungs, if inhaled.

Alkaloids tend to be bitter-tasting and to have marked pharmacological actions. They, therefore, are rarely consumed intentionally in foods. Exceptions include the monoamines, such as tyramine, present in cheese and beer. Where contamination of food occurs, this is often evident from the taste. Alkaloid-containing plants, on the other hand, are frequently taken as medicines or herbs or for their psychoactive effects. These are perhaps loose statements, as the division between herbs, food, and medicines is often blurred, the words having no precise scientific meaning, although they may have precise legal meanings. The concepts are not exclusionary. Few would think of a cup of Earl Grey tea made with sugar and milk or cream as being a medicine, but tea is psychoactive, one of the great writers of the twentieth century describing it as "the reviewing brew." To give someone a sweetened cup of tea is one of the great British panaceas. Early Grey is the infusion of the leaves of one herb, *Camellia sinensis*, flavored with the extract of another herb, the carcinogenic bergamot (*Citrus aurantium*). Earl Grey is certainly nutritious, especially if the consumer had opted for the cream rather than the milk. So this common beverage partakes of the qualities of all three of the categories listed. The uses of alkaloid-containing plants as foods, herbs, remedies, or recreation thus blend into each other.

People can be affected by alkaloids in the foods or herbs they use for a number of reasons: intentionally, if a plant is ingested for the pharmacological properties of the alkaloids it contains, as with coffee, khat, peyote or tobacco; or accidentally (Huxtable, 1990a). Accidental exposure to alkaloids can occur because of food contamination; because an alkaloid-containing plant was taken deliberately without the consumer being aware of the danger; or because a misidentified plant was consumed.

There has been a marked and continuing increase in the number of alkaloid-containing plants sold as teas, herbs, herbal remedies, food additives, and food supplements in North America. Of the 200 species Siegel reported as being sold as smoking mixtures and the 400 species being sold as teas or food supplements, many were alkaloidal (Siegel, 1976). The species included *Corynanthe yohimbe* (yohimbine), *Cola* spp. (methylxanthines), *Lobelia inflata* (lobeline), *Argemone mexicana* (berberine), *Nicotiana* spp. (nicotine), *Ilex paraguayensis* (caffeine), *Ephedra* spp. (pseudoephedrine or ephedrine, depending on whether the plant derives from the New World or Old), *Passiflora incarnata* (harmine alkaloids), *Catharanthus roseus* (indoles), *Rauwolfia serpentina* (reserpine), and *Datura* spp. (tropane alkaloids). At least in the United States, these substances are largely unregulated; if they are not sold as food or drugs, but as food additives, food supplements, or herbal remedies, they escape regulation by the Food and Drug Administration. An indication of the kind of public health problems associated with the widespread use of herbs is a Swedish study showing a correlation between herb use and hepatitis (Carlsson, 1990). Liver function tests normalized in 52 of 53 patients when herb use was stopped for 6 weeks.

II. MISIDENTIFICATION OF A PLANT SPECIES

Commercially sold plants are not infrequently misidentified. *Atropa belladonna* (deadly nightshade) has been sold as comfrey (*Symphytum* species) (Anonymous, 1983; Galizia, 1983; Routledge and Spriggs, 1989). Tropane alkaloid poisonings, probably as a result of contamination with *Atropa* species, have occurred following the consumption of plants purporting to be burdock, comfrey, mallow, and nettle (Awang and Kindack, 1989). A death was reported in England of a person supposedly drinking maté (*Ilex paraguayensis*), but which, judging from the clinical picture, was probably in fact a pyrrolizidine-containing species (McGee et al., 1976). In the western United States, two species of Compositae, *Senecio longilobus* and *Gnaphalium macounii*, had been commercially sold under the same herbal name, gordolobo yerba, for many years. The *Senecio* species is toxic, and has been responsible for a number of deaths and illnesses (Stillman et al., 1977; Fox et al., 1978; Huxtable, 1980a). *Gnaphalium* is apparently nontoxic. Some believe the two plants may have been confused, due to their similar phenotype.

Misidentification can also occur in self-collected, or noncommercially collected, plants. *Digitalis* is frequently mistaken for comfrey (*Symphytum*), with deaths resulting (Cooper et al., 1977; Dickstein and Kunkel, 1980; Bain, 1985). A team on a desert survival course in southern California became ill, one member dying, after a salad was prepared from a *Datura* species (jimsonweed), mistaken for an innocent species (Huxtable, 1980a).

III. STEROIDAL ALKALOIDS

Among the numerous botanical gifts of the New World to the Old were the tomato and the potato. These two solanaceous species have become so embedded in the cuisines of Europe and their derivatives around the world that the one is as inseparable from Italian pasta as the other from the Englishman's meat and two veg. Worldwide, 300 million tons of potatoes (*Solanum tuberosum*) and 20 million tons of tomatoes (*Lycopersicon esculentum*) are consumed yearly. Potato production worldwide is exceeded only by that of wheat and rice (Harvey et al., 1985). In the United States, the consumption of tomatoes ranks second only to that of potatoes. For 1970, U.S. production of potatoes was 16.3 million tons and of tomatoes 6.0 million tons. Sweet corn was a poor third among edible plants at 2.5 million tons (Jadhav et al., 1981). Despite the world's appetite for the tomato and the potato, these two solanaceous species, along with many others in their family (Kingsbury, 1964), contain alkaloids that are severely toxic above a certain level.

The major alkaloids in potato are α-solanine and α-chaconine (Fig. 2), steroidal glycosides differing only in their glycoside composition. These two alkaloids constitute around 95% of total alkaloid content (Harvey et al., 1985). Alkaloids are found in all parts of the potato plant, but concentrations are highest in unripe, green potatoes, damaged potatoes, and potatoes stored inappropriately. Light exposure also increases the level of alkaloids, which, past a certain point, produce a bitter or musty taste in the potato (Jadhav et al., 1981; Dalvi and Bowie, 1983). The control of potato alkaloids includes avoiding mechanical damage and protecting potatoes form light by means of colored bags.

The approximate concentrations of alkaloids found in various parts of the potato plant are (mg/100 g fresh weight): flowers, 300–500; sprouts, 200–400; leaves, 40–100; skin, 30–60; and flesh, 1.2–5. However, concentrations vary widely among the enormous number of cultivars that have been developed. Assays of 165 samples in Sweden showed alkaloid levels ranging from 2 to 30 mg/100 g (Johnsson and Hellenas, 1983). Other studies showed ranges of

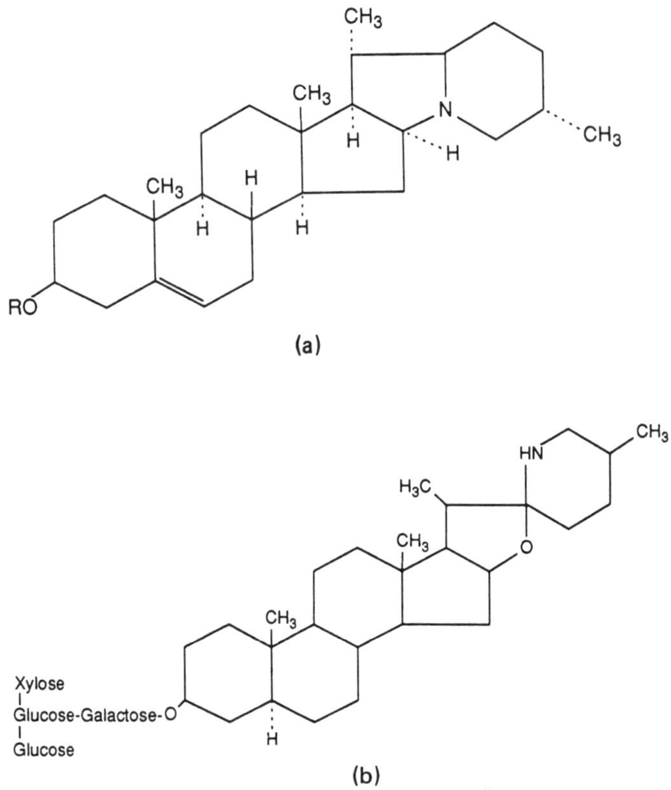

Figure 2 Steroidal alkaloids of the Solanaceae: (a) α-solanine [R: -D-galactose-(D-glucose)-L-rhamose] and α-chaconine [R: -D-glucose-(L-rhamnose)-L-rhamnose] from potatoes (*Solanum tuberosum*), and (b) α-tomatine from tomatoes (*Lycopersicon esculentum*).

4.6–3.5 mg/100 g in 39 cultivars, 1.8–13 in 32 cultivars, and 1.9–7.6 in 15 cultivars (see Sharma and Salunkhe, 1989). Levels in fresh tubers can vary 10-fold. As well as genetic differences, geographic differences produce differing alkaloid levels in the same strain. The alkaloids appear to be involved in disease and insect resistance. Damaged or poorly stored potatoes can contain up to 160 mg alkaloids/100 g (Sharma and Salunkhe, 1989).

Given an average level of 2–5 mg alkaloid/100 g potato tuber, world consumption of potato alkaloids is somewhere in the range of 5–14 × 10^6 kg per annum (5500–15,400 tons). Alkaloid content is not appreciably reduced by cooking or steeping in water, as the alkaloids are insoluble. A major action of the alkaloids is that of cholinesterase inhibition. They are also cardiotoxic, having digitalislike actions. In addition, there are repeated, disputed, claims that these alkaloids are teratogens (Ames, 1983). Doses in excess of 2–8 mg/kg produce hyperesthesia and drowsiness. Higher doses cause vomiting and diarrhea. Numerous cases of poisoning from potato alkaloids are known. These have been reviewed (McMillan and Thompson, 1979; Jadhav et al., 1981). A typical case involved 78 boys at a London school who fell ill after lunch (McMillan and Thompson, 1979). Seventeen were admitted to hospital. The steak pie, gravy, cabbage, tinned carrots, syrup sponge pudding, and custard were all eliminated as suspects, leaving the mashed potato. An extract of this was found to inhibit cholinesterase activity.

It is normally assumed that potatoes with alkaloid levels below 20 mg/100 g fresh weight are safe for consumption (Johnsson and Hellenas, 1983). However, the ratio between levels at which toxicity has been observed and levels deemed for human consumption is rather low. Also, study subjects given potatoes containing 20–30 mg alkaloid/100 g daily for a week showed no ill effects (Harvey et al., 1985). This has led to suggestions that other factors may be involved in potato poisoning. Potato alkaloids are normally poorly absorbed from the gastrointestinal tract. It is possible that an increase in alkaloid content is associated with an increase in related steroidal saponins or sapogenins and that these may increase the degree of absorption of the alkaloids. People with atypical serum cholinesterase are less susceptible to cholinesterase inhibition than people with typical activity. There could, therefore, also be a genetic component in potato toxicity.

A related alkaloid is found in tomatoes and has been christened α-tomatine (Fig. 2) (Jadhav et al., 1981). This triglycoside is found in all parts of the plant, being particularly high in leaves. Here the levels may be 10–50 times the level in the fruit. Analogous to the potato, levels fall as the fruit ripens. Tomatoes left on the vine after ripening lose almost all their alkaloid within 2–3 days. Artificially ripened fruit, however, the kind available at your local supermarket, contain higher levels.

Other solanaceous species, such as eggplant (*Melongena*), also contain steroidal alkaloids (Dalvi and Bowie, 1983).

IV. AN ISOQUINUCLIDINE

Yams (*Dioscorea* spp.) are another group of solanaceous plants comprising a major food source, in this case for tropical countries. Worldwide production is about 20 million tons per annum (Jadhav et al., 1981). In certain West African communities, yams may supply half the calories. Many wild species are highly toxic due to their content of isoquinuclidine alkaloids such as dioscorine (Fig. 3). This alkaloid, which has convulsant, picrotoxinlike effects on the central nervous system, can be partially removed by soaking and leaching the yams in water.

V. PYRROLIZIDINE ALKALOIDS

Pyrrolizidine alkaloids are abundant in the plant kingdom. It has been estimated that about 3% of all plants contain such alkaloids (Smith and Culvenor, 1981). They have been isolated from more than 60 genera in at least 13 families. Pyrrolizidines are major causes of human and animal poisoning, partly because of their geographical and botanical ubiquity, and partly because

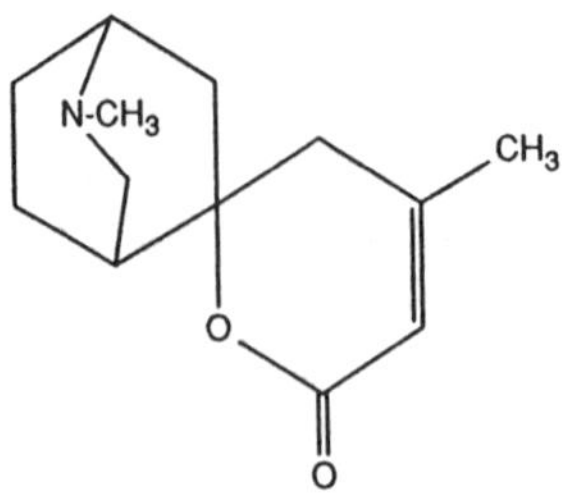

Figure 3 Dioscorine, a major alkaloid in yams (*Dioscorea* spp.).

of the chronic and cumulative nature of pyrrolizidine toxicity (Huxtable, 1980b). Pyrrolizidine-containing plants are frequently used as herbs, vegetables, and dietary supplements (Huxtable, 1990a). Contamination of grains with the seeds of pyrrolizidine-containing plants has on a number of occasions produced epidemics of pyrrolizidine poisoning (Huxtable, 1989a).

1,2-Unsaturated pyrrolizidine alkaloids produce veno-occlusive disease of the liver as a consequence of bioactivation in that organ (Huxtable, 1979, 1990b). Such disease is highly characteristic of pyrrolizidine poisoning, its only other known occurrence being a consequence of chemotherapy with drugs related to cytarabine. The three stages of veno-occlusive disease are shown in Figure 4. An acute phase of hepatomegaly and ascites may either resolve or progress to the subacute phase. In the chronic phase, cirrhosis of the liver develops (Huxtable, 1989a). As cirrhosis is a late consequence of exposure, even a large contribution of pyrrolizidines to the incidence of cirrhosis in a population will not be recognized unless specifically looked for.

Certain pyrrolizidine alkaloids, such as the *Crotalaria* alkaloids, monocrotaline and fulvine (Fig. 5), also cause pulmonary arterial hypertension and right ventricular hypertrophy in experimental and farm animals. Other pyrrolizidine alkaloids are teratogenic (Green and Christie, 1967; Peterson and Jago, 1980).

Finally, many pyrrolizidine alkaloids are carcinogenic. These include alkaloids from plants that are widely consumed, such as those of the *Senecio, Petasites, Tussilago, Crotalaria*, and *Symphytum* genera (Green and Christie, 1967; Bull et al., 1968; McLean, 1970; IARC, 1975; Mattocks, 1986). The high rate of primary liver cancer in South Africa has been ascribed to chronic low level exposure to pyrrolizidines (Schoental, 1968).

Epidemics of pyrrolizidine poisoning have occurred in many parts of the world. Genera implicated have been *Heliotropium, Trichodesma, Senecio*, and *Crotalaria*. The largest documented outbreak occurred in Afghanistan, affecting some 7200 people as a result of grain being contaminated with the seeds of *Heliotropium popovii* (Mohabbat et al., 1976). Some 2000 people died. Other outbreaks have occurred in India, Uzbekistan, South Africa, and the Caribbean nations (Huxtable, 1989a). Estimations of doses have proved difficult. For the Afghanistan outbreak, consumption levels of 2 mg/day for periods of up to 2 years have been estimated. It appears that contamination of food grains is most likely in arid climates in areas with poor irrigation facilities, weak regulations,

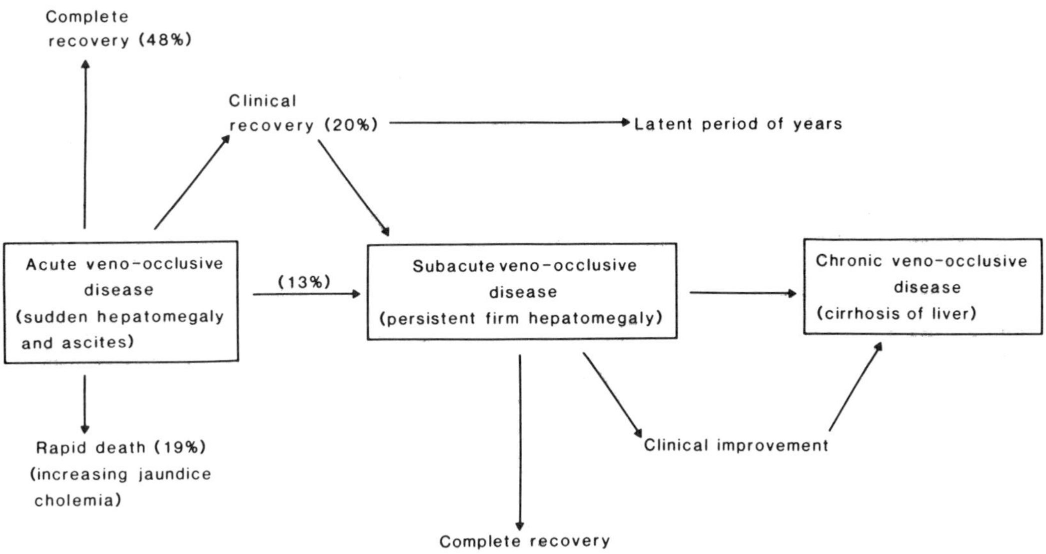

Figure 4 The major stages of veno-occlusive disease induced by pyrrolizidine alkaloid. (Adapted from Stuart and Bras, 1957.)

and underdeveloped health services, i.e., areas of the world where most of the population resides (United Nations, 1988).

Reports of veno-occlusive disease are legion. It can be safely assumed that the majority of these indicate exposure to a dietary source of pyrrolizidine alkaloids. Many of these reports have been recently summarized (Huxtable, 1989a).

Pyrrolizidine-containing plants are widely consumed in various forms all over the world. In Africa, for example, the use of *Senecio gigas* in Ethiopia has been associated with the development of ascites (Watt and Breyer-Brandwijk, 1962). Many *Crotalaria* species are used throughout Africa. In Japan, *Tussilago farfara* is commonly consumed under the name *kan-to-ka*, despite its known carcinogenicity due to its senkirkine content (Fig. 5) (Hirono et al., 1976, 1979). Other pyrrolizidine-containing plants consumed in North America, Europe, or Japan include *Petasites japonicus* Maxim, *Farfugium japonicum*, and *Senecio cannabifolius* (United Nations, 1988). However, the speed and volume of travel, and the mass migration of peoples who take customs and culture with them make the world a unity in terms of exposure to pyrrolizidines. Alkaloid poisoning has occurred in the United States following the consumption of teas imported from Europe and Asia, and pyrrolizidine poisoning has occurred in Europe following the use of teas imported from South America.

A. *Symphytum* Alkaloids

Symphytum (comfrey) species present a particular problem. *Symphytum* species are grown commercially in Europe, North America, Japan, and

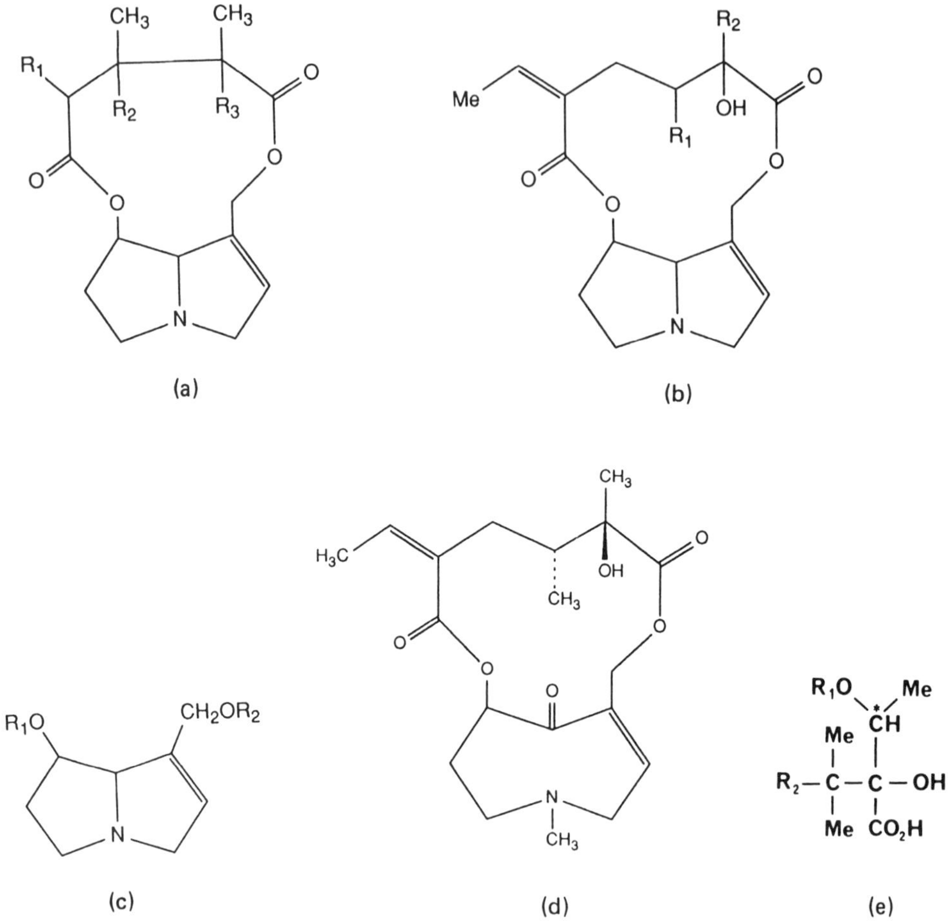

Figure 5 A selection of pyrrolizidines: (a) monocrotaline (R_1: CH_3, R_2; OH, R_3: OH); fulvine (R_1: CH_3, R_2: OH, R_3: H); trichodesmine (R_1: $(CH_3)_2CH$, R_2: OH, R_3: OH); incanine (R1: $(CH_3)_2CH$, R_2: H, R_3: OH); (b) retrorsine (R_1: CH_3, R_2: CH_2OH); senecionine (R_1: CH_3, R_2: CH_3); (c) echimidine (R_1: angeloyl [*cis*-2-methyl-2-butenoyl], R_2: echimidinoyl); symlandine (R_1: angeloyl, R_2: viridifloroyl); symphytine (R_1: tisloyl [2-methyl-but-2-enoyl], R_2: viridifloroyl); heliotrine (R_1: H, R_2: trachelanthoyl); (d) senkirkine. Esterifying acids: angelic $CH_3CH{:}C(CH_3)COOH$; (e) echimidinic (R_1: H, R_2: OH), trachelanthic and viridifloric (stereoisomers of (e) at the position indicated by *, R_1: H, R_2: H).

Australia (Furuya and Araki, 1968), and are widely consumed in the form of vegetables, salads, herbal teas, and herbal remedies, even though they have long been known to contain hepatotoxic and carcinogenic pyrrolizidine alkaloids (Svoboda and Reddy, 1972; Hirono et al., 1979, 1978; Culvenor et al., 1980). Confusion between the hybrids and species of *Symphytum* is frequent (Huxtable and Awang, 1970). There are at least 25 species of *Symphytum*. Common comfrey is *S. officinale*. The literature has been confused by the use of the term Russian comfrey to refer to *S. officinale* (Hirono et al., 1978). This term is correctly associated with *S. asperum* or its hybrids, such as *S. x uplandicum* Nym. The detection of the pyrrolizidine alkaloid, echimidine (Fig. 5), in a sample indicates the presence of *S. asperum* or its hybrids (Culvenor et al., 1980). Echimidine is significantly more toxic than other comfrey alkaloids (Mattocks, 1986). Inaccurate botanical labeling is common for herbal products and is not limited to *Symphytum*.

Alkaloid content of *Symphytum* can vary widely. Leaves can contain between 30 and 1150 mg/kg of alkaloid, with young leaves containing more than old (Mattocks, 1980). Roots contain considerably more alkaloid than the leaves. *S. asperum* roots contain between 1400 and 4000 mg/kg alkaloid (Roitman, 1981). Depending on the material and its preparation, Roitman (1981) has calculated that up to 26 mg of pyrrolizidine alkaloids per cup of comfrey tea could be consumed.

The safety of *Symphytum* has been a contentious issue between scientists and the herb industry. It is true that the number of documented cases of *Symphytum* poisoning is low. Acute toxicity is low. Thus, in rats, the acute LD_{50} for mixed *Symphytum* alkaloids has been determined to be around 550 mg/kg (Culvenor et al., 1980). However, the toxic actions of pyrrolizidines are cumulative—the total dose being more important than the length of time it takes to reach this dose (Shubat et al., 1989)—and clinical symptoms that eventually appear, such as cirrhosis, may be nonspecific and not associated with the ingestion of a herb. Furthermore, to find an association requires that an association be looked for, and this has yet to be done on any consistent basis with pyrrolizidine-containing herbs. Even where a herb is suspected, dose calculations are often difficult. It may be impossible to get a sample of the actual herb consumed, a sample taken at a given time may not accurately reflect the average level of exposure over a longer period (as with the Afghan epidemic, in which samples of food were taken on one occasion during the 6 months to 2 years of exposure), and there may be difficulty in getting estimates of how much contaminated food was consumed, how often, and over what period of time. In an outbreak of veno-occlusive disease in India, poor correlation was found in the affected villages between the pyrrolizidine content of grain in households and the presence of veno-occlusive disease in the household; i.e., the sample of grain taken was not truly representative of the family's exposure over a period of time (Tandon et al., 1976; Krishnamachari et al., 1977; Arora et al., 1981). The true incidence of pyrrolizidine poisoning is probably orders of magnitude greater than the established cases (Culvenor et al., 1980).

Several cases of comfrey poisoning have been described (Ridker et al., 1985; Weston et al., 1987; Abbott, 1988; Bach et al., 1989; Huxtable, 1989a; Jones and Taylor, 1989; Yeong et al., 1990). A 47-year-old woman developed ascites and liver disease after drinking up to 10 cups of comfrey tea per day, and consuming comfrey pills in addition, over a period of 1 year (Bach et al., 1989). A 13-year-old boy given comfrey root and comfrey leaf tea for the supposed treatment of Crohn's disease developed ascites and hepatomegaly (Weston et al., 1987). A 49-year-old woman suffered portal hypertension and veno-occlusive disease after taking comfrey-pepsin capsules daily for 6 months (Ridker et al., 1985). A 23-year-old man, a vegetarian, died of veno-occlusive disease in New Zealand after eating comfrey leaves over a period of time (Yeong et al., 1990).

In the United States, a major source of exposure to *Symphytum* alkaloids is the widespread use of comfrey-pepsin capsules as digestive aids. Typically, these are consumed with each meal. Some brands are prepared from *Symphytum* root and some from leaves, although frequently no information is given as to the source. Alkaloid content varies widely (Huxtable et al., 1986). We have, for example, found one preparation with a total alkaloid content of 270 mg/kg and another containing 2900 mg/kg (Huxtable et al., 1986). In both cases, the alkaloids found were symphytine and symlandine (Fig. 5), and the isomeric pairs, 7-acetylintermedine plus 7-acetyllycopsamine and intermedine and lycopsamine. Analysis of one batch of comfrey-pepsin capules being taken by an elderly woman with veno-occlusive disease, portal hypertension, and cirrhosis showed a pyrrolizidine content of 988 mg/kg (Huxtable, 1989a). As each capsule contains 500–600 mg of the preparation, and as numbers of capules are consumed daily for periods of months, comfrey-pepsin capsules are clearly a major source of exposure to carcinogenic and hepatotoxic alkaloids.

B. *Senecio* Alkaloids

Senecio is a many-membered, widely distributed genus in the Compositae. In excess of 100 *Senecio* species are known to contain pyrrolizidines (Mattocks, 1986). Despite this, worldwide, there are numerous uses of *Senecio* as food or medicine (Rose, 1972; Mattocks, 1986; Huxtable, 1989a). In Paraguay, for example, flower heads of *S. grisebachii* are added to maté tea. Retrorsine (12.7 mg), a highly toxic alkaloid (Fig. 5), has been found in a drink prepared in such a manner (Hirschmann and Cespedes, 1986). Retrorsine was also the major alkaloid involved in the poisoning of children in Arizona with teas prepared from *S. longilobus* (Huxtable, 1980a). Two cases of veno- occlusive disease have been reported from Switzerland following the ingestion of *Senecio* teas (Margalith et al., 1985). Numerous herbal usages of other pyrrolizidine-containing species have been reported (Huxtable, 1989a).

The first description of pyrrolizidine poisoning of humans involved poisoning with bread contaminated with the seeds of *S. ilifolius* and *S. burchelli* in South Africa (Willmot and Robertson, 1920). Deaths, primarily of children, occurred within 10 days to 2 years of exposure. An alarming aspect of this outbreak was that the symptoms of pyrrolizidine poisoning had been known in the area for at least 10 years prior to the investigations of Willmot and Robertson (1920). Underreporting of pyrrolizidine poisoning is typical, due to the unspecific nature of the symptoms (pains in the abdomen, bloating, wasting), and the chronic nature of the poisoning, symptoms developing gradually over a prolonged period. The association with ingestion of pyrrolizidine-containing plants is not readily made. Thus, 30 years after the first investigation, another series of deaths from *Senecio* contamination of grain was reported in South Africa (Selzer and Parker, 1950). Again, the investigators report that the disease was well known to the population of the district. Fifteen years ago, we described pyrrolizidine poisoning as being an iceberg disease, a characterization we feel is still descriptive (Stillman et al., 1977). Other outbreaks of poisoning due to food contamination by *Senecio* alkaloids are known (Al-Hasany and Mohamed, 1970; Rose, 1972). The epidemic of veno-occlusive disease in the West Indies that extended from at least the 1930s (and probably much earlier) until the early 1960s was caused by consumption of bush teas prepared from both *Senecio* and *Crotalaria* species. This epidemic has been reviewed recently (Huxtable, 1989a).

Poisonings, including deaths, from the use of commercially available herbal teas prepared from *S. longilobus* have been reported for the United States (Stillman et al., 1977; Fox et al., 1978; Huxtable, 1989a). For some of these cases, reasonably accurate calculations of consumption could be made. One 6-month old girl developed veno-occlusive disease progressing to cirrhosis after being fed herbal tea over a 2-week period. The quantity of tea used contained about 150 mg pyrrolizidines (primarily retrorsine *N*-oxide), but when tea was prepared according to the recipe used it was found that only about 70 mg were extracted. A 2-month old boy died after being given a similar herbal tea for 4 days. In this case, the amount of alkaloid estimated as having been consumed was 66 mg over a 4-day period (Huxtable, 1980a). Other cases of poisoning from *S. longilobus* in the United States have been described (Huxtable, 1980a). Poisonings from the use of *Senecio* teas have been reported for other countries (e.g., Margalith et al., 1985).

Senecio alkaloids are excreted in the milk of animals grazing on *S. jacobaea* and are found in the honey of bees grazing on the same plant. There is a possibility that dairy products, meat, and honey may contain traces of these alkaloids.

C. *Crotalaria* Alkaloids

Crotalaria species have been frequently used as food plants in various parts of the world, including the West Indies and Africa (Huxtable, 1989a). Large-scale outbreaks of veno-occlusive disease have been reported from Jamaica due to the use of pyrrolizidine-containing *Crotalaria* and *Senecio* species in so-called "bush teas," commonly used in large quantities to treat various childhood ailments (Hill et al., 1951, 1953) (reviewed in Huxtable, 1989a). Vigorous public health measures have, apparently, much reduced the incidence of veno-occlusive disease in recent years. Similar outbreaks for similar reasons have occurred in other countries, including Egypt and India (see Huxtable, 1989a).

Contamination of millet seed with the seeds of *C. nana* has led to epidemics of poisoning in India (Tandon et al., 1976; Krishnamachari et al., 1977). In one outbreak in Mahya Pradesh, 28 of 67 affected people died. A survey a year later found up to 9% of the population of a village suffering from ascites. The difference in size between *C. nana* seeds and the larger millet seeds allow winnowing or sieving techniques to be used in cleaning food seed.

D. *Heliotropium* Alkaloids

Heliotropium species are used medicinally, herbally, or as foodstuffs in most areas of the world (Schoental, 1968; Ford, 1975; Morton, 1981; Mattocks, 1986). Their use has been associated with an increased incidence of liver cancer. Thus, the higher cancer rates among desert-living Bedouin as compared to their town-living relatives may be connected with the consumption of *H. ramossisimium* by the former (Schoental, 1982). Poisonings by *Heliotropium* due to contamination of barley have been common in central Asia (cf. McLean, 1970; Huxtable, 1989a). The biggest documented outbreak of pyrrolizidine poisoning in modern times occurred in the Herat province of Afghanistan. This was caused by the consumption of bread prepared from grain contaminated with *H. popovii* (Mohabbat et al., 1976; Tandon et al., 1976). Heliotrine (Fig. 5) was the alkaloid primarily responsible. Thousands of people were affected.

H. eichwaldii is commonly used in Ayurvedic medicine. Deaths have been reported from the use of this plant, which may, indeed, contribute significantly to the incidence of veno-occlusive disease in India (cf. Huxtable, 1989a). Other cases of *Heliotropium* poisoning have been reported (Tandon et al., 1978; Kumana et al., 1983, 1985; Culvenor et al., 1986).

E. *Trichodesma* Alkaloids

The *Trichodesma* alkaloids, trichodesmine and incanine (Fig. 5), are closely related to monocrotaline. They are, however, much more toxic and are also unusual in that they produce neurological damage in humans, if Soviet reports are to be credited (Ismailov, 1970; cf. Huxtable, 1998a). An outbreak of *Trichodesma* poisoning occurred in the Samarkand region of Uzbekistan in the 1950s as a result of contamination of grain. At least 44 people died.

F. Thresholds for Pyrrolizidine Alkaloids

No threshold for safe exposure to pyrrolizidine alkaloids has been established (United Nations, 1988). However, the levels at which toxicity in humans has been documented has drifted steadily downwards over the years as investigators become more aware of the delayed and cryptic hazards of these substances. It appears that humans are more susceptible to pyrrolizidine poisoning than are rats. Toxicity is exacerbated when repeated small doses are given over a period of time. Babies appear to be particularly vulnerable to the dangers of low-level exposure, despite their relative deficiency of the liver P_{450} mixed function oxidase systems responsible for bioactivating pyrrolizidine alkaloids to the toxic, alkylating pyrroles (Huxtable, 1990b).

An estimate of human toxicity can be obtained by calculating exposures in terms of "rat LD_{50} units." This normalizes exposure in terms of measurements on a readily studied species. If this is done for the cases in which estimations of consumption are available, the data of Table 1 are obtained. As tenuous as the data are, the table suggests that total intake of pyrrolizidine alkaloids to levels approximating 0.05–0.1 of the rat LD_{50} can be toxic to humans.

Table 1 Estimated Intakes of Pyrrolizidine Alkaloids Causing Toxicity in Humans

			Daily intake			Total dose			
Plant	Principal alkaloid(s)[a]	Exposure	mg/kg[b]	rat LD_{50}[c] units	Period (days)	mg/kg	rat LD_{50} units	Toxic effect[d]	Ref.
Heliotropium popovii	Heliotrine	Grain	0.033	1×10^{-4}	180[c]	6	0.02	VOD, death	Mohabbat et al., 1976
					730[c]	24	0.08	VOD, death	Mohabbat et al., 1976
H. eichwaldii	Heliotrine	Herb	3.3,	0.01	20	67	0.22	Death	Datta et al., 1978
			3.3		50	167	0.55	Death	
H. lasiocarpum	Heliotrine	Herb	0.59,	0.002	45	27	0.09	VOD	
			0.49,	0.0017	46	23	0.08	Death	Kumana et al., 1983, 1985
			0.60,	0.002	19	11	0.04	VOD	Culvenor et al., 1986
			0.71	0.0023	21	15	0.05	VOD	
Senecio longilobus	Riddelliine, retrorsine	Tea	0.8–1.7[b]	0.016–0.034	14	12–25	0.24–0.50	VOD	Stillman et al., 1977 Huxtable, 1980a
S. longilobus	Riddelliine, retrorsine	Tea	3.0[b]	0.06	4	12	0.24	Death	Fox et al., 1978
Crotalaria nana	Crotananine, cronaburmine	Herb	0.66	0.007	60[e]	40	0.4	VOD, death	Tandon, et al., 1976 Tandon, R. K., et al., 1976 Krishnamachari et al., 1977
Symphytum sp.	Mixed	Capsule	0.015	3×10^{-5}	120	1.76	0.0035–0.014	VOD	R. J.Huxtable, unpublished
Symphytum sp.	Mixed	Capsule	0.06	1.2×10^{-4}	180	11.3	0.087	Cirrhosis	

[a]The principal alkaloid is recorded as the free base even if there was evidence of its presence in the plant mostly as *N*-oxide.
[b]Calculated for a 60-kg adult, unless definite information available. The *S. longilobus* cases were infants.
[c]Estimates vary as to period of exposure.
[d]Death was a consequence of severe liver damage. VOD = veno occlusive disease.
[e]Intake would be lower if extraction into water was incomplete, as occurred with the *Senecio* teas.

A minimum daily intake of 15 μg/kg/day of pyrrolizidine alkaloids was calculated for a middle-aged woman with veno-occlusive disease (Ridker et al., 1985). There may have been other, unknown, sources of exposure. This, however, compares with the 30 μg/kg/day calculated for the Afghanistan epidemic (Mohabbat et al., 1976), although this estimate has been disputed, and it has been claimed that alkaloid intake could have been as high as 1300 mg/day (Anderson, 1981).

If the identification of senecionine (Fig. 5) as the intoxicating agent in the Swiss case discussed in Section X is accurate (Roulet et al., 1988), the maximum dose the child received in utero could have been no more than 0.125 mg/kg body weight, or 0.0025 rat LD_{50} units (Huxtable, 1989b). Problematic as this value is, it is not out of line with the data of Table 1. The high values for the *S. longilobus* poisonings (Huxtable, 1989a) are probably a reflection of supra-toxic doses being administered to small children over a comparative short period of time.

In one well-investigated case of *Heliotropium* poisoning of four women in Hong Kong, seeds were grown from an herb sample and identified as *H. lasciocarpum* (Kumana et al., 1985). Reliable evidence of total alkaloid consumption was obtained in this case, helped by one patient who continued taking the herb against medical advice. She died.

VI. TROPANE ALKALOIDS

Tropane alkaloids, such as atropine (Fig. 6), scopolamine, or *l*-hyoscyamine, are found in plants such as *Atropa belladonna, Datura stramonium*, and *Hyocyamus niger*. Atropine itself is an artefact of isolation, being formed from the racemization of *l*-hyoscyamine. These plants are consumed as a result of commercial contamination of other plants (Awang and Kindack, 1989), misidentification or lack of knowledge of their toxicity by persons collecting for themselves, and, most frequently, by intentional use of plants for their central nervous system action. An accidental poisoning occurred when *D. suaveolens* seeds were added to hamburger (Anonymous, 1984). Occasionally, children are poisoned through eating *Datura* berries (Taha and Mahdi, 1984). Cases on poisoning following intentional consumption of *Datura* species, commonly called jimsonweed or moonflower, are legion (e.g., Urich et al., 1982 and references therein). A single Poison Control Center in the United States has reported 73 cases of intentional ingestion of *Datura* in a 5-year period (Klein-Schwartz and Oderda, 1984). Jimson is a corruption of Jamestown, the name referring to a mass intoxication by *Datura* in that Virginian town in 1676, when those who consumed it "turned fools upon it for several days" according to one early author. This is in keeping with Shakespeare's description of *A. belladonna* as "the insane root which takes the reason prisoner." Tropane alkaloids are anticholinergic, and toxicity is primarily a consequence of this. The intoxicated individual is described in mnemonic phrases as hot as a hare, dry as a bone, blind as a bat, mad as a hatter, red as a beet.

D. stramonium is sold as an asthma medication, and poisonings have frequently occurred as a result (Feenaghty, 1982). All parts of the plant are

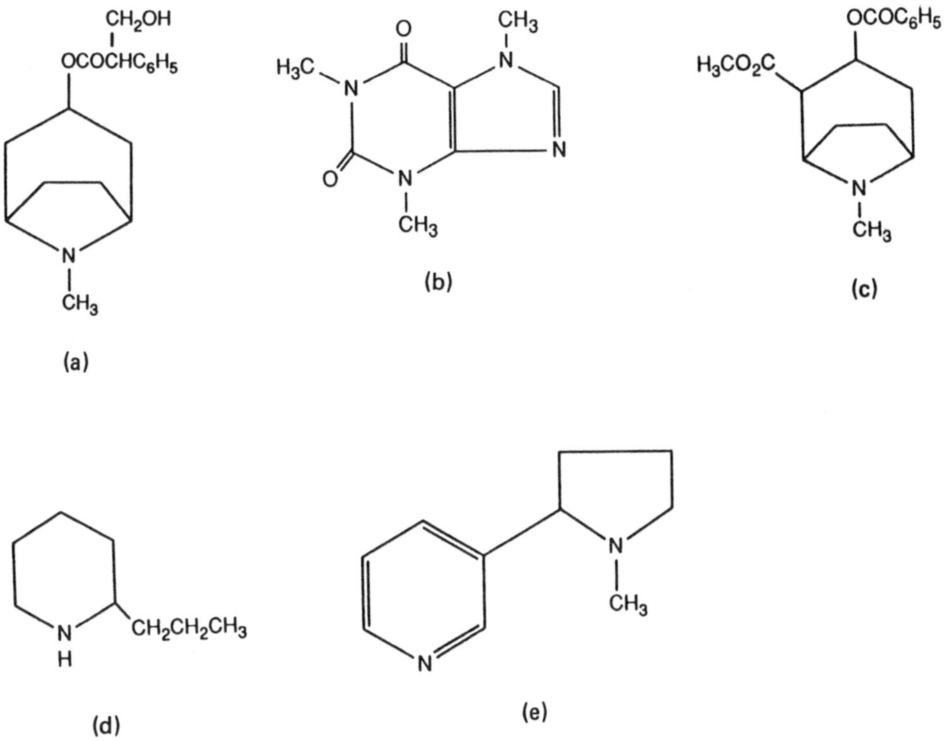

Figure 6 (a) Atropine from jimsonweed (*Datura* spp.) and deadly nightshade (*Atropa belladonna*); (b) caffeine from coffee (*Coffea* spp.), tea (*Camellia sinensis*), and maté (*Ilex paraguayensis*); (c) cocaine from *Erythroxylum coca*; (d) coniine from hemlock (*Conium maculatum*); (e) and nicotine from tobacco (*Nicotiana tabacum*).

toxic, the highest amounts being found in the roots and leaves. The alkaloids are readily absorbed through mucous membranes.

VII. METHYLXANTHINES

The most widely consumed alkaloids worldwide are, without a doubt, the methylxanthines. Of these, caffeine (Fig. 6) is far and away the leader. Worldwide caffeine consumption has been estimated to be 70 mg/day/person, or some 1.1×10^8 kg per annum (120,000 tons) (Spiller, 1984; Max, 1986). Caffeine is contained in tea, coffee, cocoa, chocolate, headache remedies, and soft drinks. Although caffeine is found in at least 63 plant species, most of the world's consumption derives from two *Coffea* species and the tea plant, *Camellia sinensis*. Of the world's consumption of caffeine, coffee accounts for 54% and tea for 43% (Max, 1986). The caffeine in soft drinks is derived from the process of decaffeinating coffee, a pharmacological illustration of the principle that what you lose on the swings you gain on the roundabouts. The average daily intake for U.S. adults is 2.5 mg/kg/day, and for Europeans, 3.5 mg/kg/day (Stavric,

1988a). The motivation for this enormous consumption is, of course, the central nervous system stimulation people get from caffeine. Theobromine, the major xanthine in chocolate, only has weak central actions, due to its low liposolubility (Stavric, 1988b). Caffeine is addictive, the withdrawal syndrome involving headaches and lassitude. Apart from this, the methylxanthines have low toxicity in adults, numerous studies failing to sustain a relationship between caffeine consumption and risk of cardiovascular disease (e.g., Grobbee et al., 1990).

The form in which caffeine is consumed varies from country to country. Tea consumption ranges from 3.44 kg/yr/capita in Ireland to 0.02 kg/yr/capita in Thailand. Coffee consumption is highest in Finland at 12.41 kg/yr/capita. In the United States, it is 4.68 kg/yr/capita. These numbers apply to 1981–1982 (Max, 1986). This represents a 54% drop since 1960, the difference being made up by the consumption of caffeine-containing soft drinks. In 1982, Americans drank 149 L/yr/person of such beverages.

Caffeine consumption is clearly within the pharmacological range. The minimum stimulant dose in humans falls between 85 and 250 mg. Average per capita daily consumption in the United Kingdom is around 165 mg, in the United States around 246 mg, and in Finland 465 mg. A considerable fraction of the populations of these countries, of course, consume much greater amounts. Thus, while the daily mean intake for the United States has been calculated as 2.6 mg/kg, the upper decile was 7.0 mg/kg (Dews, 1984). There is no doubt, therefore, that caffeine is the world's most widely consumed behaviorally active alkaloid. It is, in the words of one investigator, a model drug of abuse (Holtzman, 1990).

Although this massive consumption of alkaloids seems relatively innocuous, mankind perhaps receiving more benefit than harm from "the reviving brew" or a fragrant cup of coffee, it may pose a developmental hazard. A noted researcher in pharmacokinetics once told me that she had never performed a plasma analysis on a baby that did not show the presence of caffeine. Even pregnant or nursing women who eschew coffee may be exposed to caffeine from a variety of other sources. Babies are exposed to caffeine both in utero and via the milk. Although the average mean intake may be low—for the United States estimated to be 0.18 mg/kg for babies under the age of 1 year (Dews, 1984)—the 16–20 times longer half-life of excretion, discussed above, due to the lack of liver metabolizing enzymes means that even a low daily intake of caffeine can lead to an accumulating body burden (Aldridge et al., 1979; Aranda et al., 1979). The developmental consequences of caffeine exposure is a generally unconsidered aspect of the wide use of this generally safe substance. Although developmental studies in humans are difficult (it is next to impossible to find a control group of unexposed babies, for one), the results of animal experiments give cause for alarm. Known developmental effects based on animal studies include increased circulating catecholamine levels in the fetus, decreased placental weight, lactate accumulation, and altered uterine perfusion. When nursing rats were given caffeine equivalent to a human consumption of approximately three cups of coffee a day (rats metabolize caffeine faster), protein concentration in the brains of the pups was significantly increased, while the levels of zinc and activities of zinc-dependent enzymes such as alkaline phosphatase decreased (Nakamoto et al., 1989). When caffeine exposure was combined with the additional stress of protein malnutrition, a different spectrum of changes obtained.

VIII. ERGOT ALKALOIDS

Perhaps the best-known examples of alkaloidal contamination of food come from the epidemics of ergotism that ravaged Europe at intervals throughout the Middle Ages. Ergot is a fungus, *Claviceps purpurea*, which grows on the ears of rye, *Secale cereale*. Ergot alkaloids are mevalonylindole (lysergic acid) derivatives, major ones being ergotamine and ergonovine (Fig. 7). These compounds have a complex pharmacology. A major action is the α-adrenergic agonism which causes profound and long-lasting constriction of vascular beds. If exposure continues long enough, gangrene results.

Ergotism has existed for as long a rye has been used as cereal. Outbreaks are recorded on Assyrian clay tablets from 600 B.C. (Tanner, 1987). The consumption of moldy bread produced the medieval epidemics known as

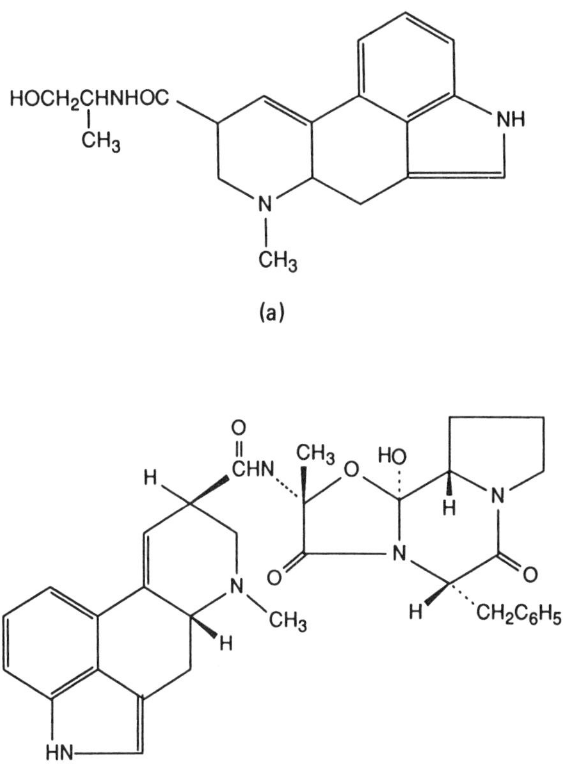

(a)

(b)

Figure 7 (a) Ergonovine and (b) ergotamine alkaloids of ergot (*Claviceps purpurea*).

St. Anthony's fire. It has been claimed that events as disparate as the Salem witch trials in New England and the lack of increase in the European population during the Middle Ages were consequences of the consumption of rye bread containing the products of the unwanted mold (Matossian, 1989). With the shift in consumption to wheat bread and better regulation of food contamination, ergotism slowly ceased to be a major public health problem. Outbreaks, however, still occur, as a result of improper storage or processing of rye. If rye is stored damp, ideal conditions obtain for the growth of these parasitic molds. In this century, major outbreaks occurred in Russia in 1926, in Ireland in 1929, and in France in 1953. In Africa, an outbreak was recorded in 1979 in Ethiopia.

Iatrogenic ergotism is not uncommon. Alkaloids such as ergotamine are used clinically in the treatment of migraine, and cases of intoxication from such usage are known (e.g., Macguire and Cassidy, 1990). Ergot alkaloids are potent oxytocins, certain of them, such as ergonovine, having been used therapeutically to induce labor. However, oxytocin itself is replacing ergonovine in current practice.

IX. OTHER ALKALOIDS

In a short chapter, it is impossible to review all the alkaloids to which humans are exposed by means of foods and herbs. The chewing of *Catha edulis* Forsk., or khat, is common in parts of Africa for the mild stimulation afford by cathinone, an alkaloid with amphetaminelike actions. The khat habit is now spreading in Europe. In the summer of 1990, I observed a man selling khat in the railway station in Amsterdam. *Sanguinaria* alkaloids are added to toothpastes, cough remedies, and mouthwashes in the United States and are used in other parts of the world as folk remedies. The use of *Nicotiana* leaves as tobacco is legion, and as consumption in the United States falls, so it rises in other parts of the world. Poisoning has occurred in the United States from the use of nicotine-containing chewing gum, and death has resulted from the consumption of the leaves of *N. glauca*, a common, naturalized plant in many parts of America (Castorena and Garriott, 1987). The quality of life for many people is also markedly affected by their dietary levels of histamine and tyramine.

X. PRINCIPLES FOR INVESTIGATION OF HERBAL POISONINGS

A recent case of pyrrolizidine poisoning in Switzerland has engendered discussion out of proportion to its intrinsic significance because some basic rules of investigation were not observed. It involves the diagnosis of hepatic veno-occlusive disease in a 5-day-old female, who died 33 days later (Roulet et al., 1988). Exposure to pyrrolizidines had occurred in utero from the mother's persistent consumption of herbal tea. According to the manufacturer, the tea in question contained 10 plant species, including 9% of *Tussilago farfara*, or coltsfoot. The authors believed this without confirming it by their own botanical analysis. Thin-layer chromatography indicated a senecionine content in the tea of 0.6 mg/kg dry weight. However, *T. farfara* contains not senecionine but the alkaloid senkirkine (Fig. 5) (Sommer, 1989). Others have concluded that the plant involved was a *Petasites* species, probably *P. hybridus*, because it grows in the area the mother lived (Anonymous, 1988). However, actual analysis of a tea sample by another laboratory showed the presence of the two pyrrolizidine-containing species, *T. farfara* and *P. officinalis* (Spang, 1989).

A number of general conclusions can be drawn from this one case. First, if possible, an actual sample of the herb consumed should be obtained. Regardless of labeling or of information from the manufacturer, botanical analysis should be done if possible on the sample and on other, separately purchased, samples of the same product. Botanical identification alone, while important, is insufficient due to the wide variability in alkaloid content from sample to sample. Chemical analysis should be done to establish (1) that pyrrolizidines are present, (2) which alkaloids are present, and (3) in what concentration they are present. Estimates can be obtained as to the quantity of material consumed, the period of time over which it was consumed, and the extraction efficiency of the alkaloids under the conditions of preparation employed. This allows mg/kg body weight exposures to be calculated, as has been done in the case of the Arizona poisonings and other intoxications (Stillman et al., 1977; Huxtable, 1980a; Ridker et al., 1985). In the Swiss case, however, no indication was given as to how the analysis was performed, and no dose calculations were done.

These, of course, are councils of perfection. Often, the material is in such a state of division or decomposition that botanical analysis is difficult (see the photographs in Huxtable, 1989a). Analytical facilities may not be available. But without these steps, it will be impossible to gauge either the true incidence of pyrrolizidine poisoning or the threshold levels of consumption posing risk (Huxtable and Awang, 1990).

Rational standards for herbs and food supplements would include (1) proper botanical identification of the plants used; (2) assays of chemical content of active ingredients, and standards for what these levels should be; (3) controls for purity, including botanical, microbiological and chemical contamination and filth levels for insect parts, animal hairs, and rat feces; and (4) appropriate storage and handling conditions.

XI. ACKNOWLEDGMENT

My own work over the years on pyrrolizidine alkaloids and herbal intoxications has been supported by USPHS grant HL-25258.

REFERENCES

Abbott, P. J. (1988). Comfrey: Assessing the low-dose health risk. *Med. J. Aust. 149*: 678–682.

Al-Hasany, M., and Mohamed, A. S. (1970). Veno-occlusive disease of the liver in Iraq. *Arch. Dis. Child 45*: 722–724.

Aldridge, A., Aranda, J. V., and Neims, A. H. (1979). Caffeine metabolism in the newborn. *Clin. Pharmacol. Ther. 25*: 447–453.

Ames, B. N. (1983). Dietary carcinogens and anticarcinogens: Oxygen radicals and degenerative diseases. *Science 221*: 1256–1264.

Anderson, C. (1981). Comfrey toxicity in perspective. *Lancet i*: 1424.

Anonymous. (1983). Celestial Seasonings halt initial offering. *Wall Street Journal*, 14 November.

Anonymous. (1984). Datura poisoning from hamburger—Canada. *MMWR 33*: 282–283.

Anonymous. (1988). Pyrrolizidinalkaloid-haltige Drogen: Wie gefährlich ist Hutflattich als Hustenstee? *Deutsche Apotheker Zeitung 43*.

Aranda, J. V., Cook, C. E., Gorman, W., Collinge, J. M., Loughnan, P. M., Outerbridge, E. W., Aldridge, A., and Neims, A. H. (1979). Pharmacokinetic profile of caffeine in the premature newborn infant with apnea. *J. Pediat. 94*: 663–668.

Arora, R. R., Pyarelal Ghost, T. K., Mathur, K. K., and Tandon, B. N. (1981). Epidemiology of veno-occlusive disease in tribal population of Madhya Pradesh and Bihar. *J. Commun. Dis. (India) 13*: 147–151.

Awang, D. V. C., and Kindack, D. G. (1989). Atropine as possible contaminant of comfrey tea. *Lancet ii*: 44.

Bach, N., Thung, S. N., and Schaffner, F. (1989). Comfrey herb tea-induced hepatic veno-occlusive disease. *Am. J. Med. 87*: 97–99.

Bain, R. J. I. (1985). Accidental digitalis poisoning due to drinking herbal tea. *Brit. Med. J. 290*: 1624.

Bull, L. B., Culvenor, C. C. J., and Dick, A. T. (1968). *The Pyrrolizidine Alkaloids: Their Chemistry, Pathogenicity and Other Biological Properties*. North-Holland, Amsterdam.

Carlsson, C. (1990). Herbs and hepatitis. *Lancet ii*: 1068.

Castorena, J. L., and Garriott, J. C. (1987). A fatal poisoning from *Nicotiana glauca*. *Clin. Toxicol. 25*: 429–435.

Cooper, L., Grunenfelder, G., Blackmon, J., Fretwell, M., Raey, J., Allard, J., and Bartleson, B. (1977). Poisoning associated with herbal teas—Washington. *MMWR 26*: 257–259.

Culvenor, C. C. J., Clarke, M., Edgar, J. A., Frahn, J. L., Jago, M. V., Peterson, J. E., and Smith, L. W. (1980). Structure and toxicity of the alkaloids of Russian comfrey (*Symphytum X uplandicum* Nyman), a medicinal herb and item of human diet. *Experientia 36*: 377–379.

Culvenor, C. C. J., Edgar, J. A., Smith, L. W., Kumana, C. R., and Lin, H. J. (1986). *Heliotropium lasiocarpum* Fisch and Mey identified as cause of veno-occlusive disease due to a herbal tea. *Lancet i*: 978.

Dalvi, R. R., and Bowie, W. C. (1983). Toxicology of solanine: An overview. *Vet. Hum. Toxicol. 25*: 13–15.

Datta, D. V., Khuroo, M. S., Mattocks, A. R., Aikat, B. K., and Chhuttani, P. N. (1978). Herbal medicines and veno-occlusive disease in India. *Postgrad. Med. J. 54*: 511–515.

Dews, P. B. (1984). *Caffeine*. Springer-Verlag.

Dickstein, E. S., and Kunkel, F. W. (1980). Foxglove tea poisoning. *Am. J. Med. 69*: 167–169.

Feenaghty, D. A. (1982). Atropine poisoning: Jimsonweed. *J. Emerg. Nurs. 8*: 139–141.

Ford, K. C. (1975). *Las Yerbas de la Gente: A Study of Hispano-American Medicinal Plants*. University of Michigan, Ann Arbor.

Fox, D. W., Hart, M. C., Bergeson, P. S., Jarrett, P. B., Stillman, A. E., and Huxtable, R. J. (1978). Pyrrolizidine (Senecio) intoxication mimicking Reye's syndrome. *J. Pediatrics 93*: 980–982.

Furuya, T., and Araki, K. (1968). Studies on constituents of crude drugs. I. Alkaloids of *Symphytum officinale* Linn. *Chem. Pharm. Bull. 16*: 2512–2516.

Galizia, E. J. (1983). Clinical curio: Hallucinations in elderly tea drinkers. *Brit. Med. J. 298*: 979.

Green, C. R., and Christie, G. S. (1967). Malformations in foetal rats induced by the pyrrolizidine alkaloid, heliotrine. *Brit. J. Exp. Pathol. 42*: 369–378.
Grobbee, D. E., Rimm, E. B., Giovannucci, E., Colditz, G., Stampfer, M., and Willett, W. (1990). Coffee, caffeine, and cardiovascular disease in men. *N. Engl. J. Med. 232*: 1026–1032.
Harvey, M. H., Morris, B. A., McMillan, M., and Marks, V. (1985). Measurement of potato steroidal alkaloids in human serum and saliva by radioimmunoassay. *Hum. Toxicol. 4*: 503–512.
Heath, D., Shaba, J., Williams, A., Smith, P., and Kombe, A. (1975). A pulmonary hypertension-producing plant from Tanzania. *Thorax 30*: 399–404.
Hill, K. R., Rhodes, K., Stafford, J. L., and Aub, R. (1951). Liver disease in Jamaican children (serous hepatosis). *West Indian Med. J. 1*: 49–63.
Hill, K. R., Rhodes, K., and Stafford, J. L. (1953). Serous hepatosis: A pathogenesis of hepatic fibrosis in Jamaican children. *Brit. Med. J. 1*: 117–122.
Hirono, I., Mori, H., and Culvenor, C. C. J. (1976). Carcinogenic activity of coltsfoot, *Tussilago farfara* L. *Gann Monograph. Cancer Res. 67*: 125–129.
Hirono, I., Haga, M., Fujii, M., Matsuura, S., Matsubara, N., Nakayama, M., Furuya, T., Hikichi, M., Takanashi, H., Uchida, E., Hosaka, S., and Ueno, L. (1979). Induction of hepatic tumors in rats by senkirkine and symphytine. *JNCI 63*: 469–472.
Hirono, I., Mori, H., and Haga, M. (1978). Carcinogenic activity of *Symphytum officinale. JNCI 61*: 865–869.
Hirschmann, G. S., and Cespedes, C. (1986). Retrosin from a Paraguayan herbal tea. *J. Ethnopharmacol. 17*: 195–196.
Holtzman, S. G. (1990). Caffeine as a model drug of abuse. *TIPS 11*: 355–356.
Huxtable, R. J. (1979). New aspects of the toxicology and pharmacology of pyrrolizidine alkaloids. *Gen. Pharmacol. 10*: 159–167.
Huxtable, R. J. (1980a). Herbal teas and toxins: Novel aspects of pyrrolizidine poisoning in the United States. *Perspect. Biol. Med. 24*: 1–14.
Huxtable, R. J. (1980b). Problems with pyrrolizidines. *TIPS 1*: 299–303.
Huxtable, R. J. (1989a). Human health implications of pyrrolizidine alkaloids and the herbs containing them. In *Toxicants of Plant Origin*, Vol. I, *Alkaloids*, P. R. Cheeke, ed. CRC Press, Boca Raton, FL, pp. 41–86.
Huxtable, R. J. (1989b). Human embryotoxicity of pyrrolizidine-containing drugs. *Hepatology 9*: 510–511.
Huxtable, R. J. (1990a). The harmful potential of herbal and other plant products. *Drug Safety 5* (Suppl. 1): 126–136.
Huxtable, R. J. (1990b). Activation and pulmonary toxicity of pyrrolizidine alkaloids. *Pharmacol. Ther. 47*: 371–389.
Huxtable, R. J., and Awang, D. V. C. (1990). Pyrrolizidine poisoning. *Am. J. Med. 89*: 547–548.
Huxtable, R. J., Luthy, J., and Zweifel, V. (1986). Toxicity of comfrey-pepsin preparations. *N. Engl. J. Med. 315*: 1095.
IARC. (1975). Pyrrolizidine alkaloids. *IARC Monograph 10*: 265–343.
Ismailov, N. I. (1970). *Heliotropic Toxicosis (Toxic Hepatitis with Ascites)*. Academy of Sciences of Uzbekistan, Tashkent.
Jadhav, S. J., Sharma, R. P., and Salunkhe, D. K. (1981). Naturally occurring toxic alkaloids in foods. *CRC Crit. Rev. Tox. 9*: 21–104.
Johnson, A. E., Molyneux, R. J., and Merrill, G. B. (1985). Chemistry of toxic range plants. Variation in pyrrolozidine alkaloid content of *Senecio, Amsinckia*, and *Crotalaria* species. *J. Agr. Food Chem. 33*: 50–55.
Johnsson, H., and Hellenas, K.-E. (1983). Total glycoalkaloid in Swedish potatoes. *Var Foda 35*: 299–314.

Jones, J. G., and Taylor, D. E. (1989). Hepatic veno-occlusive disease and herbal remedies. *Ann. Rheum. Dis. 48*: 791.

Kingsbury, J. M. (1964). *Poisonous Plants of the United States and Canada*. Prentice-Hall, Inc., Englewood Cliffs, NJ.

Klein-Schwartz, W., and Oderda, G. M. (1984). Jimsonweed intoxication in adolescents and young adults. *AJDC 138*: 737–739.

Krishnamachari, K. A. V. R., Bhat, R. V., Krishnamurthi, D., Krishnaswamy, K., and Nagarajan, V. (1977). Aetiopathogenesis of endemic ascites in Surguja district of Madhya Pradesh. *Ind. J. Med. Res. 65*: 672–678.

Kumana, C. R., Ng, M., Lin, H. J., Ko, W., Wu, P.-C., and Todd, D. (1983). Hepatic veno-occlusive disease due to toxic alkaloid in herbal tea. *Lancet ii*: 1360–1361.

Kumana, C. R., Ng, M., Lin, H. J., Ko, W., Wu, P.-C., and Todd, D. (1985). Herbal tea induced hepatic veno-occlusive disease: Quantification of toxic alkaloid exposure in adults. *Gut 26*: 101–104.

Macguire, A. M., and Cassidy, J. T. (1990). Modern ergotism. *Am. Fam. Phys. 30*: 179–193.

Margalith, D., Heraief, E., Schindler, A. M., Birchler, R., Mosimann, F., Aladjem, D., and Gonvers, J. J. (1985). Veno-occlusive disease of the liver due to the use of tea made from Senecio plants. A report of two cases. *J. Hepatology 1* (Supp. 2): S280.

Matossian, M. K. (1989). *Poisons of the Past: Molds, Epidemics and History*. Yale University Press, New Haven, CT.

Mattocks, A. R. (1980). Toxic pyrrolizidine alkaloids in comfrey. *Lancet ii*: 1136.

Mattocks, A. R. (1986). *Chemistry and Toxicology of Pyrrolizidine Alkaloids*. Academic Press, London.

Max, B. (1986). This and that: Please the patient and pass the coffee. *TIPS 7*: 12–14.

Max, B. (1988). This and that: Thanatomimetics, bradychronotoxins, osmocides and ototoxins. *TIPS 9*: 353–356.

McGee, J. O'D., Patrick, R. S., Wood, C. B., and Blumgart, L. H. (1976). A case of veno-occlusive disease of the liver in Britain associated with herbal tea consumption. *J. Clin. Path. 29*: 788–794.

McLean, E. K. (1970). The toxic actions of pyrrolizidine (*Senecio*) alkaloids. *Pharm. Rev. 22*: 429–483.

McMillan, M., and Thompson, J. C. (1979). An outbreak of suspected solanine poisoning in schoolboys: Examination of criteria of solanine poisoning. *Q. J . Med. XLVIII*: 227–243.

Mohabbat, O., Younos, M. S., Merzao, A. A., Srivastava, R. N., Sedig, G. G., and Aram, G. N. (1976). An outbreak of hepatic veno-occlusive disease in North-Western Afghanistan. *Lancet ii*: 269–271.

Morton, Julia F. (1981). *Atlas of Medicinal Plants of Middle America: Bahamas to Yucatan*. Charles C. Thomas, Springfield, IL.

Nakamoto, T., Hartman, A. D., and Joseph, F. Jr. (1989). Interaction between caffeine intake and nutritional status on growing brains in newborn rats. *Ann. Nutr. Metab. 33*: 92–99.

Peterson, J. E., and Jago, M. V. (1980). Comparison of the toxic effects of dehydroheliotridine and heliotrine in pregnant rats and their embryos. *J. Pathol. 131*: 339–355.

Ridker, P. M., Ohkuma, S., McDermott, W. V., Trey, C., and Huxtable, R. J. (1985). Hepatic veno-occlusive disease associated with the consumption of pyrrolizidine-containing dietary supplements. *Gastroenterology 88*: 1050–1054.

Roitman, J. N. (1981). Comfrey and liver damage. *Lancet i*: 944–944.

Rose, E. F. (1972). Senecio species: Toxic plants used as food and medicine in the Transkei. *Afr. Med. J. 46*: 1039–1043.

Roulet, M., Laurini, R., Rivier, L., and Calame, A. (1988). Hepatic veno-occlusive disease in newborn infant of a woman drinking herbal tea. *J. Pediatrics 112*: 433–436.

Routledge, P. A., and Spriggs, T. L. B. (1989). Atropine as possible contaminant of comfrey teas. *Lancet i*: 963–964.

Schoental, R. (1968). Toxicology and carcinogenic action of pyrrolizidine alkaloids. *Cancer Res. 28*: 2237–2246.

Schoental, R. (1982). Health hazards of pyrrolizidine alkaloids: A short review. *Toxicol. Lett. 19*: 323–326.

Selzer, G., and Parker, R. G. F. (1950). Senecio poisoning exhibiting as chiari's syndrome. *Am. J. Pathol. 27*: 885–907.

Sharma, R. P., and Salunkhe, D. K. (1989). Solanum glycoalkaloids. In *Toxicants of Plant Origin*, Vol. I, *Alkaloids*, P. R. Cheeke, ed. CRC Press, Boca Raton, FL, pp. 179–236.

Shubat, P. J., Hubbard, A. K., and Huxtable, R. J. (1989). Dose-response relationship in intoxication by the pyrrolizidine alkaloid monocrotaline. *J. Toxicol. Environ. Health 28*: 445–460.

Siegel, R. K. (1976). Herbal Intoxication: Psychoactive effects from herbal cigarettes, tea and capsules. *JAMA 236*: 473–476.

Smith, L. W., and Culvenor, C. C. J. (1981). Plant sources of hepatotoxic pyrrolizidine alkaloids. *J. Natural Prod. 44*: 129–152.

Sommer, M. (1989). Hepatic veno-occlusive disease and drinking of herbal teas. *J. Pediatr. 115*: 659–660.

Spang, R. (1989). Toxicity of tea containing pyrrolizidine alkaloids. *J. Pediatr. 115*: 1025.

Spiller, G. A. (1984). *The Methylxanthine Beverages and Food: Chemistry, Consumption and Health Effects*. A.R. Liss, New York.

Stavric, B. (1988a). Methylxanthines: Toxicity to humans. 2. Caffeine. *Food Chem. Toxicol. 26*: 645–662.

Stavric, B. (1988b). Methylxanthines: Toxicity to humans. 3. Theobromine, paraxanthine and the combined effects of methylxanthines. *Food Chem. Toxicol. 26*: 725–733.

Stillman, A. E., Huxtable, R., Consroe, P., Kohnen, P., and Smith, S. (1977). Hepatic veno-occlusive disease due to pyrrolizidine poisoning in Arizona. *Gastroenterology 73*: 349–352.

Stuart, K. L., and Bras, G. (1957). Veno-occlusive disease of the liver. *Quart. J. Med. 26*: 291–315.

Svoboda, D. J., and Reddy, J. K. (1972). Malignant tumors in rats given lasiocarpine. *Cancer Res. 32*: 908–912.

Taha, S. A., and Mahdi, A. H. (1984). Datura intoxication in Riyadh. *Trans. R. Soc. Trop. Med. Hyg. 78*: 134–135.

Tandon, B. N., Tandon, R. K., Tandon, H. D., Narndranathan, M., and Joshi, Y. K. (1976a). An epidemic of veno-occlusive disease of liver in central India. *Lancet ii*: 271–272.

Tandon, H. D., Tandon, B. N., and Mattocks, A. R. (1978). An epidemic of veno-occlusive disease of the liver in Afghanistan. *Am. J. Gastroenterology. 70*: 607–613.

Tandon, R. K., Tandon, B. N., Tandon, H. D., Bhatia, M. L., Bhargava, S., Lal, P., and Arora, R. R. (1976b). Study of an epidemic of venoocclusive disease in India. *Gut 17*: 849–855.

Tanner, J. R. (1987). St. Anthony's fire, then and now: A case report and historical review. *Can. J. Surg. 30*: 291–293.

United Nations Environment Programme, International Labour Organization, and World Health Organization. (1988). *Environmental Health Criteria 80: Pyrrolizidine Alkaloids*. World Health Organization, Geneva.

Urich, R. W., Bowerman, D. L., Levisky, J. A., and Pflug, J. L. (1982). Datura stramonium: A fatal poisoning. *J. Forensic Sci 27.*: 948–954.
Watt, J. M., and Breyer-Brandwijk, M. G. (1962). *Medicinal and Poisonous Plants of Southern and Eastern Africa*. Livingstone, Edinburgh.
Weston, C. F. M., Cooper, B. T., Davies, J. D., and Levine, D. F. (1987). Veno-occlusive disease of the liver secondary to ingestion of comfrey. *Brit. Med. J. 295*: 183.
Willmot, F. C., and Robertson, G. W. (1920). Senecio disease, or cirrhosis of the liver due to senecio poisoning. *Lancet*: 848–849.
Yeong, M. L., Swinburn, B., Kennedy, M., and Nicholson, G. (1990). Hepatic veno-occlusive disease associated with comfrey ingestion. *J. Gastroenterol. Hepatol. 5*: 211–214.

11

Toxicology of Plant Lectins

Werner G. Jaffé and Dinah S. Seidl

Universidad Central de Venezuela, Caracas, Venezuela

I. INTRODUCTION

The presence of heat-labile toxic factors in plant products, mainly legume seeds, makes them unsuitable for human consumption unless they are properly cooked. Among the antinutritional factors that are inactivated by cooking are the lectins or phytohemagglutinins (PHA), which are subject of this chapter.

Lectins were discovered in the last century when Stillmark (1889) presented evidence that the extreme toxicity of castor beans (*Ricinus communis*) could be attributed to a protein fraction which agglutinated red blood cells and which he called "ricin." Ehrlich (1891) compared it with the toxic abrin from the jeriquinty seeds (*Abrus precatorus*) and thus initiated his immunological research on the specificity of antisera obtained by the use of these lectins. This research meant the initiation of many fundamental advances in the knowledge of immunological reactions (Ford, 1913; Lis and Sharon, 1977; Jaffé, 1977; Sharon, 1989).

Landsteiner and Raubitscheck (1908) observed that extracts of many edible crude legume seeds would likewise agglutinate red blood cells, but no toxic action was detected at that time. Probably this was due to the relative low toxicity as compared to the very high activity of the above-mentioned lectins.

Today the widespread occurrence of lectins in plant and animal tissues is well known (Gold and Balding, 1975; Goldstein and Hayes, 1978). Lectins have been reported in more than 800 plant species (Lis and Sharon, 1973).

II. GENERAL PROPERTIES

The term "lectin," derived from the Latin *legere* to choose, was proposed by Boyd and Reguera (1949) to indicate the selectivity of their interaction with specific blood cells. Etzler (1985) discusses the various definitions of lectins. Besides the polyvalent, agglutinating protein molecules, the definition should also include the monovalent ones, which bind reversibly to complex carbohydrates in cell surfaces without clumping and are structurally and genetically related to agglutinating lectins.

Lectins possess specific affinity for certain carbohydrate residues. Since sugars are structural features of most animal cell membranes, lectins may attach to these receptor groups, if the specific structure of the latter fits the former. As this name indicates, hemagglutinins can be characterized and detected by their activities on red blood cells, while other cells can be agglutinated as well. In many cases the binding may occur without visible clumping. The receptor site of the cell surface must exist in an exposed position in order to be able to react with a specific lectin. For detecting hemagglutination in some cells like cow red blood cells (RBC), this may be achieved by partial proteolysis. Trypsin and pronase are often used for this purpose.

Hemagglutination is only one of the numerous detectable consequences of the lectin-receptor interaction. They play a key role in the control of various normal and pathological processes in living organisms. In addition to plants, lectins are commonly present in animal and bacterial cells (Sharon and Lis, 1989).

III. WHAT RENDERS FOOD TOXIC?

The definition of toxins is especially critical when it is applied to food. A snake may be toxic or nontoxic—the bite is a single definite event. Food is ingested daily, and with time harmful effects may accumulate and produce undesirable consequences for the health of the consumer.

Cultures and tradition have given way to habits that are strongly influenced by etiological factors—the food available in a certain environment. The availability of limited choices of food products may have obscured hidden health damage.

The definition of toxicity for a food ingredient is therefore a rather subtle problem. Many normal food ingredients can cause harm when consumed in high amounts. Saturated fats, salt, and cholesterol are well-known examples. Practically any food if consumed in excess may be harmful, but it will not be considered toxic.

Toxicology is concerned with biological effects characterized by distinct dose-response relationships. A substance may be lethal beyond a certain level of intake. The toxicity may be assessed in terms of an LD_{50}, which is the dose that causes the death of 50% of the tested animals. Tests of toxicity are normally performed with laboratory or farm animals. Unfortunately, animals and humans do not react equally to many stress situations like an intoxication.

Lack of exact toxicological evidence of natural foodstuffs or ingredients is generally taken as evidence for safety. The term "generally recognized as safe" (GRAS) expresses this belief and is applied to food legislation (WHO, 1967). It is accepted that there must exist some finite level below which no food compound is toxic. The definition of what this level may be has great practical importance. It may vary according to the physiological condition of the consumer, age, sex, etc. Some of the many plant lectins are known to be sources of hazard; the implications of their prolonged consumption are, however, unknown. Some lectins may kill experimental animals when ingested in sufficient amounts or may interfere with the bioavailability of nutrients. The term "antinutritional" is usually used for this situation (Liener, 1983).

Antinutritional activity of a compound or food may remain unrecognized under conditions of a normal and varied diet, but may exert harmful effects under stress situations, malabsorption syndromes, malnutrition, etc. It is therefore surprising that very little research has been done on "toxicological insignificance" (Goldberg, 1970). The fact that a food ingredient has been consumed for generations without apparent harm is certainly no proof that it is safe under any condition. Control groups are never available for comparison, like populations with identical consumption habits with the only difference, for example, that one consumes tomatoes and the other does not.

No animal species consumes foods as varied as humans do. The great variability probably has resulted in a certain adaptation to the digestion and absorption of different food components (Waterlow, 1990). It is only a guess whether such a capacity for adaptation may also exist for the ingestion of antinutritional factors.

In this chapter, we shall therefore mention some lectins of common foods for which no toxic activity has been demonstrated.

IV. LECTINS IN FOODS

Plant lectins have been found in a great variety of constituents of human diets. A thorough survey on the presence of lectins in commonly consumed foods in the United States was reported by Nachbar and Oppenheim (1980). They tested 88 food items with respect to their ability to agglutinate human erythrocytes of three blood groups, natural and enzyme treated, and also to clump several bacterial strains. Positive results were found in 29 food extracts. Moreover, they list literature on 53 edible plants in which phytohemagglutinins have been identified. Great variations in agglutinating activity were observed in the same food items purchased from different stores or on different days, a fact that may obscure the detection of positive samples. It can be concluded that human exposure to lectins is a widespread event notwithstanding the fact that cooking and contact with digestive enzymes may blunt or abrogate activity. Andersen and Ebbesen (1986) detected lectin activity in 40 of the 75 foods tested. Several papers review the nutritional significance of lectins (Liener, 1976, 1978, 1983, 1986; Jaffé, 1980, 1983; McPherson, 1989).

Liener (1989) in his latest comprehensive review points out the fact that legumes and some cereal grains of primary concern in human nutrition are rich in phytoagglutinins. He also includes a list of edible plants in which lectins have been detected. A slightly modified version is presented in Table 1.

Legumes are an important ingredient of the diets of most developing countries (Aykroyd and Doughty, 1964). In the future an increased consumption can be anticipated as a cheap and nutritious source of protein. Already, cereal–bean mixtures, which can be prepared locally in rural areas, are recommended as weaning food (King et al., 1966).

Following the observation that some legume lectins distinguish between different human and animal blood groups, a great number of extracts from this vegetable family were tested for agglutination (Krüpe, 1956; Makela, 1957; Tobiska, 1964). Toms and Western (1971) list nearly 500 legume species and varieties, the seeds of which show some blood agglutinating activity. It must be

Table 1 Edible Plants That Contain Lectins

CEREAL GRAINS			
Avena sativa	Oats	*Secale cereale*	Rye
Hordeum vulgare	Barley	*Triticale* spp.	Triticale
Oryza sativum	Rice	*Triticum vulgare*	Wheat
Sorghum bicolor	Sorghum	*Amaranthus caudatus*	Amaranth
		Zea mays	Corn
VEGETABLES			
Abelmoschus esculentus	Okra	*Cucurbita maxima*	Pumpkin
Apium graveolens	Celery	*Cucurbita sativus*	Cucumber
Asparagus officinalis	Asparagus	*Ipomea batatas*	Sweet potato
Beta vulgaris	Swiss chard	*Lactuca scariole*	Prickly lettuce
Brassica camapestris rapa	Turnip/Beet	*Lycopersicon esculentum*	Tomato
Brassica napobrassica	Rutabaga	*Medicago sativum*	Alfalfa
Capsicum annum	Sweet pepper	*Petrosecinum hortense*	Parsley
Solanum tuberosum	Potato	*Rheum rhapontium*	Rhubarb
FRUITS			
Carica papaya	Papaya	*Malus species*	Apple
Citrus aurantium	Orange	*Musa paradisiaca*	Banana
Citrullus vulgaris	Watermelon	*Prunus americana*	Plum
Citrus medica	Grapefruit	*Prunus avium bigarreaus*	Cherry
Cucumis melo cantalupensis	Cantaloupe	*Ribees rubrum*	Currant
Cydonia oblonja	Quince	*Rubus idacus*	Raspberry
Fragaria versa	Strawberry	*Rubus fructicosus*	Blackberry
SPICES			
Allium sativum	Garlic	*Myristica fragrans*	Nutmeg
Labiacea origanum	Marjoram	*Menta piperita*	Peppermint
Pimienta officialis	Allspice		
OTHERS			
Agaricus bisporus	Mushroom	*Juglans regia*	Walnut
Carum carvi	Caraway seeds	*Helianthus annus*	Sunflower seeds
Cocos nucifera	Coconut	*Sesamum indicum*	Sesame seeds
Coffee arabica	Coffee	*Theobroma cacao*	Cocoa
Corylus avellania	Hazelnut		

remembered that negative results may be due to the fact that the right blood type was not used.

In agglutination studies of 54 species of legumes on 18 different blood types, only 6 samples gave positive results with trypsin-treated cow erythrocytes. However, these RBC are the best for detection of the toxic bean varieties (Casotto et al., 1984).

V. ANIMAL GROWTH ASSAYS

Lectin toxicity is usually evaluated by injection or by oral ingestion. The latter is obviously of primary concern in relation to the corresponding plant products as food. Most toxic lectins are more or less heat labile. Therefore, cooking of lectin-containing food products will have a beneficial effect on the nutritive value. Despite this apparent association, one cannot assume that this effect can be attributed solely to the inactivation of toxic lectins. Enzyme inhibitors, other thermolabile compounds, and increase of digestibility may also be responsible.

In order to distinguish the effect of trypsin inhibitors, amino acid deficiency, and toxic lectins in beans, the addition of predigested casein (casitone) and methionine to the experimental diets for growing rats has been useful (Jaffé and Vega-Lette, 1968). Poor growth performance of rats consuming beans with low lectin activity could be restored to normal with this procedure. In contrast, animals given a diet of toxic beans did not respond with growth improvement. They grew well, however, on a diet of autoclaved beans supplemented with methionine. The oral toxicity of common beans (*Phaseolus vulgaris*) was recognized by Everson and Heckert (1944), Jaffé (1949), Jaffé et al. (1955), Jaffé and Gaede (1959), Honavar et al. (1962), Wagh et al. (1963), DeMuelenaere (1964, 1965), Evans et al. (1973), and confirmed by Pusztai et al. (1975), Bender and Reaidi (1982), Lojolo and Mancini (1988), and others.

The fact that purified bean lectin is highly toxic for rats was demonstrated by adding it to an experimental diet. It produces growth inhibition and will kill the animals within a few days, depending on the level and origin of the lectin as shown in Table 2 (Honavar et al., 1962). The opposite experiment with delectinized bean diet showed disappearance of toxicity as measured by normal growth of animals (Pusztai and Palmer, 1977).

VI. DIGESTIBILITY OF LECTINS

In order to exert toxic or antinutritional actions, lectins must resist digestion, in cooked foods be thermo-stable, and interact with the brush-border membrane of the intestinal mucosa. In the case of raw toxic beans given to experimental animals, the hemagglutinating activity and the specific precipitation of thyroglobulin can easily be detected in extracts of feces. These results indicate that at least part of the ingested lectins have resisted digestion (Jaffé and Vega-Lette, 1968). Similar observations have been reported for winged bean agglutinin (Higuchi et al., 1989).

In vitro experiments with pepsin and trypsin corroborate the resistance toward digestion of these proteins from beans (Jaffé and Hannig, 1965). Soybean lectins, on the other hand, have been found to be digested by gastrointestinal enzymes (Liener, 1958). Very little is known about many other lectins that may be present in our daily diet, as in cucumbers, melons, and other fruits that are eaten raw.

Tomato lectin resists digestion by rats. It can be detected bound to intestinal villi and in the feces of the experimental animals after consumption of a lectin-containing diet. ^{125}I-Labeled tomato lectin was found in human blood,

Table 2 Effect of Purified Hemagglutinin Fractions from the Black Bean and Kidney Bean on Growth of Rats

Source of hemagglutinin	Purified hemagglutinin in diet (%)	Gain in weight (g/day)	Mortality[a] (days)
Black bean	0	+2.51	
	0.5	+1.04	
	0.5[b]	+2.37	
	0.75	+0.20	
	1.2	−0.91	15–19
	2.3	−1.61	12–17
	4.6	−1.72	5–7
Kidney bean	0	+2.31	
	0.5	−0.60	13–16
	0.5[b]	+2.29	
	1.0	−0.87	11–13
	1.5	−1.22	4–7

[a]100% mortality observed during the period recorded. Blank space indicates no deaths observed.
[b]Solution of hemagglutinin boiled for 30 min and dried coagulum was fed at level indicated. Hemagglutinating activity was completely destroyed by this treatment.
Source: Honavar et al., 1962.

indicating that it also resists digestive breakdown in man (Kilpatrick et al., 1985). Nevertheless, tomatoes are often consumed raw, and no antinutritional effects have been reported, as far as we are aware.

VII. EFFECT OF HEAT TREATMENT

Cooking of beans does not necessarily destroy their toxic properties. Autoclaving at 118°C for 30 min of beans previously soaked in water for 2–3 h abolished toxicity completely (Jaffé and Vega-Lette, 1968). Contradictory opinions have been reported in the literature on whether soaking prior to cooking is essential for the improvement of the nutritional quality of beans. Pack et al. (1978) concluded that soaking was not necessary for detoxification of bean meal and whole beans. Overnight soaking was applied by Lowgren and Liener (1986) in their bean-cooking tests. Soaking alone caused a 10–15% loss of hemagglutinating activity. No significant advantage was observed by Kakade and Evans (1966) or by El-Nahry et al. (1977) for attaining complete elimination of agglutinating and toxic properties. These differences may be due to the so-called "hard-to-cook" phenomenon (Jackson and Varriano-Marston, 1981), a consequence of poor drying and storage conditions of seeds used in the assays.

The effect of cooking at relatively low temperatures, as in so-called "slow cookers" or "crockpots" on the hemagglutinating action of kidney beans, was studied by Lowgren and Liener (1986). As most previous works had been conducted at fixed temperatures, these authors determined the disappearance of the agglutinating activity, taking into account the lag of temperature rise and the rate of heat penetration into the bulk of the beans in the slow cooking vessel. After 5 h of heating, when the temperature had almost reached 80°C, over 90% inactivation was achieved, while heating to 100°C for 20 min abolished hemagglutinin activity completely.

Coffey et al. (1985) applied a sensitive electronic cell counter for measuring the hemagglutinating activity in slowly cooked beans. They observed some activity after 12 h of heating at 82°C. (This is the boiling temperature of water in Mexico City.) Moreover, energy shortage is an economic reason for applying slow cooking. Addition of sodium bicarbonate to cooking water shortens cooking time.

Dry heating had little effect on hemagglutinating activity of certain varieties of *P. vulgaris*, and some activity was still detectable after several hours of heating (DeMuelenaere, 1964). Heintze (1950) found dry heating or high frequency treatment ineffective for the cooking of beans. However, the heating of soaked beans was fully effective. Too much heating reduces the growth induced by bean diets, probably due to the impairment of the nutritive value of the proteins (Kakade and Evans, 1965).

Another procedure to prepare edible pulses is sprouting or germination, which may lower, but does not eliminate, lectin activity (Chen et al., 1977; Nielsen and Liener, 1988).

VIII. DIFFERENCES IN LECTIN CONTENT, TYPE, AND TOXICITY IN COMMON BEANS

Large differences in toxicity of lectins have been observed. Compared with the extremely toxic ricin, the LD_{50} of the toxic bean lectin is about 1/1000 times smaller. Some bean cultivars and lectins are known to be nontoxic (Jaffé and Gomez, 1975; Pusztai et al., 1979). This may be due to the lectin concentration in the seed or to the nature or type of lectins present.

In relation to specificity, there are at least four clearly distinguishable groups of bean lectins (Jaffé et al., 1972). The most abundant type A will agglutinate both rabbit and trypsinized cow blood cells. Type B is more active on rabbit than on cow blood. Type C is specific for cow blood, and type D does not agglutinate either but will agglutinate pronase-treated hamster blood (Table 3).

When extracts of the different bean types were tested by injection into mice (Jaffé et al., 1972) or by feeding the ground seeds to rats (Jaffé and Vega-Lette, 1968), it was established that only the A- and C-type beans were toxic, whereas types B and D were of low toxicity. Only the toxic beans showed mitogenic activity on human leucocytes (Jaffé et al., 1972; Jaffé, 1973) (Table 4).

Some samples of cow blood are inactive, probably due to different blood group specificities. Pronase-activated hamster blood is very sensitive to all types of bean lectins and several others, too.

Lectins of the kidney bean seed groups show remarkable differences when submitted to heat treatment. The toxic lectins which agglutinate trypsinized cow blood cells (A and C) will not lose either this ability or its toxicity after 90

Table 3 Hemagglutinating Activity of Extracts of Beans on Different Blood Samples[a]

	Bean cultivar							
	Saxa (A)		Cubagua (B)		Porillo (C)		Mountan. half runner (D)	
Type of blood	nat.	pron.[b]	nat.	pron.[b]	nat.	pron.[b]	nat.	pron.[b]
Rabbit	8	11	9	11	0	2	0	2
Cow[c]	0	12	0	2	0	12	0	1
Swine	11	12	9	12	0	0	0	0
Mouse	6	12	3	8	3	7	1	5
Rat	6	11	2	8	0	9	0	4
Hamster	8	12	7	11	6	12	3	7
Cat	12	12	5	12	0	5	0	4
Cock	6	12	6	11	0	9	0	3
Sheep	4	12	3	6	2	7	0	1
Human blood group AB	6	12	6	12	0	4	0	3
Human blood group O	6	12	6	12	0	3	0	3

[a]The highest dilution step of the crude seed extracts (1 g of ground seeds + 10 ml physiological saline) producing visible agglutination within 1 h is indicated. Only 12 dilution steps were tested.
[b]Pronase-treated RBC.
[c]Cow RBC were treated with trypsin, instead of pronase.
Source: Jaffé et al., 1972.
(A), (B), (C), (D) refer to the four lectin specificity groups.

min heating at 80°C. Under these conditions the activity toward rabbit blood is strongly diminished or completely abolished (Brucher et al., 1969; Jaffé et al., 1972). This observation should be an alert that the results of an in vitro agglutinin test must be interpreted with caution when used as evidence of the persistence for toxicity (Table 5).

The existence of these different lectin types has been confirmed by several authors. Lima et al. (1980) studied 16 Brazilian bean varieties. They found that those active as agglutinins of rabbit and trypsinized cow RBC and as mitogens were toxic, although some nontoxic samples had mitogenic activity. Mancini and Lajolo (1981) established the existence of four bean lectin types similar to those described by Jaffé et al. (1972). Koehler et al. (1986) screened 24 samples of American beans and found three of the four lectin types. The toxic lectins were detected by hemagglutination of trypsinized cow blood and also by SDS electrophoresis. Pusztai et al. (1979) found 11 of 13 cultivars of kidney beans to be active in hemagglutination and toxicity, while 2 low-lectin bean varieties had no appreciable effect on the intestine and were nontoxic in rats. Extensive variation in bean lectin types has also been observed by two-dimensional electrophoretic patterns (Brown et al., 1982). Lectin-free bean cultivars were described by Osborn et al., 1985).

Table 4 Correlation of Specific Hemagglutinating Activity with Intraperitoneal Toxicity in Mice of Extracts of Different Varieties and Cultivars of *P. vulgaris* and Their Mitogenic Action

Variety	Rabbit blood	Trypsinated cows' blood	Toxicity (no. of injected mice/ no. dead mice)	Mitogenic activity
Balin de albenga (A)	+	+	5/4	+
Merida (A)	+	+	9/9	+
Negro Nicoya (A)	+	+	5/4	+
Saxa (A)	+	+	5/5	+
Peruvita (B)	+	–	5/0	–
Palleritos (B)	+	–	6/0	–
Juli (B)	+	–	5/0	–
Cubagua (B)	+	–	5/0	–
Porillo (C)	–	+	5/5	+
Negra No. 584 (C)	–	+	5/3	+
Vainica Saavega (C)	–	+	10/6	+
Hallado (D)	–	–	5/0	–
Madrileno (D)	–	–	5/0	–
Alabaster (D)	–	–	5/0	–
Triguito (D)	–	–	6/0	–

Source: Jaffé et al., 1974.

Table 5 Hemagglutinating Activity of Extracts of Different Bean Cultivars to Rabbit and Trypsin-Treated Cows' Red Blood Cells Before and After Heating at 80°C for 90 min

	Agglutination titer			
	before heating		after heating	
Bean cultivar	rabbit	cow	rabbit	cow
Saxa (A)	9	11	4	11
Balin de albenga (A)	9	10	5	10
Guateian (A)	11	9	2	9
Juli (B)	8	3	1	0
Cubagua subline (B)	9	2	0	0
San Fernando (B)	8	3	0	0
Porillo (C)	0	9	0	9
Ecuador 4A (C)	0	11	0	11
Rabuda (C)	0	9	0	9
Mountaneer half runner (D)	0	0	0	0
Great northern (D)	0	0	0	0
Kaiser Wilhelm (D)	0	0	0	0

The highest dilution step producing visible agglutination in 1 h is indicated. The extracts were heated in presence of the ground beans used for extraction.
Source: Jaffé, 1972.

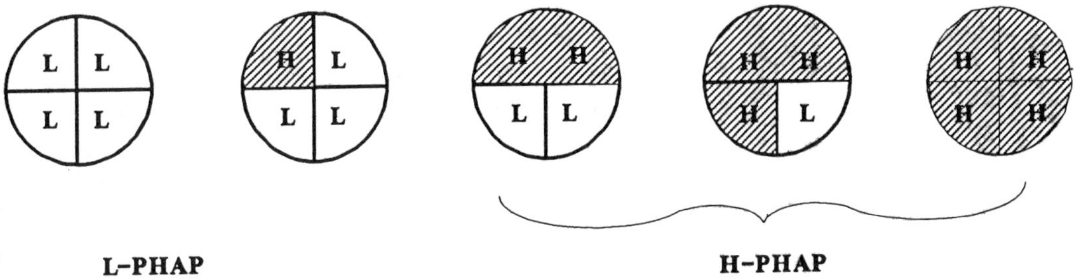

Figure 1 Tetrameric structures of bean agglutinins. L = leukoagglutinating mitogenic unit. H = hemagglutinating unit.

Field fertilization can effect the lectin content of beans (Tobiska and Lhotecka-Brazdova, 1960). It was also shown that the seeds of one bean variety grown and harvested under various environmental conditions differed in lectin activity (Fernandez et al., 1981).

The hemagglutinating and mitogenic activities have been explained by the tetrameric structure of bean lectins. They have been separated by dissociation in 8.0 M urea (Rigas and Head, 1969). Two different subunits, which can produce five combinations, have been recognized. One of the subunits has high affinity for lymphocyte membrane receptors but low or no affinity for rabbit and human RBC (Allen et al., 1969; Miller et al., 1973, 1975). This so-called leukoagglutinin has been isolated from commercial phytohemagglutinin by Weber et al. (1972). It will agglutinate trypsin-treated cow RBC and pronase-treated hamster cells (Jaffé et al., 1974) (Fig. 1).

IX. SOYBEANS

Soybeans and garden beans aroused the most interest in relation to the toxicity of the lectins. Osborne and Mendel (1917) observed the growth-promoting effect of heating on soybean meal, which pointed to the presence of heat-labile antinutritional compounds in these seeds. Among these, protease inhibitors and lectins have been studied most. Liener (1953) presented evidence that the growth inhibition observed in rats on a raw soybean diet could not fully be explained by the trypsin inhibitors. When purified soya lectin was added to the heated soybean meal diet, some growth depression was apparent. This could be attributed to decreased food intake of the experimental animals.

Soybean proteins may be freed of lectin by affinity chromatography. This delectinized material did not support better growth than the original lectin-containing extract (Turner and Liener, 1975a). Soybean lectin is digested by pepsin (Liener, 1958). This may account for the little, if any, direct effect on the nutritional properties of soybean proteins.

When injected into rats, the isolated lectins resulted toxic (Liener and Pallansch, 1952). Grant et al. (1987a) reported toxic manifestation in rats when 0.75% of soybean lectin were added to the diet, an amount higher than would be provided by a diet with 10% protein derived from soy, which is commonly used.

Loss of brush-border enterocytes, atrophy of intestinal villi, and other toxic effects in rats fed soybean lectin were described by Jindal et al. (1984). Growth was, however, not significantly impaired in the 28-day assay. In our laboratory it was observed that mice are more susceptible than rats to the ingestion of raw soybean meal and that hemagglutination can be detected in the feces of the corresponding animals.

X. WINGED BEANS

Winged beans (*Psophocarpus tetragonolobus*) are legumes of nutritional importance in Asian-tropical countries, where seeds, roots, and immature pods are commonly consumed. Diets prepared with 10% protein derived from winged beans are toxic for rats. The experimental animals will not survive for more than 10 days. Autoclaved beans are nontoxic. Their extracts will agglutinate rabbit erythrocytes (Jaffé and Korte, 1976).

Higuchi and Iwai (1985) purified winged-bean lectin by affinity chromatography. Kortt and Caldwell (1987) observed two distinct lectins in the roots of winged beans. They were essentially identical to the ones found in the seeds.

XI. FIELD BEANS

Ground field beans (*Dolichos lablab*) as part of rat diet reduced growth significantly and caused the death of the experimental animals (Jaffé, 1950). Autoclaving, but not germination, abolished toxicity (Salgarkar and Sohonie, 1965).

The isolated lectin from field beans is toxic when injected into rats (Manage et al., 1972). When fed at a level of 2.5% in the diet, it inhibits normal growth of rats (Salgarkar and Sohonie, 1965).

XII. JACK BEAN SEEDS

The nutritional value of jack bean (*Canavalia ensiformis*) meal improves markedly with heat treatment. It contains several antinutritional factors, such as trypsin and amylase inhibitors, canavanin—an arginine analog—canalin, the lectin concanavalin A (ConA), and canatoxin.

Although ConA can easily be isolated from the meal extract by affinity chromatography, much more is known about its structure than about its toxicity. Similar to other legume lectins, ConA can interact and damage cells lining the gastrointestinal tract (Weaver and Bailey, 1987).

A toxic protein named canatoxin has been isolated from jack bean seeds and separated from the hemagglutinating ConA. It is considered to be a monovalent or hemi-lectin. The presence of similar proteins has been demonstrated in several other legume seeds by immunological methods (Carlini et al., 1988).

XIII. OTHER LEGUME LECTINS

Salgarkar and Sohonie (1965) also isolated lectins from horse gram (*Dolichos biflorus*). Manage et al. (1972) observed retarded growth in rats fed this lectin, which was nontoxic when injected into rats and mice. These results contrast those obtained by the above authors with lima bean (*Phaseolus lunatus*) lectins, which were growth inhibiting when fed and toxic when injected. Levy et al. (1985) fed diets prepared with raw or autoclaved lima beans and garden beans. The diet of raw garden beans was lethal within 1 week; the raw lima bean diet did not support any growth in 28 days but did not cause death. Both permitted normal growth performance after heat treatment.

The nutritive value of peas (*Pisum sativum*) measured in rats is not enhanced by heat treatment (Schneider and Miller, 1954). The isolated lectin is slightly toxic when injected into rats (Manage et al., 1972).

Peanut lectin has been used for fractionation of thymocyte subpopulations into mature and immature cells (Reisner et al., 1976). No toxic action of this phytoagglutinin has been reported.

XIV. CEREAL LECTINS

In cereal grains such as oats, barley, rice, rye, sorghum, and wheat, lectins are present mainly in the germ (Stinissen et al., 1983; Peumans, 1985; Liener, 1989). Wheat germ agglutinin survives the digestive process of the human body and can reach the colon in biologically intact form (Brady et al., 1978). Lectin activity is also present in endosperm and can be traced to albumin, globulin, zein, and glutelin fractions. Some of the endosperm lectins are heat stable (Newburg and Concon, 1985). It has been proposed that the pathogenesis of celiac disease, an intolerance toward wheat products, is related to lectinlike activity of wheat gliadin (Kottgen et al., 1983). Nevertheless Colyer et al. (1986) did not observe any agglutination of normal and celiac human enterocytes or mammalian erythrocytes. The authors suggest, therefore, that in celiac disease there is probably no interaction of gliadin with intestinal cells in polyvalent lectinlike manner.

Lectin activity in rice is concentrated in the germ fraction and is heat labile (Barber and Barber, 1978).

XV. ANTINUTRITIONAL AND TOXIC ACTIVITIES

Based on evidence available in the 1950s, Jaffé (1960) proposed that a possible explanation for the toxic action of lectins, resistant to gastric and intestinal digestion, is that they combine with cells lining the intestinal wall, causing lesions and nonspecific interference with the absorption of nutrients. Since then several groups of researchers have produced direct evidence to substantiate the fact that bean lectins interact specifically with intestinal epithelium cells (Etzler and Brandstator, 1974), damage, and even kill them both in vivo and in vitro (King et al., 1980; Sotello et al., 1980; Pusztai et al., 1981). Etzler

(1984) described the specific lectin receptors (carbohydrate residues) on the small intestinal cell surface for several plant agglutinins.

Since surface-bound lectins are able to produce profound physiological effects on the cells, with which they interact, their capacity to absorb nutrients from the gut may be impaired, causing growth inhibition and even death. Rats switched from a toxic bean diet to a commercial diet recovered weight quickly, but histological studies showed severe ulceration and necrosis of intestinal villi in the surviving animals (Oliveira et al., 1989). The rapid loss of body weight may be explained by the observed doubling of the mucosal protein synthesis rate, which uses up large amounts of N and thus starves the body of its amino acid supply (Pusztai, 1987).

In addition, dietary lectins are specifically taken up into the systemic circulation of rats, either through the disrupted intestinal wall or by breaching the gut absorptive barrier. The concentration of toxic bean PHA in blood is higher than that of nontoxic tomato agglutinin. Up to 10% of bean lectin was detected in blood vs. 0.1% of the tomato lectin (Pusztai, 1989).

The latter, taken up at a lower level of the intestinal villi by endocytosis than PHA, is retained in the liver and detoxified. The former can act on various organs of the body, carried by the blood circulation (A. Pusztai and S. Bardocz, personal communication, 1991).

Dietary exposure to lectins or toxic lectin-containing beans produces polyspecific antibodies against the major bean proteins in rats (Grant et al., 1985), pigs (Begbie and King, 1985), and steers (Williams et al., 1984/85). The binding of PHA to the membrane receptors and its endocytosis by epithelial cells of the small intestine stimulates cellular metabolism, protein, and glycoprotein synthesis and increases DNA and RNA content. This hyperplasia is accompanied by an elevated polyamine concentration. PHA may utilize similar polyamine-dependent pathways as used by mucosal growth-stimulating signals during adaptive growth (Pusztai et al., 1988).

Consumption of kidney beans induces depletion of lipid and glycogen reserves, loss of protein, and reduction of circulating insulin. The interaction of the absorbed lectins on the pancreas could have suppressed insulin secretion and caused some of the catabolic changes observed. Several hormonal and metabolic changes were also detected in soybean-fed rats (Grant et al., 1987b).

Grant et al. (1985) conclude that the toxicity of *Phaseolus vulgaris* lectins are independent of age or maturity of the experimental animals after pair feeding rats aged between 30 and 123 days with bean diets. No significant differences between age groups could be detected in protein utilization, food intake, disruption of intestinal lining, or circulating antilectin antibodies.

In vivo studies using ConA in neonatal guinea pigs show mucosal damage in stomach, crypt cells, and villi. A substantial increase in urinary lactulose: mannitol excretion ratio, indicative of a loss of mucosal integrity, was detected. According to the authors, these findings may "have implications for the pathogenesis of childhood celiac disease" (Weaver and Bailey, 1987).

ConA binding disturbs the functional formation of brush-border response to dietary alterations (Nakata and Kimura, 1986). Similar effects of the brush-border cells were observed for the wing bean lectin (Kimura et al., 1986).

ConA given to rats at a level of 0.3 and 0.5% in the diet prevented normal adaptive changes of sucrase, alkaline phosphatase, and amino-peptidase (Nakata and Kimura, 1985).

According to Rouanet et al. (1982), of several intestinal hydrolases only alkaline phosphatase is not inhibited by bean lectin in vitro. However, in pair-fed rats receiving diets with and without PHA, the total activity of intestinal hydrolases decreases in similar proportion (Rouanet et al., 1985). Jindal et al. (1984) found loss of brush-border cells and atrophy of the villi in albino rats fed soybean lectins. They also observed a decrease in both disaccharidases and proteases, but report an increase in alkaline and acid phosphatases and Ca^{2+}-ATPase.

Lectins were shown to interact with human intestinal hydrolases (Triadou and Audran, 1983). Purified brush-border aminopeptidase and dipetidylpeptidase recognize sepharose-bound bean lectins (Erickson and Kim, 1983).

The in vivo binding of navy bean lectins to the brush-border cells decreases the rate of glucose absorption to one half of its normal value (Donatucci et al., 1987). These results definitely confirm the observations reported by Jaffé et al. (1955) and Jaffé and Camejo (1961) on the effect of kidney bean lectin on intestinal absorption.

In vitro studies revealed noncompetitive inhibition of pancreatic and salivary amylases by red kidney bean lectins. Thompson and Gabon (1987) therefore suggest that lectins may play a role in reducing the rate of starch digestion.

The oral toxicity of raw kidney beans in rats involves, in addition to hypertrophy of the pancreas, due in part to trypsin inhibitors, atrophy of the thymus and doubling in weight of the small intestine. Changes in tissue composition include protein, carbohydrate, and DNA increases. Mineral content, urea concentration, and some enzyme activities in serum and urine were also changed (Greer et al., 1985).

On the mammary gland level, ConA was shown to specifically inhibit milk secretion in minced tissue (Patton et al., 1980). The cobalamine transport to liver and kidney in vivo was inhibited by ConA. It affected the binding of the transcobalamin II-cobalamin to its receptor, interfering with the tissue uptake of the vitamin (Ramasamy et al., 1990).

Despite the considerable body of evidence on the harmful effects of the ingestion of active lectins, it has nevertheless been suggested that they may serve to protect against colon cancer by causing hypersecretion of intestinal mucus or by exerting direct toxic effect on tumor cells (Freed and Green, 1975). Indeed many lectins agglutinate and damage neoplastic cells in preference to their normal equivalents (Raedler and Raedler, 1985).

Another toxic effect in animals, observed upon ingestion of lectin-containing diets, is the decrease of food intake. Donatucci et al. (1987) and Rouanet et al. (1985) describe the phenomenon in rats, Leon et al. (1991) in chicks, Williams et al. (1984/85) in fast-growing steers, and Begbie and King (1985) in pigs. The mechanism of the above effect is still unknown. Its remarkable feature is its velocity, for food intake decreases within 30 min after ingestion of lectin diet (Leon et al., 1991).

The real importance of these findings is still obscure. It is obvious, though, that lectins from legumes may damage the intestinal structures and interfere with their normal functions.

XVI. BACTERIOLOGICAL CONSEQUENCES OF LECTIN INGESTION

Germ-free animals are better able to tolerate lectin-containing diets than conventional ones. An overgrowth or colonization of coliform bacteria has been observed in the small intestines of experimental animals. Banwell et al. (1985) found that, in addition to structural damage, the mucous layer of the jejunal, ileal, and cecal surfaces were heavily colonized by bacteria and protozoa in weanling rats fed 0.5% PHA in the diet.

There is a clear increase in lectin toxicity in conventional quail (Jayne-Williams and Burgess, 1974), chicks (Hewitt et al., 1973), and rats (Rattray et al., 1974) as compared to germ-free ones. The binding of lectins to the cells lining the intestine may interfere with their defense mechanism, which prevents the normally innocuous bacteria from passing from the lumen to lymph, blood, and other animal tissues. The ulcerative disruption of the gut may also have allowed bacteria to invade tissues.

Several lectins clump some bacteria specifically. They may act on adherence of bacteria to the intestinal wall. *Salmonella typhimurium* adherence is promoted by ConA but not by the lectins from beans, groundnut, and wheat germ. This activity may enhance bacterial colonization and infection (Abud et al., 1989).

XVII. HUMAN INTOXICATION

Several cases of intoxication in humans by the consumption of partially cooked beans have been reported. A paper by Faschingbauer and Kofler (1929) was probably the first to describe this occurrence. During the blockade of Berlin in 1948, preheated bean flakes were air-lifted to the city. They caused gastrointestinal distress among many consumers (Griebel, 1950). Acute gastroenteritis, nausea, and diarrhea following the consumption of soaked beans as part of a salad or of slow-cooked beans have been reported from England (Noah et al., 1980; Bender and Reaidi, 1982).

Korte (1972) assayed agglutination of trypsin-treated cow erythrocytes by extracts from weaning food used in Tanzania. Locally produced corn and beans were ground and heated in open vessels on three stone fireplaces to palatability. Of 91 samples tested, 20 showed positive agglutinin reaction, indicating remaining active lectins.

The possible role of bean lectins in the ethyology of protein-energy malnutrition has been analyzed in a comprehensive paper by McPherson (1989).

XVIII. INHERITANCE OF LECTINS

The presence or absence of the toxic lectin was shown to be inherited as a single gene in wild beans (*Phaseolus aborigeneus*) (Brücher et al., 1969) and also in kidney beans (Jaffé et al., 1972) (Table 6). Osborn et al. (1985) studied 46 bean

Table 6 Hemagglutinating Activity in the F_2 Generation of Types A and D Bean Plant

No.	Types of cross	Agglutination of rabbit and trypsin-treated cow RBC — Number of seeds +	−
1	A/D	23	13
2	A/D	76	28
3	A/D	22	14
4	D/A	30	6
5	D/A	55	22
6	D/A	241	81
7	D/A	231	77
Total		678	241
		73.7%	26.3%

Source: Jaffé et al., 1972.

cultivars and observed significant differences with respect to lectin type and quantity. The F_2 plants of crosses segregated in a Mendelian fashion for two paternal lectin types, indicating single gene inheritance. It is, therefore, possible to remove seed lectins genetically by backcross-breeding (Osborn and Bliss, 1985).

The occurrence of a certain soybean lectin has been attributed to a single dominant gene (Orf et al., 1978). Later Tsien et al. (1983) were able to show the presence of very small amounts of this lectin in soybean cultivars, which had previously been considered inactive. The quantities present were 1000 to 10,000 times less than those found in a reference cultivar.

XIX. ASSAY METHODS

The detection of seed lectins is most commonly performed by serial dilution. In a microtiter dish, constant amounts of normal or protease-treated RBC are added and clumping is visually determined. The acceptance of this method is widespread, among other considerations, because of the small amounts of lectin samples it requires. Screening of single seeds or seed parts is feasible with the above technique.

RBC of different species, animal and human, should be used, since lectins could be overlooked due to inactivity toward some erythrocytes. Burger (1974) has critically evaluated this procedure. In addition to blood agglutination, clumping of bacterial strains have been used (Nachbar and Oppenheim, 1980).

To overcome the semiquantitative nature of the serial dilution test, Liener (1955) devised a photometric measurement of the RBC that are left unagglutinated by the lectin. Stabilization of RBC with glutaraldehyde rendered the above method more sensitive and reproducible for the detection of nanograms of soybean agglutinin (Turner and Liener, 1975b). More recently, an electronic particle counter was applied to count the nonagglutinated cells in the microtiter wells, to give a quantitative measure of lectin activity (Koehle and Kauss, 1980; Coffey et al., 1985).

Screening of lectins in foods has been realized by a combination of line-dive immunoelectrophoresis and hemadsorption lectin test. Both methods could detect about 0.2 μg purified lectin (Andersen and Ebbesen, 1986). Osborn and Bliss (1985) prepared antibodies against isolated bean lectins, incorporated them into gels, and applied rocket immunoelectrophoresis for the quantitative determination of agglutinins in inbred backcross lines.

Nanogram quantities of castor bean lectins were detected by a technique based on the interaction of the lectin with sugar immobilized to lysozyme and the measurement of the remanent lytic effect of *Micrococcus luteus* cells. In this case the preparation of antibodies was unnecessary (Ghosh et al., 1979). Jaffé and Gómez (1975) used an intradermic test in mice to compare partially purified lectins from different bean cultivars.

XX. CHEMICAL CHARACTERISTICS

The structures of some legume lectins have been studied in detail. Many, but not all, are glycoproteins that contain different *N*-linked glycosyl residues. These are probably not essential for sugar binding. Bivalent metal ions—Ca^{2+} and Mn^{2+}—are often found as ligands in specific sites. Their removal abolishes activity. Lectins frequently contain hydrophobic regions, which may be related to cell-binding properties. They are a family of homologous proteins and quite different in composition and structure from ricin and abrin. Complete amino acid sequence has been established for some 15. The homologies are particularly striking between lectins of the same tribe. About 10% of the amino acids are invariant in all legume lectins (Sharon and Lis, 1990).

Oligomeric structures of two or four equal or different subunits are common, as mentioned in Chapter 8. This feature explains the existence of isolectins in plant tissues (Fig. 1). They may possess varying degrees of toxicity. Each subunit has one carbohydrate-binding site. Monomeric or hemi-lectins are, therefore, nonagglutinating molecules (Etzler, 1985).

ConA was the first lectin to be crystallized by Sumner. The three-dimensional structure of its carbohydrate complex was studied by high-resolution X-ray crystallography by Derewenda et al. (1989). The configuration of a few other lectins and lectin–carbohydrate complexes has been solved by this method (see Sharon and Lis, 1990).

XXI. TOXIC LECTINS IN NONEDIBLE PLANTS

Besides being found in the legume plant family, toxic lectins have been detected mostly in *Euphorbiaceae* since the last century: in *Ricinus communis* (Stillmark, 1889), *Croton triglium* (Elfstrand, 1897), *Jatropha curcas* (Siegel, 1893), and *Hura crepitans* (Richet, 1909). The body of evidence that relates edible-plant lectins to antinutritional effects observed in experimental animals is large. However, the mechanism by which they influence or damage the organisms and the cells has not been as thoroughly studied.

On the other hand, interesting details on the action of the lectins, ricin, abrin, modeccin from *Adenia digitata*, and viscumin from the mistletoe (*Viscum album*) derived from nonedible plants, and which possess different molecular structures than most legume agglutinins, are known. They exert cytotoxicity by a mechanism similar to bacterial diphtheria toxin (see Olsnes and Sandvig, 1988).

Ricin is synthesized as a single polypeptide in maturing castor beans, where it accumulates in the storage granules of the seeds (Youle and Huang, 1976). Unlike most agglutinins, ricin and abrin are cleaved afterwards into two disulfide-linked glyco-polypeptides, termed the A- and B- chains.

Chain B acts as a galactose-specific lectin that interacts with cell membrane glycoproteins and glycolipids and thus permits the translocation of chain A into the cytosol. The A-chain has enzyme activity that is basically responsible for killing the infected cell. It is a highly specific *N*-glycosidase that removes adenine from a single adenosine residue located in a conserved region near the 3′-end of 28-S RNA. This cleavage inactivates the 60S ribosomal unit required for protein synthesis (see van Deurs et al., 1990) (Fig. 2).

The inhibition of in vitro synthesis in a rabbit reticulocyte cell-free system by toxic trypsic peptides from ricin has been described by Lugnier et al. (1974).

Lethal doses of abrin and ricin are about 1 μg toxin/kg body weight in mouse, rat, and dog. Rabbits are 10 times more sensitive to these toxins, while goats are more resistant (Field, 1910). However, due to a selective effect of ricin and abrin on malignant cells, they have been assayed in treatment of human cancer (Hsu et al., 1974). The cytostatic phenomenon may be explained by the fact that malignant cells are more efficient in internalizing the toxins (Nicolson et al., 1975). The inhibitory effect on the growth of human cancer in nude mice has been demonstrated by Fodstad et al. (1977).

Cases of intoxication of operators handling press cake from the castor oil industry (Cooper et al., 1964) and of children who swallowed ricinus seeds (Alstalf, 1963) have been reported.

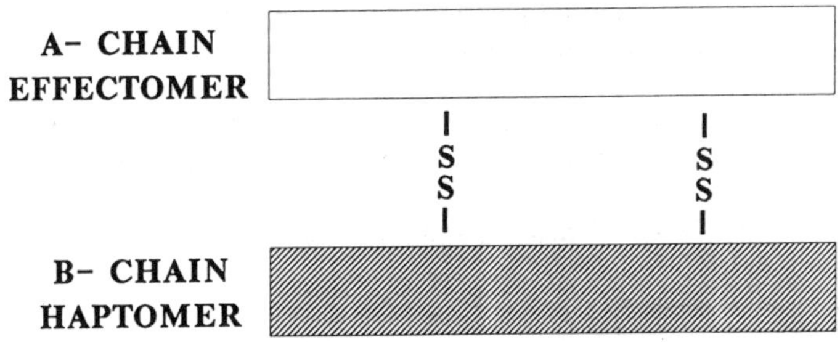

Figure 2 Schematic structure of ricin and abrin.

XXII. FINAL COMMENTS

Given the significant exposure of the consumers to dietary lectins and the diversity of their biological activities, it is rather surprising that the weight of scientific research directed to these interesting compounds has been focused mostly on chemical and biochemical aspects with little attention given to their possible antinutritional and toxicological role. It is evident that complete destruction of lectins is not always achieved by all the possible conditions of culinary preparations. What does it mean when a lectin is labeled nontoxic? Nontoxic for whom? Rats, chicks, humans?

Much more research is needed to evaluate any nutritional or physiological implications of the long-term consumption of low levels of toxic lectins and also of those until now considered nontoxic, or even those not yet detected.

ACKNOWLEDGMENT

We wish to thank Dr. Andrés Carmona for his help in the elaboration of the manuscript.

REFERENCES

Abud, R. L., Lindquist, B. L., Ernst, R. K., Merrik, J. M., Lebenthal, E., and Lee, P. C. (1989). Concanavaline A promotes adherence of *Salmonella typhimurium* to small intestinal mucosa in rats. *Proc. Soc. Exptl. Biol. Med. 192*: 81–86.

Allen, L. W., Svenson, R. H., and Yachnin, S. (1969). Purification of mitogenic proteins derived from *Phaseolus vulgaris*. Isolation of potent and weak phytohemagglutinins possessing mitogenic activity. *Proc. Natl. Acad. Sci. USA 63*: 334–337.

Andersen, M. M., and Ebbesen, K. (1986). Screening for lectins in common foods by line-dive immunoelectrophoresis and hemadsorption lectin test. Lectins: *Biol. Biochem. Clin. Biochem. 5*: 95–108.

Alstalf, E. (1963). Problemas de envenenamiento en niños. *Semana med.* (Buenos Aires) *123*: 1670–1674.

Aykroyd, W. R., and Doughty, J. (1964). Legumes in human nutrition. *FAO Nutritional Studies 19*. Rome.

Banwell, J. G., Howard, R., Cooper, D., and Costerton, J. W. (1985). Intestinal microbial flora after feeding phytohemagglutinin lectins (*Phaseolus vulgaris*). *Applied and Environmental Microbiology 50*: 68–80.

Barber, C. B., and Barber, S. (1978). Constituyentes toxicos del salvado de arroz. II. Actividad hemaglutinante del salvado crudo y tratado termicamente. *Rev. Agroquim. Tecnol. Aliment. 18*: 89–94.

Begbie, R., and King, T. P. (1985). The interaction of dietary lectins with porcine small intestine and production of lectin-specific antibodies. Lectins: *Biol. Biochem. Clin. Biochem. 4*: 15–27.

Bender, A. E., and Reaidi, G. B. (1982). Toxicity of kidney beans (*Phaseolus vulgaris*) with particular reference to lectins. *J. Plant Foods 4*: 15–22.

Boyd, W. S., and Reguera, R. M. (1949). Specificity of phytohemagglutinins. *J. Immunol. 62*: 333–401.

Brady, P. G., Vannier, A. M., and Banwell, J. G. (1978). Identification of the dietary lectin, wheat germ agglutinin in human intestinal contents. *Gastroenterology 75*: 236–239.

Brown, J. W. S., Osborn, T. C., Bliss, F. A., and Hall, T. C. (1982). Bean lectins 1. Relationship between agglutinating activity and electrophoretic variation in the lectin containing G2/albumin seed proteins of French beans (*Phaseolus vulgaris*). *Theor. Appl. Genet. 62*: 263–271.

Brucher, O., Wechsler, M., Levy, A., Palozzo, A., and Jaffé, W. G. (1969). Comparison of phytohemagglutinins in wild beans (*Phaseolus aborigineus*) and their inheritance. *Phytochemistry 8*: 1739–1743.

Burger, M. M. (1974). Assays for agglutination with lectins. *Meth. Enzymol. 32*: 615–621.

Carlini, C. R., Grace, B. S., Barcellos, A., Baeta-Nevis, D. V., and Guimaraes, J. E. (1988). Immunoreactivity for canatoxin and concanavalin A among proteins of leguminous plants. *Phytochem. 23*: 25–30.

Casotto, M., Palozzo, A., Agostini, G., and Levy, A. (1984). Estudio de las lectinas presentes en semillas de *Papilionoideae (Leguminosae)* de Venezuela. *Acta Cient. Venezol. 35*: 248–252.

Chen, L. M., Thacher, R. A., and Pan, S. H. (1977). Effect of germination and sprouting on hemagglutinating activity of pea and bean seeds. *J. Food Sci. 42*: 1666–1669.

Coffey, D. G., Uebersax, M. A., Hosfield, E. L., and Brunner, J. R. (1985). Evaluation of the hemagglutinating activity of low-temperature cooked kidney beans. *J. Food Sci. 50*: 78–87.

Colyer, J., Farthing, M. J. G., Kumar, P. J., Clark, M. L., Ohannesian, A. D., and Waldron, N. M. (1986). Reappraisal of the "lectin hypothesis" in the ethiopathogenesis of celiac disease. *Clin. Sci. 71*: 105–110.

Cooper, W. C., Perone, V. B., Scheel, L. D., and Keenan, R. G. (1964). Occupational hazard from castor bean pomace, test for toxicity. *Am. Ind. Hyg. Assoc. J. 25*: 431–439.

DeMuelenaere, A. J. H. (1964). Effect of heat treatment on the hemagglutinating activity of legumes. *Nature 201*: 1029–1030.

DeMuelenaere, A. J. H. (1965). Toxicity and hemagglutinating activity in legumes. *Nature 206*: 827–828.

Derewenda, Z., Yariv, J., Helliwell, J. R., Kalb, A. J., Dodson, E. J., Papiz, M. W., Wan, T., and Campbell, J. (1989). The structure of the saccharide-binding site of concanavaline A. *EMBO J. 8*: 2189–2193.

Donatucci, D. A., Liener, I. E., and Gross, C. J. (1987). Binding of navy bean (*Phaseolus vulgaris*) lectin to the intestinal cells of the rat and its effect on the absorption of glucose. *J. Nutr. 117*: 2154–2160.

Ehrlich, P. (1891). Experimentelle Untersuchungen über Immunität II. Über Abrin. *Deut. Med. Wochenschr. 17*: 218–221.

Elfstrand, W. (1897). Über blutkörperchen-agglutinierende Eiweisskörper. *Gorbersdorfer Veroeffentl. 1*: 1–8.

El-Nahry, F., Darwich, N. M., and Tharwat, S. (1977). Effect of preparation and cooking on the value of local kidney beans (*Phaseolus vulgaris*). *Qual. Plant. Plant Foods Hum. Nutr. 27*: 141–146.

Erickson, R. H., and Kim, Y. S. (1983). Interaction of purified brush border membrane aminopeptidase N and dipeptidylpeptidase IV with lectin Sepharose derivatives. *Biochim. Biophys. Acta 743*: 37–41.

Etzler, M. E. (1984). Lectin receptors on the cell intestinal surface. *Attachment Org. Gut Mucosa, [Pap. Res. Workshop], 2*: 147–156.

Etzler, M. E. (1985). Plant lectins: Molecular and biological aspects. *Ann. Rev. Plant Physiol. 36*: 209–234.

Etzler, M. E., and Brandstator, M. L. (1974). Differential localization of cell surface and secretory components in rat intestinal epithelium by use of lectin. *J. Cell Biol. 62*: 329–343.

Evans, R. J., Pusztai, A., Watt, W. B., and Bauer, D. H. (1973). Isolation and properties of protein fractions from navy beans (*Phaseolus vulgaris*) which inhibit growth of rats. *Biochim. Biophys. Acta 303*: 175–184.

Everson, G., and Heckert, A. (1944). The biological value of some leguminous sources of protein. *J. Am. Diet. Assoc. 20*: 81–82.

Faschingbauer, H., and Kofler, R. (1929). Über die Giftwirkung von Bohnen. *Wien. Klin. Wochenschr. 42*: 1069–1073.

Fernandez, R., Elias, L. G., and Bressani, R. (1981). Genetic and environmental variability and their effects on trypsin inhibitors and hemagglutinin compounds of common beans (*Phaseolus vulgaris*) from Central America and Colombia. *Turrialba 31*: 153–161.

Field, C. K. (1910). A study of an extremely pure preparation of ricin. *J. Exptl. Med. 12*: 525–555.

Fodstad, O., Olsnes, S., and Pihl, A. (1977). Inhibitory effect of abrin and ricin on the growth of transplantable murine tumors and of abrin on human cancers in nude mice. *Cancer Res. 37*: 4559–4567.

Ford, W. W. (1913). On hemagglutinins. *Zentralbl. Bacteriol. Parasitenk. 58*: 129–161, 193–222.

Freed, D. L. J., and Green, F. H. Y. (1975). Do lectins protect against colonic cancer? *Lancet 2*: 1261–1262.

Ghosh, M., Bachhawat, B. K., and Surolia, A. (1979). A rapid and sensitive assay for detection of nanogram quantities of castor-bean (*Ricinus communis*) lectins. *Biochem. J. 183*: 185–188.

Gold, E. R., and Balding, P. (1975). *Receptor Specific Proteins: Plant and Animal Lectins*. Elsevier, New York.

Goldberg, L. (1970). Chemical and biochemical implications of human and animal exposure to toxic substances in food. *Pure and Appl. Chem. 21*: 309–330.

Goldstein, I. J., and Hayes, C. E. (1978). The lectins: Carbohydrate-binding proteins in plants and animals. *Adv. Carbohydr. Chem. Biochem. 35*: 127–340.

Grant, G., Greer, F., McKenzie, N. H., and Pusztai, A. (1985). Nutritional response of mature rats to kidney bean (*Phaseolus vulgaris*) lectins. *J. Sci. Food Agric. 36*: 409–414.

Grant, G., Watt, W. B., Stewart, J. C., and Pusztai, A. (1987). Effects of dietary soybean (*Glycine max*) lectin and trypsin inhibitor upon pancreas of rats. *Med. Sci. Res. 15*: 1197–1198.

Grant, G., de Oliveira, J. T. A., Dorward, P., Annand, M. G., Waldron, M., and Pusztai, A. (1987). Metabolic and hormonal changes in rats resulting from consumption of kidney bean (*Phaseolus vulgaris*) or soybean (*Glycine max*). *Nutr. Rep. Intl. 36*: 763–772.

Greer, F., Brewer, A. C., and Pusztai, A. (1985). Effect of kidney bean (*Phaseolus vulgaris*) toxin on tissue weight and composition and some metabolic functions of rats. *Br. J. Nutr. 54*: 95–103.

Griebel, C. (1950). Erkränkungen durch Bohnenflocken (*Phaseolus vulgaris*) und Platterbsen (*Lathyrus tingitanus*). *Z. Lebensm. Untersuch. Forsch. 90*: 191–197.

Heintze, K. (1950). Über die Hitzebehandlung von Leguminosen und ihre Wirkung auf Geschmack, proteolytische Inhibitoren und biologische Wertigkeit. *Z. Lebensm.-Untersuch. Forsch. 91*: 100–116.

Hewitt, D., Coates, M. E., Kakade, M. L., and Liener, I. E. (1973). A comparison of fractions prepared from navy (haricot) beans (*Phaseolus vulgaris L.*) in diets for germ-free and conventional chicks. *Br. J. Nutr. 29*: 423–435.

Higuchi, M., and Iwai, K. (1985). Purification and some properties of the basic lectin from winged bean seeds. *Agric. Biol. Chem. 49*: 391–398.

Higuchi, M., Kawada, T., and Iwai, K. (1989). *In vivo* binding of winged bean basic lectin labeled with iodo-2-14-acetic acid to the intestinal epithelial cells of the rat. *J. Nutr. 119*: 490–495.

Honavar, P. M., Shih, C. V., and Liener, I. E. (1962). Inhibition of the growth of rats by purified hemagglutinin fractions isolated from *Phaseolus vulgaris*. *J. Nutr. 77*: 109–114.

Hsu, C. T., Lin, J-Y., and Tung, T-C. (1974). Further report on therapeutic effect of abrin and ricin on human cancers. *J. Formosan Med. Assoc. 73*: 526–542.

Jackson, M., and Varriano-Marston, E. (1981). Hard-to-cook phenomenon in beans: Effects of accelerated storage on water absorption and cooking time. *J. Food Sci. 46*: 799–803.

Jaffé, W. G. (1949). Toxicity of raw kidney beans. *Experientia 15*: 81–90.

Jaffé, W. G. (1950). Estudio de la inhibicion del crecimiento de ratas causada por algunas semillas de leguminosas. *Acta Cient. Venezol. 1*: 62–64.

Jaffé, W. G. (1960). Über Phytotoxine aus Bohnen. *Arzneimittel-Forschung 10*: 1012–1016.

Jaffé, W. G. (1973). Factors affecting the nutritional value of beans. In *Nutritional Improvement of Beans*, M. Milner, ed. Protein Advisory group of U.N. System, New York.

Jaffé, W. G. (1977). Immunology of plant lectins. In *Immunological Aspects of Food*, N. Catsimpolas, ed. John Wiley and Sons, New York.

Jaffé, W. G. (1980). Hemagglutinins (lectins). In *Toxic Constituents of Plant Foodstuffs*, 2nd ed., I. E. Liener, ed. Academic Press, New York, pp. 78–102.

Jaffé, W. G. (1983). Nutritional significance of lectins. In *Handbook of Naturally Occurring Food Toxins*, M. Rechcigl, ed. CRC Press, Boca Raton, FL.

Jaffé, W. G., and Camejo, G. (1961). La accion de una proteina toxica aislada de caraotas negras (*Phaseolus vulgaris*) sobre la absorcion intestinal en ratas. *Acta Cient. Venezol. 12*: 59–61.

Jaffé, W. G., and Gaede, K. (1959). Purification of a toxic hemagglutinin from black beans (*Phaseolus vulgaris*). *Nature 183*: 1329–1330.

Jaffé, W. G., and Gómez, M. J. (1975). Beans of high or low toxicity. *Qual. Plant. 24*: 359–365.

Jaffé, W. G., and Hannig, K. (1965). Fractionation of proteins from kidney beans. *Arch. Biochem. Biophys. 109*: 80–91.

Jaffé, W. G., and Korte, R. (1976). Nutritional characteristics of the winged beans in rats. *Nutr. Rep. Intl. 14*: 449–450.

Jaffé, W. G., and Vega-Lette, C. L. (1968). Heat-labile growth inhibiting factors in beans. *J. Nutr. 94*: 203–210.

Jaffé, W. G., Planchart, A., Paez-Pumar, J. I., Torrealba, R., and Franceschi, N. (1955). Nuevos estudios sobre un factor toxico de la caraota cruda (*Phaseolus vulgaris*). *Arch. Venezol. Nutr. 6*: 195–205.

Jaffé, W. G., Brucher, O., and Palozzo, A. (1972). Detection of four types of specific phytohemagglutinins in different lines of beans (*Phaseolus vulgaris*). *Z. Immun-Forsch. 142*: 439–447.

Jaffé, W. G., Levy, A., and Gonzales, I. D. (1974). Isolation and partial characterization of bean phytohemagglutinins. *Phytochem. 13*: 2685–2693.

Jayne-Williams, D. J., and Burgess, C. D. (1974). Further observations on the toxicity of navy beans (*Phaseolus vulgaris*) for Japanese quail (*Coturnix coturnix japonica*). *J. Appl. Bact. 37*: 149–169.

Jindal, S., Soni, G. L., and Singh, R. (1984). Biochemical and histopathological studies in albino rats fed on soybean lectin. *Nutr. Rep. Intl. 29*: 95–106.

Kakade, M. L., and Evans, R. J. (1965). Nutritive value of navy beans (*Phaseolus vulgaris*). *Brit. J. Nutr. 19*: 269–276.

Kakade, M. L., and Evans, R. J. (1966). Effect of soaking and germination on the nutritive value of navy beans. *J. Food Sci. 31*: 781–783.

Kilpatrick, D. C., Pusztai, A., Grant, G., Graham, C., and Ewen, S. T. (1985). Tomato lectin resists digestion in the mammalian alimentary canal and binds to intestinal villi without deleterious effects. *FEBS Lett. 185*: 299–305.

Kimura, T., Nakata, S., Herada, Y., and Yoshida, A. (1986). Effects of ingested winged beans lectin on gastrointestinal function in the rat. *J. Nutr. Sci. Vitaminol. 32*: 101–110.

King, K. W., Fougere, W., Foucauld, J., Dominique, G., and Beghin, N. D. (1966). Response of pre-school children to high intake of Haitian cereal-bean mixtures. *Arch. Latinoam. Nutr. 16*: 53–63.

King, T. P., Pusztai, A., and Clarke, E. M. W. (1980). Kidney bean (*Phaseolus vulgaris*) lectin-induced lesions in rat small intestine. I. Light microscope studies. *J. Comp. Pathol. 90*: 585–595.

Koehle, H., and Kauss, H. (1980). Improved analysis of hemagglutination assays for quantitation of lectin activity. *Anal. Biochem. 103*: 227–229.

Koehler, H. H., Herrick, E. H., and Burke, D. W. (1986). Differentiating the lectin activity in twenty-four cultivars of dry beans *Phaseolus vulgaris*. *J. Food Sci. 51*: 471–475.

Korte, R. (1972). Heat resistance of phytohemagglutinins in weaning food mixtures containing beans (*Phaeolus vulgaris*). *Ecol. Food. Nutr. 1*: 303–307.

Kortt, A. A., and Caldwell, J. B. (1987). Isolation and properties of the lectins from tuberous roots of winged beans (*Psophocarpus tetragonolobus*). *J. Sci. Food Agr. 39*: 47–57.

Kottgen, E., Kluge, F., Volk, B., and Gerok, W. (1983). The lectin properties of gluten as the basis of the patho-mechanism of gluten-sensitive enteropathy. *Klinische Wochenschrift 61*: 111–112.

Krüpe, M. (1956). *Blutgruppenspezifische pflänzliche Eiweisskörper (Phytoagglutinine)*. F. Enke, ed., Stuttgart.

Lajolo, F. M., and Mancini, F. J. (1988). Glycoproteinas com atividade antinutricional. An. 12 Simposio anual de ACIESP, Sao Paolo 1, pp. 62–101.

Landsteiner, K., and Raubitscheck, H. (1908). Beobachtungen über Hämolyse und Hämagglutination. *Zentr. Bakteriol. Parasitenk. 45*: 660–669.

Leon, A., Caffin, J. P., Plassart, M., and Picard, M. (1991). Role of concanavaline A from jack bean seeds on short term food intake regulation in chicken. *Animal Feed Sci. Technol 32*: 297–311.

Levy, A., Stein, R. I., Marquez, C. G., and Jaffé, W. G. (1985). El valor bioquimico y nutricional de las semillas de haba de lima (*Phaseolus lunatus*) en comparacion con las del frijol comun (*Phaseolus vulgaris*). *Arch. Latinoam. Nutr. 25*: 70–79.

Liener, I. E. (1953). Soyin a toxic protein from soybean flour. *J. Biol. Chem. 197*: 29–36.

Liener, I. E. (1955). The photometric determination of the hemagglutinating activity of soyin in crude soybean extracts. *Arch. Biochem. Biophys. 54*: 223–227.

Liener, I. E. (1958). Inactivation studies of the soybean hemagglutinin. *J. Biol. Chem. 233*: 401–405.

Liener, I. E. (1976). Phytohemagglutinins (phytolectins). *Ann. Rev. Plant Physiol. 27*: 291–319.

Liener, I. E. (1978). The nutritional significance of the plant lectins. In *Antinutrients and Natural Toxicants in Foods*, R. L. Ory, ed. Food and Nutrition Press, Inc., Westport, CT, pp. 143–157.

Liener, I. E. (1983). Naturally occurring toxicants in foods and their significance in the human diet. *Arch. Toxicol. Suppl. 6*: 153–166.

Liener, I. E. (1986). Lectins in food. In *The Lectins, Properties, Functions, and Applications in Biology and Medicine*, I. E. Liener, N. Sharon, and L. Goldstein, eds. Academic Press, New York.

Liener, I. E. (1989). The nutritional significance of lectins. In *Food Proteins*, J. E. Kinsella and W. G. Soucie, eds. Am. Oil Chem. Soc., Champaign, IL, 329–353.

Liener, I. E., and Pallansch, M. J. (1952). Purification of a toxic substance from defatted soybean flour. *J. Biol. Chem. 197*: 29–36.

Lima, A. L., Mancini Filho, J., Domingues, J. B., and Lajolo, F. M. (1980). Propriedades hemaglutinantes, mitogenicas e toxicas de variedades brasileiras de feijoles (*Phaseolus vulgaris*). *Rev. Farm. Bioquim. Univ. S. Paulo 16*: 145–153.

Lis, H., and Sharon, N. (1973). The biochemistry of plant lectins (phytohemagglutinins). *Ann. Rev. Biochem. 42*: 541–574.

Lis, H., and Sharon, N. (1977). Lectins: their chemistry and application to immunology. In *The Antigens*, M. Sela, ed. Academic Press, New York.

Lowgren, M., and Liener, I. E. (1986). The effect of slow-cooking on the trypsin inhibitor, hemagglutinating activities and *in vitro* digestibility of brown beans *Phaseolus vulgaris* var. Stella and kidney beans *Phaseolus vulgaris* var. Montcalm. *Qual. Plant. Foods Hum. Nutr. 36*: 147–154.

Lugnier, A. A. J., Le Meur, M. A., Gerlinger, P., and Dirheimer, G. (1974). Inhibition of *in vitro* synthesis in a rabbit reticulocyte cell-free system by toxic trypsic peptides from ricin. *Biochimie 56*: 1287–1289.

Makela, O. (1957). Studies in hemagglutinins of legume seeds. *Ann. Med. Exptl. Biol. Fenn. 35* (Suppl. 11): 1–133.

Manage, L., Joshi, A., and Sohonie, K. (1972). Toxicity to rats and mice of purified phytohemagglutinins from four Indian legumes. *Toxicon 10*: 89–91.

Mancini, Filho J., and Lajolo, F. M. (1981). Factores antinutricionales em diferentes variedades de feijoes. *Ciencia e Cultura* (Rio de Janeiro) *33*: 94–97.

McPherson, L. (1989). Lectins in the etiology of protein-energy malnutrition. *J. Royal Soc. Hyg. 2*: 66–68.

Miller, J. B., Noyes, C., Heinrikson, R., Kingdon, H. S., and Yachnin, S. (1973). Phytohemagglutinin mitogenic proteins. *J. Exptl. Med. 138*: 939–950.

Miller, J. B., Noyes, C., Heinrikson, R., Kingdon, H. S., and Yachnin, S. (1975). Bean mitogens. *Proc. Natl. Acad. Sci. USA 72*: 1388–1391.

Nachbar, M. S., and Oppenheim, J. D. (1980). Lectins in the United States diet: A survey of lectins in commonly consumed foods and a review of the literature. *Am. J. Clin. Nutr. 33*: 2338–2345.

Nakata, S., and Kimura, T. (1985). Effect of ingested toxic bean lectins on the gastrointestinal tract in the rat. *J. Nutr. 115*: 1621–1629.

Nakata, S., and Kimura, T. (1986). Behavior of ingested concanavalin A in the gastrointestinal tract of the rat. *Agr. Biol. Chem. 50*: 645–649.

Newburg, D. S., and Concon, J. M. (1985). Lectins in rice and corn endosperm. *J. Agr. Food Chem. 33*: 685–687.

Nicolson, G. L., Lacorbiere, M., and Hunter, T. R. (1975). Mechanism of cell entry and toxicity of an affinity-purified lectin from *Ricinus communis* and its differential effect on normal and transformed fibroblasts. *Cancer Res. 35*: 144–155.

Nielsen, S. S., and Liener, I. E. (1988). Effects of germination on trypsin inhibitor and hemagglutinating activities in *Phaseolus vulgaris*. *J . Food Sci. 53*: 298–301.

Noah, N. D., Bender, A. E., Reaidi, G. B., and Gilbert, R. J. (1980). Food poisoning from raw red kidney beans. *Br. Med. J. 6234*: 236–240.

Oliveira, A. C., Vidal, B., and Sgabieri, V. C. (1989). Lesions of intestinal epithelium by ingestion of bean lectins in rats. *J. Nutr. Sci. Vitaminol. 35*: 315–322.

Olsnes, S., and Sandvig, K. (1988). How protein toxins enter and kill cells. In *Immunotoxins*, A. E. Frankel, ed. Kluwer Academic Publishers.

Orf, J. H., Hymowitz, T., Pull, S. P., and Pueppke, S. G. (1978). Inheritance of a soybean seed lectin. *Crop Sci. 18*: 899–900.

Osborn, T. C., and Bliss, F. A. (1985). Effects of genetically removing lectin seed protein on horticultural and seed characteristics of common beans. *J. Am. Soc. Hort. Sci. 110*: 484–488.

Osborn, T. C., Brown, J. W. S., and Bliss, F. A. (1985). Bean lectins. 5. Quantitative genetic variation in seed lectins in (*Phaseolus vulgaris*) and its relation to qualitative lectin variation. *Theor. Appl. Genet. 70*: 22–31.

Osborne, T. B., and Mendel, M. (1917). The use of soybean as food. *J. Biol. Chem. 32*: 369–387.

Pack, N., Mateluna, A., and Araya, H. (1978). Efecto de diversos tratamientos termicos en el contenido de hemaglutininas y en la calidad proteica del frijol. *Arch. Latinoam. Nutr. 28*: 184–195.

Patton, S., Stemberger, B. H., Horton, A., and McCarl, R. L. (1980). Suppression of milk secretion (exocytosis) by concanavalin A *in vitro*. *Biochim. Biophys. Acta 630*: 530–536.

Peumans, W. J. (1985). Recent advances in biochemistry, cell biology, physiology, biosynthesis and genetics of *gramineae* lectins. *Biochem. Physiol. Pflanz. 180*: 85–106.

Pusztai, A. (1987). Plant lectins-biological functions. *Biochim. Biophys. Hung. 22*: 355–375.

Pusztai, A. (1989). Specific uptake of dietary lectins into the systemic circulation of rats. *Biochem. Soc. Transactions 17*: 481–482.

Pusztai, A., and Palmer, R. (1977). Nutritional evaluation of kidney beans (*Phaseolus vulgaris*): The toxic principal. *J. Sci. Food Agr. 28*: 620–623.

Pusztai, A., Grant, G., and Palmer, R. (1975). Nutritional evaluation of kidney beans (*Phaseolus vulgaris*). Isolation and partial characterization of toxic constituents. *J. Sci. Food Agr. 26*: 149–156.

Pusztai, A., Clarke, E. M. W., King, T. P., and Steward, J. C. (1979). Nutritional evaluation of kidney beans (*Phaseolus vulgaris*): Chemical composition, lectin content and nutritional value of selected cultivars. *J. Sci. Food Agr. 30*: 843–848.

Pusztai, A., Clarke, E. M. W., Grant, G., and King, T. P. (1981). The toxicity of *Phaseolus vulgaris* lectins. *J. Sci. Food Agr. 32*: 1037–1046.

Pusztai, A., Grant, G., Brown, D. S., Ewen, S. W. B., and Bardocz, S. (1988). *Phaseolus vulgaris* lectin induces growth and increases the polyamine content of rat small intestine *in vivo*. *Med. Sci. Res. 16*: 1283–1284.

Raedler, A., and Raedler, E. (1985). The use of lectins to study normal differentiation and malignant transformation. *J. Cancer Res. Clin. Oncol. 109*: 245–251.

Ramasamy, M., Alpers, D. H., Saxena, V., and Seetharam, B. (1990). Effect of lectins on cobalamin-protein binding reactions: Implications for the tissue uptake of cobalamin. *J. Nutr. Biochem. 1*: 213–219.

Rattray, E. A., Palmer, R., and Pusztai, A. (1974). Toxicity of kidney beans (*Phaseolus vulgaris*) to conventional and gnotobiotic rats. *J. Sci. Food Agric. 25*: 1035.

Reisner, Y., Linker-Israeli, M., and Sharon, N. (1976). Separation of mouse thymocytes into two subpopulations by the use of peanut agglutinin. *Cell Immunol. 25*: 129–134.

Richet, C. (1909). Etude sur la crepitine. *Ann. Inst. Pasteur 23*: 745–750.

Rigas, D., and Head, L. (1969). The dissociation of phytohemagglutinin of *Phaseolus vulgaris* by 8.0 M urea and the separation of the mitogenic from the erythroagglutinating activity. *Biochem. Biophys. Res. Commun. 34*: 633–641.

Rouanet, J. M., Mahamat-Silaye, O., and Beçanson, P. (1982). Effets d'une lectine purifiée de haricot (*Phaseolous vulgaris*) sur l'invertase, l'aminopeptidase et la phosphatase alcaline de l'intestin de rat. *Sci. Alim. 2, Hors série II*: 183–187.

Rouanet, J. M., Lafont, J., Chalet, M., Creppy, A., and Beçanson, P. (1985). Effects of dietary kidney bean (*Phaseolus vulgaris*) lectins in growing rats. *Nutr. Rep. Intl. 31*: 237–244.

Salgarkar, S., and Sohonie, K. (1965). Hemagglutinins of field bean (*Dolichos lablab*). Effect of feeding field bean hemagglutinin A on rat growth. *Ind. J. Biochem. 2*: 197–199.

Schneider, B. H., and Miller, D. J. (1954). The biological value of Alaska pea proteins. *J. Nutr. 52*: 581–590.

Sharon, N. (1989). A century of lectins: impact on immunology. In *Cellular Basis of Immune Modulation*. A. Liss, New York, pp. 609–620.

Sharon, N., and Lis, H. (1989). Lectins as cell recognition molecules. *Science 246*: 227–234.

Sharon, N., and Lis, H. (1990). The legume lectins. A large family of homologous proteins. *FASEB J. 4*: 3198–3208.

Siegel, S. (1893). Über Giftstoffe zweier Euphorbeacean. Dissertation, Universität Dorpat.

Stillmark, H. (1889). Über Ricin. *Arch. Pharmakol. Dorpat 3*: 59–70.

Sotello, A., Arteaga, M. E., Frias, M. I., and González-Garza, M. T. (1980). Cytotoxic effect of two legumes in epithelial cells of small intestine. *Qual. Plant. Plant Food Hum. Nutr. 30*: 79–85.

Stinissen, H. M., Peumans, W. J., and Carlier, A. R. (1983). Occurrence and immunological relationship of lectins in gramineous species. *Planta 159*: 105–111.

Thompson, L. U., and Gabon, J. E. (1987). Effect of lectins on salivary and pancreatic amylase activities and the rate of starch digestion. *J. Food Sci. 52*: 1050–1053.

Tobiska, J. (1964). *Die Phytohamagglutinine*. Akademie-Verlag, Berlin.

Tobiska, J., and Lhotecka-Brazdova, A. (1960). Einfluss der künstlichen Dungung auf den Phytoagglutiningehalt der Bohnen. *Z. Immunitatsf. 119*: 225–231.

Toms, G. C., and Western, A. (1971). *Phytohemagglutinins in chemotaxonomy of the Leguminosae*, J. B. Harborne and D. Boulter, eds. Academic Press, New York.

Triadou, N., and Audran, E. (1983). Interaction of the brush-border hydrolases of the human small intestine with lectins. *Digestion 27*: 1–7.

Tsien, H. C., Michele, A., Jack, E. L., Schmidt, E. L., and Wold, F. (1983). Lectin in five soybean cultivars previously considered to be lectin-negative. *Planta 158*: 128–133.

Turner, R. H., and Liener, I. E. (1975a). The effect of the selective removal of hemagglutinins on the nutritive value of soybeans. *J. Agr. Food Chem. 23*: 481–485.

Turner, R. H., and Liener, I. E. (1975b). The use of glutaraldehyde-treated erythrocytes for assaying the agglutinating activity of lectins. *Anal. Biochem. 68*: 651–653.

van Deurs, B., Sandvig, K., Petersen, O. W., and Olsnes, S. (1990). Endocytosis and intracellular sorting of ricin. In *Trafficking in Bacterial Toxins*, C. B. Saelinger, ed. CRC Press, Boca Raton, FL.

WHO (1967). Procedures for investigating intentional and unintentional food additives. World Health Organization Technical Report, Series 348.

Wagh, P. V., Klaustermeier, D. F., Waibel, P. E., and Liener, I. E. (1963). Nutritive value of red kidney beans (*Phaseolus vulgaris*) for chicks. *J. Nutr. 80*: 191–195.

Waterlow, J. C. (1990). Nutrition adaptation in men: General introduction and concepts. *Am. J. Clin. Nutr. 51*: 259–262.

Weaver, L. T., and Bailey, D. S. (1987). Effect of the lectin concanavalin A on the neonatal guinea pig gastrointestinal mucosa in vivo. *J. Pediatr. Gastroenterol. Nutr. 6*: 445–453.

Weber, T. H., Aro, H., and Nordman, C. T. (1972). Characterization of lymphocyte-stimulating blood-cell agglutinating glycoproteins from red kidney beans (*Phaseolus vulgaris*). *Biochim. Biophys. Acta 263*: 94–105.

Williams, P. E. V., Pusztai, A. J., Macdearmid, A., and Innes, G. M. (1984/85). The use of kidney beans (*Phaseolus vulgaris*) as protein supplements in diets for young rapidly growing beef steers. *Animal Feed Science and Technology 12*: 1–10.

Youle, R. J., and Huang, A. H. (1976). Protein bodies from the endosperm of castor beans. Subfractionation, protein components, lectins, and changes during germination. *Plant Physiol. 58*: 703–710.

12

Mycotoxins in Foods

Suresh S. Dhumal* and Dattajirao K. Salunkhe

Utah State University, Logan, Utah

I. INTRODUCTION

Mycotoxins are secondary fungal metabolites with diverse structures and toxicological properties that induce a variety of toxic effects in humans and animals when foods contaminated with these compounds are ingested. Although fungal contamination of foods is a constantly recurring phenomenon, the attitude towards it has been far from consistent. For many years, a tendency to regard fungi as harmless was common; mild fungal growth was treated as a regrettable nuisance, detracting from the appearance of the product and perhaps causing degrees of losses or spoilages. In the 1850s, human and animal health hazards of toxigenic fungi were recognized when a distinct disease called "ergotism" was shown to be associated with the ingestion of rye and other cereals infected with the fungus *Claviceps purpurea*. An incident in 1960 changed the general

**Present affiliation*: Kalyani Agro Corporation, Pune (Maharashtra), India attitude toward the fungal contamination of food and prompted an awareness of the scope of the problem. The discovery of aflatoxin in 1961 led to a vast amount of research in chemistry, biochemistry, mycology, toxicology, nutrition, and food technology.

The term "mycotoxicosis" introduced in 1962 by Forgacs and Carll is defined as "poisoning of the host following entrance into the body of toxic substances of fungal origin." This term is usually limited to those pathological entities associated with ingestion of food on which the fungi proliferate and give rise to toxic products. The first recorded mycotoxicosis is probably the bread-staggering syndrome reported by Woronin in 1981, which was attributed to *Gibberella zeae*. At the turn of the last century, equine encephalitis was reported in the state of Maryland (Buckley, 1901). Several years later, a fetal hemorrhagic afebrile disease of cattle was shown to be a case of mycotoxicosis (Schofield, 1924). Later, in 1954, Forgacs et al. isolated a toxigenic *Aspergillus clavatus*, which produced hemorrhage and hyperkeratosis in calves. Likewise, a hemorrhagic syndrome caused significant losses of chicken in Delaware and West Virginia (Forgacs et al., 1958). These investigators were able to reproduce the toxic syndrome in chickens using grains inoculated with selected strains of the genera *Aspergillus, Penicillium*, and *Alternaria*. Facial eczema of ruminants was shown to be of fungal origin (Percival, 1959), which is presently known as sporidesmin. One mycotoxicosis reported in Russia is a human disease known as aseptic angina and later as alimentary toxic aleukia (ATA) caused by *Fusarium sporotrichoides* (Joffe, 1971). ATA may also affect cattle, sheep, chickens, horses, and swine (Mayer, 1953).

Mycotoxicoses or injuries attributable to a mycotoxin have been demonstrated mostly in domestic animals and poultry with few human incidences with the possible exception of liver cancer in certain populations. Research on mycotoxins has revealed potential hazards of mycotoxin contamination of many important agricultural products (Table 1).

The occurrence of mycotoxins in agricultural commodities depends on such factors as region, season, and the conditions under which a particular crop is grown, harvested, and stored. Crops grown under warm and moist weather in the tropical and subtropical countries are especially more prone to mycotoxin contamination than those in temperate zones. However, certain toxigenic fungi such as *Fusarium* species can proliferate at low temperature and produce toxins. Over 100 fungal species have been shown to produce mycotoxins associated with naturally occurring diseases in animals and humans throughout the world (Knight, 1981). Although toxigenic fungi and their spores are ubiquitous, mycotoxicoses is primarily a problem in areas that have high rainfall and relative humidity, and temperatures that favor fungal growth and mycotoxin production. In addition to specific growth conditions, the fungal spoilage of crops and their grains is enhanced by drought, insect damage, cracked kernels during harvesting, and the presence of excessive chaff in the harvested grain. During the entire postharvest period, food crops are essentially in a state of storage, and fungal growth on them is avoidable only by careful regulation of moisture content, temperature, and

Table 1 Commonly Encountered Toxigenic Fungi, Their Toxins, and Important Agricultural Commodities They Damage

Toxin	Fungus	Commodities damaged
Aflatoxins	*A. flavus* *A. parasiticus*	Groundnut, tree nuts, cereals, cottonseed, soybean, spices, fruits
Ochratoxins	*A. ochraceus* *P. viridicatum*	Legumes, cereals, coffee beans
Zearalenone	*Fusarium* spp., e.g. F. roseum	Fungal-infested corn, wheat, barley, etc.
Trichothecenes, T-2 toxin, Vomitoxin	*Fusarium* spp., e.g. *F. tricinctum*	Fungal-infested corn, wheat
Rubratoxins	*P. rubrum* *P. purpurogenum*	Fungal-infested corn
Citrinin	*P. viridicatum* *P. citrinum* *A. ochraceus*	Barley, wheat, rye, oat, rice
Tremorgens	*P. cyclopium* *P. palitans* *Aspergillus* spp.	Fungal-infested feeds, peanuts, rice
Patulin	*Penicillium* spp. *Aspergillus* spp.	Fungal-infested fruits such as apples, plums, peaches, pears, apricots, etc.
Ergotoxins	*C. purpurea* *C. paspali*	Fungal-infested grains and grasses

other environmental conditions. Mature fruits and vegetables are also highly susceptible to invasion of toxigenic fungi, because they are high in moisture and nutrient content. In addition, many fruits become more easily injured as they approach full maturity and therefore are vulnerable to fungal attack. Postharvest losses of fresh fruits and vegetables due to microbial decay have been reported (Table 2). Thus fungal infection of foods not only results in economic losses but is a potential health hazard to man and animals. Some economically important mycotoxins contaminating human foods in the world are listed in Table 1.

This chapter encompasses both human food and animal feeds, and since meat is consumed by humans as a form of food which may be contaminated through the feed, the word "feed" is avoided in the text.

Table 2 Postharvest Losses of Fresh Fruits and Vegetables due to Microbial Decay

Fruits/Vegetables	% Loss	Ref.
Oranges	15–30	Smoot, 1969
Peaches	15–24	Wells and Harvey, 1970
Strawberry	14–18	Harris et al., 1967
Pineapple	40–50	Ramsey, 1938
Mango	20–33	Singh, 1960
Yam	50	Burton, 1970
Lettuce	10–15	Ceponis, 1970

II. MYCOTOXINS CONTAMINATING FOODS

Species of toxigenic fungi can be found in all major taxonomic groups of fungi. Most of the mycotoxins known have been recognized as metabolic products of genera such as *Aspergillus, Penicillium*, and *Fusarium*. In addition to the above, other genera such as *Claviceps* and other *Ascomycetes* are known to produce various mycotoxins. Important toxigenic fungi belonging to several taxonomic groups and their mycotoxins are given in Tables 3, 4, and 5. Toxins and their sources are listed in Table 6.

A. Mycotoxins of *Aspergillus*

1. *Aflatoxins*

The discovery of aflatoxin has revolutionized research on molds and mold metabolites because of its potency as a toxin and carcinogen, its worldwide distribution, and the various important commodities in which it has been found. More information is available about aflatoxins than any other single

Table 3 Important Mycotoxins Produced by *Aspergillus* Spp.

Mycotoxin	Producing organisms
Aflatoxins	*A. flavus*, etc.
Sterigmatocystins	*A. versicolor*
Ochratoxins	*A. ochraceus*
Fumigatin	*A. fumigatus*
Aspergillic acid	*A. flavus*
Kojic acid	*A. fumigatus*, etc.
Terreic acid	*A. terreus*
Helvolic acid	*A. fumigatus*
Fumagillin	*A. fumigatus*
Tryptoquivaline	*A. clavatus*
Fumitremorgins	*A. fumigatus*

Table 4 Mycotoxins Produced by *Penicillium* Spp.

Mycotoxin	Producing organism
Citreoviridin	*P. citreoviride*
Citrinin	*P. citrinum*, etc.
Penicillic acid	*P. puberculum*, etc.
Rubratoxins	*P. rubrum*
Griseofulvin	*P. janczewski*
Luteoskyrin	*P. islandicum*
Islanditoxin	*P. islandicum*
Mycophenolic acid	*P. brevicompactum*
Decumbin	*P. decumbens*
Viridicatin	*P. viridicatum*
Cyclopiazonic acid	*P. cyclopium*
Patulin	*P. patulum*, etc.
Brevianamide A	*P. viridicatum*
Penitrems	*P. cyclopium*, etc.
Verruculogen	*P. verruculosum*

group of mycotoxins. A renaissance in mycotoxin research developed as a direct result of concurrent outbreaks of disease in poultry and fish during the 1960s in diverse geographic locations. The most prominent development was the report of severe losses of turkey poult in Britain (Blount, 1961). The disorder was named "Turkey-X Disease" because the etiological agent involved in the disease was not known. Blount (1961) conducted the histological examinations of the diseased birds and found an acute hepatic necrosis associated with bile duct proliferation. Utilization of Brazilian groundnut (peanut) in the feed source was the common factor in the outbreak of the disease (Blount, 1961; Sargeant et al., 1961). Allcroft and Carnaghan (1963) subsequently studied the groundnut meal from various producing countries and found that 13 of the

Table 5 Mycotoxins Produced by Other Genera

Mycotoxin	Producing organism
Zearalenone	*Gibberella zeae*
Trichothecenes	*Fusarium*,
Psoralens	*Myrothecium*, etc.
	Sclerotinia sclerotiorum
Miscellaneous Mycotoxins	
Ergotoxins	*Claviceps purpurea*
Mushroom toxins	*Amanita* spp.
Monoacetoxyscirpenol	*Fusarium roseum*

Table 6 Fungal Toxins, Corresponding Fungi-Producing Toxins, and Their Effects

Toxin	Fungal species	Major toxic effects
Aflatoxins	*A. flavus* *A. parasiticus*	Hepatotoxicity, carcinogenesis
Aspergillic acid	*A. flavus*	Convulsions
Kojic acid	*A. flavus* *A. parasiticus*	Convulsions
β-Nitropropionic	*A. flavus* *A. parasiticus*	Apnea, incoordination
Terreic acid	*A. terreus*	Antibiotic effects
Helvolic acid	*A. fumigatus*	Liver lesions
Fumigatin	*A. fumigatus*	Antibiotic effects
Fumagillin	*A. fumigatus*	Dermal toxicity
Fumitremorgens	*A. fumigatus*	Neurotoxicity
Sterigmatocystin	*A. versicolor*	Hepatotoxicity
Ochratoxins	*A. ochraceus*	Nephropathy
Penicillic acid	*Penicillium* spp.	Liver lesions
Cyclopiazonic acid	*P. cyclopium*	General tissue necrosis
Griseofulvin	*P. griseofulvum*	Dermal, carcinogenic
Citreoviridin	*P. citreoviride*	Paralysis, convulsions
Mycophenolic acid	*P. brevicompactum*	Nonspecific
Decumbin	*P. decumbens*	Nonspecific
Citrinin	*Penicillium* spp.	Nephrotoxicity
Rubratoxin	*P. rubrum*	Hepatotoxicity
Viridicatin	*P. viridicatum*	Toxicity unknown
Penitrems	*Pencillium* spp.	Tremors
Luteoskyrin	P. islandicum	Carcinogenic

Table 6 (Continued)

Toxin	Fungal species	Major toxic effects
Patulin	*Pencillium* and *Aspergillus* spp.	Edema, convulsions
Zearalenone	*F. roseum*	Estrogenic syndrome
Trichothecenes	*Fusarium, Myrothecium*	Digestive disorders, hemorrhage, edema
Psoralens	*Sclerotinia sclerotiorum*	Dermatitis
Mushroom toxins	*A. phalloides*	Hepatic and renal lesions
Ergotoxins	*C. purpurea* *C. paspali*	Neurotoxicity

samples from diverse locations contained the toxin. Researchers at the Tropical Products Institute in London, the Central Veterinary Laboratory at Weybridge, and Unilever Laboratories in Holland and Britain are credited with the initial successes in narrowing the etiological agent of Turkey-X Disease to groundnut meal and the isolation of the toxic material (Sargeant et al., 1961; Carnaghan and Allcroft, 1962; Van der Zidjen et al., 1962). The discovery that a characteristic blue fluorescence parallels the toxicity observed in duckling tests eased the isolation of the toxins (Sargeant et al., 1961; Smith and McKernan, 1962). The toxic factors were later separated into distinct compounds (Sargeant et al., 1961; Nesbitt et al., 1962; Van der Zidjen et al., 1962). The name aflatoxin was given to these components with identification of their generic origin. Chemically, the aflatoxins are highly substituted coumarin and contain a fused dihydrofurofuran configuration, which is peculiar to a limited number of compounds of natural origin. The compounds occur in two series, aflatoxin B_1 and derivatives and aflatoxin G_1 and derivatives. These include B_1, B_2, G_1, G_2, M_1, M_2, GM_1, GM_2, GM_{2a}, B_{2a}, G_{2a}, M_{2a}, R_0, B_3, P_1, and Q_1 (Fig. 1).

Investigations of feed contaminated with *A. flavus* established that a typical toxicity syndrome involved liver damage in many mammals, fish, and birds (Kraybill and Shimkin, 1964; Lancaster, 1968). After aflatoxin treatment, the injured livers demonstrated a routine pattern of cellular changes, including peripheral zone necrosis and biliary proliferation (Kraybill and Shimkin, 1964). In addition to hepatomas, aflatoxin has also been implicated in the induction of neoplasms in the glandular stomach, kidney, lung, salivary gland, lachrymal gland, colon, and skin (Butler and Barnes, 1964, 1966; Wogan and Newberne, 1967; Lancaster, 1968). Since the initial implication of *A. flavus* in Turkey-X Disease, aflatoxin production by this organism and by *A. parasiticus* has been well documented. Not all strains of *A. flavus* produced aflatoxins. Other fungi have also been reported to produce aflatoxins, but confirmatory

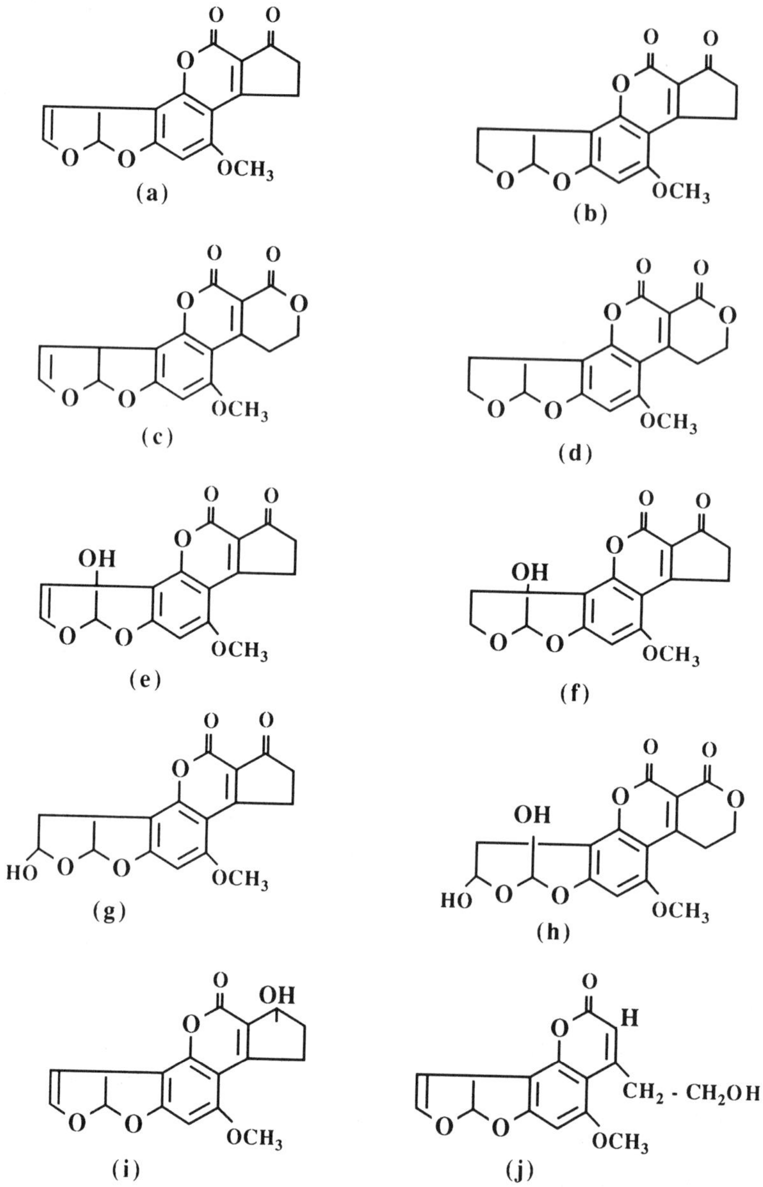

Figure 1 Chemical structures of various aflatoxins: (a) B_1, (b) B_2, (c) G_1, (d) G_2, (e) M_1, (f) M_2, (g) B_{2a}, (h) G_{2a}, (i) aflatoxicol R_0, (j) parasiticol B_3.

studies are lacking. Under a given set of conditions, two or three aflatoxins are produced by the toxin-producing organisms. Aflatoxin B_1 is the major food contaminant of all the aflatoxins, and has the highest potency of the group as a toxin and as a carcinogen. In general, fewer occurring aflatoxins B_2, G_1, and G_2 have also been reported in contaminated products in the presence of B_1.

The production of aflatoxins by *A. flavus* strains on agricultural crops such as groundnut, cottonseed, wheat, rice, barley, coconut, corn, dried peas, oat, sweet potato, millet, and cassava is well known. The natural occurrence of aflatoxin in peanuts and peanut meals has been reported by several investigators (Allcroft and Carnaghan, 1962; Allcroft and Lewis, 1963). High levels of aflatoxin have been reported in fermented peanut press cake samples in Indonesia (van Veen et al., 1967). In Taiwan, dried sweet potato was found to be heavily contaminated with *A. flavus* and contained 0.01–0.18 ppb aflatoxin (Tung and Ling, 1968). Grape wine has also been found to contain aflatoxins (Schuller et al., 1967).

Corn is by far the most susceptible crop to aflatoxin contamination of all grains grown in the United States. Aflatoxin has been found in corn samples at all stages of development and maturity from the late milk stage until harvest (Anderson et al., 1975). Insect damage has also associated with aflatoxin contamination of grains. LaPrade and Manwiller (1977) reported that 39% of naturally infested corn ears had detectable levels of aflatoxin B_1.

Dry figs imported into the United States are sometimes rejected because of contamination with aflatoxin (Anonymous, 1974). Its presence in foreign-produced figs suggest that aflatoxin could, under certain conditions, be present in domestic figs and pose a threat to domestic production. Buchanan et al. (1975) showed that immature fig fruits did not support colonization and aflatoxin production by *A. flavus* but become susceptible when ripe. While sun-drying on the tree, fruits were particularly vulnerable to fungal infection and colonization. Colonization by the *A. flavus* and aflatoxin contamination in harvested almonds in California has also been reported (Phillips et al., 1976). Aflatoxin has also been shown to occur in Indian chili powder, cayenne pepper, capsicum pepper (Scott and Kennedy, 1973), nutmeg (Beljaars et al., 1975), and dried chili peppers (Shank et al., 1972).

Aflatoxin M_1 has been noted to appear in the milk of cows that have ingested aflatoxin B_1 through the feed (Stoloff, 1980). A study using more sensitive chemical techniques in which aflatoxin B_1 was incorporated into the rations of laying hens indicated that aflatoxin could be detected in eggs (Jacobson and Wiseman, 1974).

2. *Sterigmatocystins*

Sterigmatocystin is a potent toxin first isolated from mycelial mats of *A. versicolor* as a yellow, high-melting crystalline compound in 1957. It was the first naturally occurring compound identified to contain the furfuran ring system (Hamasaki and Hatsuda, 1977). The most economically important member of the group is sterigmatocystin from *A. versicolor*. Other species producing this toxin include aspertoxin (3-hydroxy-6,7-dimethoxy-difuroxanthone) (Rodricks et al., 1968a,b; Waiss et al., 1968) *o*-methylsterigmatocystin (Burkhardt and Forgacs, 1968) and dihydro-*o*-methylsterigmatocystin (Cole and Kirksey, 1970) from *A. flavus*, 5-methoxysterigmatocystin (Holker and Kagal, 1968), 6-demethylsterigmatocystin (Elsworthy et al., 1970), dihydrosterigmatocystin (Hatsuda et al., 1972), and dihydrodemethylsterigmatocystin (Hatsuda et al., 1972) from *A. versicolor*. The major differences among the various sterigmatocystins are the presence or absence of unsaturation in the difurano ring system (similar to aflatoxin B_1 and B_2) and the substitution

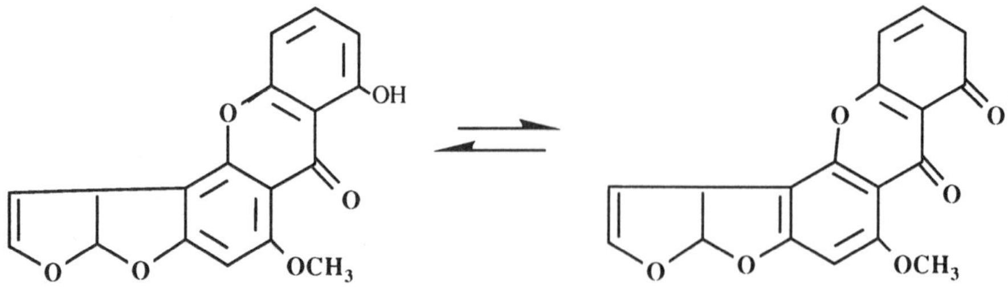

Figure 2 Chemical structure of sterigmatocystin.

pattern on positions 6, 7, and 10 of the xanthone ring system and/or position 3 of the difurano system (Fig. 2).

The toxicity of sterigmatocystin analogs on primary cell culture was greater for the compounds containing the $\Delta^{1,2}$-furobenzofuran-ring system than those containing a saturated furobenzofuran-ring system (Englebrecht and Altenkirk, 1972). The carcinogenicity of sterigmatocystin has been well documented (Dickens et al., 1966; Purchase and Van Der Watt, 1968, 1970). A carbonyl group unsaturated in the a,b position and a unsaturated bond in the $\Delta^{1,2}$ position are required for carcinogenicity according to Englebrecht and Altenkirk (1972). Also, a methoxy group at position 6 enhanced toxicity of these compounds, and a methoxy group at position 7 decreased toxicity.

Since sterigmatocystins and aflatoxin B_1 are similar in their structure, it suggests that these mycotoxins have a common biogenetic pathway or that the aflatoxins may be derived from sterigmatocystin and/or vesicolorin-type precursors (Holker and Underwood, 1964; Holker and Mulheirn, 1968; Rodricks, 1969; Biollaz et al., 1970). Hsieh et al. (1973) and Singh and Hsieh (1976) reported that sterigmatocystin was converted to aflatoxin B_1 by *A. parasiticus* and proposed a pathway for the biosynthesis of aflatoxin B_1 to be acetate → averufin → versiconal acetate → versicolorin A → sterigmatocystin → aflatoxin B_1.

Sterigmatocystin has been found in a sample of heavily fungal-infected wheat (Scott et al., 1972), green coffee beans (Purchase and Pretorius, 1973), pistachio nuts (Sommer et al., 1976), and in-shell pecans (Schroeder and Hein, 1977). The occurrence of sterigmatocystin in processed food (Gouda cheese) has also been reported by Northolt et al. (1980).

3. *Ochratoxins*

The ochratoxins are a group of seven closely related fungal metabolites produced by various species of *A. ochraceus* isolated from cereals and legumes. Ochratoxin A, the 7-carboxy-5-chloro-8-hydroxy-3-R-methyl isocoumarinamide of L-β-phenylalanine (Fig. 3), is the most toxic of the ochratoxins and is produced in highest yield (Neshiem, 1969). The LD_{50} for rats is about 22 mg/kg for ochratoxin A.

The acute and subacute toxicological properties of the ochratoxins have prompted an examination of foods for their possible presence. *Penicillium*

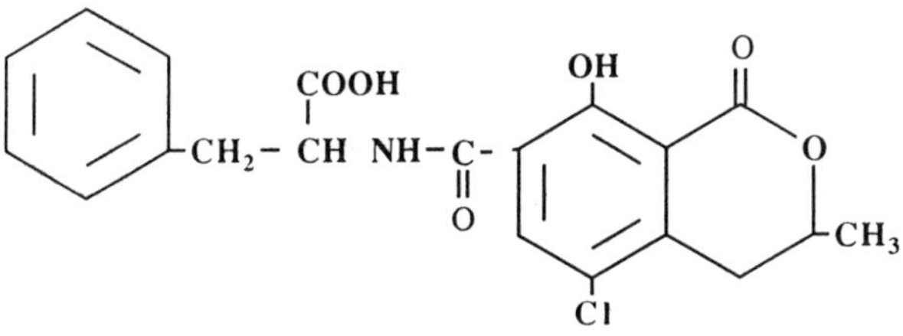

(a)

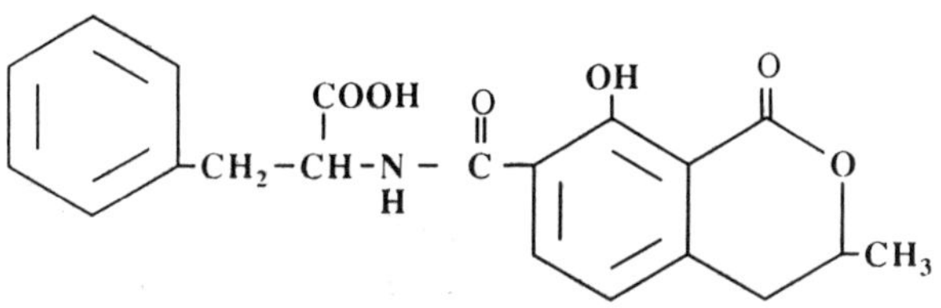

(b)

Figure 3 Chemical structure of (a) ochratoxin A, (b) ochratoxin B.

viridicatum has also been identified as a producer of ochratoxin (Van Walbeek et al., 1969; Krogh et al., 1973) and has been associated with the natural occurrence of ochratoxin A in most situations where an association could be made. Both species are widely distributed and frequently encountered on grain, legumes, and other commodities usually protected by a reduction of water activity. Residues of ochratoxin have also been found in kidneys of pigs at slaughter when fed with contaminated grain. Ochratoxin has also been found in green coffee beans.

4. *Fumigatin*

Fumigatin (Fig. 4) was first noted to be a product of *A. flavus* isolated from Indian soil which was responsible for pH color changes in the culture broth of the strain (Anslow and Raistrick, 1938). Fumigatin was also found to be produced by *A. fumigatus* (Anslow and Raistrick, 1938; Pettersson, 1963). Fumigatin has been shown to have marked in vitro inhibitory properties against several gram-positive and gram-negative bacteria. The effective range is approximately the same for both types.

5. *Aspergillic Acid*

Aspergillic acid was first discovered and named by White (1940) and White and Hill (1943). It is the first of a number of closely related pyrazine fungal metabolites reported. Aspergillic acid is the major metabolite of certain strains of *A. flavus* and other *Aspergillus* species. It is acutely toxic to mice at LD_{50} values of 100–150 mg/kg, i.p., but has no chronic effects at sublethal dosages (White and Hill, 1943). Toxicity of aspergillic acid is related to the hydroxamic

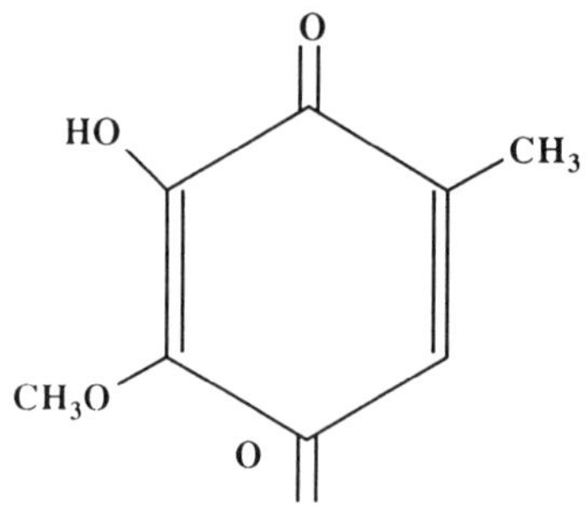

Figure 4 Chemical structure of fumigatin.

acid functionality, and little effect on toxicity was observed for differences in the 3- and 6-positioned side-chain substitutes. Aspergillic acid can exist in either the hydroxamic acid form (2-hydroxy-pyrazine-1-oxide) or the 1-hydroxy-2-pyrazinone form (Fig. 5). Chelation of physiologically important ions such as calcium by aspergillic acid appears to be the likely mechanism of its toxic action.

6. *Kojic Acid*

Kojic acid is a common metabolite of *Aspergillus flavus* with the chemical structure 5-hydroxy-2-(hydroxymethyl)-4H-pyran-4-one (Fig. 6). It is characterized by a γ-pyrone nucleus substituted at positions 2 and 5 with a hydroxymethyl and a hydroxy group, respectively. Classified as a convulsant, a relatively large quantity is required to produce severe intoxication or death in animals. A large number of microorganisms are capable of producing large amounts of kojic acid. The LD_{50} in 17-g mice was 30 mg i.p. injection (Morton et al., 1945). Kojic acid also showed toxicity in plant cells at 10^{-1} M (Gaumann and Von Arx, 1947).

7. *Terreic Acid*

Terreic acid produced by *A. terreus* was first discovered by Wilkins and Harris in 1942. Its LD_{50} of 70–119 mg/kg for mice by i.v. injection (Kaplan et al., 1954) has shown to be highly toxic. Terreic acid produced by *A. terreus*

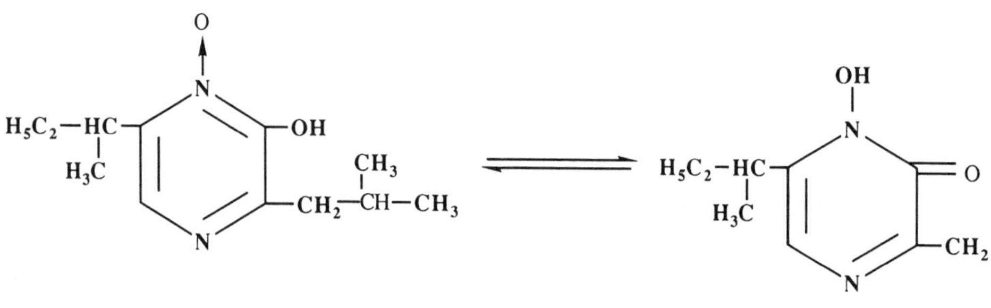

Figure 5 Chemical structure of aspergillic acid.

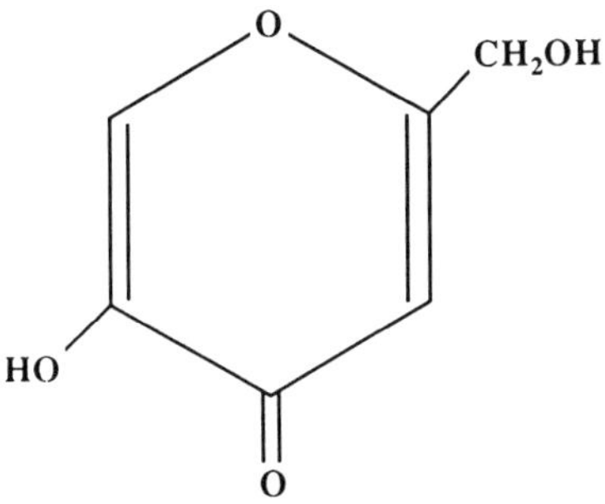

Figure 6 Chemical structure of kojic acid.

has been shown to have in vitro activity against several bacteria and fungi as well as a protozoan (*Trichomonas vaginalis*) infecting the human vaginal tract. The chemical structure of terreic acid (Fig. 7) was proposed by Sheehan et al. (1958) as 2,3-epoxy-6-hydroxy-toluquinone.

8. Helvolic Acid

Previously known as fumigacin, helvolic acid is a toxic secondary metabolite found in some isolates of *A. fumigatus: Cephalosporium caerulens* and *Emericellopsis terricola* (Cole and Cox, 1981). Helvolic acid, a toxic antibiotic of *A. fumigatus* was reported by Waksman et al. (1943) and Chain et al. (1943) at almost the same time. In 1964, Okuda and his associates determined the correct structure of helvolic acid (Fig. 8). Repeated intraperitoneal injections to 20-g mice caused peritonitis and superficial liver lesions, with minimal effects seen in the kidneys. Helvolic acid was absorbed from the subcutaneous tissues and gastrointestinal tract and was excreted in an active form of the urine and bile.

9. Fumagillin

Fumagillin (Fig. 9), a metabolite of *A. fumigatus*, is known for its anti-bacteriophage and amebicidal properties (McCowen et al., 1951). However, because of toxic side effects encountered in human clinical trials (Schindel,

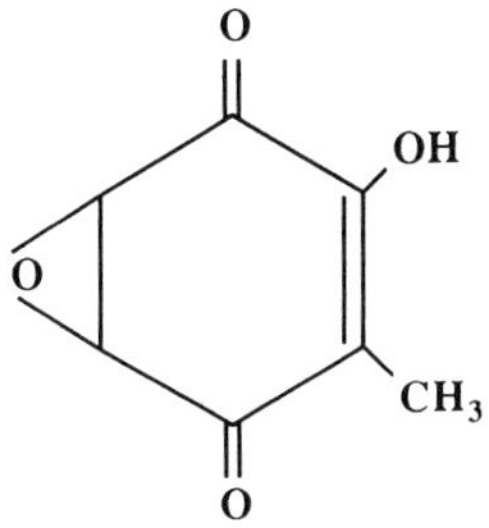

Figure 7 Chemical structure of terreic acid.

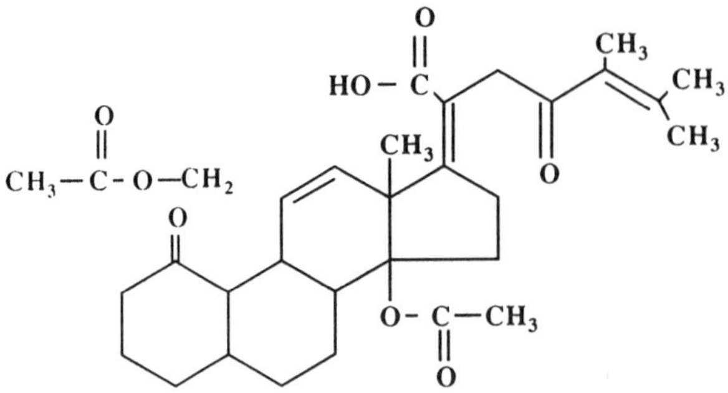

Figure 8 Chemical structure of helvolic acid.

1954), medical applications of fumagillin are restricted to its use by apiarists (Katznelson and Jamieson, 1952; Bailey, 1953) and to the veterinary profession (Field et al., 1956). An isolate of *A. fumigatus* from country-cured ham has been shown to be highly toxic to chick embryos (Wu et al., 1974b). Yokota et al. (1977) isolated a hemolytic toxin from mycelia and culture filtrates of *A. fumigatus*. Fumagillin is not a highly toxic substance since orally dosed mice can tolerate doses up to 2000 mg/kg body weight.

B. Mycotoxins of *Penicillium*

1. *Citreoviridin*

This mycotoxin (Fig. 10) was first isolated from *P. citreoviride* growing on rice and later from many other species of *Penicillium* (Hirata, 1947; Ueno, 1985). Yellowed rice infected by fungi is the major source of this mycotoxin. Ueno (1985) reported the presence of citreoviridin in corn infected by fungi. It is a neurotoxin and causes paralysis in the extremities of laboratory animals, followed by convulsions and respiratory arrest (Ueno and Ueno, 1972). Acute signs observed in mice include early onset of progressive paralysis in the hind legs and flank followed by vomiting, convulsions, and respiratory arrest.

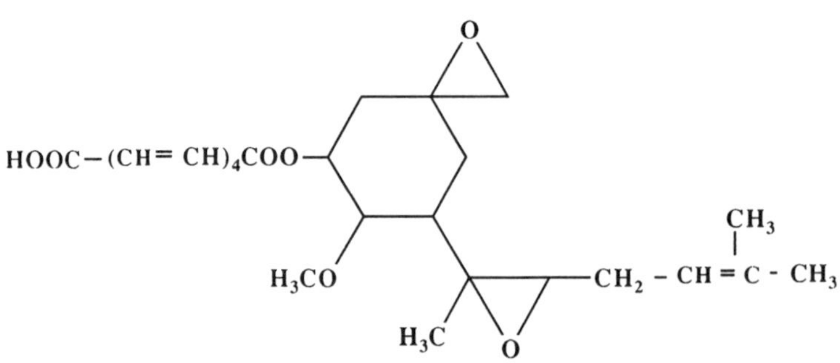

Figure 9 Chemical structure of fumagillin.

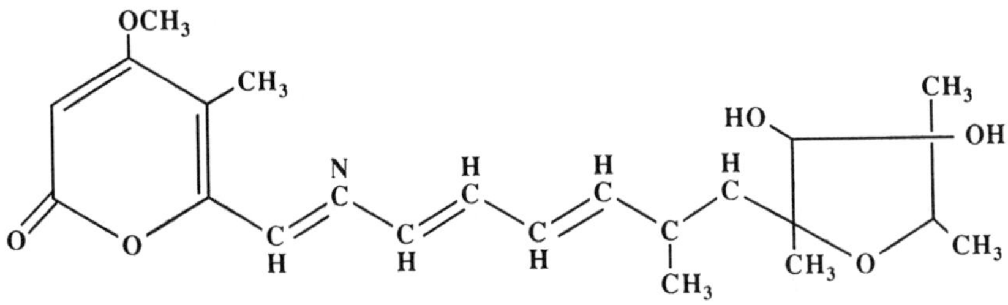

Figure 10 Chemical structure of citreoviridin.

Similar signs of poisoning can be seen in other species such as cats and dogs. Some of these toxic manifestations may be attributed to inhibition of mitochondrial ATPase activity by citreoviridin (Gause et al., 1981).

2. *Citrinin*

Citrinin (Fig. 11), an antibiotic and nephrotoxin, is produced by many species of penicillia and aspergilli (Pollock, 1947; Betina et al., 1964). After being recognized as a powerful antibiotic, it was later found to damage the kidneys of test animals, retard growth, and eventually cause death (Ambrose and Deeds, 1964; Carlton and Tuite, 1969, 1970). Citrinin-producing isolates of *P. citrinum* have been obtained from yellow-colored rice of the type associated with toxic symptoms in Japan (Saito et al., 1971). In the Danish survey of grains associated with swine nephropathy, citrinin was determined at 0.16, 1.0, and 2.0 mg/kg in three of the 22 samples of barley in which ochratoxin had been detected (Krogh et al., 1973). Wu et al. (1974a) reported that seven strains of *P. viridicatum* isolated from country-cured ham produced citrinin on artificial media and country-cured ham. Thus, it is possible that both ochratoxin A and citrinin are involved in the mycotoxicosis that has affected up to 7% of the pigs in Denmark (Krogh, 1969). Natural occurrence of citrinin in wheat, barley, rye, and oats in Canada and Denmark has been reported by Hesseltine (1976).

Citrinin has been detected in trace amounts in two naturally rotten apples containing *P. expansum* and patulin (Harwig et al.,1973). Citrinin has also

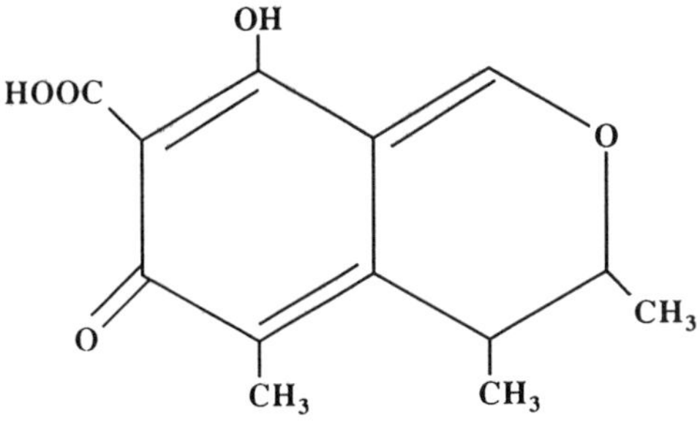

Figure 11 Chemical structure of citrinin.

been found in groundnuts from India infected with *A. flavus, P. citrinum,* and *A. terreus*, and natural contaminant of peanuts (Diener, 1960) and corn (Mislivec and Tuite, 1970).

3. *Penicillic Acid*

Penicillic acid (Fig. 12) was first isolated from a mold culture in 1913 as part of a study of corn deterioration (Alsberg and Black, 1913). Penicillic acid is toxic to animals with a LD_{50} for mice of 100 mg/kg (Spector, 1957). Ciegler and Kurtzman (1970) studied the conditions for the production of penicillic acid on different agricultural commodities and observed that the toxigenic strains found on corn could produce substantial amounts of penicillic acid in rice, barley, sorghum, and oats. Penicillic acid has been reported to occur naturally in Swiss cheese (Bullerman, 1976). Many fungus species that commonly cause storage rots in grain and other foodstuffs produce good yields of penicillic acid.

4. *Rubratoxins*

A disease in pigs and cattle caused by consumption of fungal-infected corn was reported by Burnside et al. (1957). Of 13 cultures of fungi isolated from such toxic corn, only two were shown to cause illness and death when fed to experimental animals. One of the cultures was found to be *P. rubrum*, which produced a mycotoxin. Forgacs et al. (1958) fed grains with *P. rubrum* and *P. purpurogenum* to chicks and observed a hemorrhagic syndrome. In 1962, Wilson and Wilson reported preliminary results of chemical and pathological studies on the toxic metabolite isolated from *P. rubrum*. Townsend et al. (1966) carried out further chemical studies of the culture broth of *P. rubrum*, and postmortem examinations of inspected mice, guinea pigs, and dogs, and subsequently isolated two toxic metabolites designated as rubratoxin A and B. Rubratoxin A and B have the same structure (Fig. 13), but with A, one of the anhydride groups is reduced to the lactol. Rubratoxin B is the major metabolite, and it is produced by the head-to-tail, head-to-tail coupling of two C_{13} units.

Oral toxicity is perhaps the most important parameter when considering the immediate implications of a toxin in food material. The LD_{50} value for rubratoxin A and B are 6.6 and 3.0 mg/kg, respectively. Rubratoxin B has been shown to be mutagenic as well as teratogenic (Hood et al., 1973; Evans et al., 1975).

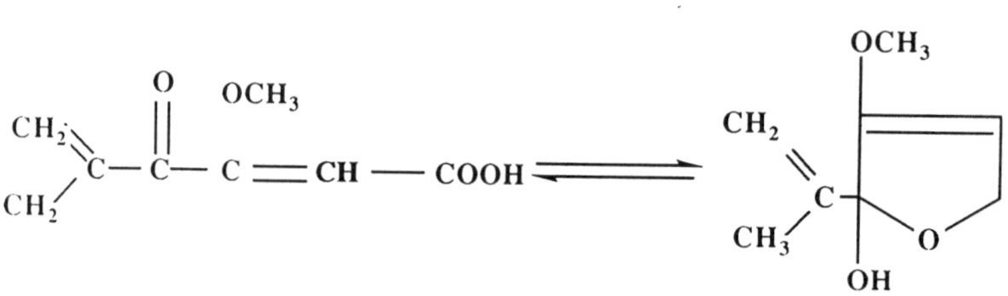

Figure 12 Chemical structure of penicillic acid.

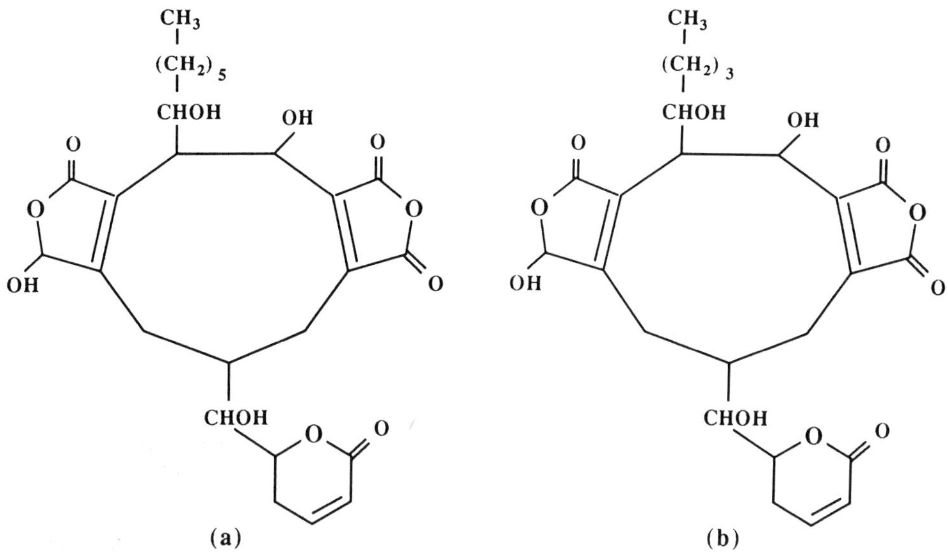

Figure 13 Chemical structure of (a) rubratoxin A, (b) rubratoxin B.

5. *Griseofulvin*

Brian et al. (1946) and McGowan (1946) isolated griseofulvin (Fig. 14) from *P. janczewski* (*P. nigricans*) and termed it "curling factor" because of a peculiar inhibitory action on hyphal development in other fungi. The identity of the compound was not recognized at that time. Griseofulvin has also been obtained from *P. patulum* (Paget and Walpole, 1958), *P. albidum, P. raciborski, P. melinii, P. urticae, P. raistrickii, P. brefeldianum, P. viridicyclopium,* and *P. brunneostoloniferum* (Rhodes, 1963). Griseofulvin has unique value as a systemic therapeutic agent for cutaneous fungal infections. In spite of the clinical effectiveness of griseofulvin and the ability of humans and animals to tolerate relatively large doses given daily for several weeks, the serious nature of toxic response observed in recent years has served to restrict its therapeutic use somewhat. Numerous toxic manifestations for griseofulvin have been reported; included are the following symptoms (Anderson, 1965):

1. In the skin–angio-neurotic edema, erythema, urticaria, vesicular and macular eruptions, photosensitivity, and lichen-planus eruptions.
2. Hematopoietic disturbances—transient leukopenia, granulocytopenia, punctate basophilia, and monocytosis.
3. Neurological manifestations—blurred vision, headaches, disorientation, and vertigo.
4. Gastrointestinal signs and symptoms—anorexia, nausea, vomiting, and diarrhea.
5. Oral changes—dry mouth, black hairy tongue, glossodynia, and angular stomatitis.
6. Miscellaneous effects—thirst, fatigue, malaise, fainting, and potentiation of alcohol effects.

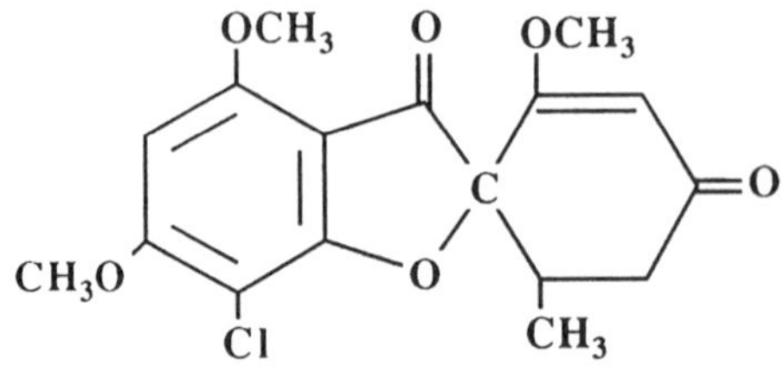

Figure 14 Chemical structure of griseofulvin.

6. Luteoskyrin and Islanditoxin

Luteoskyrin is a yellow anthraquinonelike pigment synthesized by *Penicillium islandicum* Sopp, contaminating rice, maize, and other cereals, especially in Eastern countries, where human malignant and nonmalignant hepatomas are more frequent. *P. islandicum* was first isolated in 1912 from skyr, a kind of yogurt produced in Iceland, and the pigments isolated from this fungus were named after the domestic name. Heavy fungal growth and accumulation of fungal pigments may color the rice yellow and render it bitter. Most contaminated rice contains toxic materials and may produce toxic symptoms upon ingestion by humans or animals. These toxic compounds have been the subject of extensive chemical, structural, and biological investigations (Pham Van Chuong et al., 1974). Strains of *P. islandicum* have produced hepatotoxic metabolites that induced liver neoplasm in rat and mice (Tsunoda, 1951). Liver cirrhosis (Fig. 15) has been noted in rats fed with diets containing cereals

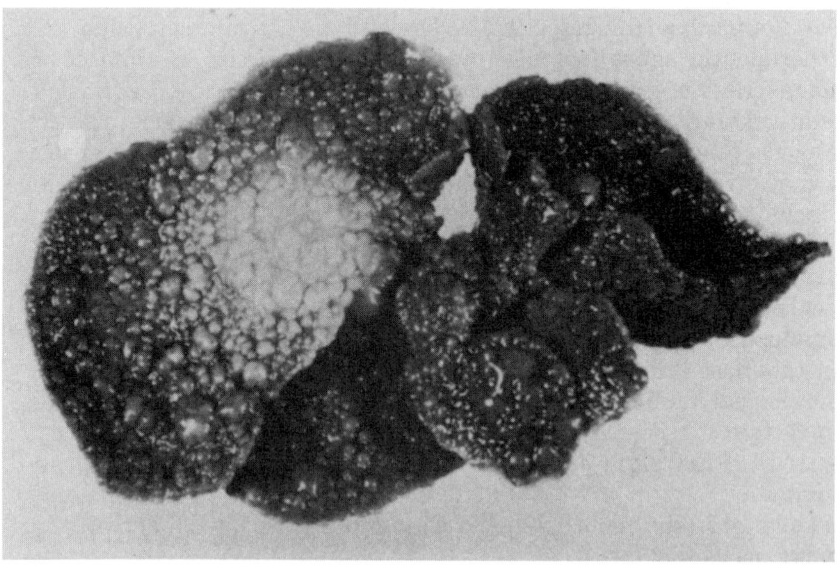

Figure 15 Liver cirrhosis.

contaminated by the fungus. Saito et al. (1971) and Miyake and Saito (1965) reported that continuous feeding of diets containing small to large percentages of the fungi produced a wide range of pathological changes in the liver of rats and mice, including acute atrophy at high levels of administration and nodular hyperplasia, bile duct hyperplasic fibrosis, and cirrhosis at lower levels. Fractionation of toxins revealed a lipophilic and a hydrophilic toxin. The yellow lipophilic toxin, luteoskyrin, is a substituted bis-polyhydroxydihydroanthraquinone (Fig. 16), and the hydrophilic toxin is islanditoxin, a toxic cyclic peptide (Fig. 17). Luteoskyrin is slow acting, and for a 10-g mouse the LD_{50} is 1.5 mg, subcutaneously, and 2.2 mg/10 g, orally. Liver damage caused by luteoskyrin is characterized by centrilobular necrosis of the liver and diffuse fatty metamorphosis of the liver cells. Islanditoxin is extremely hepatotoxic, causing severe liver damage, hemorrhaging, and death. LD_{50} values for 10-g mice range from 4.75 μg, subcutaneously, to 65.5 μg, orally. It is suggested that toxin interferes with carbohydrate metabolism by causing the disappearance of glycogen granules in the injured liver.

A chlorine-containing peptide (cyclochlorotine) was also one of the yellowed rice toxins isolated from the culture filtrate, cultured fungal mat of *P. islandicum* Sopp, and cultured fungal rice grain (Tatsuno et al., 1955). The peptide is a quick-acting hepatotoxin, causing the disappearance of glycogen granules in injured liver (Saito, 1959). The chlorine-containing peptide causes hepatic damage of the so-called acinus peripheral cytotoxic pattern characterized by vacuolation of liver and endothelial cells in the perilobular region, followed by the appearance of hyaline droplets (Saito et al., 1971). Results of long-term feeding experiments with this peptide revealed that it acts as a cirrhogenic agent.

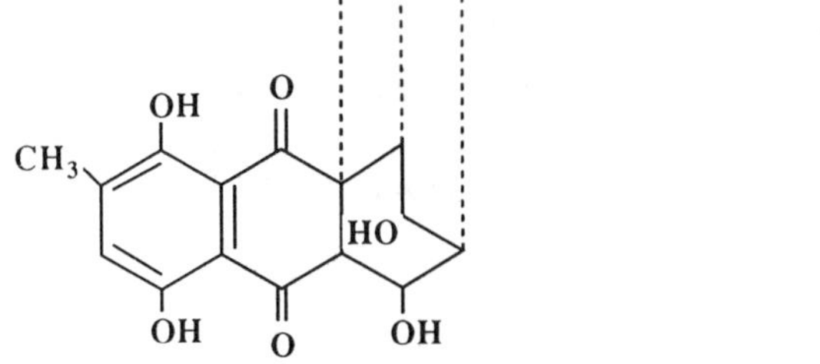

Figure 16 Chemical structure of luteoskyrin.

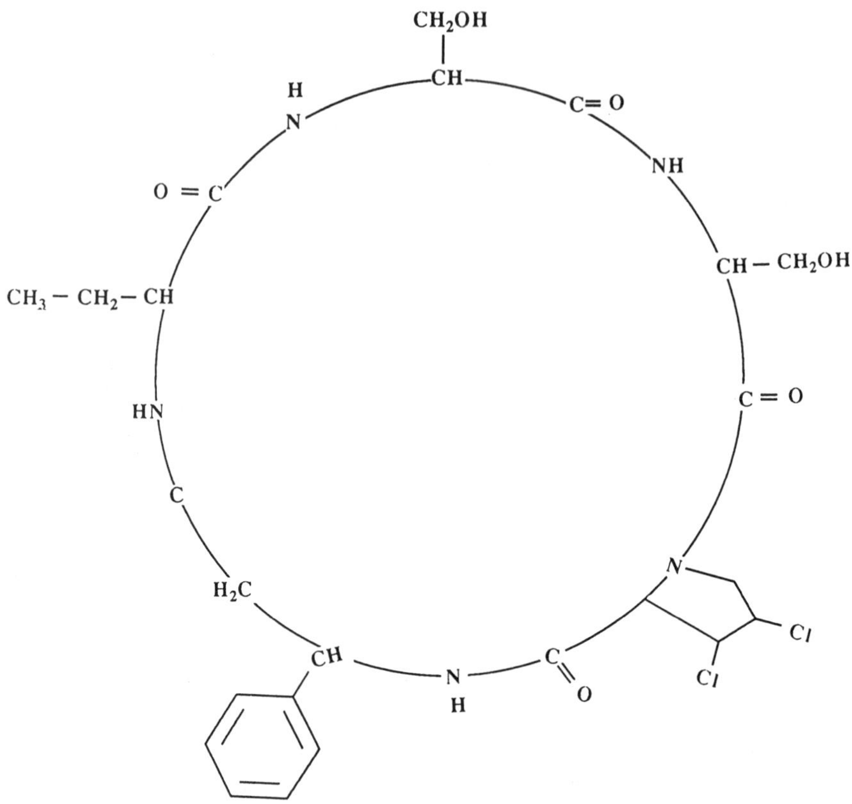

Figure 17 Chemical structure of islanditoxin.

7. *Mycophenolic Acid*

Mycophenolic acid, a product of several *Penicillium* species, *P. stoloniferum* Thom, *P. brevicompactum* (Wilson, 1971), *P. viridicatum* and *P. bialowiezense* (Burton, 1949), contains a five-membered lactone ring fused to a benzene moiety (Fig. 18) (Birkinshaw et al., 1952; Shibata et al., 1964). It is a relatively less toxic fungal metabolite. Its oral and intravenous LD_{50} values for mice have been reported to be 2.5 g/kg and 550 mg/kg, respectively, and those for rats 700 mg/kg and 450 mg/kg, respectively (Carter et al., 1969). A rhesus monkey given oral doses of 150 mg/kg/day developed abdominal colic, loss of body weight, and bloody diarrhea after 2 weeks of dosing. The compound exhibits antibacterial, antifungal, antiviral, and antitumor activity (Wilson, 1971; Cole and Cox, 1981). In food, mycophenolic acid has so far been reported only in blue cheese and starter cultures of *P. roqueforti* (Lafont et al., 1979).

8. *Decumbin*

Decumbin is a toxic metabolite of *Penicillium decumbens* which was isolated by Singleton et al. (1958) from corn spoiled in storage. The compounds,

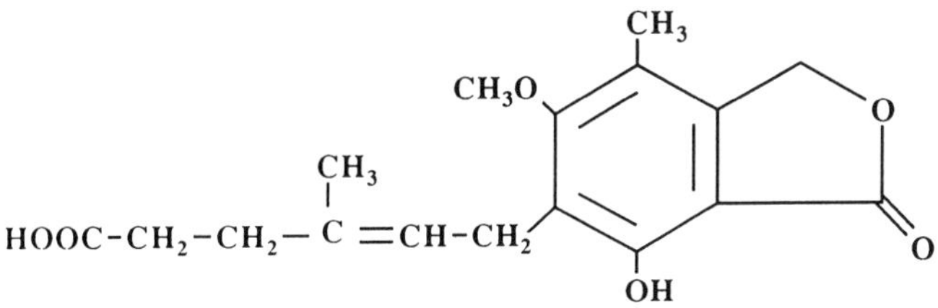

Figure 18 Chemical structure of mycophenolic acid.

brefeldin A (Fig. 19), which was isolated from the culture filtrate of *P. brefeldianum* (Harri et al., 1963), and cyanein, which was obtained from a culture of *P. cyaneum* (Betina et al., 1965), *P. simplicissimum* (Betina et al., 1966) were later found to be identical substances of decumbin. Administration of the toxin at levels of 400, 300, and 250 mg/kg with food to fasted rats resulted in 37 deaths among 38 fed, 8 deaths among 10 fed, and no death among 5 fed rats, respectively. The young rats showed signs of illness in about 2 hours in the form of loss of appetite, followed by diarrhea, lethargy, labored breathing, cyanosis, stupor, and death in about 24 hours. During autopsy there was evidence of slight nasal bleeding and congestion of the auricles and associated blood vessels. Goldfish (*Carassius auratus*) of about 1.7 g body weight were killed in water containing 0.6 mg/L. Seed germination of wheat (*Triticum aestivum*) was reduced by contact with the toxin.

Cyanein was found to be effective in inhibiting growth of *Candida albicans, C. pseudotropicalis. A. fumigatus*, and *Saccharomyces cerevisiae*, but ineffective with bacteria and protozoa. It has also been reported as cytostatic for HeLa cells (Betina et al., 1964). No inhibition of glycosis was obtained in yeasts or animal cells exposed to cyanein. However, inhibition of both microbial cells and animal cells has been demonstrated (Betina et al., 1966).

9. *Viridicatin*

Cunningham and Freeman (1953) isolated viridicatin (Fig. 20) from the mycelium of *Penicillium viridicatum* obtained from Argentine corn causing poisoning of swine and horses. This compound has also been isolated from five strains of *P. cyclopium* (Bracken et al., 1954). The toxin showed in vitro

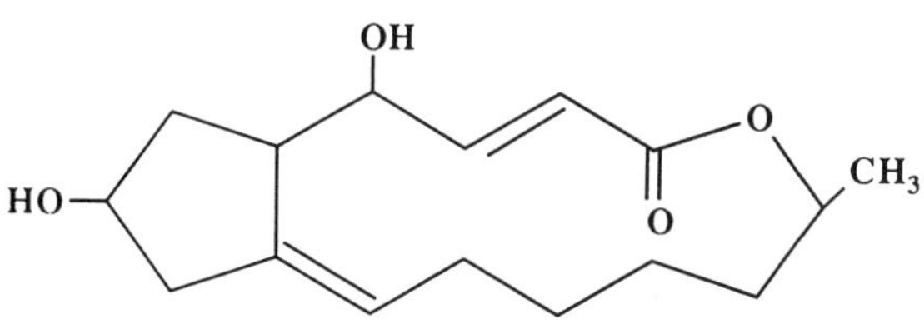

Figure 19 Chemical structure of decumbin.

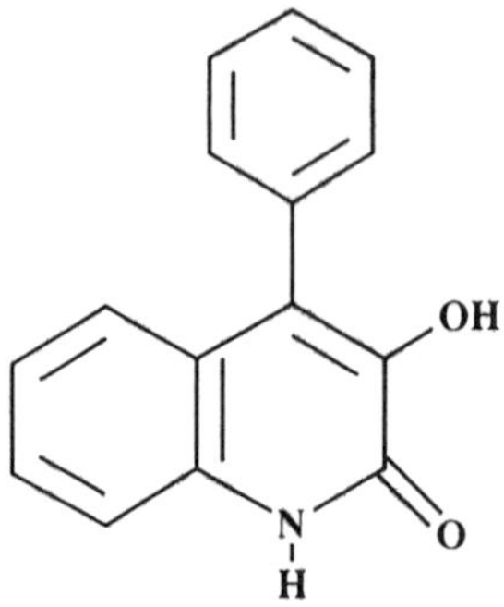

Figure 20 Chemical structure of viridicatin.

antibacterial activity against *Mycobacterium tuberculosis* at a 1:15,000 dilution; however, not much is known about its vertebrate toxicity.

10. Cyclopiazonic Acid

Cyclopiazonic acid (Fig. 21) is a toxic metabolite of penicillium species *P. cyclopium* and *P. puberulum*. In addition, it can be produced by certain species of *A. flavus* (Yates et al., 1987). Cyclopiazonic acid is a hydrophilic, colorless compound (Holzapfel, 1968). Acute mycotoxicosis in ducklings and rats has been shown to be caused by a strain of *P. cyclopium*. Toxicity of cyclopiazonic acid has been studied in many other species including chickens, rabbits, dogs, and pigs (Yates et al., 1987). The reported clinical signs of toxicity include inactivity, diarrhea, anorexia, rough hair coats, tremors, and death.

11. Patulin

This compound was discovered in a long, intensive search for new antibiotics. It was first isolated in crystalline form as *P. claviforme* and given the name "clavicin." Identical materials from other fungal species were isolated

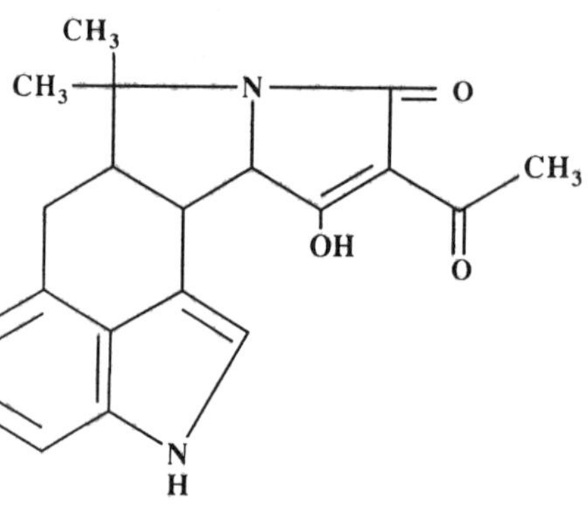

Figure 21 Chemical structure of cyclopiazonic acid.

by other investigators, each one given a name based on the fungal source. Therefore, the literature contains many synonyms for patulin, including clavicin, expansin, mycoin, penicidin, leukopin, and tercinin. The name "patulin" was finally accepted with elucidation of the correct chemical structure by Woodward and Singh in 1949.

Patulin, 4-hydroxy-4H-furo(3,2C)pyran-2(6H)one is a lactone metabolite (Fig. 22) of several species of *Penicillium, Aspergillus, Gymnoascua*, and *Byssochlamys*. This compound has carcinogenic, mutagenic, as well as teratogenic properties (Dickens and Jones, 1961; Mayer and Legator, 1969; Ciegler et al., 1976).

Intravenous injection of patulin into mice and rats produces LD_{50} values varying from 0.3 to 0.7 mg patulin/20 g body weight, and 1 mg per mouse was always lethal (Broom et al., 1944; Stansfeld et al., 1944). Patulin-producing penicillia come mainly from fruits and vegetables (Atkinson, 1943). The patulin-producing fungus *P. expansum*, has been isolated from apricots, crab apples, persimmons, pears, grapes (Sommer et al., 1974), in-shell pecans (Schindler et al., 1974), and apples (Harwig et al., 1973; Wilson and Nuovo, 1973; Sommer et al., 1974). Scott (1965) isolated the patulin-producing molds *A. clavatus, A terreus, P. expansum*, and P. urticae from cereal grains and legumes. Patulin-producing fungi such as *A. clavatus, A. terreus, P. expansum, P. urticae*, and *P. patulum* have been isolated from cereals, legumes, and dried fish and fruits. Patulin-producing strains of fungi isolated from foods generally make up a low percentage of the total isolates. Patulin is found in fruits with spontaneous brown rot, such as bananas, pineapples, grapes, peaches, and apricots. Existence of patulin in apple juice has also been reported by Scott et al. (1972). An extensive survey in terms of geography and type of pack for the presence of patulin in apple juice was carried out by the U.S. Food and Drug Administration in 1973 (Bureau of Foods, 1974). Patullin was detected in 50 of 126 consumer packs of apple juice taken in the open market from all the sections of the country. The presence of patulin in apple juice is evidence that rotted apples are being used. Scott and Sommers (1968) showed that patulin was relatively stable in grape and apple juice, but not in orange juice, possibly due to the presence of thiols. Thus apple products appear to be the foods most likely to be contaminated with patulin, whereas a lesser chance of contamination exists for grain products.

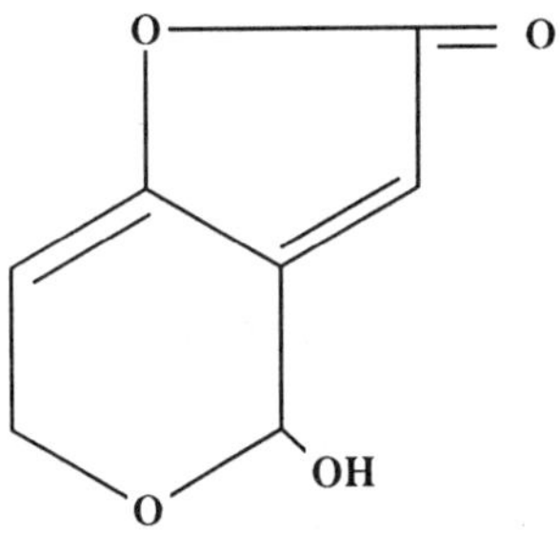

Figure 22 Chemical structure of patulin.

C. Tremorgenic Mycotoxins of *Aspergillus* and *Penicillium*

Fungal metabolites capable of causing sustained tremors, convulsions, and death in animals have been isolated from several fungi. These tremorgenic mycotoxins include several compounds that cause sustained trembling in animals. These tremorgens can be separated according to their nitrogen content into three groups: Group A consists of penitrems A, B, and C, which contain only one nitrogen atom per molecule (Fig. 23); Group B consists of fumitremorgens A, B, and C (Fig. 24) and verrucologens TR-1 and TR-2 (Fig. 25) containing three nitrogens per molecule (Cole and Kirksey, 1973); Group C consists of tryptoquivaline and tryptoquivalone containing four nitrogens per molecule (Fig. 26). The metabolites penitrems A, B, and C have been isolated from *P. cyclopium, P. crustosum, P. palitans*, and *P. puberulum*. Of these three toxins, penitrem A is the most toxic (Cysewski, 1978). The above organisms are capable of producing penitrem A on various agricultural commodities with low temperatures favoring toxin accumulation (Hou et al., 1971a). Penitrems B and C are two closely related tremorgens produced by most of the penitrem A producers (Hou et al., 1971b). Perceptible tremors have shown to be caused in mice at 250 μg of penitrem A per kg of body weight, whereas penitrem B required 1.3 mg/kg for a similar response. The mechanism of tremor production is thought to inhibit the interneurons that inhibit the α-motor cells of the anterior horn of the spinal column (Stern, 1971). *P. crustosum*, a good producer of tremorgens, is a contaminant of various refrigerated foods, grains, and cereal products and causes a soft brown rot in apples. Penitrem C is considered less toxic than penitrems A and B, but literature on its properties and toxicity are still meager (Ciegler et al., 1976).

Verruculogen TR-1, a product of *P. verruculosum*, was isolated from moldy peanuts as a result of improper storage conditions (Cole et al., 1972). LD_{50} values for mice is 2.4 mg/kg and 15.2 mg/kg in cockerels, i.p., and 126.7 mg/kg in mice and 365.5 mg/kg in cockerels when administered orally. Verruculogen TR-2, a product of verruculogen TR-1 conversion, is observed only under certain conditions (Cole and Kirksey, 1973). It appears that TR-2 is also of natural origin since it was not a photodegradation product and may be a biosynthetic precursor to TR-1 (Ciegler et al., 1976).

Fumitremorgens include three closely related toxins, namely, fumitremorgens A, B, and C, all produced by *A. fumigatus*, with the first two also produced by certain strains of *A. caespitosus* (Cole and Cox, 1981). Fumitremorgen A is a potent neurotropic toxin which causes tremors and generalized tonic-clonic convulsions in experimental animals upon intravenous injection (Nishiyama and Kuga, 1989). The structure of fumitremorgen A and B have recently been determined (Yamazaki et al., 1974). Fumitremorgen A when injected at 1 mg/kg in mice caused more severe sustained trembling than fumitremorgen B at a similar dose. Similarly, fumitremorgens B and C are known to be tremorgenic in mice and in day-old cockerels, respectively (Cole and Cox, 1981).

The tremorgenic compounds tryptoquivaline and tryptoquivalone are apparently not as toxic as the other tremorgenic compounds. These two compounds injected into weanling rats at 500 mg/kg caused tremoring that

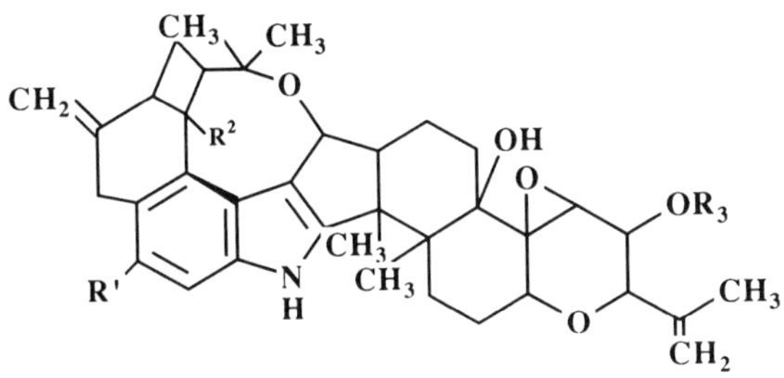

Penitrem A, R' = Cl, R2 =OH, R3 = H
Penitrem B, R' = H, R2 =H, R3 = H

(a)

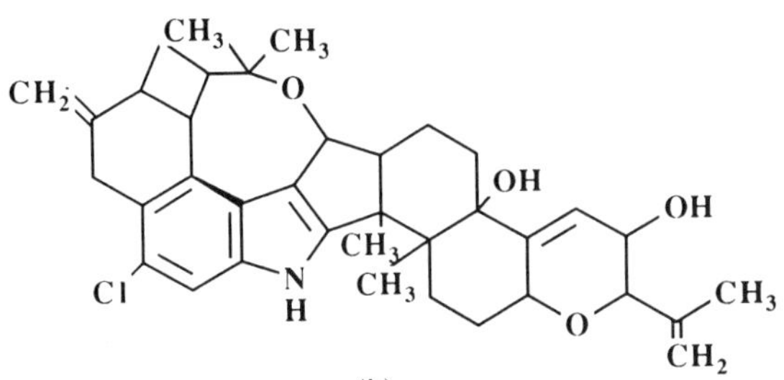

(b)

Figure 23 Chemical structure of (a) penitrems A and B, (b) penitrem C.

persisted for 5 days, and the animals died by day 8 with no observable histopathological changes (Glinsukon et al., 1974).

D. Mycotoxins of Other Genera

1. Zearalenone

Zearalenone (Fig. 27), also known as F-2 toxin, is produced by several *Fusarium* species and is a frequent contaminant of corn, wheat, barley, and grain sorghum in the United States. Generally, zearalenone concentrations are well below 1 ppm in processed cereal foods (Morehouse, 1985). In the United States and Canada, contamination of grains by zearalenone is frequently encountered. In Japan, high concentrations of zearalenone sometimes occur as a co-contaminant with deoxynivalenol and nivalenol (Jelinek, 1987). A thorough review of the hazard from zearalenone and the risk from zearalenone levels found in Canadian foods has been developed by the Health and Welfare Canada group (Kuiper-Goodman et al., 1987). Zearalenone, a isolate from maize infected with the fungus *Gibberella zeae*, the peripheral stage of *Fusarium graminearum* (Stob et al., 1962), exhibits uterotrophic and anabolic

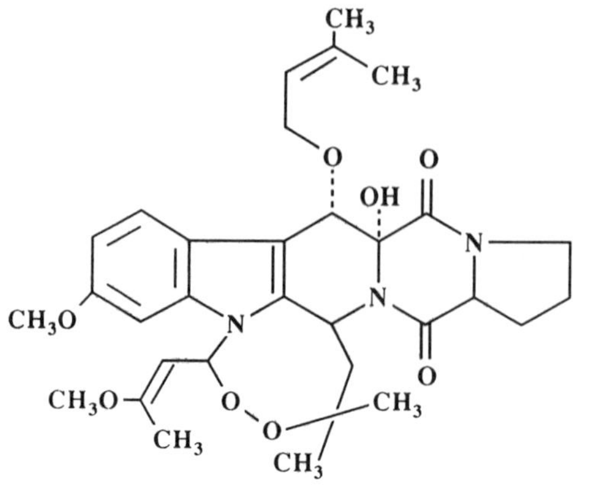

(a)

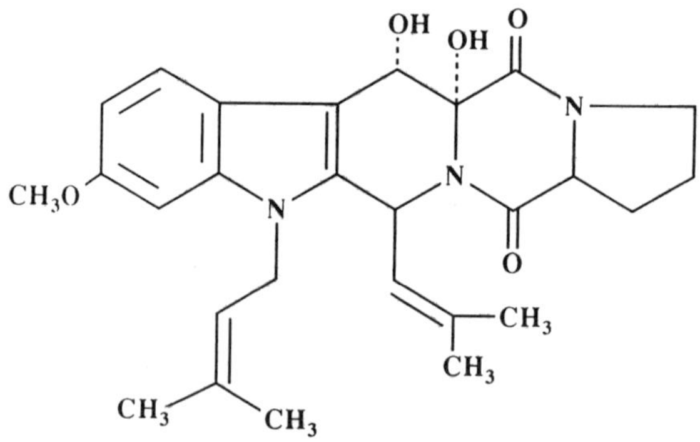

(b)

Figure 24 Chemical structure of (a) fumitremorgen A, (b) fumitremorgen B.

activity. Zearalenone and its derivatives has estrogenic effects on pigs, rabbits, and deer (Lasztity and Woller, 1975).

Invasion of grain by *G. zeae* is also related to species such as *F. tricinctum* and *F. moniliforme* (Mirocha et al., 1967, 1969; Caldwell et al., 1970). Developing corn at the silking stage is invaded by these organisms during heavy rainfall, and they proliferate on mature grains that have not dried because of wet weather at harvest or on grains that are stored wet (Caldwell and Tuite, 1970, 1974; Tuite et al., 1974). During surveys of 1967 corn crops (Shotwell et al., 1970) and of corn for export during 1968–1969 (Shotwell et al., 1971), zearalenone was found in six of the 576 samples at an average level of 624 mg/kg (range 450–800 mg/kg). Zearalenone in U.S. and Canadian foods is most commonly found in corn-based products such as breakfast cereals and cornmeal.

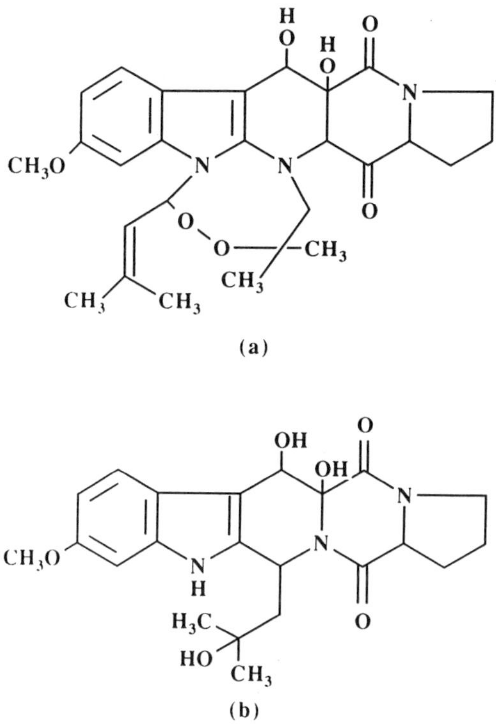

Figure 25 Chemical structure of (a) verruculogen TR-1, (b) verruculogen TR-2.

2. *Trichothecenes*

The ability of fungi to produce a large number of secondary metabolites is striking in the case of the trichothecenes. Trichothecenes (Fig. 28) are produced by various species of *Fusarium, Myrothecium, Trichoderma, Cephalosprium, Verticimonosporium, Cylindrocarpon*, and *Stachybotrys*. Over 40 trichothecene metabolites are known, of which some are extremely potent toxins. Combinations of some of the trichothecenes are thought to be involved in the human disease known as alimentary toxic aleukia, presumably from ingestion of bread made from fungal-infected wheat, which affected people in parts of the Soviet Union during World War II. This disease was characterized by severe hemorrhage, leukopenia, necrotic angina, and exhaustion of bone marrow. These symptoms have been seen in victims of "yellow rain," an alleged chemical warfare episode in Southeast Asia in which trichothecene mycotoxins are implicated (Watson et al., 1984). The most prevalent trichothecenes found in commodities in the northern United States are deoxynivalenol and nivalenol. They are implicated in a veterinary problem known as fungal- infected corn toxicosis of swine, the symptoms of which include a refusal to eat, digestive disorders, and diarrhea, ultimately leading to death. Frequently observed symptoms in humans are dermatitis, cough, rhinitis, and hemorrhage in the nose and throat.

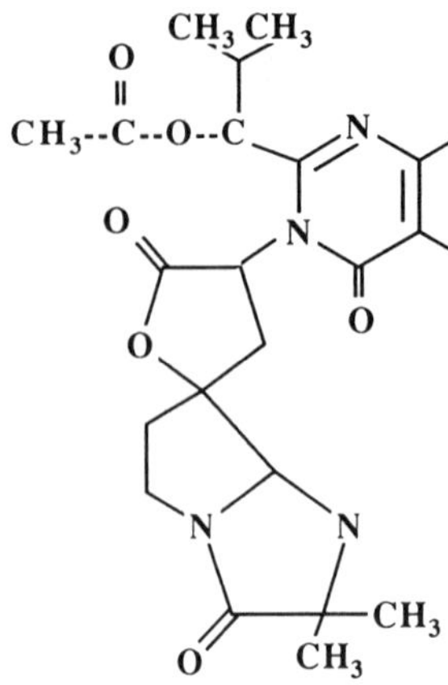

(a)

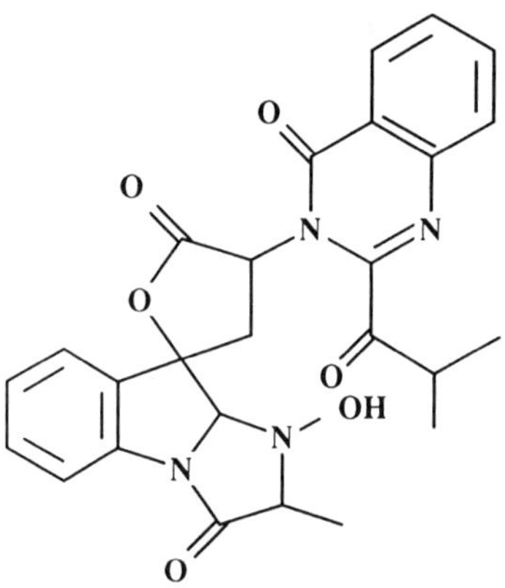

(b)

Figure 26 Chemical structure of (a) tryptoquivaline, (b) tryptoquivalone.

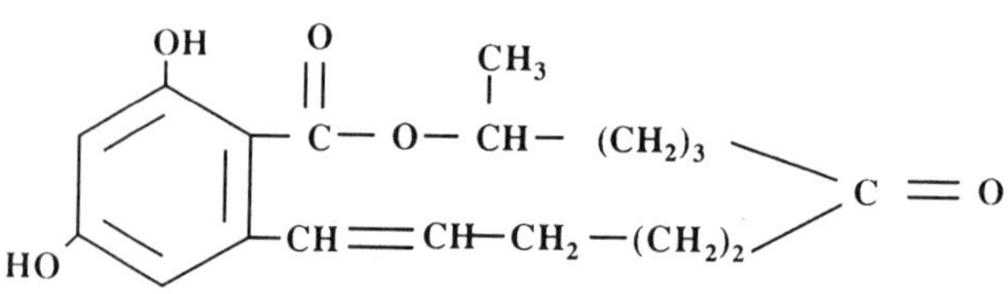

Figure 27 Chemical structure of zearelenone.

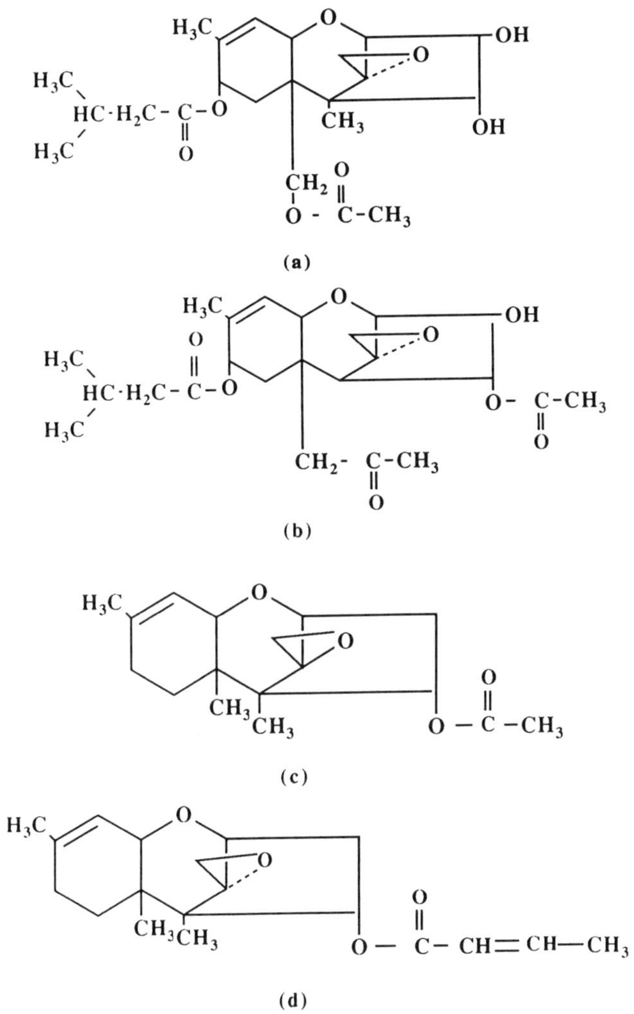

Figure 28 Chemical structure of trichothecenes (a) HT-2, (b) T-2, (c) trichodermin, (d) trichothecin.

3. Psoralens

A number of naturally occurring furanocoumarins have phototoxic activity, and much research has been done on the simplest member of the group, psoralen. Psoralens are characterized by a linearly annulated structure (Fig. 29) formed by the fusion of a furan ring in the 2 and 3 positions with carbon atoms 6 and 7, respectively, of the coumarin structure. Photosensitizing psoralens occur as natural constituents of many plants belonging principally to the botanical families *Umbelliferae, Rutaceae, Leguminosae*, and *Morraceae* (Pathak et al., 1962). The fungus *Sclerotinia sclerotiorum* growing on the celery plant has been reported to result in the biosynthesis of two phototoxic

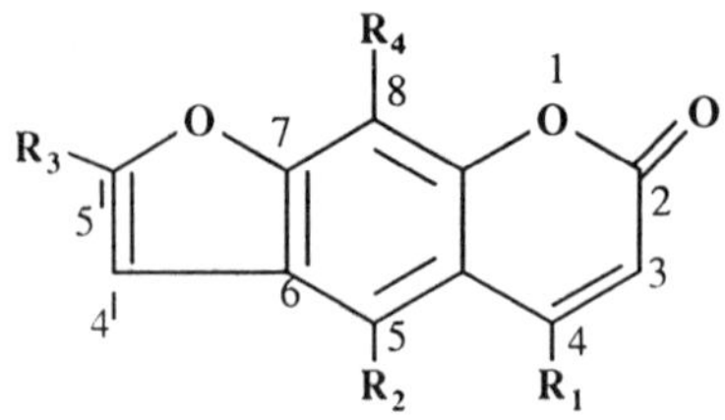

Furanocoumarin	R1	R2	R3	R4
Psoralen	H	H	H	H
Xanthotoxin	H	H	H	OCH_3
4,5′,8 - Trimethyl psoralen	CH_3	H	CH_3	CH_3

Figure 29 Chemical structure of fouranocoumarins.

derivatives, xanthotoxin and 4,5′,8-trimethylpsoralen, in the affected area of this plant (Scheel et al., 1963). These compounds possessing phototoxic properties have been associated with bullous dermatitis suffered by workers handling celery parasitized by the fungus. These compounds are not detected in healthy celery tissue. Xanthotoxins also occur naturally in a number of plants. The outbreak of the cutaneous lesions occurred only when exposure to sunlight or ultraviolet radiation having wavelengths in the 320 to 370 nm region followed contact with diseased plant. Ancient Egyptians, Hindus, and Turks used furanocoumarins extracted from plants to treat leukoderma. Research has shown that the side effects associated with its use are erythema, edema, and scabbing.

4. *Ergotoxins*

Ergot is the oldest known mycotoxin. It was known as "St. Anthony's fire" in the 1500s and 1600s. Despite people suffering from many regions of Europe for several years from severe epidemics of peripheral gangrene and convulsions due to the consumption of ergot-infested rye and other grains, it was not until 1850 or so that a distinct association between the ingestion of rye infected with *Claviceps purpurea* and ergotism was established. In 1934 toxic substances from ergot grains were isolated and purified as six derivatives of lysergic acid (Groger, 1972). Cereal grains and pasture grasses under high moisture conditions are invaded by the fungus-producing sclerotia, approximately 2–20 mm long and purple-black in color, that contain many toxic alkaloids (Lorenz, 1979). Ergot alkaloids are derivatives of lysergic acid (ergotamine), isolysergic acid (ergocristine), or dimethyl ergoline (agroclavine), of which L-tryptophan and mevalonic acid are precursors (Berry, 1988). Figure 30 illustrates the general structure of peptide-type ergot alkaloids derived from lysergic acid. The effects of ergot can be divided into three groups depending on the site of action: (1) peripheral effects, (2) neurohumoral effects, and (3) effects on the central nervous system.

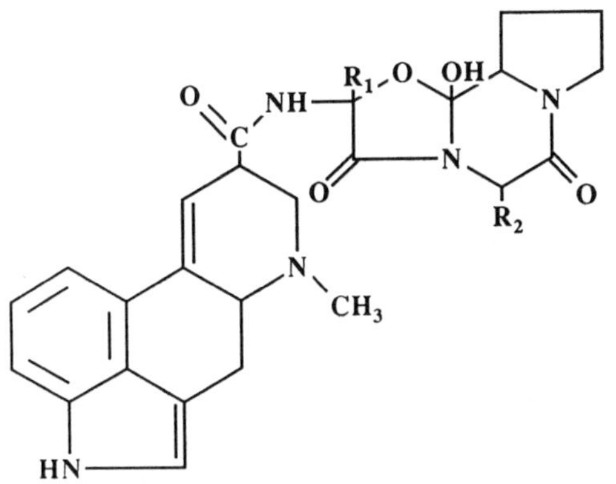

Alkaloid	R1	R2
Ergotamine	CH_3-	$C_6H_5CH_2-$
Ergosine	CH_3-	$(CH_3)_2CH-CH_2-$
Ergostine	CH_3CH_2-	$C_6H_5CH_2-$
Ergocristine	$(CH_3)_2CH-$	$C_6H_5CH_2-$

Figure 30 Chemical structure of ergot alkaloids derived from lysergic acid.

Hallucination is one of the most famous effects of ergot. Typical gangrenous ergotism was described in an Ethiopian epidemic in 1978 after human consumption of grains contaminated with *C. purpurea* infected wild oats (Demeke et al., 1979; King, 1979; Pokrovsky and Tutelyan, 1982). While approximately 50% of the affected individuals died, others revealed dry gangrene of the limbs, swollen limbs, skin desquamation, and loss of limbs. Common symptoms were weakness, burning sensations, nausea, vomiting, and diarrhea. Incidences in India have been reported following human ingestion of pearl millet infected with *C. fusiformis* (Krishnamachari and Bhat, 1976). Van Rensburg (1977) stated that as little as 0.2% (by weight) ergot in grain could cause mild symptoms or signs of ergotism in humans, and death from gangrene could follow consumption of about 100 g of ergot over a few days. The suggested maximum level of 0.05% of ergot particles by count in flour may be acceptable (Peace and Harwig, 1982).

5. *Mushroom Toxins*

The group of toxins produced in the poisonous mushrooms of the *Amanita* species, including green *Amanita phalloides*, white *Amanita verna, Amanita virosa, Amanita tenuifolia,* and *Amanita bisporigera,* are known as Amanita toxins. Although mushroom poisoning is encountered infrequently in animals and humans, often it is serious, especially with *Amanita* species. Most mushroom poisoning in humans occurs in children under 5 years of age (Wilson and

Holladay, 1987) whereas that in animals has been reported in cattle, cats, and dogs (Wilson and Holladay, 1987; Kallet et al., 1988). The toxic compounds of the most troublesome mushroom species of the genus *Amanita*, generally *A. phalloides*, are cyclopeptides, which are protoplasmic poisons, ibotinic acid and muscarine, which exert their toxic effects on the central nervous system, and gastrointestinal irritants such as the amatoxin.

6. Others

Buchi et al. (1977) have isolated new mycotoxins from *A. clavatus*: hydroxylamine, nortryptoquivaline, and three secondary amines, deoxytryptoquivaline, deoxynortryptoquivaline, and deoxynortryptoquivalone. Brevianamide A, a product of *Penicillium brevicompactum*, *P. ochraceum*, and *P. viridicatum* (Birch and Wright, 1969, 1970; Robbers et al., 1973, 1975; Wilson et al., 1973), has been shown to cause renal and hepatic lesions (Carlton et al., 1972). Monoacetoxyscirpenol, a new mycotoxin produced by *Fusarium roseum* Gibb., has been isolated from corn suspected of causing illness and death in several dairy cattle (Pathre et al., 1976). Recently a significant breakthrough was made with the isolation and characterization of a mycotoxin named Fumonisins from *Fusarium moniliforme* in South Africa in 1988. This most prevalent fungus is associated with maize throughout the world and has been shown to cause liver cancer in rats and leukoencephalomalacia (LEM), a neurotoxic disease in horses and donkeys. Two toxins, fumonisin B_1 and B_2, have been isolated, and fumonisin B_1 has been shown to be the causative factor of LEM in horses. Esophageal cytological abnormalities in humans in South Africa appear to be associated with the high prevalence of toxin of the fungus *F. moniliforme* in maize (Diener, 1990).

III. CONTROL OF MYCOTOXINS IN FOODS

The deleterious effects of fungal spoilage on many grain, fruit, and vegetable crops results in serious economic consequences. Consumption of contaminated foods with mycotoxins produced during fungal growth is a serious health problem. The toxicity syndromes known as mycotoxicoses have posed direct or indirect health hazards to humans.

Mycotoxin contamination is either a field problem, a storage problem, or a combination of the two. Preventive management of mycotoxins in crops has been attempted through recommended practices for growing, harvesting, handling, storage, processing/manufacturing, and sampling and analysis. Significant contamination may still occur in spite of preventive measures that have been established to prevent mycotoxin contamination in crops (USDA, 1968a,b; Anderson, 1983). Mycotoxigenic fungi can be prevented in field-grown crops through proper management of crop residues, moisture and plant nutrition, crop rotation, and use of resistant varieties. Crop residues often provide the basic inoculum for the fungi when susceptible crops are grown. The fungi may produce the spores early in the season in the crop residues, as in the case of ergot. The crop residues have sclerotia which germinate and provide the primary inoculum. Sclerotia of mycelium of *A. flavus* may be present in the crop residue or soil and may germinate and provide early *A. flavus* inoculum, thus increasing the probability of aflatoxin contamination (Wicklow and Wilson, 1986). Proper management of crop residues, therefore, may be an important factor in reducing mycotoxin contamination in the field. Moisture has been determined to play an important role in the contamination of field crops by mycotoxigenic fungi. Drought during the growing season has been shown to produce high risk of aflatoxin contamination in peanuts. Cole et al. (1985) have shown that in field-grown peanuts adequate calcium in peanuts helped to reduce aflatoxin contamination. Crop rotation plays a beneficial role in lowering the primary inoculum of fungi. Use of resistant varieties may help in reducing the fungal infection and inhibit toxin synthesis through genetic resistance. Certain environmental conditions in the field at preharvest favor mycotoxin contamination. Factors such as soil temperatures, wet, cool, warm seasons, and insect damage play important roles in mycotoxin contamination.

Grain and oilseed crops that are susceptible to fungal damage should be harvested at their optimum maturity when the moisture content is the lowest. Delay in harvesting of many crops influences mycotoxin contamination, creating loss of yield and quality. During harvesting, damage to the crop should be avoided. Damaged portions of the crop should be removed during the harvesting process. Drying of the crop should be carried out to reduce the moisture content so as not to allow any fungal growth. The moisture content on drying depends on the type of crop and the climatic conditions in which it is to be stored. When the product is stored after prolonged drying to avoid any fungal growth, and it is stored without any insect and rodent activity or moisture invasion in storage through leaks and condensation, no further deterioration will occur. Control of storage insects should be given more attention, because these storage insects cause activity in stored products, creating a favorable microclimate for fungal growth. The water of metabolism from the fungus, when fungal growth starts, provides sufficient water for further growth and mycotoxin development (Marasas and Nelson, 1987).

Processing of agricultural products into foods for humans should involve careful selection of raw materials, and high-quality control practices should be employed from the source to final preparation of the food. Commodities like nuts, kernels, or oilseeds should be visibly checked for any damage before processing because they create highly favorable conditions for fungal growth. Agricultural products should be monitored in varying degrees depending on the crop and its environment for possible mycotoxin contamination. In commodities, such as peanuts, processors and manufacturers follow strict quality control standards of the Peanut Advisory Council and the USDA Peanut Marketing Agreement regarding aflatoxin contamination. To confirm that the levels of aflatoxin contamination are below those required by the FDA, additional analyses are performed before the product is consumed as food.

Detoxification of mycotoxin-contaminated foods is carried out through the use of physical, chemical, and biological methods. Several strategies for detoxification of mycotoxin-contaminated foods have been reported (Goldblatt and Dollear, 1977, 1979; Diener et al., 1979; Marth and Doyle, 1979; Anderson, 1983). More information on detoxification of aflatoxins is available than on any other mycotoxin. The physical methods of detoxification are: (1) thermal inactivation, (2) irradiation, (3) solvent extraction, and (4) adsorption from solutions.

Aflatoxins are not totally destroyed by boiling water, autoclaving, and a variety of food-processing procedures, because aflatoxins are heat resistant (Christensen et al., 1977). Reduction in aflatoxin content of nuts and oilseed meals on roasting has been reported by Marth and Doyle (1979). Feuell (1977) reported that gamma irradiation did not degrade aflatoxin in contaminated peanut meal, and UV light produced an observable change in fluorescence or toxicity of the treated sample. Extraction of aflatoxins from different foods with minimal effects on protein content and nutritional quality can be achieved by using various solvents (Rayner et al., 1977; Goldblatt and Dollear, 1979). Use of solvents for extraction of aflatoxins appears to be expensive and impractical compared to other methods of physical separation (Shantha, 1987). Removal of aflatoxins in aqueous solutions through binding with adsorbent materials like activated charcoal (Decker, 1980) and clays (Masimanco et al., 1973) has been reported.

Biological methods of detoxification include the use of microorganisms to inactivate aflatoxins. Microorganisms including yeasts, fungi, and bacteria have been identified for their ability to modify or inactivate aflatoxins. Ciegler et al. (1966) reported the use of *Flavobacterium aurantiacum* (NRRL B-184) to significantly remove aflatoxin from liquid medium without producing toxic by-products. To structurally degrade and/or inactivate aflatoxins, many chemicals have tested positive, including acids, bases, aldehydes, sodium hypochlorite (NaOCl), bisulfite, oxidizing agents, and various gases including ammonia (Goldblatt and Dollear, 1979; Anderson, 1983). Toxicity of mycotoxins can be strongly influenced by dietary nutritional components such as protein, fat, vitamins, and trace elements. The use of chemisorbents to tightly bind and immobilize mycotoxins in the gastrointestinal tracts of animals is a new approach to detoxifying mycotoxins.

IV. SUMMARY

Toxic fungal metabolites, known as mycotoxins, have chemically diverse structures and toxicological properties, which induce a variety of toxic effects in humans and animals on ingestion. The mycotoxin-producing fungi invade foods during production, harvesting, storage, and processing. Factors influencing mycotoxin production by fungi include substrate, moisture, temperature, pH, other environmental factors, and associated growth of other fungi. The three major genera of mycotoxin-producing fungi are *Aspergillus, Penicillium*, and *Fusarium*. Many agricultural products have revealed potential hazards of mycotoxin contamination. Crops grown during warm and moist weather in the tropical and subtropical countries are more prone to mycotoxin contamination than those grown in temperate zones. More than 100 fungal species have been shown to produce mycotoxins associated with human and animal diseases throughout the world. The toxicity of mycotoxins to animals ranges from acute death to chronic disease and interference with reproductive efficiency.

Contamination of foods by mycotoxins causes economic losses, involving direct crop and livestock losses through reduced health and production efficiency. Regardless of efforts to control the occurrence of mycotoxins in foods, they do occur, and therefore detoxification/decontamination of mycotoxins are carried out through physical, chemical, and biological methods.

REFERENCES

Allcroft, R., and Carnaghan, R. B. A. (1962). Groundnut *Aspergillus flavus* toxin (aflatoxin) in animal. *Vet. Record 74*: 863.

Allcroft, R., and Carnaghan, R. B. A. (1963). Groundnut toxicity: An examination for toxin in human food products and animal fed toxic groundnut meal. *Vet. Record 75*: 259.

Allcroft, R., and Lewis, G. (1963). Groundnut toxicity in cattle: Experimental poisoning of calves and a report on clinical effect in older cattle. *Vet. Record 75*: 487.

Alsberg, C. L., and Black, O. F. (1913). Contributions to the study of maize deterioration. *U.S. Dept. Agr. Bull. Bur. Plant Ind. 270*: 7.

Ambrose, A. M., and Deeds, F. (1964). Some toxicological and pharmacological properties of citrinin. *J. Pharmacol. Exp. Ther. 88*: 173.

Anderson, D. W. (1965). Griseofulvin, biology and clinical usefulness. *Ann. Allergy 23*: 103.

Anderson, H. W., Nehring, E. W., and Wichser, W. R. (1975). Aflatoxin contamination of corn in the field. *J. Agr. Food Chem. 23*: 775.

Anderson, R. A. (1983). Detoxification of aflatoxin contaminated corn. In *Aflatoxin and Aspergillus flavus in Corn*, Diener, U., Asquith, R., and Dickens, J., eds. Southern Coop. Series Bull. 279, Auburn University, Auburn, AL.

Anonymous, (1974). Imported figs recalled because of aflatoxin. *Food Chem. News 16*: 17.

Anslow, W. K., and Raistrick, H. (1938). Studies in the biochemistry of micro-organisms. LVII. Fumigatin (3-hydroxy-4-methoxy-2:5-toluquinone) and spinulosin (3:6-dihydroxy-4-methoxy-2:5-toluquinone), metabolic products respectively of *Aspergillus fumigatus* Fresenius and *Penicillium spinulosum* Thom. *Biochem. J. 32*: 687.

Atkinson, M. (1943). Antibacterial substances produced by some common Penicillia. *Aust. J. Expt. Biol. and Med. Sci. 21*: 15.

Bailey, L. (1953). Effects of fumagillin upon *Nosema* pigs (Zander). *Nature. 171*: 212.

Beljaars, J. C., Schumans, H. M., and Koken, P. J. (1975). Quantitative fluorodensitometric determination and survey of aflatoxins in nutmeg. *J. Assoc. Anal. Chem. 58*: 263.

Berry, C. (1988). The pathology of mycotoxins. *J. Pathol. 154*: 301.

Betina, V., Drobnica, L., Nemec, P., and Zemanova, M. (1964). The antifungal activity of the antibiotic, cyanein. *J. Antibiotics* (Tokyo) *17*: 93.

Betina, V., Nemec, P., Kovak, S., Kjaer, A., and Shapiro, R. H. (1965). The identity of cyanein and brefeldin A. *Acta. Chem. Scand. 19*: 519.

Betina, V., Fuska, J., Kjaer, A., Kutkova, M., Nemec, P., and Shapiro, R. H. (1966). Production of cyanein by *Penicillium simplicissimum. J. Antibiotics* (Tokyo) *19*: 115.

Biollaz, M., Buchi, G., and Milne, G. (1970). The biosynthesis of the alfatoxins. *J. Am. Chem. Soc. 92*: 1035.

Birch, A. J., and Wright, J. J. (1969). The breveanamides: A new class of fungal alkaloid. *Chem. Commun. 25*: 644.

Birch, A. J., and Wright, J. J. (1970). Studies in relation to biosynthesis XLII. The structural elucidation and some aspects of the biosynthesis of the brevianamides A and E. *Tetrahedron 26*: 2329.

Birkinshaw, J. H., Raistrick, H., and Ross, D. J. (1952). Studies in the biochemistry of microorganisms. 86. The molecular constitution of mycophenolic acid, a metabolic product of *Penicillium brevicompactum* Dierekx. Part 3. Further observations on the structural formula for mycophenolic acid. *Biochem. J. 50*: 630.

Blount, W. T. (1961). Turkey "X" disease. *Turkeys 9*: 53, 58, 61, 77.

Bracken, A., Pocker, A., and Raistrick, H. (1954). Studies in the biochemistry of microorganisms. 93. Cyclopenin, a nitrogen-containing metabolic product of *Penicillium cyclopium* Westling. *Biochem. J. 57*: 587.

Brian, P. W., Curtis, P. J., and Hemming, H. J. (1946). A substance causing abnormal development of fungal hyphae produced by *Penicillium janczewskii* Zal. I. Biological assay, production and isolation of "curling factor." *Br. Mycol. Soc. Trans. 29*: 173.

Broom, W. A., Bulbring, E., Chapman, C. J., Hampton, J. W. F., Thompson, A. M., Ungar, J., Wien, R., and Woolfe, G. (1944). The pharmacology of patulin. *Br. J. Exp. Pathol. 25*: 195.

Buchanan, J. R., Sommer, N. F., and Fortlage, R. J. (1975). *Aspergillus flavus* infection and aflatoxin production in fig fruits. *Appl. Microbiol. 30*: 238.

Buchi, G., Luk, K. C., Kobbe, B., and Townsend, J. M. (1977). Four new mycotoxins of *Aspergillus clavatus* related to tryptoquivaline. *J. Org. Chem. 42*: 244.

Buckley, S. S. (1901). Acute hemorrhagic encephalitis prevalent among horses in Maryland. *Am. Vet. Review 25*: 99.

Bullerman, L. B. (1976). Examination of swiss cheese for incidence of mycotoxin producing molds. *J. Food Sci. 41*: 26.

Bureau of Foods. (1974). Evaluation of results from FY-73 Compliance Program, Mycotoxins in Foods, U.S. Food and Drug Administration, Washington, D.C.

Burkhardt, H. J., and Forgacs, J. (1968). *o*-Methylsterigmatocystin, a new metabolite from *Aspergillus flavus*, Link Ex Fries. *Tetrahedron 24*: 217.

Burnside, J. E., Sippel, W. L., Forgacs, J., Carll, W. T., Atwood, M. B., and Doll, E. R. (1957). A disease of swine and cattle caused by eating moldy corn. II. Experimental production with pure cultures of molds. *Am. J. Vet. Res. 18*: 817.

Burton, C. L. (1970). Diseases of tropical vegetables on the Chicago market. *Trop. Agr.* (Trinidad) *47*: 303.

Burton, H. S. (1949). Antibiotics from *Penicillia*. *Br. J. Exptl. Pathol. 30*: 151.

Butler, W. H., and Barnes, J. M. (1964). Toxic effect of groundnut meal containing aflatoxin to rats and guinea pigs. *Br. J. Cancer 17*: 699.

Butler, W. H., and Barnes, J. M. (1966). Carcinoma of the glandular stomach in rats given diets containing aflatoxin. *Nature 209*: 90.

Caldwell, R. W., and Tuite, J. (1970). Zearalenone production in field corn in Indiana. *Phytopathol. 60*: 1696.

Caldwell, R. W., and Tuite, J. (1974). Zearalenone in freshly harvested corn. *Phytopathol. 64*: 752.

Caldwell, R. W., Tuite, J., Stobb, M., and Baldwin, R. (1970). Zearalenone production by *Fusarium* species. *Appl. Microbiol. 20*: 31.

Carlton, W. W., and Tuite, J. (1969). Toxicosis in miniature swine induced by corn cultures of *Penicillium viridicatum. Toxicol. Appl. Pharmacol. 14*: 636.

Carlton, W. W., and Tuite, J. (1970). Mycotoxicosis induced in guinea pigs and rats by corn cultures of *Penicillium viridicatum. Toxicol. Appl. Pharmacol. 16*: 345.

Carlton, W. W., Tuite, J., and Caldwell, R. W. (1972). Mycotoxicosis induced in mice by *Penicillium ochraceum. Toxicol. Appl. Pharmacol. 21*: 130.

Carnaghan, R. B. A., and Allcroft, R. (1962). Groundnut toxicity. *Vet. Record 74*: 925.

Carter, S. B., Franklin, T. J., Jones, D. F., Leonard, B. J., Mills, S. D., Turner, R. W., and Turner, W. B. (1969). Mycophenolic acid: An anti-cancer compound with unusual properties. *Nature 223*: 848.

Ceponis, M. J. (1970). Diseases of California head lettuce on the New York market during the spring and summer months. *Plant Disease Reptr. 54*: 964.

Chain, E., Florey, H. W., Jennings, M. A., and Williams, T. I. (1943). Helvolic acid, an antibiotic produced by *Aspergillus fumigatus*, mut. helvola Yuill. *Br. J. Exp. Pathol. 24*: 108.

Christensen, C. M., Mirocha, C. J., and Meronuck, R. A. (1977). *Molds, mycotoxins, and mycotoxicoses*. Ag. Exp. Stn. Miscellaneous Report 142. University of Minnesota, St. Paul, MI.

Ciegler, A., and Kurtzman, C. P. (1970). Penicillic acid production by blue-eye fungi on various agricultural commodities. *Appl. Microbiol. 20*: 761.

Ciegler, A., Lillehoj, E. B., Peterson, R. E., and Hall, H. H. (1966). Microbial detoxification of aflatoxin. *Appl. Microbiol. 14*: 934.

Ciegler, A., Beckwith, A. C., and Jackson, L. K. (1976). Teratogenecity of patulin and patulin adducts formed with cysteine. *Appl. Environ. Microbiol. 31*: 644.

Cole, R. J., and Cox, R. H. (1981). (Eds.) *Handbook of toxic fungal metabolites*. Academic Press, Inc., New York.

Cole, R. J., and Kirksey, J. W. (1970). Dihydro-o-methylsterigmatocystin, a new metabolite from *Aspergillus flavus. Tetrahedron Lett. 35*: 3109.

Cole, R. J., and Kirksey, J. W. (1973). The mycotoxin verruculogen: A 6-0-methylindole. *J. Agr. Food Chem. 21*: 927.

Cole, R. J., Kirksey, J. W., Moore, J. H., Blankenship, B. R., Diener, U. L., and Davis, N. D. (1972). Tremorgenic toxin from *Penicillium verruculosum. Appl. Microbiol. 24*: 248.

Cole, R. J., Csinos, A. S., Blankenship, P. D., Sanders, T. H., Gaines, T. P., Davidson, J. I. (1985). Evaluation of soil calcium as methods of prevention of preharvest aflatoxin contamination of peanuts. *Proc. Am. Peanut Res. Educ. Soc. 17*: 71.

Cunningham, K. G., and Freeman, G. G. (1953). The isolation and some chemical properties of viridicatin, a metabolic product of *Penicillum viridicatum* Westling. *Biochem. J. 53*: 328.

Cysewski, S. J . (1978). The effects of tremorgenic mycotoxins in laboratory animals. In *Mycotoxic Fungi, Mycotoxins, Mycotoxicoses*, Vol. 2. T. D. Wyllie and L. G. Morehouse, eds. Marcel Dekker, New York, pp. 472.

Decker, W. J. (1980). Activated charcoal absorbs alflatoxin B1. *Vet. Human Toxicol. 22*: 388.

Demeke, T., Kidane, Y., and Wuhib, E. (1979). Ergotism: A report on an epidemic. *Ethiop. Med. J. 17*: 107.

Dickens, F., and Jones, H. E. H. (1961). Carcinogenic activity of a series of reactive lactones and related substances. *Br. J. Cancer 15*: 85.

Dickens, F., Jones, H. E. H., and Waynforth, H. B. (1966). Oral, subcutaneous, and intratracheal administration of carcinogenic lactones and related substances: The intratracheal administration of cigarette tar in the rat. *Br. J. Cancer 20*: 134.

Diener, U. L. (1960). The mycoflora of stored peanuts. *J. Alabama Acad. Sci. 30*: 5.

Diener, U. L., ed. (1990). *Mycotoxicology Newsletter*, Vol. 1, Auburn University, Auburn, AL.

Diener, U. L., Hesseltine, C. W., Ayres, J. C., Carlton, W. W., Cole, R. J., Goldblatt, L. A., Hamilton, P. B., Hsieh, D. P. H., Marth, E. H ., Mirocha, C. J., Pier, A. C., Sinnhuber, R. O., and Wallin, J. R. (1979). *Aflatoxins and other mycotoxins: An agricultural perspective*. Cast Task Force Report No. 80. Council for Agricultural Science and Technology, Ames, IA.

Elsworthy, G. C., Holker, J. S. E., McKeown, J. M., Robinson, J. B., and Mulheirn, L. J. (1970). The biosynthesis of the aflatoxins. *Chem. Commun. 26*: 1069.

Englebrecht, J. C., and Altenkirk, B. (1972). Comparison of some biological effects of sterigmatocystin and aflatoxin analogues on primary cell cultures. *JNCI 48*: 1647.

Evans, M. A., Wilson, B. J., and Harbison, R. D. (1975). Toxicity and mutagenic effects of rubratoxin B. *Pharmacologists 17*: 399.

Feuell, A. J. (1977). Aflatoxin in groundnuts. IV. Problems of detoxification. *Trop. Sci. 8*: 61.

Field, J. B., Filler, D. A., Bascoy, L. T., Costa, F., and Boryczka, A. (1956). Antibiotics as sources of anticarcinogens. *Fed. Proc. 15*: 250.

Forgacs, J. and Carll, W. T. (1962). Mycotoxicosis. *Adv. Vet. Sci. 7*: 274.

Forgacs, J., Carll, W. T., Herring, A. S., and Mahlandt. (1954). A toxic *Aspergillus clavatus* isolated from feed pellets. *Am. J. Hyg. 60*: 15.

Forgacs, J., Koch, H., Carll, W. T., and White-Stevens, R. H. (1958). Additional studies on the relationship of mycotoxicoses to the poultry hemorrhagic syndrome. *Am. J. Vet. Res. 19*: 744.

Gaumann, E., and Von Arx, A. (1947). Antibiotica als pflanzliche plasmagifte. II. Ber. Schweiz. *Botan. Ges. 57*: 174.

Gause, E. M., Buck, M. A., and Douglas, M. G. (1981). Binding of citreoviridin to the beta subunit of yeast F-ATPase. *J. Biol. Chem. 256*: 557.

Glinsukon, T., Yuan, S. S., Wightman, R., Kitaura, Y., Buchi, G., Shank, R. C., Wogan, G. N., and Christensen, C. M. (1974). Isolation and purification of cytochalasin E and two tremorgens from *Aspergillus clavatus. Plant Foods Man. 1*: 113.

Goldblatt, L. A., and Dollear, F. G. (1977). Detoxification of contaminated crops. In *Mycotoxins in Human and Animal Health*, J. V. Rodricks, C. W. Hesseltine, and M. A. Mehlman, eds. Pathotox Publishers, Inc., Park Forest South, IL.

Goldblatt, L. A., and Dollear, F. G. (1979). Modifying mycotoxin contamination in feeds—use of mold inhibitors, ammoniation, roasting. In *Interactions of Mycotoxins in Animal Production*. National Academy of Sciences, Washington, DC.

Groger, D. (1972). Ergot. In *Microbial Toxins*, VIII. Kadis, S., Ciegler, A., and Ajl, S. J., eds. Academic Press, New York.

Hamasaki, T., and Hatsuda, Y. (1977). Sterigmatocystin and related compounds. In *Mycotoxins in Human and Animal Health*, J. V. Rodricks, C. W. Hesseltine, and M. Mehlman, eds. Pathotox Publishers, Inc., Park Forest South, IL.

Harri, E., Loeffler, W., Sigg, H. P., Stahelin, H., and Tamm, C. (1963). Über die Isolierung neuer Stoffwechselprodukte aus *Penicillium brefeldianum* Dodge. *Helv. Chim. Acta 46*: 1235.

Harris, C. M., Porter, F. M., and Harvey, J. M. (1967). Freight shipment of California strawberries in mechanically refrigerated cars, test shipments. 1967. *U.S. Dept. of Agr., ARS 51.*

Harwig, J., Chen, Y. K., Kennedy, B. P. C., and Scott, P. M. (1973). Occurrence of patulin and patulin-producing strains of *Penicillium expansum* in natural rots of apple in Canada. *Can. Inst. Food Sci. Technol. J. 6*: 22.

Hatsuda, Y., Hamasaki, T., Ishida, M., Matsui, K., and Hara, S. (1972). Dihydrosterigmatocystin and dihydrodemethylsterigmatocystin, new metabolites from *Aspergillus versicolor. Agr. Biol. Chem. 36*: 521.

Hesseltine, C. W. (1976). Mycotoxins other than aflatoxins. In *Proc. 3rd Int. Biodegradation Symp*, J. M. Sharpley and A. M. Kaplan, eds. Applied Science Publishers Ltd., London.

Hirata, Y. (1947). On the products of mould. I. Poisonous substance from moldy rice (Part I) extraction. *J. Jpn. Chem. Soc. 68*: 63.

Holker, J. S. E., and Kagal, S. A. (1968). 5-Methoxysterigmatocystin, metabolite from a mutant strain of *Aspergillus versicolor. Chem. Commun. 24*: 1574.

Holker, J. S. E., and Mulheirn, L. J. (1968). The biosynthesis of sterigmatocystin. *Chem. Commun. 24*: 1576.

Holker, J. S. E., and Underwood, J. G. (1964). A synthesis of cyclopentenocoumarin structurally related to aflatoxin B. *Chem. Ind.* 1865.

Holzapfel, C. W. (1968). The isolation and structure of cyclopiazonic acid, a toxic metabolite of *Penicillium cyclopium* westling. *Tetrahedron 24*: 2101.

Hood, R. D., Innes, J. E., and Hayes, A. W. (1973). Effects of rubratoxin B on prenatal development in mice. *Bull. Env. Contam. Toxicol. 10*: 200.

Hou, C. T., Ciegler, A., and Hesseltine, C. W. (1971a). Tremorgenic toxins from Penicillia. III. Tremortin production by *Penicillium* species on various agricultural commodities. *Appl. Microbiol. 21*: 1101.

Hou, C. T., Ciegler, A., and Hesseltine, C. W. (1971b). Tremorgenic toxins from penicillia. II. A new tremorgenic toxins, tremortin B, from *Penicillium palitans. Can. J. Microbiol. 17*: 599.

Hsieh, D. P. H., Lin, M. T., and Yao, R. C. (1973). Conversion of sterigmatocystin to aflatoxin B1. *Biochem. Biophys. Res. Commun. 52*: 992.

Jacobson, W. L., and Wiseman, H. G. (1974). The transmission of aflatoxin B_1 into eggs. *Poultry Sci. 53*: 1743.

Jelinek, C. F. (1987). *Distribution of Mycotoxin—An Analysis of Worldwide Commodities Data Including Data from FAO/WHO/UNEP Food Contamination Monitoring Programme*. Joint FAO/WHO/UNEP second Intl. Conf. on mycotoxins, Bangkok, Thailand.

Joffe, A. Z. (1971). Alimentary toxic aleukia. In *Microbial Toxins*, Vol. 7: *Algal and Fungal Toxins*, Kadis, S., Ciegler, A., and Ajl, S. J., eds. Academic Press, New York.

Kallet, A., Sousa, C., and Spangler, W. (1988). Mushroom (*Amanita phalloides*) toxicity in dogs. *Calif. Vet.* (Jan./Feb.): 9.

Kaplan, M. A., Hooper, I. R., and Heinemann, B. (1954). Antibiotic producing properties of *Aspergillus terreus. Antibiot. Chemotherapy 4*: 746.

Katznelson, H., and Jamieson, C. A. (1952). Control of Nosema disease of honeybees with fumagillin. *Science 115*: 70.

King, B. (1979). Outbreaks of ergotism in Wollo, Ethiopia. *Lancet 1*: 1411.

Knight, A. P. (1981). Mycotoxicoses of food animals. *Compend. Cont. Educa. Pract. Vet. 3*: S112.

Kraybill, H. F., and Shimkin, M. B. (1964). Carcinogenesis related to foods contaminated by processing and fungal metabolites. *Adv. Cancer Res. 8*: 191.

Krishnamachari, K. A. V. R., and Bhat, R. V. (1976). Poisoning of ergoty bajra (pearl millet) in man. *Indian J. Med. Res. 64*: 1624.

Krogh, P. (1969). The pathology of mycotoxicoses. *J. Stored Prod. Res. 5*: 259.

Krogh, P., Hald, B., and Pedersen, J. (1973). Occurrence of ochratoxin A and citrinin in cereals associated with mycotoxic porcine nephropathy. *Acta. Path. Microbiol. Scand. B. 81*: 689.

Kuiper-Goodman, T., Scott, P. M., and Watanabe, H. (1987). Risk assessment of the mycotoxin, zearalenone. *Reg. Toxicol. Pharmacol.* 7: 253.

Lafont, P., Siriwardana, M. G., Combemale, I., and Lafont, J. (1979). Mycophenolic acid in marketed cheese. *Food Cosmet. Toxicol. 17*: 147.

Lancaster, M. C. (1968). Comparative aspects of aflatoxin induced hepatic tumors. *Cancer Res. 28*: 2288.

LaPrade, J. C., and Manwiller, A. (1977). Relation of insect damage, vector, and hybrid reaction to aflatoxin B1 recovery from field corn. *Phytopathol. 67*: 544.

Lasztity, R., and Woller, L. (1975). Effects of zearalenone and some derivatives on animals fed on contaminated fodder. *Acta Alimentaria 4*: 189.

Lorenz, K. (1979). Ergot on cereal grains. *CRC Crit. Rev. Food Sci. Nutr. 11*: 311.

Marasas, W. F. O., and Nelson, P. E. (1987). *Mycotoxicology*. Pennsylvania State University Press, University Park, PA.

Marth, E. H., and Doyle, M. P. (1979). Update on molds: Degradation aflatoxin. *Food Technol. 33*: 81.

Masimanco, N., Remacle, J., Ramaut, J. (1973). Elimination of aflatoxin B_1 by absorbent clays in contaminated substrates. *Ann. de Nutr. et Alimen. 23*: 137.

Mayer, C. F. (1953). Endemic panmyelotoxicosis in the Russian grain belt. Part I. The clinical aspects of alimentary toxic aleukia (ATA). A comprehensive review. *Military Surgeon 113*: 173.

Mayer, V. W., and Legator, M. S. (1969). Production of petite mutan of *Saccharomyces cerevisiae* by patulin. *J. Agr. Food Chem. 17*: 454.

McGowan, J. C. (1946). A substance causing abnormal development of fungal hyphae produced by *Penicillium janczewskii* Zal. II. Preliminary notes on the chemical and physical properties of "curling factor." *Brit. Mycol. Soc. Trans. 29*: 188.

McCowen, M. C., Callender, M. E., and Lawlis, J. F., Jr. (1951). Fumagillin (H-3), a new antibiotic with amebicidal properties. *Science 113*: 202.

Mirocha, C. J., Christensen, C. M., and Nelson, G. H. (1967). Estrogenic metabolite produced by *Fusarium gramainearum* in stored corn. *Appl. Microbiol. 15*: 497.

Mirocha, C. J., Christensen, C. M., and Nelson, G. H. (1969). Biosynthesis of the fungal estrogen F-2 and a naturally occurring derivative (F-3) by *Fusarium moniliforme. Appl. Microbiol. 17*: 482.

Mislivec, P. B., and Tuite, J. (1970). Species of *Penicillium* occurring in freshly harvested and in stored dent corn kernels. *Mycologia 62*: 67.

Miyake, M., and Saito, M. (1965). Liver injury and liver tumors induced by toxins of *Penicillium islandicum* growing on yellowed rice. In *Mycotoxins in foodstuffs*, G. N. Wogan, ed. M.I.T. Press, Cambridge, MA.

Morehouse, L. G. (1985). Mycotoxins of veterinary importance in the United States. In *Trichothecenes and Other Mycotoxins*, J. Lacey, ed. Proc. of Intl. Mycotoxin Symp., Sydney, Australia, John Wiley & Sons, New York.

Morton, H. E., Kocholaty, W., Junowicz-Kocholaty, R., and Kelner, A. (1945). Toxicity and antibiotic activity of kojic acid produced by *Aspergillus luteovirescens. J. Bacteriol. 50*: 579.

Nesbitt, B. F., O'Kelly, J., Sargeant, K., and Sheridan, A. (1962). Toxic metabolites of *Aspergillus flavus. Nature 195*: 1062.

Nesheim, S. (1969). Isolation and purification of ochratoxins A and B and preparation of their methyl and ethyl esters. *J. AOAC 52*: 975.

Nishiyama, M., and Kuga, T. (1989). Central effects of the neorotropic mycotoxin fumitremorgin A in the rabbit. (I). Effects on the spinal cord. *Jap. J. Pharmacol. 50*: 167.

Northolt, M. D., van Egmond, H. P., Soentoro, P., and Deijll, E. (1980). Fungal growth and presence of sterigmatocystin in hard cheese. *J. Assoc. Off. Anal. Chem. 63*: 115.

Okuda, S., Iwasaki, N., Tsuda, K., Sano, Y., Hata, T., Uda-Gawa, S., Nakayama, Y., and Yamaguchi, H. (1964). Helvolic acid. *Chem. Pharm. Bull. 12*: 121.

Paget, G. E., and Walpole, A. I. (1958). Some cytological effects of griseofulvin. *Nature 182*: 1320.

Pathak, M. A., Daniels, F., Jr., and Fitzpatrick, T. B. (1962). The presently known distribution of furocoumarins (psoralens) in plants. *J. Invest. Dermatol. 39*: 225.

Pathre, S. V., Mirocha, C. J., Christensen, C. M., and Behrens, J. (1976). Monoacetoxysirpenol, a new mycotoxin produced by *Fusarium roseum* Gibbosum. *J. Agr. Food Chem. 24*: 97.

Peace, D. M., Harwig, J. (1982). Screening for ergot particles in grain products by light microscopy. *Can. Inst. Food Sci. Technol. J. 15*: 147.

Percival, J. C. (1959). Photosensitivity diseases in New Zealand. XVII. The association of *Sporidesmium bakeri* with facial eczema. *NZ J. Agr. Res. 2*: 1040.

Pettersson, G. (1963). Toluquinones from *Aspergillus fumigatus. Acta Chem. Scand. 17*: 1771.

Pham Van Chuong, P., Bouchet, J. C., Schneider, C. R. L., and Fromageot, P. (1974). Magnetic circular dichroism of quinones and hydroxyquinones. Two related carcinogenic compounds, luteoskyrin, rugulosin and their complexes with nucleic acids. *J. Chim. Phys. Physiochim. Biol. 71*: 401.

Phillips, D. J., Uota, M., Monticelli, D., and Curtis, C. (1976). Colonization of almond by *Aspergillus flavus. J. Am. Soc. Hort. Sci. 101*: 19.

Pokrovsky, V. I., and Tutelyan, V. A. (1982). Ergotism: A companion of natural disaster. *Ter. Ark.*: 108.

Pollock, A. V. (1947). Production of citrinin by five species of *Penicillium. Nature 160*: 331.

Purchase, I. F. H., and Pretorious, M. E. (1973). Sterigmatocystin in coffee beans. *J. Assoc. Off. Anal. Chem. 56*: 225.

Purchase, I. F. H., and Van Der Watt, J. J. (1968). Carcinogenicity of sterigmatocystin. *Food Cosmet. Toxicol. 6*: 555.

Purchase, I. F. H., and Van Der Watt, J. J. (1970). Carcinogenicity of sterigmatocystin. *Food Cosmet. Toxicol. 8*: 289.

Ramsey, G. B. (1938). Fruit and vegetable diseases on the Chicago market in 1937. *Plant Disease Reptr. Suppl. 106*: 62.

Raynor, E. T., Koltun, S. P., and Dollear, F. G. (1977). Solvent extraction of aflatoxins from contaminated agricultural products. *J. Am. Oil Chem. Soc. 54*: 242A.

Rhodes, A. (1963). Griseofulvin: production and biosynthesis. Progr. *Ind. Microbiol. 4*: 165.

Robbers, J. E., Marcello, M. J., Carlton, W. W., and Tuite, J. F. (1973). The isolation and identification of brevianamide A from corn cultures of *Penicillium viridicatum* (Abstract). *Lloydia 36*: 440.

Robbers, J. E., Strauss, J. W., and Tuite, J. (1975). The isolation of brevianamide A from *Penicillium ochraceum. Lloydia 38*: 355.

Rodricks, J. V. (1969). Fungal metabolites which contain substituted 7,8-dihydrofuro-(2,3-b)furan (DHFF) and 2,3,7,8-tetrahydrofuro (2,3-b), furans (THFF). *J. Agr. Food Chem. 17*: 457.

Rodricks, J. V., Lustig, E., Campbell, A. D., and Stoloff, L. (1968a). Aspertoxin, a hydroxy derivative of o-methylsterigmatocystin from aflatoxin-producing cultures of *Aspergillus* flavus. *Tetrahedron Lett. 25*: 2975.

Rodricks, J. V., Henery-Logan, K. R., Campbell, A. D., Stoloff, L., and Verett, M. J. (1968b). Isolation of a new toxin from cultures of *Aspergillus flavus. Nature 217*: 668.

Saito, M. (1959). Liver cirrhosis induced by metabolites of *Penicillium islandicum. Acta Pathol.* (Japan) *9*: 785.

Saito, M., Enomoto, M., and Tatsuno, T. (1971). Yellow rice toxins. Luteoskyrin and related compounds, chlorine-containing compounds and citrinin. In *Microbial Toxins*, Vol. VI. *Fungal Toxins*, A. Ciegler, S. Kadis, and S. J. Ajl, eds. Academic Press, New York.

Sargeant, K., Sheridan, A., O'Kelly, J., and Carnaghan, R. B. A. (1961). Toxicity associated with certain samples of groundnuts. *Nature 192*: 1096.

Scheel, L. D., Perone, V. B., Larkin, R. L., and Kupel, R. E. (1963). The isolation and characterization of two phototoxic furanocoumarins (psoralens) from diseased celery. *Biochemistry 2*: 1127.

Schindel, L. (1954). Treatment of amebiasis with fumagillin. *J. Am. Med. Assoc. 155*: 903.

Schindler, A. F., Abadie, A. N., Gecan, J. S., Mislivec, P. B., and Brickey, P. M. (1974). Mycotoxins produced by fungi associated from in shell pecans. *J. Food Sci. 29*: 213.

Schofield, F. W. (1924). Damaged sweet clover: The cause of a new disease in cattle simulating hemorrhagic septicemia and blackleg. *Am. Vet. Med. Assoc. J. 64*: 553.

Schroeder, H. W., and Hein, H. Jr. (1977). Natural occurrence of sterigmatocystin in in-shell pecans. *Can. J. Microbiol. 23*: 639.

Schuller, P. L., Ockhuizen, T., Werringloer, J., and Marquardt, P. (1967). Aflatoxin B_1 und Histamin in Wein. *Arzneimettel-Forsch. 17*: 888.

Scott, De. B. (1965). Toxigenic fungi isolated from cereal and legume products. *Mycopathol. Mycol. Appl. 25*: 213.

Scott, P. M., and Kennedy, B. P. C. (1973). Mycotoxins in stored grain, feeds, and other cereal products. In *Grain Storage: Part of a system*, R. N. Sinha and W. E. Muir, eds. Avi Publishing Co., Westport, CT.

Scott, P. M., and Sommers, E. (1968). Stability of patulin and penicillic acid in fruit juices and flour. *J. Agr. Food Chem. 16*: 483.

Scott, P. M., Miles, W. F., Toft, P., and Dube, J. G. (1972). Occurrence of patulin in apple juice. *J. Agr. Food Chem. 20*: 450.

Shank, R. C., Bhamarapravati, N., Gordon, J. E., and Wogan, G. N. (1972). Dietary aflatoxins and human liver cancer. IV. Incidence of primary liver cancer in two municipal populations of Thailand. *Food Cosmet. Toxicol. 10*: 171.

Shantha, T. (1987). Detoxification of groundnut seed and products in India. In *Summary and recommendations of the international workshop on aflatoxin contamination of groundnut*. ICRISAT Center, Hyderabad, India.

Sheehan, J. C., Lawson, W. B., and Gaul, R. J. (1958). The structure of terreic acid. *J. Am. Chem. Soc. 80*: 5536.

Shibata, S., Natori, S., and Udagana, S. (1964). *List of Fungal Products*. University of Tokyo Press, Tokyo.

Shotwell, O. L., Hesseltine, C. W., Goulden, M. L., and Vandegraft, E. E. (1970). Survey of corn for aflatoxin, zearalenone and ochratoxin. *Cereal Chem. 47*: 700.

Shotwell, O. L., Hesseltine, C. W., Vandegraft, E. E., and Goulden, M. L. (1971). Survey of corn from different regions for aflatoxin, ochratoxin and zearalenone. *Cereal Sci. Today 16*: 266.

Singh, L. B. (1960). *The Mango*. Interscience Publishers, New York.

Singh, R., and Hsieh, D. P. H. (1976). Enzymatic conversion of sterigmatocystin into aflatoxin B1 by cell-free extracts of *Aspergillus parasiticus*. *Appl. Environ. Microbiol. 31*: 743.

Singleton, V. L., Bohonos, N., and Ullstrup, A. J. (1958). Decumbin, a new compound from a species of *Penicillium*. *Nature 181*: 1072.

Smith, R. H., and McKernan, W. (1962). Hepatotoxic action of chromatographically separated fractions of *Aspergillus flavus* extracts. *Nature 195*: 1301.

Smoot, J. J. (1969). Decay of Florida citrus fruits stored in controlled atmospheres and in air. *Proc. 1st Intern. Citrus Symp., Univ. Calif.* (Riverside) *3*: 1285.

Sommer, N. F., Buchanan, J. R., and Fortlage, R. J. (1974). Production of patulin by *Penicillium expansum*. *Appl. Microbiol. 28*: 589.

Sommer, N. F., Buchanan, J. R., and Fortlage, R. J. (1976). Aflatoxin and sterigmatocystin contamination of pistachio nuts in orchards. *Appl. Environ. Microbiol. 32*: 64.

Spector, W. S. (1957). *Handbook of Toxicology*, Vol. II. Sanders, Philadelphia, PA.

Stansfeld, J. M., Francis, A. E., and Stuart-Harris, C. H. (1944). Laboratory and clinic trials of patulin. *Lancet 247*: 370.

Stern, P. (1971). Pharmacological analysis of the tremor induced by Cyclopium toxin. *Yugoslav. Physiol. Pharmacol. Acta 7*: 187.

Stob, M., Baldwin, R. S., Tuite, J., Anderson, F. N., and Gillette, K. G. (1962). Isolation of an anabolic, uterotrophic compound from corn infested with *Gibberella zeae*. *Nature 196*: 1318.

Stoloff, L. (1980). Aflatoxin M_1 in perspective. *J. Food Prot. 43*: 226.

Tatsuno, T., Sukioka, M., Sakai, Y., Suzuki, Y., and Asami, Y. (1955). The toxic substance in yellowed rice. *Pharm. Bull.* (Japan) *3*: 476.

Townsend, R. J., Moss, M. O., and Peck, H. M. (1966). Isolation and characterization of hepatatotoxins from *Penicillium rubrum. J. Pharm. Pharmacol. 18*: 471.

Tsunoda, H. (1951). Studies on a poisonous substance produced on the cereals by a *Penicillium* spp. under storage. *Jap. J. Nutr. 8*: 185.

Tuite, J., Shaner, G., Rambo, G., Foster, J., and Caldwell, R. W. (1974). The *Gibberella* ear rot epidemics of corn in Indiana in 1965 and 1972. *Cereal Sci. Today 19*: 238.

Tung, T. C., and Ling, K. H. (1968). Study on aflatoxin of foodstuffs in Taiwan. *J. Vitaminol. 14*: 48.

Ueno, Y. (1985). The toxicology of mycotoxins. *CRC Crit. Rev. Toxicol. 14*: 99.

Ueno, Y., and Ueno, I. (1972). Isolation and acute toxicity of citreoviridin, a beurotoxic mycotoxin of *Penicillium citreoviride* Biourge. *Jpn. J. Exp. Med. 42*: 91.

U.S. Department of Agriculture. (1968a). *Preventing mycotoxins in farm commodities.* Agricultural Research Service 20, Washington, D.C.

U.S. Department of Agriculture. (1968b). Guideines for mold control in high moisture corn. *Farmers Bull.*: 2238, Washington, D.C.

van Der Zidjen, A. S. M., Koelensmid, W. A. A. B., Boldingh, J., Varett, C. B., Ord, W. Q., and Philp, J. (1962). *Aspergillus flavus* and turkey "X" disease. *Nature 195*: 1060.

van Rensburg, S. J. (1977). Role of epidemiology in the elucidation of mycotoxin health risks. In *Mycotoxins in Human and Animal Health*, J. V. Rodricks, C. W. Hesseltine, and M. A. Mehlman, eds. Pathotox Publishers, Inc., Park Forest South, IL.

van Veen, A. G., Graham, D. C. W., and Steinkraus, K. H. (1967). Fermented peanut presscake. *Cereal Sci. Today 12*: 109.

Van Walbeek, W., Scott, P. M., Harwig, J., and Lawrence, J. W. (1969). *Penicillium viridicatum* Westling: a new source of ochratoxin A. *Can. J. Microbiol. 15*: 1281.

Waiss, A. C., Jr., Wiley, M., Black, D. R., and Lundin, R. E. (1968). 3-Hydroxy-6,7-dimethoxydifuroxanthone—a new metabolite from *Aspergillus flavus. Tetrahedron Lett. 28*: 3207.

Waksman, S. A., Horning, E. S., and Spencer, E. L. (1943). Two antagonistic fungi, *Aspergillus fumigatus* and *Aspergillus clavatus*, and their antibiotic substances. *J. Bacteriol. 45*: 233.

Watson, S. A., Mirocha, C. J., and Hayes, A. W. (1984). Analysis for trichothecenes in samples from Southeast Asia associated with "yellow rain." *Fund. Appl. Toxicol. 4*: 700.

Wells, J. M., and Harvey, J. M. (1970). Combination heat and 2,6-dichloro-4-nitroaniline treatments for control of *Rhizopus* and brown rot of peaches, plums, and nectarines. *Phytopathol. 60*: 116.

White, E. C. (1940). Bactericidal filtrate from a mold, culture. *Science 92*: 127.

White, E. C., and Hill, J. H. (1943). Studies on antibacterial products formed by molds. I. Aspergillic acid, a product of a strain of *Aspergillus flavus. J. Bacteriol. 45*: 433.

Wicklow, D. T., and Wilson, D. M. (1986). Germination of *Aspergillus flavus* sclerotia in a Georgia maize field. *Trans. Br. Mycol. Soc. 87*: 651.

Wilkins, W. H., and Harris, G. C. M. (1942). Investigation into the production of bacteriostatic substances by fungi. I. Preliminary examination of 100 fungal species. *Br. J. Expt. Path. 28*: 166.

Wilson, B. J. (1971). Miscellaneous Penicillium toxins. In *Microbial Toxins*, Vol. VI, A. Ciegler, R. Radis, and S. J. Ajl, eds. Academic Press, New York.

Wilson, B. J., and Holladay, J. A. (1987). Mushroom poisoning. *Compd. Cont. Educat. Pract. Vet. 9*: 791.

Wilson, B. J., and Wilson, C. H. (1962). Extraction and preliminary characterization of a hepatotoxic substance from cultures of *Penicillium rubrum*. *J. Bacteriol. 84*: 283.

Wilson, B. J., Yang, D. T. C., and Harris, T. M. (1973). Production, isolation and preliminary toxicity studies of brevianamide A from cultures of *Penicillium viridicatum*. *Appl. Microbiol. 26*: 633.

Wilson, D. M., and Nuovo, E. J. (1973). Patulin production in apples decayed in *Penicillium expansum*. *Appl. Microbiol. 26*: 124.

Wogan, G. N., and Newberne, P. M. (1967). Dose response characteristics of aflatoxin B1 carcinogenesis in the rats. *Cancer Res. 27*: 2370.

Woodward, R. B., and Singh, G. (1949). The structure of patulin. *J. Am. Chem. Soc. 71*: 758.

Woronin, M. (1981). Uber das "Taumel-getreide" in Sud-Ussurien. *Bot. Z. 49*: 81.

Wu, M. T., Ayres, J. C., and Koehler, P. E. (1974a). Production of citrinin by *Penicillium viridicatum* on country-cured ham. *Appl. Microbiol. 27*: 427.

Wu, M. T., Ayres, J. C., and Koeher, P. E. (1974b). Toxigenic aspergilli and penicillia isolated from aged cured meats. *Appl. Microbiol. 28*: 1094.

Yamazaki, M., Sasago, K., and Miyaki, K. (1974). The structure of fumitremorgin B (FTB), a tremorgenic toxin from *Aspergillus fumigatus* Fres. *Chem. Commun 30*: 408.

Yates, I. E., Cole, R. J., Giles, J. L., and Dorner, J. W. (1987). Interaction of aflatoxin B1 and cyclopiazonic acid toxicities. *Mol. Toxicol. 1*: 95.

Yokota, K., Shimada, H., Kamaguchi, A., and Sakaguchi, O. (1977). Studies on the toxin of *Aspergillus fumigatus*. Purification and some properties of hemolytic toxin (asp-hemolysin) from culture filtrates and mycelia. *Microbiol. Immunol. 21*: 11.

IV

ALLERGY

13

Food Allergies

Tracy J. Bargman,* Steve L. Taylor, and John H. Rupnow

University of Nebraska, Lincoln, Nebraska

**Present affiliation*: General Mills, Inc., Minneapolis, MN.

I. INTRODUCTION

It has been estimated that the average gastrointestinal (GI) system will handle approximately 100 tons of material during a lifetime (Johansson et al., 1984). While food is essential for life, it also represents the largest antigenic load faced by the human immune system. Therefore, the intestine has a primary role in host defense (Lessof, 1989).

The GI tract possesses an elaborate barrier system, which engages both immunological and nonimmunological mechanisms in protection against dietary allergens and other toxic agents that it may encounter (Haddad, 1982; Sampson, 1988; Lessof, 1989; Schreiber and Walker, 1989a). Among the nonimmunological factors is the endothelial lining of the intestine, which prevents invasions of large foreign molecules by acting as a mechanical barrier. Peristalsis determines the transit time and, therefore, limits the time of exposure to the antigen. Stomach acid and digestive enzymes reduce the potential antigenicity of ingesta by denaturing and degrading large macromolecules into smaller subunits. The immunological component of the barrier system is termed the gut-associated lymphoid tissue and is the largest lymphoid organ in the body. Included in this lymphoid tissue are Peyer's patches, macrophages, mast cells, plasma cells, and lymphocytes. When an antigenic molecule traverses the endothelium, this immune system responds and ultimately prevents further absorption of the antigen and clears that which has already penetrated the endothelium. Any inherent abnormality or disruption of this mucosal barrier can lead to the development of food allergy (Haddad, 1982; Schreiber and Walker, 1989a).

A. Definitions

The term food allergy has been used by consumers and some physicians to describe many types of individual adverse reactions to foods. However, in recent years it has become widely recognized that many different diseases fall into the category of adverse reactions to foods, and that true food allergy represents only one type of illness. This confusion resulted from a lack of standardization of the terminology used to describe adverse reactions to foods. In recognition of this problem, the American Academy of Allergy and Immunology (Anderson and Sogn, 1984) recommended a standard terminology, which is outlined in Table 1. The term adverse reaction refers to any abnormal response attributed to ingestion of a food or food additive. Adverse reactions are categorized as either food intolerance or food hypersensitivity (food allergy). A food intolerance is any abnormal physiological response to a food that is not immunologically mediated. Several types of food intolerances are known to occur and together constitute a majority of the adverse reactions to foods. Food hypersensitivity or true food allergy refers to those reactions to foods or food

Table 1 Standard Terminology Used to Describe Adverse Reactions to Foods

Food hypersensitivity (immunological)	Food intolerances (nonimmunological)
IgE-mediated	Food toxicity
Non IgE-mediated	Anaphylactoid reactions
	Idiosyncratic reactions
	Metabolic reactions
	Pharmacological reactions

components (usually proteins) that are immunologically mediated. Food hypersensitivity reactions can be further categorized as Types I–IV, but are more frequently referred to as IgE (immunoglobulin E)-mediated or non–IgE-mediated food allergy.

IgE-mediated food allergy is also called immediate food hypersensitivity because the symptoms usually develop within minutes following ingestion. Non–IgE-mediated reactions are more difficult to identify because the symptoms may not appear for hours or even days following ingestion (Altman, 1981). For this reason, these reactions are often described as delayed food hypersensitivity.

1. *Food Intolerances*

The symptoms of food hypersensitivity and some food intolerances are remarkably similar. This makes diagnosis challenging and reaffirms the need to understand the mechanisms responsible for the different reactions. While the bulk of this review will focus on food allergies, this section will be devoted to a brief description of some food intolerances (Anderson, 1984).

"Food toxicity" or food-poisoning reactions are caused by the direct action of a food or food additive without the involvement of the immune system. The substance responsible for the reaction may be a natural or intentionally added component of the food or may be a contaminant, such as spoilage organisms or parasites. This type of reaction may involve the ingestion or release of chemical mediators, such as histamine, that are normally associated with an immune response. A classical example of food toxicity is histamine intoxication, caused occasionally by ingestion of some cheeses or spoiled fish (Taylor et al., 1989b).

"Anaphylactoid reactions" are anaphylaxislike reactions that result from the nonimmune release of histamine from lymphoid cells by substance contained within the food. Histamine poisoning is sometimes referred to as an anaphylactoid reaction because of the associated anaphylactic symptoms. "Strawberry allergy" is also considered an anaphylactoid reaction (Panush and Webster, 1985).

"Idiosyncratic reaction" is used to describe a variety of food intolerance thought to have nonimmunological but unknown mechanisms. Sulfite-induced asthma is a well-established idiosyncratic reaction (Taylor and Nordlee, 1988).

Many other food additives (e.g., tartrazine and other azo-dyes, BHA, BHT, and monosodium glutamate, among others) have also been implicated in adverse reactions. While these reactions are loosely classified as idiosyncratic, poor documentation and lack of controlled studies have cast doubt on the role of food additives in many of the cases reported (Simon, 1986).

"Metabolic food reactions" result from the effect of a food or food component on the metabolism of the individual. A classic example of a metabolic disorder is lactose intolerance. This disease afflicts a large portion of the Hispanic, black, and Southeast Asian populations as well as older Caucasians and is the result of a deficiency in intestinal lactase, the enzyme necessary for proper metabolism of the milk sugar lactose (Anonymous, 1988). Phenylketonuria, another metabolic disorder, results from the inability to properly metabolize phenylalanine. Individuals with this disease frequently follow a restricted diet and must avoid foods that contain aspartame, the artificial sweetener in which phenylalanine is a major constituent (Koch and Wenz, 1984). Celiac disease, also known as gluten-sensitive enteropathy, may also be a metabolic disorder. Yet, the mechanism of this illness is uncertain; it may even be a form of true food allergy (Mike and Asquith, 1987).

"Pharmacological reaction" is used to describe a response to a food or food additive that produces a druglike effect. These reactions are frequently included under the food idiosyncrasy category. Biogenic amines, such as tyramine and phenylethylamine, have been reported to produce pharmacological reactions (headaches) in predisposed subjects (Finn, 1987). These compounds are found in many common foods such as chocolate, wine, and some cheeses.

Most food allergies and food intolerances are the result of some genetic predisposition and are termed primary food sensitivities. However, adverse reactions to foods may develop following an initial event such as illness or drug therapy. These reactions are referred to as secondary food sensitivities (Institute of Food Technologists' Expert Panel, 1985).

B. Prevalence

The public perceives food allergies as a major health concern. A recent survey of women's opinions found that about 30% of the women polled felt that someone in their family had a food sensitivity or food allergy (Sloan and Powers, 1986). While the actual prevalence of food allergy is unknown, it is probably much less than is perceived (Anderson and Sogn, 1984). In a study of 480 infants conducted by Bock (1987), 28% were suspected by their parents as having adverse reactions to foods. Yet, reactions were confirmed by food challenges in just 8% of the 480 children. Similar results were reported in a study of Finnish children conducted by Kajosaari (1982). While the actual incidence of immune-mediated reactions was not determined in either study, true food allergies probably accounted for fewer reactions than other non–immune-mediated food intolerances (Anderson, 1984; Anderson and Sogn, 1984).

An accurate estimate of the actual prevalence of food allergy is difficult due to the lack of standardization of diagnostic criteria, materials, methods, and terminology. While reports in the literature vary widely, food allergy probably afflicts less than 1% of the adult population (Golbert, 1972; Breneman, 1979; Bahna and Gandhi, 1983; Anderson and Sogn, 1984). Prevalence among the pediatric population is greater and is believed to be closer to 2–3% (Sampson and Valentine, 1990). Food allergy is more common among children with certain diseases, such as atopic dermatitis, and appears more frequently in male versus female children (Burks et al., 1988; Schreiber and Walker, 1989a).

Several factors contribute to the predisposition and development of food allergy. Included among these factors are genetics, age, gastrointestinal absorption, and food or allergen exposure (Sampson, 1988; Van Hooser and Crawford, 1989). A study conducted by Atkins suggests a strong link for genetics in food allergy in which 80% of the individuals with food allergy had a family history of atopy (allergic disease) (Atkins et al., 1985a). The occurrence of food allergy decreases with age and is probably associated with an increase in gut maturity (Schreiber and Walker, 1989b; Van Hooser and Crawford, 1989). Children often outgrow allergies to egg and milk (Bock, 1982; Ford and Taylor, 1982). However, allergies to other foods such as peanut and fish usually last through adulthood (Bock, 1982; Ford and Taylor, 1982). Frequency of exposure to the allergen and age at the time of initial exposure will also influence the development or incidence of allergy. The most common food allergens among infants and children are milk, eggs, soy, peanuts, wheat, and tree nuts, most of which are introduced into the diet early in life (Sloan and Powers, 1986; Burks et al., 1988; Van Hooser and Crawford, 1989). Alternatively, peanuts, tree nuts, soy, fish, and crustacea and molluscs appear to be the most common allergens in adults (Taylor, 1985; Burks et al., 1988). The occurrence of allergy to specific foods will also vary between societies and ethnic populations, based on differences in eating habits (Van Hooser and Crawford, 1989). For example, fish allergies are more common in Sweden, while the Japanese experience a higher incidence of rice and soybean allergy.

The overall occurrence of atopic disease has been reported to be on the rise, apparently as a result of increased exposure to allergens due to changes in living habits (Wuthrich, 1990). However, the importance of food allergy in this increase is not clear (Wuthrich, 1990).

II. MECHANISMS

The pathogenesis of food hypersensitivity is complex and not completely understood. Many factors contribute to the development of the disease. The intestinal mucosal barrier, through regulation of uptake of dietary antigen, appears to play an important role (Schreiber and Walker, 1989a). Antigenic peptides that traverse the mucosal barrier elicit an immune response leading to the secretion of antigen specific antibodies (secretory IgA) that complex with the antigen, thus preventing further absorption. Circulating antibodies then clear the antigens that have penetrated the mucosa (Sampson, 1988). In animals, the production of IgA is accompanied by a suppression of IgG and IgE antibodies, which reduces the likelihood of an immune reaction in organs outside the GI tract (Wershil and Walker, 1988). This phenomenon of reduced immunological reaction is termed "oral tolerance," and any abnormality or disruption of this elaborate barrier system (e.g., immaturity of the gut during infancy, intestinal infection) could lead to the development of hypersensitivity (Walker, 1987; Wershil and Walker, 1988).

Genetic predisposition is also an important factor in the development of food allergy. Children born to atopic parents have a greater chance of developing allergic disease including food allergies. Also, it appears that some individuals may inherit a suppressor cell defect which leads to the inability to suppress the IgE response (Geha, 1984). The role of IgE and other immune mechanisms in food allergy will be described further in the following section.

A. Immunological Mechanisms

1. *Gell and Coombs Classification*

Gell et al. (1975) categorized hypersensitivity reactions into four types, based on differences in the immune response. While our understanding of the disease has grown, this classification system remains useful. These four types of reactions are not considered mutually exclusive, and more than one may be involved in a given allergic reaction. In addition, it is not clear whether all types of reactions are involved in the pathogenesis of food allergy (Wright and Robertson, 1987).

Type I sensitivity is also referred to as anaphylactic or IgE-mediated hypersensitivity. These reactions are produced by the release of pharmacologically active substances from certain effector cells caused by interaction of allergen with specific IgE that is bound to the surface of these cells. These reactions are commonly implicated in food allergy and will be discussed in more detail later.

Type II or cytotoxic hypersensitivity occurs when antibodies (usually of the M or G isotype) attach to an antigen on a cell surface and cause cellular destruction through one of many pathways. To date there is no evidence to suggest that Type II reactions are important in food allergy.

Type III reactions result from tissue deposition of immune complexes (allergen or antigen with antibody), which provokes an inflammatory reaction and tissue damage. Circulating immune complexes in allergic individuals following ingestion of allergen are both qualitatively and quantitatively different than those found in nonallergic individuals (Brostoff et al., 1979; Paganelli et al., 1979). While the prevalence of type III reactions is not known, they have been shown to cause gastrointestinal abnormalities in animals and might to be linked to delayed enteropathy in humans (Stern and Walker, 1985; Wright and Robertson, 1987).

Type IV or delayed hypersensitivity is a cellular response to antigen as opposed to the humoral responses of Types I–III. The antigen or allergen binds to a sensitized T lymphocyte, which induces lymphokine synthesis, lymphocyte proliferation, and generation of cytotoxic T cells. These reactions are slow to develop and usually begin 18–24 hours after exposure to the allergen and dissipate in 72–96 hours. The importance of type IV hypersensitivity in food allergy is not clear primarily due to the lack of adequate immunological methods for investigation (Wright and Robertson, 1987). Nevertheless, these reactions are thought to be important in cows' milk allergy and may contribute to the pathogenesis of celiac disease (Brandtzaeg et al., 1987; Wright and Robertson, 1987; Scott and Brandtzaeg, 1989).

2. IgE-Mediated Reactions

IgE-mediated hypersensitivity in food allergy is well documented (Gell et al., 1975; Altman, 1981; Sampson, 1988). These reactions begin with the formation of allergen-specific IgE by plasma cells upon initial exposure. This IgE becomes bound to tissue mast cells and circulating basophils via Fc_{ε} receptors on the cells' surface. These "sensitized" cells will degranulate and release a number of mediators when the surface IgE becomes cross-linked by allergen upon subsequent exposure (Fig. 1). While more than 20 substances have been identified as mediators of allergic disease released by mast cell and basophil mediators, histamine is responsible for most of the immediate effects that usually appear minutes after exposure (Altman, 1981). Some mediators are preformed in the mast cells and basophils, and others are synthesized following activation of arachidonic acid metabolism in the cell membranes (Altman, 1981; Scott and Brandtzaeg, 1989). These newly formed mediators, usually prostaglandins and leukotrienes, cause the slower-developing reactions (ca. 4–6 h after exposure) observed in some food allergies (Altman, 1981).

Mediator release from other cells (monocytes, eosinophils, platelets, and lymphocytes) bearing low affinity Fc_{ε} receptors, as opposed to the high affinity receptors on mast cells and basophils, are also thought to contribute to these

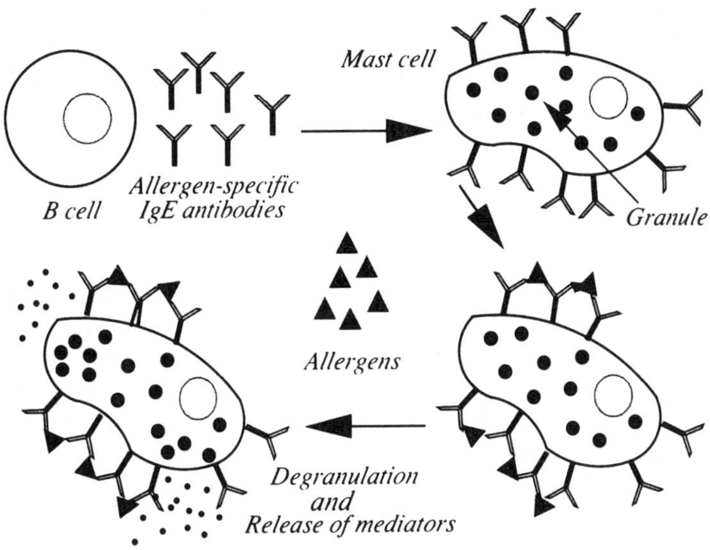

Figure 1 Mechanisms of an IgE-mediated food hypersensitivity reaction. Allergen-specific IgE antibodies are produced by plasma cells in response to exposure to allergen and attach to the surface of mast cells. Upon subsequent exposure, these surface-bound antibodies may be cross-linked by the allergen, which leads to degranulation of the mast cell and release of mediators. (From Taylor et al., 1989b.)

late-phase reactions (Turner, 1989; Sampson et al., 1989). Sampson et al. (1989) suggested that the histamine releasing factors (HRF), released by allergen stimulated monocytes, could be important in the prolonged reactivity of some organs (e.g., the skin in atopic dermatitis or the lung in asthma).

B. Other Mechanisms

It has been suggested that a subclass of the immunoglobulin G isotype, IgG_4, plays a role in some food allergies. Elevated IgG_4 levels were found in individuals with atopic eczema to egg and/or milk (Merrett et al., 1984; Shakib et al., 1984). It was also discovered that these immunoglobulins could bind to basophils. However, the allergen could not mediate release of histamine from IgG_4-bound basophils (Van Toorenenbergen and Aalberse, 1982). Other studies have demonstrated the presence of food-specific IgG_4 in the sera of nonallergic individuals making the clinical significance of this antibody questionable (Merrett et al., 1983; Layton and Stanworth, 1984).

In a recent report, Shakib suggested that IgE-mediated hypersensitivity could be an autoimmune disease, mediated in part by anti-IgE autoantibodies (Shakib, 1990). This speculation is based on the detection of human autoantibodies to IgE in atopic individuals. While no studies have been performed to confirm or disprove such a hypothesis, the presence of these autoantibodies does provide ground for further investigation.

Recently, recognition has been given to the phenomenon of exercise-induced anaphylaxis, which may be a form of IgE-mediated food allergy. While the mechanism is not known, in some individuals, allergylike symptoms appear only when exercise precedes or follows ingestion of certain foods. Cases involving celery, wheat, shellfish, and peaches have been reported (Maulitz et al., 1979; Buchbinder et al., 1983; Kidd et al., 1983; Kushimoto and Aoki, 1985). Most cases of exercise-induced anaphylaxis, however, do not involve food ingestion.

III. SYMPTOMS

Many clinical manifestations of food allergy have been reported, and these vary in location, severity and time of onset (Sampson et al., 1987; Schreiber and Walker, 1989a). Symptoms vary between individuals and can range from slight urticaria (hives) to fatal anaphylaxis and may appear within minutes of ingestion. The age of the individual, the quality and quantity of food ingested, and the extent of associated medical problems can also influence the expression of symptoms (Sampson et al., 1987). The primary organs affected include the skin, the gastrointestinal tract (GI), and the respiratory system. Effects on the central nervous system are less well documented but are thought to be manifested as migraine headaches (Monro, 1987). The most common target organs and clinical symptoms are given in Table 2 (Sampson et al., 1987; Taylor, 1987; Sampson and Valentine, 1990). In addition to these frequently observed symptoms, food allergy has been suggested as a causative factor in a variety of other disorders or disease states. Lagrue et al. (1989) suggested a

Table 2 Common Symptoms of Food Allergy

Oropharyngeal/Gastrointestinal symptoms	
	Nausea and abdominal pain
	Vomiting
	Diarrhea
	Colic
Cutaneous symptoms	
	Urticaria
	Angioedema
	Atopic dermatitis
Respiratory symptoms	
	Rhinitis
	Laryngeal edema
	Asthma
Neurological symptoms	
	Migraine headaches
Systemic symptoms	
	Anaphylaxis

role for food allergy in some individuals with idiopathic nephrotic syndrome. Matteo and Sarles (1990) attributed several cases of acute pancreatitis to food allergy. Certain behavioral disorders, such as hyperactivity, have also been associated with food allergy. However, conclusive immunological data for any of these relationships is lacking (Pearson and Rix, 1985).

The oropharynx and GI system are generally the first sites of exposure to the allergen and, therefore, may be the first to exhibit symptoms. Symptoms that are limited to the mouth and throat are referred to as "oral allergy syndrome" and are most frequently reported following ingestion of fresh fruits and vegetables (Sampson and Valentine, 1990). Passage of the allergen into the stomach and intestines may induce the acute onset of abdominal cramping, nausea, vomiting, and diarrhea. While these manifestations usually appear minutes to hours following ingestion, some delayed symptoms may also occur. Slow onset reactions are often a result of intestinal mucosal damage caused by continual exposure to the allergen (Walker-Smith, 1989; Schreiber and Walker, 1989a). A classic example is the protein-losing enteropathy (usually accompanied by diarrhea and anemia) in some infants with cows' milk allergy (Walker-Smith, 1989).

Cutaneous symptoms in food allergy are common and are evidenced by acute urticaria, angioedema, or both (Hannuksela, 1983; Sampson et al., 1987). The extent to which food can induce atopic dermatitis (AD) is controversial (Goldenhersh, 1990). However, children with AD have a high frequency of positive skin reactions to foods and high levels of circulating food-specific IgE

(Barnetson, 1980; Turner et al., 1980). Studies by Sampson and coworkers have demonstrated a pathogenic role for food hypersensitivity in 60% of patients with AD (Sampson, 1983; Sampson and McCaskill, 1985).

Respiratory manifestations, such as rhinitis, wheezing, and/or sneezing, frequently result from inhalant allergy but have also been attributed (although less frequently) to food allergy, especially in infants (Atkins et al., 1985b; Novembre et al., 1988). Such symptoms are almost always accompanied by other clinical manifestations such as skin disorders and gastrointestinal distress (Novembre et al., 1988). Although less frequent, asthma has also been associated with food hypersensitivity (Onorato et al., 1986; Novembre et al., 1988). In many asthmatics, symptoms appear only when ingestion of the food allergen is coupled with a cofactor (e.g., exercise, certain drugs, cross-reactive foods) that increases bronchial reactivity (Novembre et al., 1988).

The role of food allergy in neurological symptoms is somewhat controversial. As stated previously, the immunological basis of behavior disorders, depression, and other similar symptoms has not been established (Pearson and Rix, 1985; Sampson et al., 1987). However, the role of food allergy in migraine headaches has been demonstrated using blinded food challenges and by measuring levels of food-specific IgE (Mansfield et al., 1985; Monro, 1987).

The most severe reaction associated with food allergies is anaphylactic shock, a systemic reaction involving multiple target organs that can be fatal if not treated immediately (Sampson et al., 1987). While drugs and venoms are the most frequent precipitators of anaphylaxis, reports of anaphylaxis attributed to food are increasing (Toft Sorensen et al., 1989). Yunginger et al. (1988) identified seven cases of fatal food-induced anaphylaxis over a 16-month period. The causative agents were identified as peanut in four cases, and pecan, crab, and fish, each in one case. Other common foods including milk, eggs, other legumes, tree nuts and seafoods, and some fruits and vegetables have also been implicated in anaphylactic reactions (Taylor, 1985; Evans et al., 1988; Miell et al., 1988; Boyd, 1989).

While a multitude of symptoms have been attributed to food allergy reactions, the most common clinical manifestations involve the skin, the GI tract, or the respiratory system. Just as individuals differ in their sensitivity to specific foods, symptoms also vary between individuals. Because these symptoms are so diverse, and are also some of the same symptoms associated with many nonallergic diseases, it is impossible to make an accurate diagnosis based on symptomology alone (Taylor, 1985).

IV. DIAGNOSIS

Accurate diagnosis of food allergies is critical to proper treatment. A number of in vivo and in vitro diagnostic tests have been developed and are currently being practiced (Sampson et al., 1987; Bock et al., 1988; Pearson, 1989; VanArsdel and Larson, 1989; Sampson and Valentine, 1990). Due to their inherent variabilities and subjectivity, it is often recommended that several methods be employed in the diagnosis and confirmation of a food allergy (Sampson et al., 1987; VanArsdel and Larson, 1989). The choice of testing materials and protocol used are based on an extensive history provided by the patient (Sampson et al., 1987; Bock et al., 1988; Pearson, 1989; Sampson and Valentine, 1990).

A. In Vivo Tests

1. Skin Tests

Skin testing has been used for over a century to identify allergens and is the basis upon which the specialty of allergy was developed (VanArsdel and Larson, 1989). Skin tests are used primarily to detect immediate (IgE-mediated) hypersensitivity to foods (Sampson et al., 1987; Bock et al., 1988; VanArsdel and Larson, 1989; Sampson and Valentine, 1990). Alternatively, the patch test is a specialized version of the skin test that is useful in diagnosis of some delayed-type hypersensitivities, especially contact dermatitis (VanArsdel and Larson, 1989). The patch test is conducted by exposing the skin to a pad containing the suspected sensitizing agent with periodic examination of the exposure site. The pad is typically left in place for 48–72 hours, unless a reaction develops sooner (VanArsdel and Larson, 1989).

Skin testing for the diagnosis of immediate-type hypersensitivity may be accomplished either by intradermal injection or an epidermal puncture with an extract made from a suspected allergenic food. Epidermal skin tests (skin prick tests) are often preferred because they incur a lower risk of severe adverse reaction and have been proven to be more reliable than intradermal injection (Bock et al., 1988; VanArsdel and Larson, 1989). While positive skin prick tests may occur in individuals with no clinical symptoms of IgE-mediated food allergy (false-positive responses), the reverse (false-negative results) occur less frequently. Thus, skin prick tests (SPT) are most useful in the negative prediction or exclusion of IgE-mediated hypersensitivity (Sampson et al., 1987; Bock et al., 1988; VanArsdel and Larson, 1989).

Skin-testing extracts are manufactured and sold commercially for a number of foods. Because extract preparation conditions vary between manufacturers, the quality and the allergen content of these extracts is variable. However, efforts are underway to standardize skin testing extracts, and some reference extracts currently exist for some inhalant allergens (Taylor, 1985; Eichler et al., 1988; Reed et al., 1989).

2. Provocation Tests

Provocation tests are designed to provoke the patient's main symptoms by limited exposure to the suspected food or substance in a controlled setting (VanArsdel and Larson, 1989). Such tests (or food challenges) may be conducted in an open manner in which no attempt is made to disguise the food or as blinded challenges in which the foods are encapsulated or otherwise disguised prior to administration (Sampson et al., 1987; Bock et al., 1988; VanArsdel and Larson, 1989). Blinded challenges may be conducted in a single-blinded manner, where only the patient is unaware of the contents of the capsule. Alternatively, in double-blinded circumstances, both patient and the administrator are unaware of the contents. When proper placebos are used, the double-blind food challenge (DBFC) is considered the most definitive procedure for diagnosis of food allergy (Sampson et al., 1987; Bock et al., 1988). However, DBFCs are not recommended for the evaluation of patients with a history of severe food allergy reactions (Taylor, 1985).

Food challenges are often used to confirm the results of other diagnostic procedures and may also be used to detect nonimmunologically mediated food intolerances (VanArsdel and Larson, 1989). Perhaps the most valuable aspect of food challenges is in the refutation of patient accounts of adverse reactions to foods. This aspect is supported by a study by Bock (1986) where less than 40% of children with reported food sensitivities had reproducible reactions when subjected to double-blinded food challenges.

In addition to food challenges, several unproven provocation testing schemes have been developed (VanArsdel and Larson, 1989). Sublingual administration of drops of food extracts, the measurement of certain physiological parameters (e.g., the pulse or muscular strength) following oral provocation with a food, and other similar practices have no proven immunological basis.

3. *Elimination Diets*

Elimination or exclusion diets operate on much the same principle but are much more tedious than food challenges (Sampson et al., 1987). Elimination diets involve removing the suspected food(s) from the diet until symptoms subside. Foods are then reintroduced, one by one, until the symptoms reappear. Generally, elimination of only a few foods from the diet is sufficient for diagnosis. However, in some cases severely restricted or elemental diets must be employed. Such diets can be expensive and difficult to sustain for long periods of time (Sampson et al., 1987; Pearson, 1989).

B. In Vitro Tests

1. *Serological Tests*

Many methods have been developed for the in vitro measurement of total and allergen-specific IgE. The PRIST (paper radioimmunosorbent test) is a method used to measure total serum IgE (Kjellman et al., 1976). However, because the level of serum IgE in allergic individuals often falls within the normal range, the PRIST and other methods of measuring total serum IgE have value mainly in research applications (Klink et al., 1990).

The RAST (radioallergosorbent test) is the most widely used technique used to measure allergen specific serum IgE. The efficacy of the RAST in predicting food allergy is similar to that of SPT, however, the RAST is more time consuming and expensive. Therefore, the RAST is used primarily in research settings and when skin testing would be unreliable (e.g., patients with generalized dermatitis) or is considered too risky (Sampson et al., 1987; VanArsdel and Larson, 1989). Newer methods, similar to the RAST, that employ different solid phases and/or labels have been reported and promise to be less expensive and time consuming than the RAST (Gleich et al., 1980; Matejtschuk et al., 1988; VanArsdel and Larson, 1989).

Other serological methods that have been described include measurement of IgG_4 and of circulating immune complexes or of serum complement (Merrett et al., 1983; Council on Scientific Affairs, 1987; Bell and Potter, 1988). However, none of these methods is considered reliable for the diagnosis of food allergy (VanArsdel and Larson, 1989).

2. Cellular Tests

The Histamine Release Test (HRT) measures antigen-induced histamine release from blood basophils. Although the procedure has been used primarily as a research tool, it may have future potential as a diagnostic tool (VanArsdel and Larson, 1989). Lymphocyte transformation measurement has found use primarily in research and in the diagnosis of drug allergy. Other diagnostic tests that have been reported include lymphocyte subset measurements and cytotoxicity testing; neither have been proven to be reliable (Sampson et al., 1987; VanArsdel and Larson, 1989).

3. Other Tests

Measurement of changes in intestinal permeability upon exposure to a food allergen has been suggested as a method of detecting food allergy. An in vivo study of intestinal permeability is accomplished by measuring the percentage of an orally administered solution of macromolecules that is excreted in the urine. This technique has been used predominantly in the evaluation of malabsorptive syndromes such as celiac disease and has not gained wide acceptance for food allergy diagnosis (Pastorello et al., 1989).

V. TREATMENT AND PREVENTION

Treatment and/or prevention of food allergy has been the subject of much study and controversy. A number of methods for treatment have been suggested and, for the most part, can be classified as: (1) dietary avoidance, (2) pharmacology (drug treatment), or (3) hyposensitization. Controlling exposure to common food allergens during infancy has been studied as a means of preventing food allergy.

A. Dietary Avoidance

Once an offending food or foods have been identified, dietary avoidance is the most effective therapy known (Taylor et al., 1987a; Norman and Van Metre, Jr., 1990; Sampson and Valentine, 1990). While in theory avoidance should be easy, actual practice of dietary avoidance can be quite difficult. In constructing a safe avoidance diet, consideration must be given to: the degree of tolerance by the individual, the possibility of cross-reacting foods, and adequate nutrition (Institute of Food Technologists' Expert Panel, 1985; Taylor, 1987; Zanussi and Pastorello, 1987).

In IgE-mediated reactions, the degree of tolerance to the offending food(s) can be extremely low, where even trace quantities of the food can cause a reaction (Institute of Food Technologists' Expert Panel, 1985; Taylor, 1987; Taylor et al., 1987a; Bernhisel-Broadbent et al., 1989). In cases where small quantities of the allergen do not cause a reaction, caution must be taken as such exposure could heighten the individual's sensitivity (Taylor et al., 1987a). The degree of tolerance or sensitivity to specific foods affects the degree of selectivity allowed in the formulation of a diet (Taylor et al., 1987a). Because the allergenic component of most foods is proteinaceous (Taylor, 1985), foods in which the protein component has been removed or those foods that have been severely processed may not be allergenic. For example, soybean oil, peanut oil, and sunflower oil failed to elicit reactions in soy-, peanut-, or sunflower-allergic individuals during double-blind food challenges (Taylor et al., 1981; Bush et al., 1985; Halsey et al., 1986). In addition, hydrolysis of proteins may eliminate their allergenicity, such as hydrolyzed casein, which is used in infant formulas for milk-allergic children (Knights, 1985; Zanussi and Pastorello, 1987; Guesry et al., 1989; Zeiger et al., 1989). It should be noted, however, that some casein hydrolysates have been shown to contain large molecular weight proteins and, therefore, may still elicit reactions in some individuals (Seban et al., 1977; Zanussi and Pastorello, 1987). Processing of food can also complicate avoidance through the use of allergenic foods as additives or processing aids. Allergic individuals must become well versed in food composition and scrutinize labels carefully to avoid inadvertent exposure (Taylor et al., 1987a).

Cross-reactivity of certain foods is also a concern and has been demonstrated among species of crustacea (e.g., shrimp and crab), legumes (e.g., soybean and peanut) and between different cereals (Goodwin and Rawcliffe, 1983; Waring et al., 1983; Waring et al., 1985; Bernhisel-Broadbent et al., 1989). Different species of avian eggs as well as cows' and goats' milk are known to cross-react in most individuals allergic to those foods (Langeland, 1982; Juntenen and Ali-Yrkko, 1983). In addition, cross-reactivity has been described between some tree pollens and certain fruits, vegetables, and nuts (Errikson et al., 1982; Moller, 1989; Zanussi and Pastorello, 1987). Because cross-reactivity varies between allergic individuals, adequate testing is necessary prior to dietary restriction (Taylor et al., 1987a; Taylor et al., 1989a).

Substitution of the offending foods with others is often important in maintaining adequate nutrition. This generally is not a problem unless many foods are implicated or when the food is a main dietary staple, as is true of infants with milk allergy (Taylor, 1987). Casein hydrolysates or soy protein are the most common substitutes for milk protein in hypoallergenic infant formulas. As previously described, some casein hydrolysates may still cause reactions (Taylor, 1987; Seban et al., 1977). In addition, nearly 20–25% of milk-allergic infants develop sensitivities to soybean if soy formulas are used as milk substitutes (Ament and Rubin, 1980; Bahna and Gandhi, 1983).

A major complicating factor in the effective use of dietary avoidance in the treatment of food allergies is self-diagnosis and use of unsupervised, uncontrolled diets (Bock et al., 1978). This is frequently practiced by parents whose offspring suffer from atopic dermatitis (Webber et al., 1989). Webber et al. (1989) studied 73 children suffering from atopic dermatitis and found that 71% had significant alterations made to their diets prior to seeking a physician's advice. The dietary alterations were questionable and in some cases dangerous (e.g., substituting unpasteurized goats' milk for cows' milk). Although less than 10% reported benefit from these unsupervised diets, most continued for fear of exacerbating the child's symptoms by reintroducing the food(s). Therefore, while dietary manipulation can be an effective method for treatment for food allergy, proper diagnosis and professional assistance in dietary planning are necessary.

B. Pharmacotherapy

The symptoms of allergic reactions are often treated with drugs such as antihistamines or, in cases of severe, life-threatening anaphylaxis, with epinephrine (Taylor, 1987; Youlten, 1987). Patients with a history of life-threatening reactions to certain foods are often advised to carry antihistamines and/or an epinephrine-filled syringe at all times (Atkins, 1983). Prophylactic uses of a number of drugs have recently been reviewed by Podleski (1989). Sodium cromoglycate (SCG), corticosteroids, ketotifen, aspirin, and other nonsteroidal, noninflammatory drugs, among others, may have potential in reducing or eliminating the allergic response in certain individuals. However, use of these drugs is still in experimental stages, and their effectiveness and mechanism of action have not been elucidated (Podleski, 1989).

C. Hyposensitization

Allergen immunotherapy or hyposensitization was first initiated with environmental allergens in the early 1900s (World Health Organization, 1989). This procedure involved the administration of gradually increasing amounts of a food or food extract (either orally or parenterally) to an allergic individual. While evidence now indicates that this procedure can be effective in treating many IgE-mediated disorders (e.g., inhalant and drug allergies), it has not been proven effective in treating those attributed to foodstuffs (Zanussi and Pastorello, 1987; Norman and Van Metre, Jr., 1990). Even when the food sensitivity appears to be related to an inhalant exposure to food-related dusts in occupational settings, hyposensitization is not effective (Moller, 1989). Moller (1989) attempted pollen immunotherapy on 72 children with cross-reactive pollen and food sensitivity. While the hay fever (pollen allergy) symptoms improved, no significant decrease in food sensitivity was found.

Unfortunately, hyposensitization for food allergy appears logical and simple and is often practiced by nonmedical practitioners (Zanussi and Pastorello, 1987). Such practices are sometimes dangerous as any dose may produce a life-threatening response in highly sensitive individuals (Zanussi and Pastorello, 1987; World Health Organization, 1989). Alternatively, enzyme potentiation, a form of hyposensitization that utilizes a β-glucuronidase–allergen mixture, has been reported to be relatively safe and effective in controlling food allergy in some patients (McEwen, 1987). Reportedly, β-glucuronidase can alter and enhance the sensitizing or desensitizing effect of an antigen. This form of immunotherapy has not been widely accepted.

D. Prevention During Infancy

A child may become exposed to food allergens via several routes. In addition to the obvious route of oral ingestion of a food, an infant may be exposed prenatally by placental transfer or through contact with allergens in breast milk that arise from the mother's diet (Kjellman, 1982; Hamburger et al., 1983; Van Aspergen et al., 1983; Bjorksten and Kjellman, 1987; Soothill, 1987; Kjellman, 1988; Zeiger, 1988). This knowledge is the basis for some avoidance methods that have become popular. Pregnant women carrying high allergy-risk babies (biparental history of atopy) have been told to avoid cows' milk, eggs, and other allergenic foods during pregnancy and lactation (Kjellman, 1982; Kjellman, 1988). While such a practice may seem logical, recent studies by Zeiger et al. (1989) and Kjellman (1988) have demonstrated that dietary avoidance of allergenic foods during pregnancy had no effect on the incidence of food allergy in infants. In addition, restrictive diets during pregnancy could compromise the well-being of both mother and fetus (Zeiger et al., 1989).

Exclusive breast feeding to at least 6 months of age has also been advocated (Kjellman, 1988; Hansson et al., 1984). This is based on the knowledge that breast milk provides antibodies (mainly secretory IgA) and gut maturation factors that are important in the protection and maturation of the infant gastrointestinal tract (Bjorksten and Kjellman, 1987). However, breast milk may also contain allergenic material from the maternal diet (Kjellman et al., 1989; Zeiger et al., 1989). While the efficacy of breast feeding as a preventative measure remains controversial, recent studies have found that maternal avoidance of commonly allergenic foods (cows' milk, egg, and peanut) during exclusive breast feeding did reduce the incidence of allergic symptoms in infants up to the first year of life (Kjellman, 1988; Hattevig et al., 1989; Zeiger et al., 1989).

Delayed introduction of allergenic foods may also reduce sensitization during infancy (Zeiger et al., 1989). While some authors have suggested that dietary avoidance during infancy merely postpones sensitization (Saarinen and Kajosaari, 1980), Zeiger et al. (1989) reported that less than 4% of infants studied became sensitized to food when exposed to solid foods between 12 and 24 months of age. This decreased incidence may be partially attributed to the reduced tendency toward sensitization with age (Bock, 1982).

VI. NATURE OF FOOD ALLERGENS

In addition to genetic, environmental, and relative exposure factors, the molecular nature of the allergen has a large influence on the development of food allergies (Aas, 1978; Taylor et al., 1987b; Van Hooser and Crawford, 1989). In IgE-mediated hypersensitivities, the allergen(s) are usually naturally occurring protein(s) in the food (Aas, 1978; Taylor et al., 1987b). In contrast, some nonproteinaceous food additives have also been reported to provoke an IgE-mediated response (Hannuksela and Haahtela, 1987). Presumably, the additive acts as a hapten and becomes allergenic by binding to a carrier protein (Hannuksela and Haahtela, 1987).

The most common food allergens tend to be regularly consumed foods with relatively high protein contents (e.g., milk, eggs, nuts, legumes, seafoods). Interestingly, some foods such as beef, pork, and chicken, that would seem to fall into this category, are rarely implicated in allergic disease (Aas, 1978; Taylor et al., 1987b). While mechanisms other than IgE-mediation are probably involved in allergic reactions to foods (see Sec. II), the study of most known food allergens has been based on their ability to produce an IgE response. Therefore, the following discussion will focus on the structural and immunological characteristics of those proteins known to be involved in IgE-mediated reactions.

It is not uncommon for multiple allergenic proteins to exist in a particular food (Taylor et al., 1987b). While one of these proteins will serve as a major allergen (one that is recognized by a majority of allergic individuals), allergen recognition patterns differ between individuals (Aas, 1978). This phenomenon of multiple allergens is not understood. It has been suggested, but not proven, that the allergenic proteins may contain identical or cross-reacting IgE binding sites (epitopes) (Taylor et al., 1987c). The factors that cause a protein to be an allergen are also unknown. The relative prevalence of a particular protein, its ability to stimulate an immune response, and its comparative stability, among other factors, may influence the potential allergenicity of a food protein (Aas, 1978; Taylor et al., 1987c).

A prerequisite for allergenic activity is the ability to stimulate an immune response. Complex proteins with numerous antigenic determinants are generally better immunogens than small proteins with few antigenic determinants (King, 1976). Yet, antigenic determinants and allergenic determinants are not necessarily identical. Therefore, an important feature is the ability of the protein to specifically induce an IgE response (Aas, 1978).

Allergens must bridge IgE molecules on the surface of a mast cell to cause degranulation and, therefore, are somewhat constrained in molecular dimensions (Aas, 1978). Bridging appears to be dependent upon the shape of the protein molecule and the availability of two or more allergenic determinants spaced at an appropriate distance for binding to the IgE on the surface of the mast cell. It is possible that the allergenic determinants involved in bridging are identical, however, there is no available evidence to make this a prerequisite (Aas, 1978). Molecular size is also important in allergenicity. Most known allergens have molecular weights between 10,000 and 70,000 daltons. While small molecules (<10,000 daltons) could act as haptens, a molecular weight of 10,000 probably represents a lower limit for an immunogenic response. The upper limit is probably a result of restricted intestinal absorption of larger molecules (Aas, 1978).

Proteins that maintain their immunogenicity through food-processing treatments and digestive mechanisms are most likely to elicit an immune response (Aas, 1978). There is variability in how different allergens are affected by common food-processing methods. For example, the coffee bean allergen is destroyed by roasting, and the allergenicity of the cocoa bean is lost during chocolate making (Fries, 1978; Lehrer et al., 1978). The apple, potato, and carrot allergens are heat labile and cannot withstand most cooking processes (Dreborg and Foucard, 1983). Although, the codfish allergen M is very resistant to heat and acid denaturation, its allergenicity can be eliminated by complete proteolysis (Aas and Elsayed, 1969; Elsayed and Aas, 1971). Condensation, evaporation, drying, heating, and other processes have no effect on cows' milk allergens (Taylor, 1986). In addition, the allergenicity of cows' milk may actually be enhanced by digestion. Haddad et al. (1979) found some cows' milk–allergic patients to be sensitive to proteolytic digests of β-lactoglobulin rather than to the undigested protein.

Structural differences may influence the relative stabilities of different food allergens (Aas, 1978). Allergenic determinants that are conformational (a specific three-dimensional structure formed by the folding of a protein) would seem to be more affected by denaturation with heat or chemical treatment than sequential epitopes (composed of a number of linear sequence of amino acids) (Baldo and Donovan, 1988). Yet, the amino acid sequence and three-dimensional structure of most food allergens is unknown, so this hypothesis cannot be proven.

Despite the many proteins from a variety of foods that are reportedly involved in allergic reactions, only a few have been isolated and/or characterized (Table 3). The properties of those that have been studied will be briefly described below.

A. Milk Allergens

The total protein content of cows' milk is approximately 3–3.5% (Swaisgood, 1985). The two major protein fractions of cows' milk, casein and whey, are comprised of several different proteins. The caseins account for 80% of the total milk protein and exist with calcium phosphate in a highly hydrated spherical complex called a micelle. The α_s-caseins are the most prevalent, followed by β, K, and γ-caseins. The molecular weights range from 11,557 daltons for γ_3-casein A to 25,228 daltons for α_{s2}-casein A (Swaisgood, 1985). The principal whey proteins are β-lactoglobulin with a molecular weight of 18,263 daltons and α-lactalbumin with a molecular weight of 14,147 daltons (Swaisgood, 1985).

Goldman et al. (1963b) evaluated the allergenicity of preparations of casein, β-lactoglobulin, α-lactalbumin, and bovine serum albumin by skin testing normal and allergic children. Positive skin tests were found to one or more of these milk protein preparations in 50 of 85 children with allergies to cows' milk, 21 of 31 children with allergies to substances other than milk, and 6 of 102 normal children. The positive skin tests in subjects without a current history of milk allergy may be a result of previous cows' milk allergy that had been outgrown. Of the 50 allergic children with positive skin tests, 34 were to casein, 22 to α-lactalbumin, 20 to β-lactoglobulin, and 21 to serum albumin (Goldman et al., 1963b). Oral challenges of 45 of these patients, using the purified protein preparations, resulted in reactions to β-lactoglobulin in 66% of the patients, to casein in 57%, and to α-lactalbumin and serum albumin in 54% (Goldman et al., 1963a). A comparative study of results of oral challenges by several investigators revealed that sensitivity to β-lactoglobulin was

Table 3 Purified Food Allergens

Source	Allergen	Molecular weight (daltons)	Comments
Milk	β-Lactoglobulin	18,263	Whey protein
	α,β,K,Y-caseins	11,557–25,228	Exist together as a Protein micelle
	α-Lactalbumin	14,174	Whey protein
Egg White	Ovomucoid (*Gal d* I)	31,500	Very heat stable
	Ovalbumin (*Gal d* II)	44,500	Major egg protein
	Conalbumin (*Gal d* III, Antigen-22)	76,000	Complexes with metal ions
Codfish	M (*Gad c* I, parvalbumin)	12,328	113 amino acids, 1 glucose
Shrimp	Antigen I	20,500	189 amino acids, 0.5% CHO*
	Antigen II	38,300	341 amino acids, 4% CHO
Soybean	Kunitz trypsin inhibitor	20,500	Probably not a major allergen
Peanut	Peanut I	—	8.7% CHO, 20,000 and 30,000 MW subunits
	Concanavlin A–reactive protein	65,000	Glycoprotein
Green Pea	Albumin (?)	1800	30% CHO
Rice	Globulin	16,000	Fairly heat stable

CHO = carbohydrate.

the most common and occurred in 82% of the patients followed by casein in 43%, α-lactalbumin in 41%, bovine immunoglobulins in 27%, and bovine albumins in 18% (Lebenthal, 1965). Another study reported that reactivity toward cows' milk proteins was β-lactoglobulin > α-lactalbumin > caseins > serum albumin using the RAST (Baldo, 1984). In addition, IgE antibodies to some minor milk proteins (e.g., lactoferrin, lactoperoxidase, alkaline phosphatase, and catalase) were identified in some individuals allergic to cows' milk (Baldo, 1984).

In conclusion, multiple allergens exist in cows' milk and some individuals react to more than one of the allergens. The major proteins are also the major allergens. While much is known about the structural properties of these proteins, the characteristics that contribute to their allergenicity remain unknown.

B. Egg Allergens

Eggs can by physically divided into the yolk and the white. The yolk contains over 50% lipid on a solids basis. A number of proteins are also present in the yolk including: (1) several forms of the lipoproteins (lipovitellin and lipovitellinin), (2) the water-soluble livetens, and (3) phosvitin, a phosphoprotein (Powrie and Nakai, 1985). While a majority of the allergenic activity is found in the egg white, some yolk proteins will also bind to serum IgE from egg-allergic individuals (Anet et al., 1985).

The egg white is composed almost entirely of proteins, several of which have been well characterized (Powrie and Nakai, 1985). Ovalbumin, conalbumin (ovotransferrin), and ovomucoid (a trypsin inhibitor) account for over 75% of egg white protein. G_1 and G_2 globulins, ovomucin, lysozyme, ovoinhibitor, and a number of trace proteins constitute the remainder of egg white protein (Powrie and Nakai, 1985).

Bleumink and Young examined the allergenicity of both boiled and raw egg white and found that ovomucoid was responsible for the majority of the positive skin test reactions (Bleumink and Young, 1969; Bleumink and Young, 1971). Chromatographic separation of water-soluble extracts from both cooked and fresh eggs yielded fractions, identified as ovomucoid, that contained a majority of the reactive material (Bleumink and Young, 1971). A purified and electrophoretically homogeneous ovomucoid protein of approximately 31,500 molecular weight was subsequently shown to be highly reactive in skin tests of egg-allergic patients (Bleumink and Young, 1971). Later studies have shown that ovomucoid is very heat stable and the IgE-binding ability remains even after heating at 100°C for 45 minutes (Gu et al., 1986).

In an attempt to determine the number and identity of all the allergens in egg white, Langeland (1982, 1985) used crossed radioimmunoelectrophoresis (CRIE) and sera from 70 egg allergic individuals. A total of 13 IgE-binding proteins were identified, with ovalbumin, ovomucoid, and an unidentified protein called antigen-22 as the major allergens. Antigen-22 was subsequently purified and identified as ovotransferrin, also known as conalbumin (Langeland and Harbitz, 1983). Other studies using CRIE or RAST with purified egg white proteins have also demonstrated that ovalbumin, ovomucoid, and conalbumin react most frequently with IgE from sera of egg allergic individuals (Hoffman, 1983; Anet et al., 1985). While differences have been observed in the CRIE patterns of different individuals, this could not be correlated with symptomology, age, total IgE level, or RAST results with egg white (Langeland, 1982; Langeland, 1983).

In summary, the most prevalent proteins in egg white (ovalbumin, ovomucoid, and conalbumin) also appear to be the major allergens. Additional allergens may also exist in the yolk fraction.

C. Legume Allergens

1. Peanuts

Peanuts (*Arachis hypogaea*) contain 25–28% protein. Peanut proteins have been broadly classified into three groups: arachin, conarachin (globulins), and albumin (Basha and Pancholy, 1981). Arachin exists in two polymeric forms, A and B. Arachin A is composed of α, β, ϒ, and δ peptide chains, while arachin B lacks the α chain (Tombs, 1965). Arachin contains a small amount of phosphorus (0.04%) and 0.5% carbohydrate (Shetty and Rao, 1974). Conarachin can be separated by ultracentrifugation into two components (Dechary et al., 1961). One of these components, termed conarachin II or β-conarachin, has a molecular weight of 295,000 and contains 0.6% carbohydrate (Dechary et al., 1961); Shetty and Rao, 1977). The albumin fraction is known to contain several biologically active proteins, many of which have been purified (Yuninger and Jones, 1985). Albumin fraction proteins include lectins, lectin-reactive glycoprotein, protease inhibitor, α-amylase inhibitor, and phospholipase-D (Yunginger and Jones, 1985). Qualitative and quantitative differences are known to occur in the storage proteins of different peanut varieties and as a function of growing area and climate (Cherry et al., 1971; Basha, 1979).

Several immunological techniques have been used to study peanut allergens. Barnett et al. (1983) identified 16 IgE-binding proteins in raw and seven in roasted peanut extracts using CRIE and sera from 10 peanut allergic individuals. Eleven IgE-binding proteins were identified by Bush et al. (1983) using CRIE. Five of these proteins were considered major allergens as they bound IgE from over half of the seven subjects used. Further studies employed immunoblotting to locate three major allergenic peptides with molecular weights of 15,000, 20,000, and 66,000, respectively (Meier-Davis et al., 1987).

Barnett et al. (1983) also examined IgE binding to specific proteins using RAST and CRIE and found that β-arachin and conarachin I exhibited IgE binding with a majority of patients. Peanut agglutinin and phospholipase D also bound to IgE but to a lesser extent (Barnett et al., 1983). In later studies the concanavalin A–reactive glycoprotein was identified as a major allergen, was purified, and shown to have a molecular weight of 65,000 and a pI of 4.6 (Kemp et al., 1985; Barnett and Howden, 1986).

Sachs et al. (1981) purified a peanut allergen from raw peanuts by ion exchange chromatography and preparative gel electrophoresis. This allergen, termed Peanut-I, produced a positive skin test in three individuals with peanut allergy. Peanut I contained 11% nitrogen and 8.7% carbohydrate. While it was homogeneous using nondenaturing polyacrylamide gel electrophoresis (PAGE) it separated into two major bands, with molecular weights of 20,000 and 30,000, and several minor bands, using sodium dodecyl sulfate-PAGE (SDS-PAGE). It was concluded that Peanut-I is an acidic glycoprotein with nonidentical subunits and may be either a fraction of arachin or conarachin (Sachs et al., 1981).

2. *Soybeans*

Soybeans (*Glycine max*) contain 32–42% protein, which can be separated into two main groups, the globulins and the whey (Catsimpoolas, 1977). The globulins are the seed storage proteins and constitute up to 80% of the total soybean protein. The globular proteins are further classified according to their sedimentation coefficients of 11S, also known as glycinin, 7S, which is primarily β-conglycinin but also contains some minor proteins (β-amylase, a lectin, and a lipoxygenase), and 2S, which contains some trypsin inhibitors and contributes only slightly to the protein content (Catsimpoolas, 1977; Murphy, 1985). Glycinin is a dodecamer of acidic and basic subunits and has a molecular weight of 309,000–363,000 daltons. Several subunits have been isolated and characterized (Murphy, 1985). β-Conglycinin is a glycoprotein of approximate molecular weight of 180,000 and is composed of three or four different polypeptide subunits, namely α, α′, β, and γ (Murphy, 1985). The soybean whey fraction has not been intensely studied but contains enzymes, protease inhibitors, and lectins (Shibasaki et al., 1980).

Although many soybean proteins have been well characterized, very few have been studied for their allergic potential. Allergenic activity has been identified in the 11S, 7S, and 2S fractions using RAST and RAST inhibition techniques with sera from five allergic individuals (Shibasaki et al., 1980). Considerable cross-reactivity was also demonstrated between these fractions (Shibasaki et al., 1980). Herian et al. (1990) identified several major IgE-binding proteins using immunoblotting and sera from seven soy-allergic individuals. This group also evaluated the IgE-binding patterns of two types of individuals, those with both soy and peanut allergy (category I) and those with soy but not peanut allergy (category II). Some similarity in binding patterns was found between category I individuals. Category II individuals reacted to a 20,000 molecular weight peptide that was not recognized by patients in category I (Herian et al., 1990). While the identity of the 20,000 dalton peptide was not known, it was not believed to be the Kunitz soybean trypsin inhibitor (SBTI) (Herian et al., 1990). However, previous studies have implicated the SBTI as a significant allergen in one patient with an occupational exposure (Moroz and Yang, 1980). Yet, RAST results in two other soybean-allergic individuals were negative, indicating that SBTI may only be a minor allergen (Moroz and Yang, 1980).

3. *Green Peas*

The allergens in green peas (*Pisum sativum*) have been characterized to some extent (Malley et al., 1975, 1976). Skin test reactivity was found in the albumin fraction and not in the legumin or vicilin fractions prepared from a crude extract of green pea (Malley et al., 1975). The allergenicity of the albumin fraction was heat stable and gave positive skin tests on individuals with allergies to soybeans and alfalfa (Malley et al., 1975). In a later study, a 1800 molecular weight pea protein containing 30% carbohydrate was purified by conventional chromatography (Malley et al., 1976). It was suggested that this substance was actually a fragment of the pea albumin and possessed some of the same allergenic epitopes (Malley et al., 1976).

D. Seafood Allergens

Allergic reactions have been reported for many species of fish and crustacea (Taylor and Bush, 1988). Only a few seafood allergens have been studied and these have been the subject of a recent review (Taylor and Bush, 1988).

1. *Fish Allergens*

Allergen M (*Gad c* I) is an allergenic protein obtained from codfish. Although it is one of the few fish allergens that has been studied, it is the most extensively characterized food allergen known (Aas, 1980). In addition, protamine sulfate, a low molecular weight protein found in the sperm of certain fishes, is believed to be responsible for some fish allergies (Caplan and Berkman, 1976).

Fish muscle contains the usual protein components: connective tissue, proteins, myofibrillar proteins, and sarcoplasmic proteins. *Gad c* I is a sarcoplasmic protein belonging to a group of proteins known as parvalbumins (Aas, 1980). It has a molecular weight of 12,328, a pI of 4.75, and is a single polypeptide consisting of 113 amino acids and one glucose molecule (Aas, 1980). The protein closely resembles the parvalbumin of other fish species, perhaps explaining some of the cross-reactivity observed between fish species (Aas, 1966). The molecule is arranged into a series of three domains that are referred to as loops AB, CD, and EF. The latter two loops can bind one calcium ion each. While two calcium ions are necessary for maintaining the tertiary structure, it is unlikely that they are part of the allergenically reactive sites (Elsayed and Apold, 1983).

Gad c I contains several IgE-binding sites (in the loops noted above) along the polypeptide chain. Using a combination of enzymatic cleavage, amino acid sequencing, and peptide synthesis, three immunoglobulin binding regions were identified which encompass amino acids 13–32, 41–64, and 88–96 (Elsayed and Apold, 1983). Region 41–64 is composed of three tetrapeptides with similar amino acid sequences (Asp-Glu-Asp-Lys and Asp-Glu-Leu-Lys) that are interspaced by six amino acids. The two tetrapeptides at each end of region 41–64 are essential for IgE binding (Elsayed and Apold, 1983). The role of the third (center) tetrapeptide is unknown. While the other two domains, 13–32 and 88–96, do not contain these tetrapeptide units, a high degree of homology exists between the overall amino acid sequences (Elsayed and Apold, 1983).

2. *Crustacean Allergens*

Two allergens have been isolated from an unspecified species of shrimp (Hoffman et al., 1981). These allergens, termed antigen I and antigen II, were isolated from raw and cooked shrimp, respectively. Antigen I has a molecular weight of 20,500, a pI of 4.75–5.0, and contains 189 amino acid residues and 0.5% carbohydrate. Its molecular weight by gel filtration chromatography was found to be 45,000, suggesting that it might exist as a dimer (Hoffman et al., 1981). Antigen I cannot be isolated from cooked shrimp and, therefore, is considered heat labile. Antigen II, isolated from cooked shrimp, has a molecular weight of 38,300, a pI of 5.4–5.8, and contains 341 amino acid residues and 4% carbohydrate. This antigen may exist in an aggregated form as the molecular weight by gel filtration was over 200,000. Antigen II is apparently heat stable as it was isolated from shrimp that had been boiled for 10–15 minutes. Antigen II bound IgE from sera from all 11 patients used, while antigen I reacted with only seven patients. Therefore, antigen II appears to be a more significant allergen (Hoffman et al., 1981).

In a study by Lehrer et al. (1985), CRIE and sera from six shrimp-allergic individuals was used to identify seven allergens, including three major allergens, in shrimp. Two of the major allergens seemed to be common crustacean allergens that could also be found in lobster, crab, and crawfish (Lehrer et al., 1985). Allergens in crawfish and lobster have also been identified by CRIE (Halmepuro et al., 1985). Later studies by Lehrer et al. (1990) found that the water that had been used to boil shrimp contained a relatively high concentration of proteins that bound IgE from sera of shrimp-sensitive individuals. Using chromatofocusing and immunoprinting, these researchers found multiple IgE binding proteins with pIs ranging from 4.0 to 6.0. By RAST inhibition these allergens were shown to be similar to those found in cooked shrimp meat extracts (Lehrer et al., 1990). Allergens have also been identified in the water used to cook crab and crayfish and are considered to be of primary concern in occupational asthma among seafood handlers (Cartier et al., 1986; Halmepuro et al., 1987).

E. Rice Allergens

Shibasaki et al. (1979) demonstrated that two of the three major rice protein fractions, glutelin and globulin, were able to bind serum IgE from five rice-allergic subjects. Three globulin fractions, separated using gel filtration chromatography, were found to bind to IgE. Heating reduced the allergenicity (determined by RAST) of these fractions (Shibasaki et al., 1979).

Matsuda et al. isolated an IgE-binding protein from rice using ion exchange and gel filtration chromatography. This protein had an approximate molecular weight of 16,000 daltons and was thought to be part of the globulin fraction. Its allergenicity was determined using an enzyme-linked immunosorbent assay (ELISA) and sera from three rice allergic individuals. Heating (at 100°C for 60 min) reduced, but did not eliminate, the IgE-binding activity (Matsuda et al., 1988).

F. Other Allergens

A water-soluble allergenic fraction was isolated from tomatoes by a series of precipitations and ion exchange chromatography (Bleumink et al., 1966, 1967). The allergenic activity was determined using skin testing of nine individuals with tomato allergy. The isolated fraction appeared to contain several glycoproteins, and the allergenic activity was stable at acid and neutral pH and relatively trypsin resistant.

Allergies have been reported to a number of cereal grains. While the etiology of celiac disease is uncertain, it is often classified as a food allergy, although it is distinct from IgE-mediated wheat allergy (Mike and Asquith, 1987). Wheat is a common allergen, especially in children, yet the major wheat allergens have not been clearly identified (Bock, 1987). Hoffman (1975) determined that wheat albumins and globulins, as opposed to gliadins and glutelins, exhibited the greatest IgE reactivity in the serum of individuals with high RAST scores to wheat. Using serum from 20 wheat-allergic children, Sutton et al. (1982) found strong IgE-binding in the globulin fraction and also in the glutelin fraction. The gliadin fraction was implicated in study of a patient with extreme hypersensitivity to wheat (Goldstein et al., 1969).

The most common allergic complaint with cereal grains is occupational asthma or baker's asthma caused by respiratory exposure to grain dusts (Baldo and Wrigley, 1984). Symptoms caused by respiratory exposure to a food allergen may not always be manifested when the allergen is ingested orally. For example, individuals with baker's asthma to wheat dust reportedly have high wheat gluten–specific IgE but rarely react when eating wheat-containing products (Aas, 1978). Occupational asthma has also been reported to many other flours or dusts from foods including soybeans, castor beans, tea, eggs, and proteolytic enzymes (Spies and Coulson, 1943; Uragoda, 1970; Bush and Cohen, 1977; Votaw and Newman, 1989).

Menendez-Arias et al. (1988) isolated the major protein in the 1.7S fraction of mustard seed. Using RAST inhibition, leukocyte histamine release and reverse-enzyme immunoassay with IgE, they determined that a majority of the allergenicity of mustard seed was located in the 1.7S fraction. Unfortunately, the mustard sensitivity of the patients used in these studies was not well documented. Characterization studies revealed that the protein contained two polypeptide chains of 39 and 88 amino acids, respectively (Menendez-Arias et al., 1988). Epitope mapping studies revealed a tyrosine-containing antigenic determinant that is reportedly important in IgE binding (Menendez-Arias et al., 1990).

Allergens from sesame seeds were also partially characterized (Malish et al., 1981). Density gradient centrifugation of sesame seed extracts revealed that the most active allergens had molecular weights in the range of 8,000–62,000 daltons. Further characterization of these proteins was not performed.

VII. SUMMARY

Less than 1% of adults are afflicted by food allergies. While this percentage is slightly higher in children, some food allergies are outgrown. The symptoms experienced as a result of an allergic reaction vary between individuals and can range from a minor skin irritation to anaphylactic shock and even death. Treatment options for food allergies are limited, with avoidance being the only proven effective therapy. While all foods have the potential to be allergenic, only a few are commonly implicated in food allergy. The etiology and pathology of the disease continues to be an area of intense study among a specialized group of medical professionals, yet, very little is known about the physicochemical and immunological properties of most of the allergens. Further research in this area could provide a greater understanding of the role foods play in provoking food allergies.

REFERENCES

Aas, K. (1966). Studies of hypersensitivity to fish. Allergological and serological differentiation between various species of fish. *Int. Arch. Allergy 30*: 257–267.

Aas, K. (1978). What makes an allergen an allergen. *Allergy 33*: 3–14.

Aas, K. (1980). The codfish allergen model. In *Advances in Allergology and Applied Immunology*, A. Oehling, I. Glaxer, E. Mathov, and C. Arbesman, eds. Pergamon Press, New York, pp. 339–344.

Aas, K., and Elsayed, S. (1969). Characterization of a major allergen (cod). Effect of enzymic hydrolysis on the allergenic activity. *J. Allergy 44*: 333–343.

Altman, L. C. (1981). Basic immune mechanisms in immediate hypersensitivity. *Med. Clin. North Am. 65*: 941–957.

Ament, M. E., and Rubin, C. E. (1980). Soy protein—another cause of the flat intestinal lesion. *Gastroenterology 62*: 399–402.

Anderson, J. A. (1984). Non-immunologically-mediated food sensitivity. *Nutr. Rev. 42*: 109–116.

Anderson, J. A., and Sogn, D. D. (1984). NIH Publication, No. 84-2442, National Institute of Allergy and Infectious Diseases and American Academy of Allergy and Immunology.

Anet, J., Back, J. F., Baker, R. S., Barnett, D., Burley, R. W., and Howden, M. E. H. (1985). Allergens in the white and yolk of hen's egg. A study of IgE binding by egg proteins. *Int. Arch. Allergy Appl. Immunol. 77*: 364–371.

Anonymous. (1988). Efficacy of exogenous lactase for lactose intolerance. *Nutr. Rev. 46*: 150–152.

Atkins, F. M. (1983). The basis of immediate hypersensitivity reactions to foods. *Nutr. Rev. 41*: 229–234.

Atkins, F. M., Steinberg, S. S., and Metcalfe, D. D. (1985a). Evaluation of immediate adverse reactions to foods in adult patients. I. Correlation of demographic, laboratory and prick skin test data with response to controlled oral food challenge. *J. Allergy Clin. Immunol. 75*: 348–355.

Atkins, F. M., Steinberg, S. S., and Metcalfe, D. D. (1985b). Evaluation of immediate adverse reactions to food in adult patients. II. A detailed analysis of reaction patterns during oral food challenge. *J. Allergy Clin. Immunol. 75*: 356–363.

Bahna, S. L., and Gandhi, M. D. (1983). Milk hypersensitivity. I. Pathogenesis and symptomology. *Ann. Allergy 50*: 218–224.

Baldo, B. A. (1984). Milk allergies. *Aust. J. Dairy Technol. 39*: 120–128.

Baldo, B. A., and Donovan, G. R. (1988). The structural basis of allergenicity: Recombinant DNA-based strategies for the study of allergens. *Allergy 43*: 81–97.

Baldo, B. A., and Wrigley, C. W. (1984). Allergies to cereals. *Adv. Cereal Sci. Technol. 6*: 289–356.

Barnetson, R. S. (1980). Hyperimmunoglobulinaemia E in atopic eczema (atopic dermatitis) is associated with "food allergy." *Acta Derm. Venereol.* (Suppl.) *92*: 94–96.

Barnett, D., and Howden, M. E. H. (1986). Partial characterization of an allergenic glycoprotein from peanut (*Arachis hypogaea* L.) *Biochim. Biophys. Acta 882*: 97–105.

Barnett, D., Baldo, B. A., and Howden, M. E. (1983). Multiplicity of allergens in peanuts. *J. Allergy Clin. Immunol. 72*: 61–68.

Basha, S. M. M. (1979). Identification of cultivar differences in seed polypeptide composition of peanuts (*Arachis hypogaea*, L.) by two dimensional polyacrylamide gel electrophoresis. *Plant Physiol. 63*: 301–306.

Basha, S. M. M., and Pancholy, S. K. (1981). Polypeptide composition of arachin and non-arachin proteins from early bunch peanut (*Arachis hypogaea* L.) seed. *Peanut Sci. 8*: 82–88.

Bell, S. J. D., and Potter, P. C. (1988). Milk whey-specific immune complexes in allergic and non-allergic subjects. *Allergy 43*: 497–503.

Bernhisel-Broadbent, J., Taylor, S. L., Sampson, H. A. (1989). Cross-allergenicity in the legume botanical family in children with food hypersensitivity. II. Laboratory correlates. *J. Allergy Clin. Immunol. 84*: 701–709.

Bjorksten, B., and Kjellman, N-I. M. (1987). Perinatal factors influencing the development of allergy. *Clin. Rev. Allergy 5*: 339–347.
Bleumink, E., and Young, E. (1969). Studies on the atopic allergen in hen's egg. I. Identification of the skin reactive fraction in egg white. *Int. Arch. Allergy Appl. Immunol. 35*: 1–19.
Bleumink, E., and Young, E. (1971). Studies on the atopic allergen in hen's egg. II. Further characterization of the skin-reactive fraction in egg-white; immunoelectrophoresis studies. *Int. Arch. Allergy Appl. Immunol. 40*: 72–80.
Bleumink, E., Berrens, L., and Young, E. (1966). Studies on the atopic allergen in ripe tomato fruits. I. Isolation and identification of the allergen. *Int. Arch. Allergy Appl. Immunol. 30*: 132–145.
Bleumink, E., Berrens, L., and Young, E. (1967). Studies on the atopic allergen in ripe tomato fruits. II. Further chemical characterization of the purified allergen. *Int. Arch. Allergy Appl. Immunol. 31*: 25–37.
Bock, S. A. (1982). The natural history of food sensitivity. *J. Allergy Clin. Immunol. 69*: 173–177.
Bock, S. A. (1986). A critical evaluation of clinical trials in adverse reactions to foods in infants and children. *J. Allergy Clin. Immunol. 78*: 165–174.
Bock, S. A. (1987). Prospective appraisal of complaints of adverse reactions to foods in children during the first 3 years of life. *Pediatr. 79*: 683–688.
Bock, S. A., Lee, W. Y., Remigio, L. K., and May, C. D. (1978). Studies of hypersensitivity reactions to foods in infants and children. *J. Allergy Clin. Immunol. 62*: 327–334.
Bock, S. A., Sampson, H. A., Atkins, F. M., Zeiger, R. S., Lehrer, S., Sachs, M., Bush, R. K., and Metcalfe, D. D. (1988). Double-blind, placebo controlled food challenge (DBPCFC) as an office procedure: A manual. *J. Allergy Clin. Immunol. 82*: 986–997.
Boyd, G. K. (1989). Fatal nut anaphylaxis in a 16-year-old male: Case report. *NER Allergy Proc. 10*: 255–257.
Brandtzaeg, P., Baklien, K., Bjerke, K., Rognum, T. O., Scott, H., and Valnes, K. (1987). Nature and properties of the human gastrointestinal immune system. In *Immunology of the Gastrointestinal Tract*, K. Miller and S. Nicklin, eds. CRC Press, Inc., Boca Raton, FL, pp. 1–85.
Breneman, J. C. (1979). Food allergy. *Contemporary Nutr. 4*(3): 1–2.
Brostoff, J., Carini, C., Wraith, D. G., Paganelli, R., and Levinsky, R. J. (1979). Immune complexes in atopy. In *The Mast Cell, Its Role in Health and Disease*, J. Pepys and A. M. Edwards, eds. Pitman Medical Pub. Co., Kent, England, pp. 380–393.
Buchbinder, E. M., Bloch, K. J., Moss, J., and Guiney, T. E. (1983). Food-dependent exercise-induced anaphylaxis. *JAMA 250*: 2973–2974.
Burks, A. W., Mallory, S. B., Williams, L. W., and Shirrell, M. A. (1988). Atopic dermatitis: Clinical relevance of food hypersensitivity reactions. *Pediatr. 113*: 447–451.
Bush, R. K., and Cohen, M. (1977). Immediate and late onset asthma from occupational exposure to soybean dust. *Clin. Allergy 7*: 369–372.
Bush, R., Voss, M., Taylor, S., Nordlee, J., Busse, W., and Yunginger, J. (1983). Detection of peanut allergens by crossed radioimmunoelectrophoresis (CRIE) (Abstract). *J. Allergy Clin. Immunol. 71*: 95.
Bush, R. K., Taylor, S. L., Nordlee, J. A., and Busse, W. W. (1985). Soybean oil is not allergenic to soybean-sensitive individuals. *J. Allergy Clin. Immunol. 76*: 242–245.
Caplan, S. N., and Berkman, E. M. (1976). Protamine sulfate and fish allergy. *New Engl. J. Med. 296*: 172.
Cartier, A., Malo, J-L., Ghezzo, H., McCants, M., and Lehrer, S. B. (1986). IgE sensitization in snow crab-processing workers. *J. Allergy Clin. Immunol. 78*: 344–348.

Catsimpoolas, N. (1977). Immunological properties of soybean proteins. In *Immunological Aspects of Food*, N. Catsimpoolas, ed. AVI Publishing, Westport, CT, pp. 37–59.
Cherry, J. P., Neucere, J. J., and Ory, R. (1971). Comparison of proteins of peanuts grown in different areas. II. Disc electrophoretic analysis of qualitative and quantitative variations. *J. Am. Peanut Res. Educ. Assoc. 3*: 63–74.
Council on Scientific Affairs (1987). In vitro testing for allergy: Report II of the Allergy Panel. *JAMA 258*: 1639–1643.
Dechary, J. M., Talluto, K. F., Evans, W. J., Carney, W. B., and Altschul, A. M. (1961). α-Conarachin. *Nature 191*: 1125–1126.
Dreborg, S., and Foucard, T. (1983). Allergy to apple, carrot and potato in children with birch pollen allergy. *Allergy 38*: 167–172.
Eichler, I., Gotz, M., Jarisch, R., Eichler, H. G., and Moss, R. (1988). Reproducibility of skin prick testing with allergen extracts from different manufacturers. *Allergy 43*: 458–463.
Elsayed, S., and Aas, K. (1971). Isolation of purified allergens (cod) by isoelectric focusing. *Int. Arch. Allergy 40*: 428–438.
Elsayed, S., and Apold, J. (1983). Immunochemical analysis of cod fish allergen M: Locations of the immunoglobulin binding sites as demonstrated by the native and synthetic peptides. *Allergy 38*: 449–459.
Errikson, N. E., Formgren, H., and Svenonius, E. (1982). Food hypersensitivity in patients with pollen allergy. *Allergy 37*: 437–443.
Evans, S., Skea, D., and Dolovich, J. (1988). Fatal reaction to peanut antigen in almond icing. *Can. Med. Assoc. J. 139*: 231–232.
Finn, R. (1987). Pharmacological actions of foods. In *Food Allergy and Intolerance*, J. Brostoff and S. J. Challacombe, eds. Bailliere Tindall, London, pp. 425–430.
Ford, R. P. K., and Taylor, B. (1982). Natural history of egg hypersensitivity. *Arch. Dis. Child. 57*: 649–652.
Fries, J. H. (1978). Chocolate: A review of published reports of allergic and other deleterious effects, real or presumed. *Ann. Allergy 41*: 195–207.
Geha, R. S. (1984). Human IgE (CME article). *J. Allergy Clin. Immunol. 74*: 109–120.
Gell, P. G. H., Coombs, R. R. A., and Lachman, D. J. (1975). *Clinical Aspects of Immunology*, 3rd ed. Lippincott, Philadelphia.
Gleich, G. J., Adolphson, C. R., and Yunginger, J. W. (1980). The mini-RAST: Comparison with other varieties of the radioallergosorbent test for the measurement of immunoglobulin E antibodies. *J. Allergy Clin. Immunol. 65*:20–28.
Golbert, T. M. (1972). Food allergy and immunologic diseases of the gastrointestinal tract. In *Allergic Diseases: Diagnosis and Management*, R. Patterson, ed. Lippincott, Philadelphia, pp. 355–379.
Goldenhersh, M. A. (1990). Atopic dermatitis and food hypersensitivity. *N. Engl. J. Med. 332*: 274–275.
Goldman, A. S., Anderson, D. W., Sellars, W. A., Saperstien, S., Kniker, W. T., and Halpern, S. R. (1963a). Milk allergy. I. Oral challenge with milk and isolated milk proteins in allergic children. *Pediatr. 32*: 425–443.
Goldman, A. S., Sellars, W. A., Halpern, S. R., Anderson, D. W., Furlow, T. E., and Johnson, C. H. (1963b). Milk allergy II. Skin testing of allergic and normal children with purified milk proteins. *Pediatr. 32*: 572–579.
Goldstein, G. B., Heiner, D. C., and Rose, B. (1969). Studies of reagins to alpha-gliadin in a patient with wheat hypersensitivity. *J. Allergy 44*: 37–50.
Goodwin, B. F. J., and Rawcliffe, P. M. (1983). Food allergies associated with cereal products. *Food Chem. 11*: 321–338.
Gu, J., Matsuda, T., and Nakamura, R. (1986). Antigenicity of ovomucoid remaining in boiled shell eggs. *J. Food Sci. 51*: 1448–1450.

Guesry, P. R., Secretin, M. C., Jost, R., Pahud, J. J., and Monti, J. C. (1989). Hypoallergenic formulas. In *Food Intolerance in Infancy: Allergology, Immunology and Gastroenterology*, R. N. Hamburger, ed. Raven Press, New York, pp. 253–265.

Haddad, Z. (1982). Clinical and immunological aspects of food hypersensitivity. *Ann. Allergy 49*: 29–34.

Haddad, Z. H., Kalra, V., and Verma, S. (1979). IgE antibodies to peptic and peptic-tryptic digests of beta-lactoglobulin: Significance in food hypersensitivity. *Ann. Allergy 42*: 368–371.

Halmepuro, L., Nuntirooj, K., Salvaggio, J. E., and Lehrer, S. (1985). Identification of crawfish and lobster allergens. *Ann. Allergy 55*: 307A.

Halmepuro, L., Salvaggio, J., and Lehrer, S. B. (1987). Studies of allergens present in crawfish and lobsters. *Int. Arch. Allergy Appl. Immunol. 84*: 165–172.

Halsey, A., Martin, M., Ruff, M., Jacobs, F., and Jacobs, R. (1986). Sunflower oil is not allergenic in sunflower seed-sensitive individuals. *J. Allergy Clin. Immunol. 78*: 408–410.

Hamburger, R. N., Heller, S., Mellon, M. H., O'Connor, R., and Zeiger, R. S. (1983). Current status of the clinical and immunological consequences of a prototype allergic disease prevention program. *Ann. Allergy 51*: 281–290.

Hannuksela, M. (1983). Food allergy and skin diseases. *Ann. Allergy 51*: 269–272.

Hannuksela, M., and Haahtela, R. (1987). Hypersensitivity reactions to food additives. *Allergy 42*: 561–575.

Hansson, L. A., Ahlstedt, S., Andersson, B., Cruz, J. R., Dahlgren, U., Falstrom, S. P., Porras, O., Eden-Svenborg, E., Soderstrom, T., and Wettergren, B. (1984). The immune response of the mammary gland and its significance for the neonate. *Ann. Allergy 53*: 567–582.

Hattevig, G., Kjellman, B. K., Sigurs, N., Bjorksten, B., and Kjellman, N.-I. M. (1989). Effect of maternal avoidance of eggs, cow's milk and fish during lactation upon allergic manifestations in infants. *Clin. Exp. Allergy 19*: 27–32.

Herian, A. M., Taylor, S. L., and Bush, R. K. (1990). Identification of soybean allergens by immunoblotting with sera from soy-allergic adults. *Int. Arch. Allergy Appl. Immunol. 92*: 193–198.

Hoffman, D. R. (1975). The specifics of human IgE antibodies combining with cereal grains. *Immunochemistry 12*: 535–538.

Hoffman, D. R. (1983). Immunochemical identification of the allergens in egg white. *J. Allergy Clin. Immunol. 71*: 481–486.

Hoffman, D. R., Day, E. D., and Miller, J. S. (1981). The major heat stable allergen of shrimp. *Ann. Allergy 47*: 17–22.

Institute of Food Technologists' Expert Panel on Food Safety and Nutrition. (1985). Food allergies and sensitivities. *Food Technol. 39*: 65–71.

Johansson, S. G. O., Dannaeus, A., and Lilja, G. (1984). The relevance of anti-food antibodies for the diagnosis of food allergy. *Ann. Allerlgy 53*: 665–672.

Juntunen, K., and Ali-Yrkko, S. (1983). Goat's milk for children allergic to cow's milk. *Kiel Milchwirt. Forschungsberg. 35*: 439–440.

Kajosaari, M. (1982). Food allergy in Finnish children aged 1 to 6 years. *Acta Paediatr. Scand. 71*: 815–819.

Kemp, A. S., Mellis, C. M., Barnett, D., Sharota, E., and Simpson, J. (1985). Skin test, RAST and clinical reactions to peanut allergens in children. *Clin. Allergy 15*: 73–78.

Kidd, J. M., Cohen, S. H., Sosman, A. J., and Fink, J. N. (1983). Food dependent exercise-induced anaphylaxis. *J. Allergy Clin. Immunol. 71*: 407–411.

King, T. P. (1976). Chemical and biological properties of some atopic allergens. *Adv. Immunol. 23*: 77–105.

Kjellman, N.-I. M. (1982). Prediction and prevention of atopic allergy. *Allergy 37*: 463–473.

Kjellman, N.-I. M. (1988). Allergy prevention: Does maternal food intake during pregnancy or lactation influence the development of atopic disease during infancy? In *Biology of Human Milk*, L. A. Hanson, ed. Raven Press, Ltd., New York, pp. 197–203.

Kjellman, N.-I. M., Johansson, S. G. O., and Roth, A. (1976). Serum IgE levels in healthy children by a sandwich technique (PRIST). *Clin. Allergy 6*: 51–59.

Kjellman, N.-I. M., Hattevig, G., Falth-Magnusson, K., and Bjorksten, B. (1989). Epidemiology of food allergy: With emphasis on the influence of maternal dietary restrictions during pregnancy and lactation on allergy in infancy. In *Food Intolerance in Infancy: Allergology, Immunology and Gastroenterology*, R. N. Hamburger, ed. Raven Press, New York, pp. 105–114.

Klink, M., Kline, M. G., Halonen, M., and Burrows, B. (1990). Problems in defining normal limits for serum IgE. *J. Allergy Clin. Immunol. 85*: 440–444.

Knights, R. J. (1985). Processing and evaluation of the antigenicity of protein hydrolysates. *Clin. Dis. Pediatr. Nutr. 4*: 105–115.

Koch, R., and Wenz, E. J. (1984). Aspartame ingestion by phenylketonuric heterozygous and homozygous individuals. In *Aspartame Physiology and Biochemistry*, L. D. Stegink and L. J. Filer, Jr., eds. Marcel Dekker, Inc., New York, pp. 593–606.

Kushimoto, H., and Aoki, T. (1985). Masked type I wheat allergy, relation to exercise induced anaphylaxis. *Arch. Dermatol. 121*: 355–360.

Lagrue, G., Laurent, J., and Rostoker, G. (1989). Food allergy and idiopathic nephrotic syndrome. *Kidney Int. 36* (Suppl. 27): S147–S151.

Langeland, T. (1982). A clinical and immunological study of allergy to hen's egg white. III. Allergens in hen's egg white studies by crossed radioimmunoelectrophoresis (CRIE). *Allergy 37*: 521–530.

Langeland, T. (1983). A clinical and immunological study of the allergy to hen's egg white. IV. Specific IgE-antibodies to individual allergens in hen's egg white related to clinical and immunological parameters in egg-allergic patients. *Allergy 38*: 493–500.

Langeland, T. (1985). Allergy to hen's egg white in atopic dermatitis. *Acta Derm. Venereol., Suppl. 114*: 109–112.

Langeland, T., and Harbitz, O. (1983). A clinical and immunological study of the allergy to hen's egg white. V. Purification and identification of a major allergen (antigen 22) in hen's egg white. *Allergy 38*: 131–139.

Layton, G. T., and Stanworth, D. R. (1984). The quantitation of IgG_4 antibodies to three common food allergens by ELISA with monoclonal anti-IgG_4. *J. Immunol. Meth. 73*: 347–356.

Lebenthal, E. (1965). Cow's milk protein allergy. *Pediatr. Clin. North Am. 22*: 827–833.

Lehrer, S. B., Karr, R. M., and Salvaggio, J. E. (1978). Extraction and analysis of coffee bean allergens. *Clin. Allergy 8*: 217–226.

Lehrer, S. B., McCants, M. L., and Salvaggio, J. E. (1985). Identification of crustacea allergens by crossed radioimmunoelectrophoresis. *Int. Arch. Allergy Appl. Immuno. 77*: 192–194.

Lehrer, S. B., Ibanez, M. D., McCants, M. L., Daul, C. B., and Morgan, J. E. (1990). Characterization of water-soluble shrimp allergens released during boiling. *J. Allergy Clin. Immunol. 85*: 1005–1013.

Lessof, M. H. (1989). Food allergy and intolerance. *Curr. Opin. Immunol. 1*: 667–671.

Malish, D., Glovsky, M. M., Hoffman, D. R., Ghekiere, L., and Hawkins, J. M. (1981). Anaphylaxis after sesame seed ingestion. *J. Allergy Clin. Immunol. 67*: 35–38.

Malley, A., Baecher, L., Mackler, B., and Perlman, F. (1975). The isolation of allergens from the green pea. *J. Allergy Clin. Immunol. 56*: 282–290.

Malley, A., Baecher, L., Mackler, B., and Perlman, F. (1976). Further characterization of a low-molecular weight allergen fragment isolated from the green pea. *Clin. Exp. Immunol. 25*: 159–164.

Mansfield, L. E., Vaughan, T. R., Waller, S. F., Haverly, R. W., and Ting, S. (1985). Food allergy and adult migraine: double-blind and mediator confirmation of an allergic etiology. *Ann. Allergy 55*: 126–129.

Matejtschuk, P., Easter, G., Thorpe, R., and Coombs, R. R. A. (1988). Experimental studies on red cell-based assays for total IgE and allergen-specific IgE. *Int. Arch. Allergy Appl. Immunol. 86*: 106–111.

Matsuda, T., Sugiyama, M., Nakamura, R., and Torii, S. (1988). Purification and properties of an allergenic protein in rice grain. *Agric. Biol. Chem. 52*: 1465–1470.

Matteo, A., and Sarles, H. (1990). Is food allergy a cause of acute pancreatitis? *Pancreas 5*: 234–237.

Maulitz, R. M., Pratt, D. S., Schocket, A. L. (1979). Exercise-induced anaphylaxis reaction to shellfish. *J. Allergy Clin. Immunol. 63*: 433–434.

McEwen, L. M. (1987). Hyposensitization. In *Food Allergy and Intolerance*, J. Brostoff and S. J. Challacombe, eds. Bailliere Tindall, London, pp. 985–994.

Meier-Davis, S., Taylor, S. L., Nordlee, J., and Bush, R. (1987). Identification of peanut allergens by immunoblotting (Abstract). *J. Allergy Clin. Immunol. 79*: 218.

Menendez-Arias, L. J., Moneo, I., Dominguez, J., and Rodrigues, R. (1988). Primary structure of the major allergen of yellow mustard (*Sinapis alba* L.) seed, Sin a I. *Eur. J. Biochem. 177*: 159–166.

Menendez-Arias, L. J., Dominguez, J., Moneo, I., and Rodriguez, R. (1990). Epitope mapping of the major allergen from yellow mustard seeds, Sin a I. *Mol. Immunol. 27*: 143–150.

Merrett, J., Burr, M. L., and Merrett, T. G. (1983). A community survey of IgG_4 antibody levels. *Clin. Allergy 13*: 397–407.

Merrett, J., Barnetson, R. S. C., Burr, M. L., and Merrett, T. G. (1984). Total and specific IgG_4 antibody levels in atopic eczema. *Clin. Exp. Immunol. 56*: 645–652.

Miell, J., Papouchado, M., and Marshall, A. J. (1988). Anaphylactic reaction after eating a mango. *Br. Med. J. 297*: 1639–1640.

Mike, N., and Asquith, P. (1987). Gluten toxicity in coeliac disease and its role in other gastrointestinal disorders. In *Food Allergy and Intolerance*, J. Bostoff and S. J. Challacombe, eds. Bailliere Tindall, London, pp. 521–548.

Moller, C. (1989). Effect of pollen immunotherapy on food hypersensitivity in children with birch pollinois. *Ann. Allergy 62*: 343–345.

Monro, J. (1987). Food-induced migraine. In *Food Allergy and Intolerance*, J. Brostoff and S. J. Challacombe, eds. Bailliere Tindall, London, pp. 633–665.

Moroz, L. A., and Yang, W. H. (1980). Kunitz soybean trypsin inhibitor. *New. Engl. J. Med. 302*: 1126–1128.

Murphy, P. A. (1985). Structural characteristics of soybean glycinin and β-conglycinin. In *World Soybean Research Conference III Proceedings*, R. A. Shibles, ed. Westview Press, Boulder, CO, pp. 143–151.

Norman, P. S., and Van Metre, Jr., T. E. (1990). The safety of allergenic immunotherapy. *J. Allergy Clin. Immunol. 85*: 522–525.

Novembre, E., de Martino, M., and Vierucci, A. (1988). Foods and respiratory allergy. *J. Allergy Clin. Immunol. 81* (Suppl. 5, part 2): 1059–1065.

Onorato, J., Merland, N., Terral, C., Michel, F. B., and Bousquet, J. (1986). Placebo-controlled double-blind food challenge in asthma. *J. Allergy Clin. Immunol. 78*: 1139–1146.

Paganelli, R., Levinsky, R. J., Brostoff, J., and Wraith, D. G. (1979). Immune complexes containing food proteins in normal and atopic subjects after oral challenge and effect of sodium cromoglycate on antigen absorption. *Lancet ii*: 1270–1272.

Panush, R. S., and Webster, E. M. (1985). Food allergies and other adverse reactions to foods. *Med. Clin. North Am. 69*: 533–546.

Pastorello, E., Stoocchi, L., Bigi, A., Pravettoni, V., Schilke, M. L., Valente, D., and Zanussi, C. (1989). Value and limits of diagnostic tests in food hypersensitivity. *Allergy 44* (suppl. 9): 151–158.

Pearson, D. J. (1989). Clinical diagnosis of food allergy. *Clin. Exp. Allergy 19*: 83–85.

Pearson, D. J., and Rix, K. J. B. (1985). Allergomimetic reactions to food and pseudo-food allergy. In *Pseudo-Allergic Reactions: 4. Idiopathic, Food-Induced and Drug-Induced Pseudo-Allergic Reactions*, P. Kukor, P. Kallos, and H. D. Schlumberger, eds. S. Karger, AG., New York, pp. 59–105.

Podleski, W. K. (1989). Pharmacotherapy of food allergy—a neglected option. *Int. J. Immunopharmacol. 11*: 311–326.

Powrie, W. D., and Nakai, S. (1985). Characteristics of edible fluids of animal origin: Eggs. In *Food Chemistsry*, 2nd ed., O. Fenema, ed. Marcel Dekker, New York, pp. 829–855.

Reed, C. E., Yunginger, J. W., and Evans, R. (1989). Qualilty assurance and standardization of allergy extracts in allergy practice. *J. Allergy Clin. Immunol. 84*: 4–8.

Saarinen, U. M., and Kajosaari, M. (1980). Does dietary elimination in infancy prevent or only postpone a food allergy. A study of fish and citrus allergy in 375 children. *Lancet i*: 166–167.

Sachs, M. I., Jones, R. T., and Yunginger, J. W. (1981). Isolation and partial characterization of a major peanut allergen. *J. Allergy Clin. Immunol. 67*: 27–34.

Sampson, H. A. (1983). Role of immediate food hypersensitivity in the pathogenesis of atopic dermatitis. *J. Allergy Clin. Immunol. 71*: 473–480.

Sampson, H. A. (1988). IgE-mediated food intolerance. *J. Allergy Clin. Immunol. 81*: 495–504.

Sampson, H. A., and McCaskill, C. C. (1985). Food hypersensitivity and atopic dermatitis: Evaluation of 113 patients. *J. Pediatr. 107*: 669–675.

Sampson, H., and Valentine, M. (1990). Diagnosing and treating adverse reactions to food ingestion. *Allergy Clin. Immunol. News 212*: 47–49.

Sampson, H. A., Buckley, R. H., and Metcalfe, D. D. (1987). Food allergy. *JAMA 258*: 2886–2890.

Sampson, H. A., Broadbent, K. R., and Bernhisel-Broadbent, K. R. (1989). Spontaneous release of histamine from basophils and histamine-releasing factor in patients with atopic dermatitis and food hypersensitivity. *New Engl. J. Med. 321*: 228–232.

Schreiber, R. A., and Walker, W. A. (1989a). Food allergy: Facts and fiction. *Mayo Clin. Proc. 64*: 1381–1391.

Schreiber, R. A., and Walker, W. A. (1989b). Gut immaturity in neonates. In *Food Intolerance in Infancy. Allergology, Immunology and Gastroenterology*, R. N. Hamburger, ed. Raven Press, New York, pp. 43–58.

Scott, H., and Brandtzaeg, P. (1989). Pathogenesis of food protein intolerance. *Acta Paediatr. Scand. Suppl. 351*: 48–52.

Seban, A., Konijn, A., and Freier, S. (1977). Chemical and immunological properties of a protein hydrolysate formula. *Am. J. Clin. Nutr. 30*: 840–846.

Shakib, F. (1990). Is IgE-mediated hypersensitivity an autoimmune disease? *Allergy 45*: 1–9.

Shakib, F., Brown, H. M., and Stanworth, D. R. (1984). Relevance of milk- and egg-specific IgG_4 in atopic eczema. *Int. Arch. Allergy Appl. Immunol. 75*: 107–112.

Shetty, K. J., and Rao, M. S. N. (1974). Studies on groundnut proteins, III. Physiochemical properties of conarachin II. *Indian J. Biochem. Biophys. 14*: 31–34.

Shetty, K. J., and Rao, M. S. N. (1977). Studies on groundnut proteins. VI. Isolation, characterization and hydrogen ion titration of conarachin II. *Int. J. Peptide Proteins Res. 9*: 11–17.

Shibasaki, M., Suzuki, S., Nemoto, H., and Kuroume, T. (1979). Allergenicity and lymphocyte-stimulating property of rice protein. *J. Allergy Clin. Immunol. 64*: 259–264.

Shibasaki, M., Suzuki, S., Tajima, S., Nemoto, H., and Kurome, T. (1980). Allergenicity of major component proteins of soybean. *Int. J. Arch. Allergy Appl. Immunol. 61*: 441–448.

Simon, R. A. (1986). Adverse reactions to food additives. *NER Allergy Proc. 7*: 533–542.

Sloan, A. E., and Powers, M. E. (1986). A perspective on popular perceptions of adverse reactions to foods. *J. Allergy Clin. Immunol. 78*: 127–139.

Soothill, J. F. (1987). Prevention of food allergy. In *Food Allergy and Intolerance*, J. Brostoff and S. J. Challacombe, eds. Bailliere Tindall, London, pp. 1005–1016.

Spies, J. R., and Coulson, E. J. (1943). The chemistry of allergens. VIII. Isolation and properties of an active protein-polysaccharide fraction, CB-1A, from castor beans. *J. Am. Chem. Soc. 65*: 1720–1725.

Stern, M., and Walker, W. A. (1985). Food allergy and intolerance. *Pediatr. Clin. North Am. 32*: 471–492.

Sutton, J., Hill, D. J., Baldo, B. A., and Wrigley, C. W. (1982). Immunoglobulin E antibodies to ingested flour components: studies with sera from subjects with asthma and eczema. *Clin. Allergy 12*: 63–74.

Swaisgood, H. E. (1985). Characteristics of edible fluids of animal origin: Milk. In *Food Chemistry*, 2nd ed., O. R. Fennema, ed. Marcel Dekker, New York, pp. 791–827.

Taylor, S. L. (1985). Food allergies. *Food Technol. 39*: 98–105.

Taylor, S. L. (1986). Immunologic and allergic properties of cows' milk proteins in humans. *J. Food Prot. 49*: 239–250.

Taylor, S. L. (1987). Allergic and sensitivity reactions to food components. In *Nutritional Toxicology*, Vol. II, J. N. Hathcock, ed., Academic Press, Inc., New York, pp. 173–198.

Taylor, S. L., and Bush, R. K. (1988). Allergy by ingestion of seafoods. In *Handbook of Natural Toxins. Marine Toxins and Venoms*, Vol. 3, A. T. Tu, ed. Marcel Dekker, Inc., New York, pp. 149–183.

Taylor, S. L., and Nordlee, J. A. (1988). Sensitivity to ingested sulfites. *ISI Atlas Sci: Immunol. 1*: 254–258.

Taylor, S. L., Busse, W. W., Sachs, M. I., Parker, J. L., and Yunginger, J. W. (1981). Peanut oil is not allergenic to peanut-sensitive individuals. *J. Allergy Clin. Immunol. 68*: 372–375.

Taylor, S. L., Bush, R. K., and Busse, W. W. (1987a). Avoidance diets—how selective should they be? In *Food Allergy*, R. K. Chandra, ed. Nutritional Research Education Foundation, St. Johns, Newfoundland, pp. 253–256.

Taylor, S. L., Lemanske, R. F., Bush, R. K., and Busse, W. W. (1987b). Chemistry of food allergens. In *Food Allergy*, R. K. Chandra, ed. Nutritional Research Education Foundation, St. Johns, Newfoundland, pp. 21–44.

Taylor, S. L., Lemanske, R. F., Bush, R. K., and Busse, W. W. (1987c). Food allergens: Structure and immunological properties. *Ann. Allergy 59*: 93–99.

Taylor, S. L., Nordlee, J. A., and Rupnow, J. H. (1989a). Food allergies and sensitivities. In *Food Toxicology. A Perspective on the Relative Risks*, S. L. Taylor and R. A. Scanlan, eds. Marcel Dekker, New York, pp. 255–295.

Taylor, S. L., Stratton, J. E., and Nordlee, J. A. (1989b). Histamine poisoning (scombroid fish poisoning): An allergy-like intoxication. *J. Clin. Toxicol. 27*: 225–240.

Toft Sorensen, H., Nielsen, B., and Ostergaard Nielsen, J. (1989). Anaphylactic shock occurring outside hospitals. *Allergy 44*: 288–290.

Tombs, M. P. (1965). An electrophoretic investigation of groundnut proteins: The structure of arachins A and B. *Biochem. J. 96*: 119–133.

Turner, K. J. (1989). The biological role of IgE bound to low affinity receptors: In and out? *Allergy Clin. Immunol. News 114*: 110–119.

Turner, M. W., Brostoff, J., Mowbray, J. F., and Skelton, A. (1980). The atopic syndrome: In vitro immunological characteristics of clinically defined subgroups of atopic subjects. *Clin. Allergy 10*: 575–584.

Uragoda, D. G. (1970). Tea maker's asthma. *Br. J. Ind. Med. 27*: 181–182.

VanArsdel, P. P., and Larson, E. B. (1989). Diagnostic tests for patients with suspected allergic disease. Utility and limitations. *Ann. Int. Med. 110*: 304–312.

Van Asperen, P. P., Kemp, A. S., and Mellis, C. M. (1983). Immediate food hypersensitivity reactions on the first known exposure to the food. *Arch. Dis. Child. 58*: 253–256.

Van Hooser, B., and Crawford, L. V. (1989). Allergy diets for infants and children. *Comprehensive Therapy 15*: 38–47.

Van Toorenenbergen, A. W., and Aalberse, R. C. (1982). IgG_4 and release of histamine from human peripheral blood leukocytes. *Int. Arch. Allergy Appl. Immunol. 67*: 117–122.

Votaw, A. L., and Newman, M. A. (1989). Occupational asthma among egg and meat processing workers. *Nat. Provisioner* (July 29): 12–13.

Walker, W. A. (1987). Pathophysiology of intestinal uptake and absorption of antigens in food allergy. *Ann. Allergy 59*: 7–16.

Walker-Smith, J. A. (1989). Intestinal manifestations of food allergy. In *Food Intolerance in Infancy. Allergology, Immunology, and Gastroenterology*, R. N. Hamburger, ed. Raven Press, New York, pp. 127–134.

Waring, N. P., de Shazo, R., Salvaggio, J. E., Daul, C., and Lehrer, S. B. (1983). Skin and RAST reactions to shell-fish antigens. *J. Allergy Clin. Immunol. 71*: 111.

Waring, N. P., Daul, C. B., de Shazo, R. D., McCants, M. L., and Lehrer, S. B. (1985). Hypersensitivity reactions to ingested crustacea: Clinical evaluation and diagnostic studies in shrimp-sensitive individuals. *J. Allergy Clin. Immunol. 76*: 440–445.

Webber, S. A., Graham-Brown, R. A. C., Hutchinson, P. E., and Burns, D. A. (1989). Dietary manipulation in childhood atopic dermatitis. *Br. J. Dermatol. 121*: 91–98.

Wershil, B. K., and Walker, W. A. (1988). Milk allergies and other food allergies in children. *Immunol. Allergy Clin. North Am. 8*: 485–504.

World Health Organization (1989). Current status of allergen immunotherapy (hyposensitization): Memorandum from a WHO/IUIS meeting. *Bulletin WHO 67*: 263–272.

Wright, R., and Robertson, D. (1987). Immunologically mediated damage—local and distant. In *Food Allergy and Intolerance*, J. Brostoff and S. J. Challacombe, eds. Bailliere Tindall, London, pp. 237–247.

Wuthrich, R. (1990). Epidemiology of the allergic diseases: Are they really on the increase? *Int. Arch. Allergy Appl. Immunol. 90*: 3–10.

Youlten, L. J. F. (1987). Drug treatment of food allergy and intolerance. In *Food Allergy and Intolerance*, J. Brostoff and S. J. Challacombe, eds. Bailliere Tindall, London, pp. 977–984.

Yunginger, J. W., and Jones, R. T. (1985). A review of peanut chemistry: Implications for the standardization of peanut extracts. In *Proceedings of the Fourth International Paul Ehrlich Seminar on Regulatory Control and Standardization of Allergenic Extracts*, Gustav Fischer Verlag, Stuttgart, Germany.

Yunginger, J. W., Sweeney, K. G., Sturner, W. Q., Giannandrea, L. A., Teigland, J. D., Bray, M., Benson, P. A., York, J. A., Biedrzycki, L., Squillace, D. L., and Helm, R. M. (1988). Fatal food-induced anaphylaxis. *JAMA 260*: 1450–1452.

Zanussi, C., and Pastorello, E. (1987). Dietary treatment of food allergy. In *Food Allergy and Intolerance*, J. Brostoff and S. J. Challacombe, eds. Bailliere Tindall, London, pp. 971–976.

Zeiger, R. S. (1988). Development and prevention of allergic disease in childhood. In *Allergy: Principles and Practice*, Vol. II, E. Middleton, Jr., C. E. Reed, E. F. Ellis, N. F. Adkinson, Jr., and J. W. Yunginger, eds. C. V. Mosby, St. Louis, pp. 930–968.

Zeiger, R. S., Heller, S., Mellon, M. H., Forsythe, A. B., O'Conner, R. D., Hamburger, R. N., and Schatz, M. (1989). Effect of combined maternal and infant food-allergen avoidance on development of atopy in early infancy: A randomized study. *J. Allergy Clin. Immunol. 84*: 72–89.

14

Cereal Allergies and Intolerances

Klaus Lorenz

Colorado State University, Fort Collins, Colorado

I. INTRODUCTION

Allergies and intolerances are abnormal reactions associated with natural substances which are harmless to most individuals. Allergies affect nearly half the population at one time or another (Baldo and Wrigley, 1984).

Cereals (especially wheat) are among the important foodstuffs which on ingestion produce respiratory, gastrointestinal, or skin manifestations in food-sensitive persons. Inhalation of dusts derived from cereals may induce symptoms of respiratory allergy—vasomotor rhinitis and bronchial asthma (Baldo and Wrigley, 1984). Cereals have also been implicated in the triggering of migraine attacks (Dickerson et al., 1978; Grant, 1980; Monro et al., 1980).

We all inhale pollens and eat cereals. Occupational groups inhale dust from the harvesting, handling, milling, and processing of these grains. Bakers and millers who work in an environment filled with grain dust often suffer from bronchial asthma. The affected person is frequently forced to leave the trade.

Ingestion of cereals has been associated with flatulence (Anderson et al., 1981) and irritable bowel syndrome (Alun-Jones et al., 1982). In such cases, celiac disease is suspected. Related to celiac disease is dermatitis herpetiformis, which produces severe skin reactions (Weinstein et al., 1974; Ross et al., 1978; Scott and Losowsky, 1978). Mental disorders have also been linked to the ingestion of cereal grains (Dohan, 1972; Singh and Kay, 1976; Rice et al., 1987; Lorenz, 1990).

Most allergens are proteins or glycoproteins, although pure polysaccharides have been shown to cause reactions (Baldo and Pepys, 1976).

II. TAXONOMIC CLASSIFICATION AND USES OF CEREALS

Avoidance of cereal allergens is virtually impossible. Cereal grains contribute about half the world's supply of dietary proteins and more than half of our energy needs. Annual production of wheat, rice, and maize combined is about 300 kg per person per year (Baldo and Wrigley, 1984).

Table 1 shows a taxonomic classification of grass species that produce grain for food and the food uses of these grains. Knowledge of the taxonomic relationship between cereals can be valuable in assessing likely cross-reactivities between cereal allergens (Baldo et al., 1980). A person with known intolerance to wheat would, for instance, be more likely to have similar problems with rye than with rice or corn. Celiac patients, who find wheat gluten the most toxic protein, are progressively less affected by rye, barley, and oats, while rice and corn appear to be safe to eat (Kasarda, 1978).

III. ALLERGIES CAUSED BY INHALATION OF CEREALS

A. Pollens and Grain Particles

Pollens are the most important cause of inhalant allergies due to cereals. Furthermore, inhalable particles are produced when cereals are harvested, transported, and processed. Dust from dry straw and grains is inhaled by farmers, particles from the bran layer of grains by grain handlers and silo operators, and flour dust by millers and bakers.

Pollens are quite small in size, ranging from 20 to 50 μm. Millions of these pollens may be released by one plant. They become airborne, since grasses are wind-pollinated, not insect-pollinated. When the pollen settles on the moist surface of the bronchial mucosa, proteins and glycoproteins may be exuded, initiating an allergic response. A person who is allergic to a certain pollen often has no adverse reaction, however, when eating grain from the same species (Baldo and Wrigley, 1984). Allergic reactions do not

Table 1 Taxonomic Classification of Cereals Presumed to be Important in Allergies and Intolerances and Their Food Uses

Taxonomic name	Common name	Major food uses
Triticanae		Bread (leavened and unleavened), pasta (spaghetti, macaroni), noodles, breakfast cereals (processed cereals, porridge, bran, and germ), cakes, biscuits, cookies, scones, chappatis, porridge, extruded snack foods, bulgur, beer, flavorings, many canned, packaged frozen and convenience foods and sweets, vegetarian foods containing gluten
Triticum aestivum	Bread wheat	
Triticum durum	Durum wheat	
Triticosecale	Triticale	
Secale cereale	Rye	Bread, crispbread, spirits
Hordeum vulgare	Barley	Porridge, cooked grains, malt, beer, spirits
Aveneae		
Avena sativa	Common oat	Porridge; cooked grains; breakfast cereals, extruded snacks, oatcakes
Avena fatua	Wild oat	
Oryzoids		
Oryza sativa	Rice	Cooked grains, breakfast cereals, extruded snacks, cakes, beer, baby food, convenience foods, sake
Zizania aquatica	Wild rice	Cooked grain
Chloridoids		
Eleusine coracana	Indian millet	
Eupanicoids		
Echinochloa spp.	Japanese millet	Cooked grains, porridge, unleavened bread, flatcakes, beer
Panicum miliaceum	Common millet	
Pennisetum americanum	Pearl millet	
Setaria italica	Italian millet	
Andropogonoids		
Sorghum bicolor	Grain sorghum	Cooked grains, porridge, unleavened bread, flatcakes, beer
Zea mays	Corn, maize	Hominy, tortillas, arretas, cornbreads, cooked grains, polenta, breakfast foods, popcorn, extruded snack foods, corn syrup, many manufactured foods

Source: Adapted from Saxelby and Venn-Brown, 1980, and Baldo and Wrigley, 1984.

always occur, however, when people with sensitivities to wheat inhale pollen or straw dust.

Lai et al. (1981) defined grain dust as the finely divided material that becomes airborne and can be removed from grain during handling. It consists of dirt from the fields, pieces of plant material, tiny pieces of grain resulting from abrasion during handling, and pieces of grain resulting from feeding by insects. Grain dusts are well known for causing respiratory problems such as chronic bronchitis, grain dust asthma, extrinsic allergic alveolitis (farmer's lung), grain fever, rhinitis, and conjunctivitis (Chan-Yeung et al., 1978) in persons handling grain at many points from harvest to mill. Occasionally, however, wheat sensitivity is not entirely due to the cereal grain, but to parasitic fungi of cereals, such as molds and smut. Urbach and Gottlieb (1943) point out the importance of these fungi in relation to asthma in workers in flour mills, in farmers, and in people living close to mills or in the country. One single smutted wheat kernel may contain from 6 to 9 million spores. Corn smut has been reported to reach a count of 1 million spores per square foot in 24 hr in parts of the country. These figures are impressive. However, the volume of the smut spore is only one-eighth that of pollen, so that the actual contact is less than the figures might indicate.

Rankin et al. (1979) concluded that chronic bronchitis and other respiratory symptoms develop more frequently in grain handlers than in comparable non–grain-handling workers. The effect of exposure to grain dust is usually greater than that of smoking. The adverse effects of grain handling on lung function are as severe as those caused by smoking.

The existence of an occupational disease resulting from exposure to grain dust was confirmed by the observations of many researchers (Pinto, 1941; Smith et al., 1941; Jimenez-Diaz and Canto, 1947), but the first systematic study of this problem was the investigation of Dunner et al. (1946), who examined lung lesions due to inhaled dust in 55 dock workers and concluded that the silica, fine hairs, starch grains, and cellular material in cereal dusts may produce lung disease.

The role of allergy in sensitization to grain dust was emphasized by Cohen and Osgood (1953), but disabling respiratory symptoms following exposure to grain dust can be induced in the absence of allergic sensitivity. An investigation into the high incidence of respiratory symptoms among grain elevator agents in Saskatchewan, Canada, revealed a higher frequency of cough, wheezing, and breathlessness than occurs in the average population (Williams et al., 1964).

Kleinfield (1974) found symptoms of cough, dyspnea, wheezing, and grain fever in a group of 55 grain handlers in New York. Tse et al. (1973) surveyed 68 grain elevator agents in southern Manitoba and found that 75% had grain dust-associated respiratory symptoms including chronic cough, sputum, and dyspnea.

A survey by DoPico et al. (1977) of respiratory abnormalities in 300 grain workers in Wisconsin and Minnesota reported exposure of the operators to large amounts of dust and contaminants and poor enforcement of occupational safety and health standards for dust in grain elevators.

Less information is available on the effects of grain dust on the health of farmers, although respiratory problems are thought to be common in this group (Bartschi and Regli, 1969; Lefcoe and Wonnacott, 1974).

Outside North America, few surveys of health hazards following exposure to grain dust have been undertaken. Gandevia and Ritchie (1966) and Gandevia (1980) studied grain-handling dock workers in a major Australian city and a country port and concluded that approximately 10% of workers frequently and heavily exposed to wheat dust became allergic.

Cereal grain dusts as a cause of respiratory allergies in South Africa were examined in some detail by Ordman (1958). Sensitivities to dusts from corn, wheat, "kaffir-corn" (*Sorghum vulgare*), oats, rye, and rice were investigated in 128 subjects. Respiratory allergies to corn dust occurred in 71.9% of the cases and to dusts from wheat, sorghum, oats, rye, and rice in 39.1, 22.7, 14.8, 7.0, and 3.9% of the cases, respectively.

Examination of the numerous health surveys conducted so far clearly reveals that exposure to grain dust is injurious to health.

B. Flour Dust (Baker's Asthma)

The inhalation of flour dust may cause allergic reactions in the nose, eyes, and airways of sensitive subjects. In one of the early studies of baker's asthma, de Besche (1929) concluded that it is an allergic industrial disease. Flour allergy occurs most common in bakers (Baagoe, 1933). Asthma and rhinitis are IgE-mediated allergic reactions in which in the first stage (sensitization), the inhalation of flour leads to the synthesis of immunoglobulin E (IgE) antibodies specific to flour. These IgE molecules, which are attached to mast cells of the bronchial mucosa, become attachment sites of flour proteins on subsequent exposure, leading to the production of mediators that cause asthmatic symptoms (Baldo and Wrigley, 1984).

Flour-induced rhinitis and asthma are frequently severe enough to cause inconvenience, discomfort, time loss, and even abandonment of the trade. In some countries, this has been recognized by including baker's asthma on the list of occupational diseases.

Numerous surveys have shown that baker's asthma and rhinitis are not uncommon afflictions, although the frequency of sensitivity to flour is decreasing because of removal of airborne flour from the workplace through modern flour-handling equipment. Findings of selected studies of baker's asthma in bakery and mill workers carried out during the past 50 years are summarized in Table 2.

Schwartz (1947) observed that the more dust generated, the greater the number of individuals who were sensitized and exhibited allergic symptoms. According to Schwartz, 44% of bakers in small bakeries became sensitized, but this figure fell to 25% in larger establishments. Observing that bakers are usually sensitized to the kind of flour with which they work most (Salen and Juhlin-Dannfeldt, 1935; Tse and Raghuprasad, 1982), Schwartz (1947) considered it impossible to distinguish whether a common cereal allergen was involved or whether each subject had allergic responses to more than one

Table 2 Selected Studies of Flour Allergies in Bakery and Mill Workers

Findings	Ref.
25 of 100 mill workers with positive skin reactions; 2 had asthma	Rastelli and Brambilla, 1937
25% of 262 workers in bakeries and mills in Amsterdam with allergic symptoms to wheat and rye flour	Van Dishoeck and Roux, 1939
25 of 115 millers in Paris with asthma	Najera and Dantin, 1939
20% of 328 workers in bakeries allergic to flour, 2/3 had nasal symptoms; 1/3 nasal and asthmatic symptoms	Linko, 1947
163 cases of flour allergy in 583 bakers; half suffered from rhinitis, half from rhinitis and asthma	Kallos and Kallos-Deffner, 1971
Asthma due to wheat and rye flours made up significant portion of total number of cases of occupational asthma of bakery employees in Finland	Keskinen et al., 1978
58 of 234 bakery employees with allergic rhinitis, asthma and/or eczema	Jarvinen et al., 1979
325 new cases of bakers' asthma per year in West Germany	Thiel and Ulmer, 1980

species. In a recent study by Thiel and Ulmer (1980), flour-dependent rhinitis was found in 5% of the apprentices, 21% of the unselected bakers, and all of the bakers with proven flour allergy. Asthma occurred in 82% of the latter group, 10% of the unselected bakers, and in only 1% of the apprentices. The data are shown in Table 3.

After symptoms of rhinitis or asthma have appeared, continued exposure does not necessarily lead to a further deterioration in the allergic condition. In a survey of 500 bakers, 93 developed baker's asthma over a 6-year period. At the end of 6 years, however, 40 of the 80 symptomatic bakers still in the study had improved, even though their exposure to flour had not been reduced (Bonnevie, 1958).

Bakers in Japan rarely seem to be affected by wheat flour asthma. Nakazawa et al. (1972) observed only two such cases, both with long-term exposure (10 and 20 years) to the allergen before the onset of asthma. The asthma attacks were typical bronchial asthma with no fever. Sera from both cases revealed weak precipitin reactions with the allergen.

Table 3 Percentage of Bakers with Occupational Complaints

	No. of subjects	Meal rhinitis	Baker's asthma	Time of occupation (mean in years)	Exposure until onset of symptoms (mean in years)
Bakers' apprentices	85	4	1	1.8 ± 0.9	1–3
Unselected bakers	29	6	3	24.8 ± 6.7	17.4 ± 9.1 (7–32)
Bakers with proven occupational disease	38	38	31	25.2 ± 8.0	17.3 ± 8.1 (1–31)

Source: Thiel and Ulmer, 1980.

1. *Diagnosis*

Crucial to diagnosing baker's asthma is knowing the patient's occupational history. An important clue to the possibility of the disease being work-related is the abrupt onset of asthma in an adult with no previous history of allergic disease. The symptoms of asthma develop after exposure at work and improve during weekends. Chest examination and chest X-ray are usually normal. Physical examination of the worker in the office may not be helpful, but examination at work during exposure may lead to diagnosis.

Certain laboratory tests are helpful in diagnosing baker's asthma (Table 4). Bronchial provocation testing, using the "occupational-type exposure," is the most specific procedure in documenting asthmatic response to suspected allergens (Baldo and Wrigley, 1984). Like the asthmatic reaction following exposures at work, immediate, late, or dual asthmatic reaction to the provocation test may occur (Tse and Raghuprasad, 1982).

Thiel and Ulmer (1980) used several of the tests mentioned in Table 4 in their study of asthma in bakers and bakers' apprentices. The results are shown in Table 5. Notable is the high percentage (21.7%) of positive acetylcholine test responses in the group of apprentices compared to only 8.3% in the controls and the increasing incidence of positive acetylcholine tests with time of exposure. The bronchial provocation tests showed the same trend.

Despite the continuing interest in baker's asthma, attempts to identify the flour allergens involved in provoking allergic reactions have only recently been initiated.

Blands et al. (1976) detected 40 different antigens in wheat flour by crossed immunoelectrophoresis. Twenty of these antigens cross-reacted with rye flour extract, and 18 bound serum IgE in sera from allergic bakers.

Studies with wheat flour fractions and purified proteins showed that the water-soluble proteins and purified albumins were approximately equally active in binding the IgE antibodies in sera from patients with baker's asthma (Baldo and Wrigley, 1978). Subsequent studies demonstrated that wheat flour

Table 4 Diagnostic Aids in Grain Dust–Induced Asthma

Laboratory test	Criteria	Clinical significance and explanation of test
Total blood eosinophils	>400/mm^3	Elevated eosinophils in peripheral blood may occur in atopic allergy and parasitic infections. Eosinophils preferentially phagocytize IgE-containing immune complexes.
Total IgE (PRIST)	>250 U/ml	This test quantitates the amount of total IgE in human serum. IgE is significantly elevated in most patients with allergic diseases, such as extrinsic asthma.
Specific IgE (RAST)	>10% binding	This test measures the amount of allergen specific IgE in serum and correlates well with clinical allergy in patients sensitive to pollens.
Skin tests	>2 + (read in 10–20 min)	The immediate skin test reaction is a result of the interaction between specific antigen and IgE skin-sensitizing antibodies bound to mast cells, which causes the release of histamine and other pharmacological mediators. It is useful in diagnosing extrinsic asthma and allergic rhinitis. If skin tests are negative or equivocal, RAST and bronchial provocation tests should be employed to confirm diagnosis.
Leukocyte histamine release	≥50%	The peripheral blood leukocytes of an allergic individual liberate histamine in the presence of specific antigens. In the diagnosis of allergies, a high correlation between histamine release and skin test response was found.
Bronchial provocation	≥20% ↓ in FEF	This test is the most accurate method of corroborating suspected natural and occupational allergens. It is also used as a standard with which to compare other tests, such as RAST or skin tests. FEF measures small airway obstruction.

↓ = decrease; FEF = forced expiratory flow between the 25th and 75th percentile of the forced vital capacity; PRIST = Paper radioimmunosorbent test; RAST = radioallergosorbent test.
Source: Adapted from Tse and Raghuprasad, 1982.

Table 5 Percentage of Positive Findings in RAST, Skin, Acetylcholine, and Provocation Tests in Bakers

	Number of subjects	Positive RAST (%)		Positive skin tests (%)		Positive acetyl-choline tests (%)	Bronchial Provocation tests (%)	
		Wheat	Rye	Wheat	Rye		Wheat	Rye
Bakers' apprentices	85	13.2	9.6	4.8	6.0	21.7	1.2	1.2
Controls	60	16.7	13.3	1.7	3.4	8.3	—	—
Unselected bakers	29	27.6	20.7	20.7	27.6	46.4	10.3	17.2
Controls	29	6.8	6.8	3.4	3.4	17.2	—	—
Bakers with proven occupational disease	18	77.8	83.3	91	91	84.2	61.3	71.0

Source: Thiel and Ulmer, 1980.

albumins are important heterogeneous allergens in baker's asthma. For example, fractionation of wheat albumins by ion exchange chromatography and preparative isoelectric focusing showed that serum IgE antibodies from different allergic bakers bind to many, and sometimes quite different, wheat proteins (Baldo et al., 1982).

2. *Treatment*

The best therapeutic approach to the management of baker's asthma is the avoidance to the allergen (Tse and Raghuprasad, 1982). However, this may not be practical, and the use of special masks or respirators is often recommended.

The pharmacological treatment of baker's asthma does not differ from that of other types of asthma. Isolated episodes of mild asthma can be treated initially with drugs having β-adrenergic activity (e.g., aerosol sympathomimetic agents such as albuterol, isoproterenol, or metaproterenol). Theophylline derivatives (aminophylline, theophylline, and oxtriphylline) or the selective β_2-stimulating agents (terbutaline, albuterol) may help diminish symptoms of baker's asthma (Brooks, 1977).

Parenteral therapy may be required for acute bronchospastic episodes. Epinephrine (1:1000) is very effective; the usual dose is 0.3 ml injected subcutaneously (Kelson et al., 1978). Terbutaline is also available for subcutaneous injection at a recommended dosage of 0.5 mg (Pang et al., 1977). If acute bronchoconstriction does not respond to the above adrenergic drugs, aminophylline 4–5 mg/kg i.v., injected slowly over a period of 10 to 15 minutes, successfully controls the majority of acute attacks in adults (Piafsky and Ogilvie, 1975; Hendeles and Weinberger, 1979).

The protective effect of cromolyn sodium on grain-dust–sensitive subjects is well documented, and it is indicated as a prophylactic medication when exposure to grain dust will induce an acute episode of asthma. A dose of 20–40 mg, given 20 minutes before the anticipated exposure or three to four times daily, will usually prevent the bronchoconstriction response (Nakazawa et al., 1976). This treatment has been shown to inhibit both the immediate and the late component of the dual response in baker's asthma. However, when asthmatic symptoms can not be controlled successfully with the above drugs, a patient may need to change professions (Tse and Raghuprasad, 1982).

IV. SKIN SENSITIVITIES

A very severe neurodermatitis lasting many years was shown to be due to inhalation of rye flour, as observed by Urbach and Gottlieb (1943). The patient was a baker's daughter whose bedroom was adjacent to the bakery. The diagnosis was based on the fact that the girl became free of symptoms when she left home.

Skin sensitivity to wheat and rye flour among new bakers' apprentices in West Berlin was reported by Herxheimer (1973). Skin tests conducted annually for 5 consecutive years showed that 9–11% of the new apprentices were initially skin positive to flour, and half of them became skin negative during the first 12 months. However, during the 5 years, other apprentices who had been skin negative became skin positive. The percentage increased gradually to about 20%. Skin sensitivity to pollen and flour often occurred simultaneously. Approximately the same percentage of flour-positive and flour-negative subjects were sensitive to house dust, indicating that an allergic disposition may facilitate sensitization to flour.

Cereal ingestant extracts of rice, rye, wheat, corn, and oats were administered intracutaneously to adults and by a prick technique to children in a study by Lewis and Imber (1975). The responses of pediatric and adult patients to rye, wheat, and corn were similar, but differed considerably with rice and oats, as shown in Table 6.

The reaction to rice and oats was low in children, whereas adults responded at a much higher level to rice and slightly higher to oats. Removal of a certain percentage of protein from polished rice may have contributed to its low level of allergenicity and population frequency in children. The low allergenicity in children to oats is difficult to explain. Lewis and Imber (1975) believe that the high reaction of adults to rice may be attributed to prolonged and enhanced sensitivity with age to the allergens present.

V. CEREAL INTOLERANCES

A. Celiac Disease

Celiac disease is a polygenic, polymorphic disorder usually with intestinal and often with psychiatric symptoms evoked by wheat, rye and barley protein

Table 6 Adult and Pediatric Patient Reactions to Cereal Preparations

	Adults			Children		
Cereal	N	Average reactivity (0 to 4+)	Reaction frequency (%) (2+ to 4+)	N	Average reactivity (0 to 4+)	Reaction frequency (%) (2+ to 4+)
Rice	1196	1.31	39.1	118	0.64	5.9
Rye	1197	0.90	26.1	274	1.04	25.2
Wheat	1197	1.00	29.8	406	1.10	18.0
Corn	1204	1.10	32.7	306	0.96	18.3
Oats	1155	1.14	32.6	132	0.71	7.6

Source: Adapted from Lewis and Imber, 1975.

fractions (Kasarda, 1975; Kasarda et al., 1976). Celiac condition is not a type I allergic reaction because it does not involve the production of IgE specific to gluten (Bjorksten et al., 1977; Baldo and Wrigley, 1978). However, an account of celiac condition is justified in this chapter because of its prominence as a type of intolerance to gluten. The disease is known under a number of different names including gluten-sensitive enteropathy, nontropical sprue, idiopathic steatorrhea, celiac disease, and sprue. In persons with this disorder, the lining of the small intestine is damaged by gliadin, which is present in wheat, rye, barley, and probably oats. Many symptoms may appear or only one of a wide range may be present: diarrhea, bloating, weight loss, anemia, chronic fatigue, weakness, bone pain, muscle cramps, the skin disorder dermatitis herpetiformis, and, in children, vomiting. Children may fail to grow at a normal rate (Hartsook, 1984). The disease is now also recognized in many without such marked symptoms by means of peroral biopsy demonstration of the characteristic histological changes of the small intestine (e.g., villous atrophy, delayed immune reaction), plus response to diet.

Celiac disease may also occur with psychiatric symptoms, which, in association with other symptoms, may be of diagnostic help. No one knows the causes of the psychiatric symptoms, however, they do not appear to be related to the long-term metabolic effects of gluten as indicated by the rapid psychic improvement in children on a gluten-free diet (Dohan, 1976). In children, psychiatric symptoms often improve a few days after starting a gluten-free diet (Townley and Anderson, 1967). Käser (1961) described celiac children as conspicuously quiet, turned inward, often weepy, often discontented, and apparently lacking all joy in living. They are outstandingly crotchety and at the slightest provocation can become unhappy, very sad, or enraged. In older patients, speech development is often markedly impaired, the vocabulary limited to a few words, and the intonation is soft and whining. Rate of occurrence of about 1 celiac in 2000 persons is often accepted for Western countries, but estimates of frequency range from 1 in 100 to 1 in 8000 (Stenhammer and Johansson, 1981).

1. *Involvement of Gluten Fractions*

The relationship between the development of symptoms of celiac disease and the feeding of wheat flour was first established by Dicke (1950) in Holland. Dicke et al. (1953) confirmed this association through feeding experiments. Anderson et al. (1952), working independently, also demonstrated this correlation and confirmed that gluten, or the protein fraction of wheat flour, was the deleterious agent causing symptoms and steatorrhea.

Rye also produces the symptoms of celiac disease and must be avoided by celiac patients. Some researchers believe that barley and oats contain the toxic factor (Frazer, 1956; Rubin et al., 1962). Research data by Moulton (1959), however, indicated that oat flakes in amounts up to 20 oz/day may be fed without ill effects. Even the highest quantity of oat flakes given in this study (169 g/day for 3 weeks) produced an increase in fecal excretion in only four celiac children. The reason for this discrepancy remains a mystery.

Corn and rice are considered nontoxic to celiac patients, although these cereals may trigger allergic responses including respiratory problems, headaches, joint pains, and hives (Kasarda, 1972).

It was thought that blood glutamine could be used as an index of the toxicity of various gluten fractions after Alvey et al. (1957) found that celiac patients show a higher average blood glutamine level after ingestion of gluten, as shown in Table 7. As can be seen, the rise in blood glutamine was three times greater in celiac patients than in control subjects. Glutamine peptides, however, did not exert toxic effects on celiac patients; this indicated that some barrier must exist in the function of the intestinal mucosa (Frazer et al., 1959; Frazer, 1962). Digestion of gliadin (the toxic fraction of gluten) with a peptic-tryptic crude pancreatic extract or a crystalline papain extract failed to destroy the toxic factor (Messer et al., 1964). However, predigestion of gliadin with crude papain or enzyme extracts from the intestinal mucosa of swine destroyed the toxic agent(s). End products of enzymatic digestion suggest that the noxious substance(s) is a peptide(s) which has L-glutamine as its N-terminal amino acid (Messer et al., 1964). Indications are that acidic peptides play a role in the toxicity of wheat protein (Bronstein et al., 1966). Also, a group of glycopolypeptides and a group of acidic polypeptides of low molecular weights were isolated from ultrafiltrates of a peptic-tryptic crude pancreatic enzyme digest of gliadin. Both groups of polypeptides were rich in glutamine or glutamine and proline, and both groups were toxic in celiac patients and nontoxic in control subjects (Kowlessar, 1972). Heiner et al. (1964) detected precipitants to the antigens of wheat in about half of their patients with well-documented cases of gluten-induced celiac disease. These authors proposed that the precipitin reaction is presumptive of celiac disease.

2. *Morphological Changes*

Morphological changes associated with the malabsorption of nutrients from the intestinal tract occur in the small bowel. Histological examinations show that the jejunal mucosa of the celiac patient is characterized by villous atrophy and changes in the structure and absorptive capacity of the epithelial cells (Rosenlund, 1970; Rubin, 1971; Kowlessar, 1972). Electron microscopy of

Table 7 Blood Glutamine Values Before and After a Test Dose of 700 mg/Gluten/kg Body Weight

		Glutamine (mg/100 ml Blood)		
		Fasting	2 hr after test dose	Increase (%)
Control subjects	1	7.5	8.1	8
	2	4.9	6.5	32
	3	7.0	8.7	34
	4	8.7	11.7	34
Celiac patients	1	4.7	7.3	55
	2	2.9	4.7	62
	3	4.1	7.0	72
	4	3.2	8.0	128

Source: Adapted from Alvey et al., 1957.

absorptive cells reveals the abnormal structure of the microvilli of the apial surface, i.e., irregularity, clubbing, and fusion (Kowlessar, 1972).

Townley et al. (1973) showed that 1 out of 10 fractions obtained by chromatography of a peptic-tryptic-pancreatinic digest of wheat gliadin disrupted rat liver lysosomes and inhibited the morphological improvement of celiac mucosa in organ cultures. Since the fraction may exceed the digestive capacity of normal surface epithelial cells and produce damage in celiac patients, it would lend support to the view that the lesions in celiac disease are caused by a deficiency of an intestinal peptidase, allowing the accumulation of peptides toxic to the mucosa.

Townley et al. (1973) found that the ultrastructures of the epithelial cells of biopsy samples from patients with untreated celiac disease improved during culture in the absence of gliadin digest or its fractions. Surface epithelial cells became taller, and microvilli, initially irregular and short, became more regular, numerous, and taller. The gliadin fraction consistently inhibited such improvement of duodenal mucosa from patients with untreated celiac disease. Reviews of the large volume of literature on celiac disease are available (Goldstein and Heiner, 1970; Hekkens and Pena, 1974; McNicholl et al., 1978; Kasarda, 1978, 1981; Lebenthal and Branski, 1981; Goodwin and Rawcliffe, 1983).

3. *Mechanisms of Celiac Disease*

There are several not mutually exclusive hypotheses for the mechanism of celiac disease (Goodwin and Rawcliffe, 1983). In the first mechanism, it is suggested (Frazer et al., 1959; Townley et al., 1973) that a specific mucosal peptidase deficiency allows accumulation of harmful amounts of a toxic partial gluten digest. This hypothesis has been modified to suggest that an abnormal, rather than deficient, peptidase is present, which catalyzes the formation of a toxic gluten peptide (Yeoman, 1974; Cordone et al., 1975). The second theory suggests that reaction to the disease is the outcome of an immunological response or cell-mediated delayed hypersensitivity to wheat gluten in the jejunal mucosa.

An additional hypothesis suggests that gluten-induced damage depends on the material acting as a lectin (Weiser and Douglas, 1976). Either of these theories may be correct and, particularly in the case of the immunological changes, it is uncertain whether they are the cause or a result of the disease (Goodwin and Rawcliffe, 1983).

4. *Treatment*

Strict, lifelong adherence to a gluten-free diet is the basic treatment. Wheat, rye, oats, barley, and their byproducts must be removed from the diet. When these grains are removed, the small intestine is able to repair most of the damage. Often, within days after gluten is removed from the diet, the cells in the intestinal lining begin to heal, symptoms become less severe, test values revert to normal, and subsequent biopsies of the small intestinal mucosa show the villi reverting to normal (Hartsook, 1984).

Celiac children gain weight rapidly after being placed on a gluten-free diet, as was shown by Shmerling (1967). Weight and height of a 22-month-old girl reached average values for her age within a relatively short period of time. Various recipes have been devised using nontoxic cereal grain products (Nilson, 1974; Nishita et al., 1976; Brümmer and Stephan, 1981). Furthermore, a range of gluten-free foods, formulated specifically for celiacs, is now generally available, distinguished by a gluten-free symbol.

5. *Breeding Nontoxic Wheat*

Assuming that α-gliadin is the most toxic protein for celiacs, Kasarda et al. (1978) produced nullisomic 6A-tetrasomic 6B Chinese Spring wheat, which lacks the genes for α-gliadin. Bread made from it was fed to celiac patients. Initial results with a few celiacs were encouraging because they were largely free of symptoms for 2 weeks. However, longer evaluation of six celiacs showed that even this genetically tailored wheat retained considerable toxicity for celiacs (Kasarda, 1981). Jos et al. (1977) provided evidence, on the basis of in vitro studies of the effects of peptides derived from purified gliadin fractions on cultured epithelial tissues from celiac patients, that both α- and β-gliadins were definitely toxic, that γ-gliadins were toxic, although possibly less so than α- and β-gliadins, and that ω-gliadins were either nontoxic or weakly toxic. If many different gliadins coded on several different chromosomes are toxic, it will be difficult to remove all toxic factors from wheat.

These experiments strengthen the likelihood that many different grain proteins are responsible for celiac condition and that breeding a wheat that lacks these proteins may be impossible. Likewise, consideration has been given to breeding cereal varieties that would not cause IgE-mediated allergies (Wrigley, 1982) by identifying the grain proteins responsible. Unfortunately, this seems unattainable at present because of the diversity of proteins involved and the variation in allergenic proteins from one individual to another (Baldo and Wrigley, 1984).

B. Schizophrenia

Schizophrenia is a psychosis characterized by a loss of contact with reality. It is accompanied by delusions, hallucinations, disturbances in thinking and communication, and deteriorating social functioning. It is *not* a "split personality." Basically, a schizophrenic cannot tell the difference between what is real and what is not real (American Psychiatric Association, 1987).

Schizophrenia usually starts to show up between the ages of 15 and 25. Epidemiological studies show that schizophrenia begins earlier in males than in females. The onset and first hospitalization for schizophrenic males peak while they are in their early twenties. Women are usually first diagnosed and hospitalized for schizophrenia in their late twenties and early thirties. Also, the lowest socioeconomic groups typically have the highest rates of schizophrenia (Garfield, 1983).

1. *Involvement of Cereal Proteins*

The causes of schizophrenia are unknown, except that genetic factors, which probably act in conjunction with environmental factors, are involved (Singh and Kay, 1976). Dohan et al. (1969) suggested that the condition may be genetically linked with celiac disease and that cereal grain proteins may be pathogenic in schizophrenics.

Celiac disease appears to occur in at least 1 in 100 schizophrenics compared to 1 in 3000 in the general population (Dohan, 1969). The evidence relating celiac disease and schizophrenia is based largely on clinical observations. Bossak et al. (1957) found 5 psychotic patients among 94 patients with nontropical sprue. Graff and Handford (1961) found a history of childhood celiac disease in 4 of 37 men entering a hospital for the first time with schizophrenia. Emotional disturbances, which occur frequently in patients with celiac disease, are alleviated when the patients are placed on a gluten-free diet (Sheldon, 1959).

Data collected by Dohan (1966) show a high statistical correlation between the annual consumption of wheat and the number of first admissions of women for schizophrenia to mental hospitals in Finland, Sweden, Norway, Canada, and the United States ($r = 0.96$; $p < 0.01$). The high correlation of the percent changes in wheat plus rye consumption with the first admissions for schizophrenia (Table 8), suggests that cereals may be involved in the pathogenesis of schizophrenia.

Standardized prevalence rates for schizophrenia derived from more than 50 published reports comparing consumption of wheat, rye, and barley are shown in Figure 1. These data (Dohan et al., 1980) are from published surveys of 45 populations. Rates from multiple studies of the same location were averaged. Schizophrenia rates were standardized using the number of individuals over 14–15 years old as the population base. Consumption data for wheat, rye, and barley were taken from national or local statistics near the time of the prevalence survey. The populations eating 51–140 kg/person/yr of wheat, rye, and barley were all located in countries with Western-type cultures except for one prevalence study in rural Korea where diet surveys indicate an intake of about 75 kg/person/yr of barley plus wheat. Populations eating

Table 8 Wheat Consumption and First Hospital Admission of Schizophrenic Women

Country	Year(s)	First hospital admission for schizophrenia	Consumption of wheat or wheat and rye flour
United States	1939	9,557	70.5[b]
	1940–1942	10,230	70.1[b]
	1943–1945	10,943	74.6[b]
Canada	1937–1939	814	84.0[b]
	1940–1942	721	75.0[b]
	1943–1945	871	84.6[b]
Sweden	1937–1939	938	732.2[c]
	1940–1942	654	481.3[c]
	1943–1945	608	458.5[c]
Norway	1936–1940	332	299.6[c]
	1941–1945	201	123.4[c]
Finland	1936–1939	1,217[a]	69.5[d]
	1940–1942	1,107[a]	60.9[d]
	1943–1945	832[a]	48.0[d]

[a]Readmissions included.
[b]Wheat and rye flour (kg/person/yr); rye flour < 1.4% of total.
[c]Wheat production plus import minus seed and export (10 million kg/country/harvest year).
[d]Wheat (kg/capita/harvest year).
Source: Adapted from Dohan, 1966.

<50 kg/person/yr of wheat, rye, and barley were located in Japan, Taiwan, Africa, and Micronesia.

In populations eating little or no wheat, rye, and barley, the prevalence of schizophrenia is quite low. Dietary studies to test this hypothesis were conducted by Dohan et al. (1969) with males in a locked psychiatric ward where strict control of access to food was possible. The number of days each patient was confined to the locked ward before release to an open ward provided an index of the rate of improvement. All patients admitted to the locked ward during study period one (175 days) were assigned to either a milk- and cereal-free diet or a high-cereal diet. During the second study period (143 days), all patients were randomly assigned to either the high-cereal diet or the cereal-free diet, to which wheat gluten (approximately 19 g/day) was secretly added. The results of this study showed that the mean length of stay in the locked ward was 17.3 days for the cereal-free group and 30.6 days for the high-cereal group. When gluten was secretly added during study period two, this difference did not occur.

Discharge from the hospital during the first 90 days after admission was more than twice as high for schizophrenics assigned to a cereal- and milk-free diet than for those on a high-cereal diet, as shown in Table 9. Dohan and Grasberger (1973) observed that the average time until discharge for the cereal- and milk-free patients (77 days) was 55% that of the high-cereal patient (139 days).

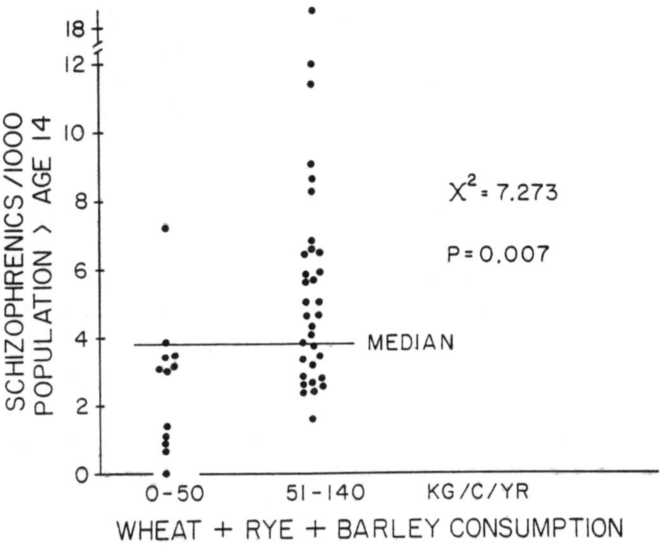

Figure 1 Standardized prevalence rates for schizophrenia vs. consumption of wheat + rye + barley. Data are from published prevalence surveys of 45 populations. Prevalence rates have been standardized using the number of individuals over 15 years old as the population base. Populations eating 51–140 kg/person/yr are from Western-type cultures—Australia, European Russia. Populations eating <50 kg/person/yr are from Japan, Taiwan, Africa, and Micronesia. (From Dohan et al., 1980.)

Table 9 Effect of Diet (Cereal- and Milk-free vs. High-Cereal) on Hospital Discharge of Schizophrenic Men

Days after admission	Cereal- and milk-free diet,[a] discharged patients (cumulative)		High-cereal diet,[b] discharged patients (cumulative)	
	Number	%	Number	%
30	6	10.2	2	3.6
60	17	28.8	7	12.5
90	22	37.2	9	16.1
120	24	40.7	12	21.4
150	26	44.1	12	21.4
180	27	45.8	15	26.8
360	30	50.8	22	39.3

[a]N = 59.
[b]N = 56.
Source: Adapted from Dohan and Grasberger, 1973.

A study by Singh and Kay (1976) with 14 schizophrenics confirmed the earlier findings of Dohan et al. (1969) and Dohan and Grasberger (1973). Patients on a cereal grain–free and milk-free diet were observed drug-free for the first 2 weeks of the study and then were placed on neuroleptic medication for 12 weeks. During the period on medication, a drink containing Kool-Aid® powder, dextrose, water, and soy flour (30 g/day) was added to the diet during weeks 3–6 and 11–14 of the study. During weeks 7–10, the test substance, wheat gluten (30–45 g/day), was substituted for soy flour. Thus, the study involved a period of wheat gluten challenge along the course of the treatment. Singh and Kay (1976) hypothesized that if wheat gluten were pathogenic to schizophrenics, the therapeutic course would be interrupted or reversed during the period of gluten challenge. Results of the study showed that wheat gluten aggravated the schizophrenic process and diminished responses to treatment. The therapeutic progress resumed its course after gluten was withdrawn and patients were returned to soy flour drinks. Schizophrenic exacerbation was particularly marked in the more seriously ill patients. Singh and Kay (1976) admit that their data do not exclude the possibility that the gluten effect was due to the inhibition of neuroleptic absorption or changes in neuroleptic metabolism, but they believe this to be unlikely.

The studies cited here support the hypothesis that ingestion of cereals may be pathogenic for those with the genotype for schizophrenia. The irregular response of celiac patients to ingestion or avoidance of gluten and the occasional severe reaction to a small amount seem to require consideration in similar studies on schizophrenic patients.

There are, however, several published studies in which no correlation between ingestion of gluten and schizophrenia could be established. Davis (1978) studied a small number of schizophrenics and detected no changes in mental state that could be attributed to either a gluten load or to a gluten-free diet. Potkin et al. (1981) failed to detect any behavioral changes after gluten challenge in eight young chronic cases of schizophrenia, who remained on a cereal-free, milk-free diet throughout the study.

Some investigators found that wheat gluten in the diet may even ameliorate the mental state of some schizophrenic patients or may have no effect (Osborne et al., 1982; Storms et al., 1982). Patients in the Storms et al. (1982) study on a locked ward were placed on a cereal- and milk-free diet. Thirteen schizophrenics were given gluten-free, peanut flour–supplemented cookies, and 13 were given virtually identical cookies with gluten added. The schizophrenics on a cereal- and milk-free diet with no gluten added to their peanut flour cookies showed no greater improvement than the schizophrenics who received 30 g of gluten daily in their cookies. In fact, the subjects with gluten added to their cookies improved significantly more ($p < 0.01$) on measures of tension-anxiety and anger-hostility. Subjects were on this diet for only 10 days, and this time may have been too short for any beneficial effects of the diet to occur.

2. *Gluten and Schizophrenia Hypothesis*

Ingested wheat gluten appears to be without psychotoxic effects in those not genetically susceptible to gluten-evoked disorders. Gluten overload, in doses

5–10 times the usual daily intake, given for weeks to healthy soldiers was not associated with significant change in mood or physical symptoms (Levine et al., 1966).

In persons genetically susceptible, there appears to be, however, a relationship between gluten and schizophrenia (Ross-Smith and Jenner, 1980). There is evidence indicating that large as well as small peptides pass the gut and other barriers in laboratory animals and humans (Matthews, 1975; Hemmings, 1978). Gluten polypeptides have been shown to be absorbed through the gut in rodents (Hemmings et al., 1976). Normal adult humans probably do not absorb such polypeptides to any significant degree (Kowlessar et al., 1970), but the possibility that such an absorption may occur in schizophrenics has been suggested (Dohan, 1978). Dohan (1980) postulated that abnormal genes responsible for an increased passage of specific peptides from glutens across the gut barrier to the gut lamina propria (a site of the enhanced immune response in celiacs) are present in schizophrenics and that these abnormal genes impairing the gut barrier to gluten peptides might, among many possibilities, code for defective cell membranes or enzymes. He proposed that neuroactive peptides produced during digestion of some food proteins are the cause of symptoms in schizophrenics and that gluten is the most important source of these neuroactive peptides. These peptides reach the brain cells of schizophrenics in symptom-producing amounts because of genetically defective gut and other barriers (e.g., membrane receptors, enzymes) to their passage from gut lumen to brain cells (Dohan, 1978, 1980) (Fig. 2). These hypotheses are not incompatible with the numerous genetically governed brain disorders (e.g., phenylketonuria) caused by food-derived substances.

The work of Huebner et al. (1984) confirmed the presence of peptides in gluten protein digests that exhibited high activity in binding to sites in brain tissues with which narcotics, such as morphine or peptides having endorphin activity, are associated. To locate the protein component that contained peptides with the highest opioid activity, they, therefore, fractionated the gluten proteins by solubility to obtain saline-soluble gliadin and glutenin fractions.

Necessary Environmental Factor	+	Abnormal Genes (Major Effect)	------->	Brain Function
Neuroactive Peptides Produced during Digestion of Food Proteins (e.g. cereal grain glutens)		Defective Gut (possibly other barrier systems; e.g. membrane receptors, enzymes)		Variety of Abnormal Behavior

Figure 2 Mode of action of polypeptides from food in producing schizophrenia. (Modified from Dohan, 1980.)

Table 10 Opioidlike Activity of Peptide Fractions from Different Wheat Proteins

Protein fraction	Peptide fraction	Sensitivity (mg peptide/nM morphine)
Glutenin	1	15.4
	2	9.0
	3	28.6
Gliadin A	1	33.3
	2	21.7
	3	2.3
Gliadin B	1	6.5
	2	2.9
	3	2.0
	4	0.31
Gliadin C	1	4.6
	2	1.7
	3	7.5

Source: Adapted from Huebner et al., 1984.

Highest activity was found in gliadin A (Table 10). There is the possibility that peptides with high activity are also present in glutenin. Earlier work by Huebner and Wall (1974) and by Bietz and Wall (1980) demonstrated that more than 40% of glutenin consists of gliadinlike alcohol-soluble proteins.

Extrapolation of these findings suggests that reduction or elimination of gluten consumption could reduce or even eliminate hospital admission for schizophrenia (Rudin, 1981). This extrapolation is predicted on the assumption that the sole or major environmental cause of schizophrenia is the consumption of gluten. Combining this assumption with genetic findings, one would modify the proposition by saying that evidently the major cause of schizophrenia is the consumption of gluten by those with genetic sensitivity to gluten.

For a comprehensive review of the relationship between cereals and schizophrenia, the reader is referred to an article by Lorenz (1990).

VI. CONCLUSION

As the world population increases, there is an ever-increasing demand for the supply of food available. Cereals will assume even greater importance in human nutrition than they do today.

Some known or alleged harmful effects are caused by cereal products; the vast majority of humans experience none of these problems. Some of the alleged intolerances to cereal have yet to be established as valid. Nevertheless, further investigation is important to help the minority of intolerant individuals and also to indirectly learn more about the chemistry and biology of cereal grains.

REFERENCES

Alvey, C., Anderson, C. M., and Freeman, M. (1957). Wheat gluten and celiac disease. *Arch. Dis. Child. 32*: 434.

Alun-Jones, V., McLaughlan, P., Shorthouse, M., Workman, E., and Hunter, J. O. (1982). Food intolerance: A major factor in the pathogenesis of irritable bowel syndrome. *Lancet 2*: 1115–1117.

American Psychiatric Association (1987). *Diagnostic and Statistical Manual of Mental Disorders*, 3rd ed., rev. The American Psychiatric Association, Washington, DC.

Anderson, C. M., Frazer, A. C., French, J. M., Gerrard, J. W., Sammonds, H. G., and Smellie, J. M. (1952). Celiac disease: Gastrointestinal studies and the effect of dietary wheat flour. *Lancet 1*: 836.

Anderson, H., Levine, A. J., and Levitt, M. D. (1981). Incomplete adsorption of the carbohydrates in all-purpose wheat flour. *New Engl. J. Med. 304*: 891–892.

Baagoe, K. H. (1933). Mehlidiosynkrasie als Ursache von vasomotorischer Rhinitis und Asthma. *Klin. Wochenschr. 12*: 792.

Baldo, B. A., and Pepys, J. (1976). Radioallergosorbent test (RAST) studies with insolubilized poplysaccharides. *Clin. Allergy 6*: 563–571.

Baldo, B. A., and Wrigley, C. W. (1978). IgE antibodies to wheat flour components. Studies with sera from subjects with bakers' asthma and coeliac condition. *Clin. Allergy 8*: 109–124.

Baldo, B. A., and Wrigley, C. W. (1984). Allergies to cereal. In *Advances in Cereal Science and Technology*, Vol. 6. Y. Pomeranz, ed. American Association of Cereal Chemists, St. Paul, MN, chapter 5.

Baldo, B. A., Krilis, S., and Wrigley, C. W. (1980). Hypersensitivity to inhaled flour allergens. Comparisons between cereals. *Allergy 35*: 45–56.

Baldo, B. A., Sutton, R., and Wrigley, C. W. (1982). Grass allergens, with particular reference to cereals. *Prog. Allergy 30*: 1–66.

Bartschi, R., and Regli, J. (1969). Chronic bronchitis in a rural area and its prognosis. *Respiration 26*: 231–238.

Bietz, J. A., and Wall, J. S. (1980). Identity of high molecular weight gliadin and ethanol soluble glutenin subunits of wheat: Relation to gluten structure. *Cereal Chem. 57*: 415–421.

Bjorksten, F., Backman, R., Jarvinen, K. A. J., Lehti, H., Savilahti, E., Yvanen, P., and Karkkainen, T. (1977). Immunoglobulin E specific to wheat and rye flour proteins. *Clin. Allergy 7*: 473–483.

Blands, J., Diamant, B., Kallos, P., Kallos-Deffner, L., and Lowenstein, H. (1976). Flour allergy in bakers. *Int. Arch. Allergy Appl. Immunol. 52*: 392–406.

Bonnevie, P. (1958). Occupational allergy in bakery. In *Occupational Allergy*, Stenfert-Kroese, Leiden, p. 161.

Bossak, E. T., Wang, C. I., and Adlersberg, D. I. (1957). Clinical aspects of the malabsorption syndrome. In *The Malabsorption Syndrome*, Adlersberg, D. I., ed. Grune and Stratton, New York, p. 112.

Bronstein, H. D., Haeffner, L. J., and Kowlessar, O. D. (1966). Enzymatic digestion of gliadin; the effect of the resultant peptides in adult celiac disease. *Clin. Chim. Acta 14*: 141.

Brooks, S. M. (1977). Bronchial asthma of occupational origin: A review. *Scand. J. Work Environ. Health 3*: 53–72.

Brümmer, J. M., and Stephan, H. (1981). Gliadinfreie Brote. *Dtsch. Lebensm. Rundsch.* 77: 60–62.

Chan-Yeung, M., Ashley, M. J., and Grzybowski, S. (1978). Grain dust and the lungs. *Can. Med. Assoc. J. 118*: 1271–1274.

Cohen, V. L., and Osgood, H. (1953). Disability due to inhalation of grain dust. *J. Allergy 24*: 193–211.

Cordone, G., Gemme, G., Comelli, A., Vianello, M. G., and Calodoni, S. (1975). Peptidase and coeliac disease. *Lancet 1*: 807–808.

Davis, C. (1978). Dietary pathogenesis of schizophrenia: An investigation into the effects of gluten. *Nursing Times 74*: 2020–2021.

De Besche, A. (1929). Serologische Untersuchugen über allergische Krankheiten. *Acta Pathol. Microbiol. Scand. 6*: 115–238.

Dicke, W. K. (1950). Coeliakie. M.D. thesis, Utrecht, Holland.

Dicke, W. K., Weijers, H. A., and van de Kamer, J. H. (1953). Celiac disease. II. The presence in wheat of a factor having a deleterious effect in cases of celiac disease. *Acta Paediatr.* (Stockholm) *42*: 34.

Dickerson, J. W. T., Ballantine, L., and Hastrop, L. (1978). Food allergy. *Lancet 1*: 773.

Dohan, F. C. (1966). Cereals and schizophrenia: Data and hypothesis. *Acta Psychiatr. Scand. 42*: 125–132.

Dohan, F. C. (1969). Is celiac disease a clue to the pathogenesis of schizophrenia? *Mental Hygiene 53*: 525–539.

Dohan, F. C. (1972). Cereal grains: A pathogenic factor common to celiac disease and schizophrenia. *Am. J. Clin. Nutr. 25*: 455–456.

Dohan, F. C. (1976). The possible pathogenic effect of cereal grains in schizophrenia. *Acta Neurol. 31*: 195–205.

Dohan, F. C. (1978). Are some food-derived polypeptides pathogenic? Coeliac disease as a model. In *The Biological Basis of Schizophrenia*, G. and W. A. Hemmings, eds. MTP Press, Lancaster, England, pp. 167–178.

Dohan, F. C. (1980). Hypothesis: Genes and neuroactive peptides from food as cause of schizophrenia. In *Neural Peptides and Neuronal Communication*, E. Costa and M. Trabucchi, eds. Raven Press, New York, pp. 535–548.

Dohan, F. C., and Grasberger, J. C. (1973). Relapsed schizophrenics: Early discharge from the hospital after cereal-free, milk-free diet. *Am. J. Psychiatry 130*: 685–688.

Dohan, F. C., Grasberger, J. C., Lowell, F. M., Johnston, H. T., and Arbegast, A. W. (1969). Relapsed schizophrenics: More rapid improvement on a milk and cereal-free diet. *Br. J. Psychiatry 115*: 595–596.

Dohan, F. C., Harper, E. H., and Lorenz, K. (1980). Schizophrenia: Variations in prevalence rates vs. differences in cereal grain consumption. Soc. Biol. Psychiatry Ann. Mtg., Boston, Sept. 5–7, 1980.

DoPico, G. A., Reddan, W., Flaherty, D., Tsiastis, A., Peters, M. E., Rao, P., and Rankin, J. (1977). Respiratory abnormalities among grain handlers. A clinical, physiologic and immunologic study. *Am. Rev. Resp. Dis. 115*: 915–927.

Dunner, L., Hermon, R., and Bagnall, D. J. T. (1946). Pneumoconiosis in dockers dealing with grain and seeds. *Br. J. Radiol. 19*: 506–511.

Frazer, A. C. (1956). Discussion on some problems of steatorrhea and reduced stature. *Proc. R. Soc. Med. 49*: 1009.

Frazer, A. C. (1962). The malabsorption syndrome with special reference to the effect to wheat gluten. *Adv. Clin. Chem. 5*: 69.

Frazer, A. C., Fletcher, R. F., Ross, C. A. C., Shaw, B., Sammonds, H. G., and Schneider, R. (1959). Gluten-induced enteropathy; the effect of partially digested gluten. *Lancet 2*: 252.

Gandevia, B. (1980). Australian experience of grain dust exposure, 1961–1962. In *Occupational Pulmonary Disease, Focus on Grain Dust and Health*, J. A. Dosman and D. J. Cotton, eds. Academic Press, New York, pp. 391–398.

Gandevia, B., and Ritchie, B. (1966). Relevance of respiratory symptoms and signs to ventilatory capacity changes after exposure to grian dust and phosphate rock dust. *Br. J. Ind. Med. 23*: 181–187.
Garfield, E. (1983). What do we know about the group of mental disorders called schizophrenia? Part I: Etiology. *Current Contents 25*: 5–11.
Goldstein, G. B., and Heiner, C. E. (1970). Clinical and immunological perspectives in food sensitivity. A review. *J. Allergy 46*: 270–291.
Goodwin, B. F. J., and Rawcliffe, P. M. (1983). Food allergies associated with cereal products. *Food Chem. 11*: 321–338.
Graff, H., and Handford, A. (1961). Celiac syndrome in the case histories of five schizophrenics. *Psychiat. Quart. 35*: 306–313.
Grant, E. C. G. (1980). Food and migraine. *Nutr. Food Sci. 65*: 10–11.
Hartsook, E. I. (1984). Celiac sprue: Sensitivity to gliadin. *Cereal Foods World 29*(2): 157–158.
Heiner, D. C., Lahey, M. E., and Wilson, J. F. (1964). Precipitins to wheat gliadin in the study of celiac disease. *Am. J. Dig. Dis. 9*: 786.
Hekkens, W. T. J. M., and Pena, A. S., eds. (1974). *Coeliac Disease*. Stenfert Kroese, Leiden.
Hemmings, W. A. (1978). The entry into the brain of large molecules derived from dietary protein. *Proc. Royal Soc. 200*: 175–192.
Hemmings, C., Hemmings, W. A., and Williams, E. W. (1976). Immunological assay for antigen in tissues following feeding of labelled alpha-gliadin to suckling and adult rats. *IRCS Med. Sci. 4*: 458.
Hendeles, L., and Weinberger, M. (1979). Guidelines for avoidiing theophylline overdose. *N. Engl. J. Med. 300*: 1217.
Herxheimer, H. (1973). The skin sensitivity to flour of bakers' apprentices. *Acta Allergol. 28*: 42–49.
Huebner, F. R., and Wall, J. S. (1974). Wheat glutenin subunits. I. Preparative separation by gel-filtration and ion-exchange chromatography. *Cereal Chem. 52*: 228–239.
Huebner, F. R., Lieberman, K. W., Rubino, R. P., and Wall, J. S. (1984). Demonstration of high opioid-like activity in isolated peptides from wheat gluten hydrolysates. *Peptides 5*(6): 1139–1147.
Jarvinen, K., Pirila, V., Bjorksten, F., Keskinen, H., Lehtinen, M., and Stubb, S. (1979). Unsuitability of bakery work for a person with atopy: A study of 234 bakery workers. *Ann. Allergy 42*: 192–195.
Jimenez-Diaz, C., and Canto, G. (1947). The allergens of mill dust. Asthma in millers, farmers and others. *Ann. Allergy 5*: 519–525.
Jos, J., Lenoir, G., De Ritis, G., and Rey, J. (1977). Isolation and characterization of the toxic fraction of wheat gliadin in coeliac disease. In *Perspectives in Coeliac Disease*, McNicholl, B., McCarthy, C. F., and Fottrell, P. E., eds. University Park Press, Baltimore, MD, pp. 75–89.
Kallos, P., and Kallos-Deffner, L. (1971). Flour allergy in bakers. In 75th Congr. Trade Union of Swedish Food Workers, Stockholm, p. 182.
Kasarda, D. D. (1972). Celiac disease. Malabsorption of nutrients induced by a toxic fractor in gluten. *Bakers Dig. 46*(6): 25.
Kasarda, D. D. (1975). Celiac disease: Malabsorption of nutrients induced by toxic fraction in gluten. In *Protein Nutritional Quality of Foods and Feeds*, Friedman, M., ed. Marcel Dekker, New York, pp. 565–593.
Kasarda, D. D. (1978). The relationship of wheat proteins to coeliac disease. *Cereal Foods World 23*: 240–244, 262.

Kasarda, D. D. (1981). Toxic proteins and peptides in coeliac disease: Relations to cereal genetics. In *Food, Nutrition and Evolution*, D. Walcher and N. Kretchmer, eds. Masson Publishing USA Inc., New York, pp. 201–216.

Kasarda, D. D., Bernardin, J. E., and Nimmo, C. C. (1976). Wheat proteins. In *Advances in Cereal Science and Technology*, Pomeranz, Y., ed. American Association of Chemists, St. Paul, MN, pp. 158–236.

Kasarda, P., Qualset, C. O., Mecham, D. K., Goodenberger, D. M., and Strober, W. (1978). A test of toxicity of bread made from wheat lacking α-gliadins coded for by the 6A chromosome. In *Perspectives in Coeliac Disease*, B. McNicholls, C. F. McCarthy, and P. F. Fottrell, eds. MTP Press, Lancaster, England, pp. 55–62.

Käser, H. (1961). Diagnose and Klinik der Coeliakie. *Ann. Paediat.* (Basel) *197*: 320–334.

Kelson, S. G., Kelson, D. P., Fleegler, B. F., Jones, R. C., and Rodman, T. (1978). Emergency room assessment and treatment of patients with acute asthma. *Am. J. Med. 64*: 622–629.

Keskinen, H., Alanko, K., and Saarinen, L. (1978). Occupational asthma in Finland. *Clin. Allergy 8*: 569–579.

Kleinfield, M. (1974). A comparative clinical and pulmonary function study of grain handlers and bakers. *Ann. N.Y. Acad. Sci. 221*: 86–96.

Kowlessar, O. D. (1972). Dietary gluten sensitivity updated. *J. Am. Diet. Assoc. 60*: 475.

Kowlessar, O. D., Warren, R. E., and Bronstein, H. D. (1970). Celiac disease: Enzyme defect or immune mechanisms. In *Progress in Gastroenterology*, Vol. II, G. B. J. Glass, ed. Grune and Stratton, New York, pp. 409–429

Lai, F. S., Pomeranz, Y., Miller, B. S., Martin, C. R., Aldis, D. F., and Chang, C. S. (1981). Status of research on grain dust. In *Advances in Cereal Science and Technology*, Vol. 4, Y. Pomeranz, ed. American Association Cereal Chemists, St. Paul, MN, pp. 237–337.

Lebenthal, E., and Branski, D. (1981). Childhood coeliac disease—A reappraisal. *J. Ped. 98*: 681–690.

Lefcoe, N. M., and Wonnacott, T. H. (1974). Chronic respiratory disease in four occupational groups. *Arch. Environ. Health 29*: 143–146.

Levine, R. A., Briggs, G. W., Harding, R. S., and Nolte, L. B. (1966). Prolonged gluten administration in normal subjects. *N. Engl. J. Med. 274*: 1109–1114.

Lewis, W. H., and Imber, W. E. (1975). Allergy epidemiology in the St. Louis, Missouri Area. V. Cereal ingestants. *Ann. Allergy 35*: 251.

Linko, E. (1947). On allergic rhinitis and bronchial asthma in bakers. *Ann. Med. Intern. Fenn. 36*: 98–111.

Lorenz, K. (1990). Cereals and schizophrenia. In *Advances in Cereal Science and Technology*, Y. Pomeranz, ed. American Association of Cereal Chemists, St. Paul, Vol. X, Chapter 7.

Matthews, D. M. (1975). Absorption of peptides by mammalian intestine. In *Peptide Transport in Protein Nutrition*, D. M. Matthews and J. W. Payne, eds. Elsevier, New York, pp. 61–146.

McNicholl, B., McCarthy, C. F., and Fottrell, P. F. (1978). *Perspectives in Coeliac Disease*. MTP Press, Lancaster, England.

Messer, M., Anderson, C. M., and Hubbard, H. (1964). Studies on the mechanism of destruction of the toxic action of wheat gluten in celiac disease by crede papain. *Gut 5*: 295.

Monro, J., Brostoff, J., Carini, C., and Zilkha, K. (1980). Food allergy in migraine. Study of dietary exclusion and RAST. *Lancet 2*: 1–4.

Moulton, A. L. (1959). The place of oats in the celiac diet. *Arch. Dis. Child. 34*: 51.

Najera, A. L., and Dantin, G. J. (1930). *Arch. Mal. Prof. Hyg. Toxicol. Ind., 2*: 337.

Nakazawa, T., Shimomura, Y., Higuchi, T., Kuramochi, G., Yamanda, M., Kobayashi, S., and Shichijo, K. (1972). Inhalative bronchial asthma caused by wheat flour. *Jap. J. Allergol. 21*: 13.

Nakazawa, T., Toyoda, T., Furukawa, M., Taya, T., and Kobayaski, S. (1976). Inhibitory effects of various drugs on dual asthmatic responses in wheat-flour sensitive subjects. *J. Allergy Clin. Immunol. 58*: 1–9.

Nilson, G., ed. (1974). *The Coeliac Handbook*. The Coeliac Society, London.

Nishita, K. D., Roberts, R. L., and Bean, M. M. (1976). Development of a yeast-leavened rice-break formula. *Cereal Chem. 53*: 626–635.

Ordman, D. (1958). Cereal grain dust as a cause of respiratory allergy in South Africa. *S. Afr. Med. J. 32*: 784–788.

Osborne, M., Crayton, J. W., Javaid, J., and Davis, J. M. (1982). Lack of effect of a gluten-free diet on neuroleptic blood levels in schizophrenic patients. *Biol. Psychiatry 17*: 627–629.

Pang, L. M., Rodriguez-Martinez, F., Davis, W. J., and Mellins, R. B. (1977). Terbutaline in the treatment of status asthmaticus. *Chest 72*: 469–473.

Piafsky, K. M., and Ogilvie, R. I. (1975). Dosage of theophylline in bronchial asthma. *N. Engl. J. Med. 292*: 1218–1222.

Pinto, S. S. (1942). Grain dust as occupational hazard. *Neb. Med. J. 26*: 60.

Potkin, S. G., Weinberger, D., Kleinman, J., Nasrallah, H., Luchins, D., Bigelow, L., Linnoila, M., Fischer, S. H., Fjornsson, R. D., Carman, J., Gillin, J., and Wyatt, R. J. (1981). Wheat gluten challenge in schizophrenic patients. *Am. J. Psychiatry 138*: 1208–1211.

Rankin, J., DoPico, G. A., Reddan, W. G., and Tsiatis, A. (1979). Respiratory disease in grain handlers. In *Proc. Int. Symp. on Grain Dust*, B. S. Miller and Y. Pomeranz, eds. Oct. 2–4, Kansas State University, Manhattan, KS, p. 91.

Rastelli, G., and Brambilla, F. (1937). *Med. Lav. 28*: 321, 357.

Rice, J. R., Ham, C. H., and Gore, W. E. (1978). Another look at gluten in schizophrenia. *Am. J. Psychiatry 135*: 1417–1418.

Rosenlund, M. L. (1970). What is celiac disease? *Cliln. Pediatr. 9*: 695.

Ross, I. N., Thompson, R. A., Montgomery, R. D., and Asquith, P. (1978). Immunoglobulin staining in the skin of patients with gastrointestinal disease: Specificity and significance of IgA depositioin in dermatitis herpetiformis. In *Perspectives of Coeliac Disease*. B. McNicholl, C. F. McCarthy, and P. R. Fottrell, eds. MTP Press, Lancaster, England, pp. 217–266.

Ross-Smith, P., and Jenner, F. A. (1980). Diet (gluten) and schizophrenia. *J. Human Nutr. 34*: 107–112.

Rubin, C. E., Brandborg, L. L., Flick, A., MacDonald, W. C., Parkins, R. A., Parmentier, C. M., Phelps, P., Sribhibhadh, S., and Trier, J. S. (1962). In *Intestinal Biopsy*, Wolsenholme, G. E. W., and Cameron, M. P., eds. Little, Brown, Boston, p. 67.

Rubin, W. (1971). Celiac disease. *Am. J. Clin. Nutr. 24*: 91.

Rudin, D. O. (1981). The choroid plexus and system disease in mental illness. III. Peptide hypothesis of mental illness. *Biol. Psychiatry 1605*: 489–512.

Salen, E. B., and Juhlin-Dannfeldt, C. (1935). Über das Vorkommen von sogenannter latenter Allergie. *Acta Med. Scand. 86*: 505–569.

Saxelby, C., and Venn-Brown, U. (1980). *The Role of Australian Flour and Bread in Health and Nutrition*. Bread Research Institute of Australia, Sydney.

Schwartz, M. (1947). Flour allergy. *J. Allergy 18*: 341–350.

Scott, B. B., and Losowsky, M. S. (1978). Gluten antibodies in coeliac disease and dermatitis herpetiformis. In *Perspectives in Coeliac Disease*, B. McNicholl, C. F. McCarthy, and P. F. Fottrell, eds. MTP Press, Lancaster, England, pp. 365–367.

Sheldon, W. (1959). Celiac disease. *Pediatrics 23*: 132.

Shmerling, D. H. (1967). Die glutenfreie Ernährung bei Coliakie. *Schweiz. Med. Wochenschr. 97*(22): 706.
Singh, M. M., and Kay, S. R. (1976). Wheat gluten as a pathogenic factor in schizophrenia. *Science 191*: 401–402.
Smith, A. R., Greenburg, L., and Siegel, W. (1941). Respiratory disease among grain handlers. *Ind. Bull. N.Y. State Dep. Labor 20*: 33–36.
Stenhammer, L., and Johansson, C. G. (1981). The incidence of coeliac disease in children in south-east Sweden. *Acta Paediatr. Scand. 70*: 379–381.
Storms, L. H., Clopton, J. M., and Wright, G. (1982). Effects of gluten on schizophrenics. *Arch. Gen. Psychiatry 39*: 323–327.
Thiel, H., and Ulmer, W. T. (1980). Bakers' asthma: Development and possibility for treatment. *Chest 78*: 4005–4055.
Townley, R. R., and Anderson, C. M. (1967). Coeliac disease—A review. *Ergebnisse in der Med. Kinderheilkunde 26*: 1–44.
Townley, R. R. W., Bhathal, P. S., Cornell, H. J., and Mitchell, J. D. (1973). Toxicity of wheat gliadin fractions in coeliac disease. *Lancet 1*: 1363–1364.
Tse, C. S. T., and Raghuprasad, P. K. (1982). Baker's asthma (grain-dust-induced asthma). *Drug Intell. Clin. Pharm. 16*: 14–18.
Tse, K. S., Warren, P., Janusz, M., McCarthy, D. S., and Cherniack, R. M. (1973). Respiratory abnormalities in workers exposed to grain dust. *Arch. Environ. Health 27*: 74–77.
Urbach, E., and Gottlieb, P. M. (1943). *Allergy*. Grune and Stratton, New York, pp. 323, 344, 355, 357, 375.
Van Dishoeck, H. A. E., and Roux, D. J. (1939). Sensitization to flour and flour illness among flour workers. *J. Hyg. 39*: 674–679.
Weinstein, W. M., Piercey, J. R. A., and Dossetor, J. B. (1974). Dermatitis herpetiformis and coeliac sprue. In Coeliac disease, *Proc. Int. Coeliac Symp.*, 2nd ed. W. T. S. M. Hekkens and A. S. Pena, eds. Stenfort Kroese, Leiden, pp. 361–373.
Weiser, M. M., and Douglas, A. P. (1976). An alternative mechanism for gluten toxicity in coeliac disease. *Lancet 1*: 567–569.
Williams, N., Skoulas, A., and Merriman, J. E. (1964). Exposure to grain dust. I. A survey of effects. *J. Occup. Med. 6*: 319–329.
Wrigley, C. W. (1982). The use of genetics in understanding protein composition and grain quality in wheat. *Qual. Plant. Plant Foods Hum. Nutr. 31*: 205–227.
Yeoman, N. D. (1974). Pathogenesis of coeliac sprue. *Lancet 1*: 843–844.

V

SEAFOOD

15

Symptoms and Treatment of Common Seafood Poisonings

Joseph I. Smith*

U.S. Army Medical Research Institute of Infectious Diseases, Fort Detrick, Frederick, Maryland

I. CIGUATOXIN

Ciguatoxin is a lipid-soluble, heat-resistant, acid-stable, nonprotein toxin that is produced by a single-celled, free-swimming marine dinoflagellate of the species *Gambierdiscus toxicus*. Reports of possible ciguatera intoxication date back to Egypt between 2700 and 2400 B.C. In 1492, Columbus reported a clinical case while exploring the Caribbean. In 1789, Captain Bligh almost succumbed to fish poisoning in Tahiti after the mutiny aboard his HMS Bounty (Halstead, 1965a).

In 1978, ciguatera intoxication in the United States accounted for 12.3% of food poisoning cases reported to the Centers for Disease Control (CDC), and it is presently the most frequent reported fishborne intoxication worldwide (CDC, 1985). From 1983 to 1987, 87 outbreaks and 332 cases were reported to the CDC with no deaths (CDC, 1990). The predominant intoxications were from semitropical areas such as Hawaii, the Virgin Islands, Puerto Rico, and Florida (Lawrence et al., 1980; CDC, 1981, 1982; Engleberg et al., 1983; Holt

*The views of the author do not purport to reflect the position of the Department of the Army or the Department of Defense.

et al., 1984). Significant outbreaks have also occurred in nontropical states due to the shipment of fish from endemic areas (CDC, 1980a, 1986a). It is not uncommon for patients living outside the high endemic areas to have ciguatera intoxication diagnosed as another disease, such as multiple sclerosis, which has signs easily confused with the acute intoxication by ciguatera. A psychosomatic/conversion disorder may also be hard to differentiate from chronic intoxication (Heimbecker, 1979; Schatz, 1989).

Over 400 species of fish, most commonly species of herbivorous and carnivorous reef fish, harbor the toxin. The toxin enters the food chain when the dinoflagellate attaches itself to marine algae, which are consumed by small, herbivorous fish. The herbivorous fish are then consumed by larger carnivorous fish. Surgeonfish, parrotfish, jackfish, barracuda, moray eel, mackerel, grouper, snapper, and sea bass commonly contain the toxin (Halstead, 1965b, 1967b, 1970; Schultz, 1983; Rodgers and Muench, 1986). The reef diver's adage "Never eat a fish bigger than your frying pan" is a sound approach to avoiding intoxication. This is based upon the toxin becoming more concentrated as it passes through the food chain. Besides the viscera, toxin is also present in the blood, flesh, gonads, gills, heart, skin, and bones of fish, yet fish do not display signs of intoxication (Vernoux et al., 1985). Cooking does not inactivate ciguatoxin or the coexisting toxins, scaritoxin and maitotoxin.

Ciguatoxin opens the voltage-dependent sodium channels in the cell membrane of nerve and muscle by competitively inhibiting calcium regulation of passive cell membrane (Rayner, 1972; Bagnis et al., 1979; Emerson et al., 1983). The sodium-potassium ATP pump is not affected.

Clinical manifestations of ciguatera intoxication usually begin within 1–6 hr after ingestion of contaminated fish; however, signs can occur within several minutes if a large quantity of toxin is consumed. Initial signs are nausea, vomiting, watery nonbloody diarrhea, abdominal pain, and cramping. Circumoral or facial paresthesia and numbness, which proceed to the extremities, may follow. In certain ethnic groups, the signs of paresthesia, which do not follow dermatomal patterns can precede the gastrointestinal signs (Bagnis et al., 1979; Sims, 1987). Cold-to-hot sensory reversal dysesthesia (cold objects are burning or painful to touch) developing 2–5 days after intoxication is considered by some to be pathognomonic. The median duration of the paresthesia and dyesthesia is 17 days. Weakness, dizziness, dry mouth, blurred vision, photophobia, transient blindness, myalgia, and arthralgia are common. Sharp, shooting pains in the extremities and sensations of looseness and pain in the teeth have also been reported. Either generalized pruritus or localized itching may present; fatigue and malaise that can last for weeks usually follow. In severe cases, fatigue may persist for years. Clinical findings can be either nonexistent or manifested as cranial nerve palsies, dilation of the pupils, strabismus, ptosis, hypotension (with or without sinus bradycardia), or varying degrees of atrioventricular block. In severe intoxication or reintoxication, circulatory collapse (shock), acute respiratory failure, and coma may occur (Bagnis et al., 1979; Sims, 1987; Lee, 1980; McGuigan, 1981a; Chretien et al., 1981; Morris et al., 1982; Withers, 1982; Pearn et al., 1982; van der Sar, 1982; Pearce et al., 1983; Johnson and Jong, 1983; Lewis, 1986; Hamburger, 1986).

Treatment is supportive. The use of emetics, gastric lavage, and activated charcoal is only effective in patients with paresthesia and with residual contaminated food products within their stomach and duodenum. Intravenous normal saline is indicated for patients who present with protracted vomiting and diarrhea or hypotension and/or shock. If severe bradycardia develops, intravenous atropine (0.01 mg/kg) is indicated. A single clinical report indicates that mannitol (20% i.v., 1 g/kg, 500 ml/hr) was effective in reversing the neurological and gastrointestinal signs (Palafox et al., 1988). Treatment may have to be repeated after several hours of observation. One explanation of the possible or probable mechanism of action of mannitol on ciguatera intoxication is competitive inhibition with the toxin in sodium channels and neutralization of the toxin (Palafox et al., 1988). Dopamine (5–20 μg/kg/min) and calcium gluconate (3–5 g/24 hr) infusions have been successful in treating severe hypotension and shock (Sims, 1987). Although no controlled clinical trials have been conducted, oral amitriptyline (25 mg twice a day) or oral tocainide (400 mg three times a day) may be useful in treating protracted paresthesia, dysesthesia, and pruritus (Bowman, 1984; Davis and Villar, 1986; Lang et al., 1988).

Management of chronic ciguatera fish poisoning has been a difficult problem. No effective drug therapy is presently available. Psychotherapy plays an important role in helping the patient live with the disability. The prevention of reintoxication is an important consideration because a small amount of toxin can cause exacerbation of the disease. A diet free of fish, shellfish, alcohol, and nuts has been advocated for 3–6 months after acute ciguatera poisoning and lifelong for patients suffering from the chronic form of the disease (Sims, 1987).

II. TETRODOTOXIN-TARICHATOXIN

Tetrodotoxin is a naturally occurring toxin found in a variety of animals; the most notable is the pufferfish (Mosher et al., 1964; Halstead, 1967a, 1978; Noguchi and Hashimoto, 1973; Kim et al., 1975; Sheumack et al., 1978).

Tetrodotoxism commonly follows the consumption of the flesh, viscera, skin, liver, and/or ovary of the pufferfish (*Diodron hystrix*), or "Fugu." Although not commonly consumed by man, the eggs of the California newt (*Taricha*), porcupine fish, ocean sunfish, triggerfish, and boxfish are also sources of tetrodotoxin. The affected fish do not suffer any obvious ill effects from carrying the toxin. It has been suggested that the toxin is secreted by the pufferfish exocrine glands, acting as a natural defense mechanism to repel predators (Kodama et al., 1985; Saito et al., 1985). In female pufferfish, the ovaries are the principal site of toxin concentration, and female fish contain more toxin than males. The level of toxin in the female also appears to be related to the spawning season. In Japan, pufferfish poisoning presents the highest risk of severe intoxication from March through June during the spawning season, when the toxin level is highest.

Severe cases of intoxication have up to a 60% mortality rate in Japan where Fugu is considered a delicacy (Sims and Ostman, 1986). Pufferfish poisoning may also become more common in the United States with the opening of a Fugu restaurant in New York City (Hill, 1982).

Accounts of pufferfish intoxication date back to the Egyptian experience in the years 2700 to 2400 B.C. (Mills and Passmore, 1988). Captain James Cook provided one of the first accounts of what some believe to be tetrodotoxism from the pufferfish (Beaglehole, 1961). The more recent Japanese clinical and management experience reports over 6000 cases over 82 years (Fuhrman, 1986).

The toxin is heat-stable and is not inactivated by cooking the affected animal flesh, viscera, gonads, liver, or skin. The toxin selectively blocks the sodium channel, thus interfering with the propagation of nerve action potential (Narahashi, 1972; Kao, 1972). It appears that tetrodotoxin receptors are located at the sodium channel of the external nerve axon cell membrane (Kao and Yeoh, 1978).

The initial signs of tetrodotoxism usually begin with circumoral paresthesia. Nonspecific signs such as nausea, vomiting, and diarrhea commonly precede the sign of paresthesia. The onset of signs usually begins within 3 hr after ingesting the toxin-containing organ, although this could vary from 10 min to 15 hr, depending on the quantity of toxin consumed. Other common complaints include headache, diaphoresis, unusual taste sensation with hypersalivation, generalized muscle weakness, myalgia, lethargy, floating sensation, and progressive numbness of the entire body. If the signs of paresthesia progress from the lip, tongue, and oropharynx to the distal extremities, this diagnosis should be considered.

Clinical signs associated with intoxication include dysarthria, dysphagia, hyperemesis, progressive weakness, ataxia, hypersalivation, progressive ascending paralysis, loss of deep tendon reflex, cranial nerve dysfunction, muscle fasciculations, cardiac arrhythmia (particularly sinus bradycardia), hypotension (shock), and acute respiratory failure with associated cyanosis, pallor, and dyspnea (Tahara, 1910; Yokoo, 1950; Goldfrank et al., 1981; Lyn, 1985; Kodama et al., 1985; Sims, 1987; Lang, 1990).

Differential diagnosis included paralytic shellfish poisoning and ciguatera fish poisoning, as well as organic phosphate intoxication. In paralytic shellfish poisoning, hypotension may be present, but is not a hallmark of the intoxication as with tetrodotoxin, which directly affects the vascular smooth muscle and the neurovascular innervation of blood vessels. In ciguatera poisoning, nausea, vomiting, diarrhea, and abdominal pain followed by paresthesia are among the first presenting signs.

Treatment is supportive. If emesis or hyperemesis has not already been induced by the toxin, an emetic should be administered. Residual toxin in the stomach can be removed by gastric lavage with particular care taken to prevent aspiration. Lavage with 2% sodium bicarbonate during the first hour of treatment may be useful in neutralizing residual toxin within the stomach (Yokoo, 1950; Kodama et al., 1985). More aggressive therapy includes endoscopy to remove ingested toxin from the proximal small bowel (Goldfrank et al., 1981). Activated charcoal is effective in binding the toxin, thus preventing further gastrointestinal absorption. Following lavage, charcoal should be administered by nasogastric tube (Tahara, 1910; Kodama et al., 1985). At present there is no commercial source of anti-tetrodotoxin-immune IgG globulin or monoclonal antibody to bind the absorbed but yet unbound toxin within the circulation (Huot et al., 1989b).

General supportive care will depend on signs and symptoms. Early intubation with ventilatory assistance and oxygen supplementation has also been reported to increase survival (Torda et al., 1973; Lyn, 1985; Lang, 1990). For hypotension (shock) and reduced cardiac output, which are results of suppression of cardiac contraction and dilatation of peripheral blood vessels, use of intravenous normal saline should first be used and if the patient is unresponsive, dopamine (Intropin) drip should be started. If the patient is unresponsive to fluids and dopamine, a trial of ephedrine (1 mg/kg) may prove beneficial (Kuno et al., 1988). Since bradycardia is commonly present, intravenous atropine (starting with a dose of 0.5 mg followed by 0.01–0.02 mg/kg every 5 min, maximum dose 1.0 mg/kg) is indicated until resolved. Edrophonium (Enlon and Tensilon), pyridostigmine (Mestinon and Regonol), calcium, and neostigmine (Prostigmin) have all been advocated, but there have been no controlled clinical trials to prove their usefulness. Antihistamine and corticosteroids have not proven useful (Lyn, 1985; Lang, 1990). If the patient survives beyond 24 hr, recovery from the intoxication can be expected.

III. SAXITOXIN-NEOSAXITOXIN-GONYATOXIN

Saxitoxin, neosaxitoxin, and gonyatoxin are heat-resistant, water-soluble neurotoxins found in shellfish contaminated with dinoflagellates. The most common cause of paralytic shellfish intoxication occurs when humans consume shellfish (mussels, clams, oysters, scallops, and univalve mollusks) contaminated with toxins stored in their hepatopancreas. Starfish and sand crabs may also contain the toxins (Halstead and Courville, 1965).

Saxidomas giganteus, the Alaska butter clam, provides the origin of the designation saxitoxin. The term gonyatoxin is derived from the dinoflagellate *Gonyaulax catanella*, a protozoan contaminating the shellfish. The habitat for the dinoflagellate ranges from tropic to polar seas. When concentrations of the protozoa in seawater become relatively high (20,000 cells/ml), a visible bloom (red tide) may occur. Some blooms may contain 50,000 or more organisms per ml. A concentration of as little as 200 protozoa/ml in seawater results in toxic shellfish. Shellfish can filter up to 20 liters of water per day and, in continuous contact with the red tide, can ingest 3.0 g dry weight of the protozoa in 24 hr and can contain as much as 180 mg of toxin per g. Levels > 8 μg of the toxin per 100 g of shellfish meat are considered unsafe for consumption (Shantz, 1975).

Paralytic shellfish poisoning is a worldwide problem in temperate coastal areas. The actual number of cases per year is unknown, but some authors suggest an estimated incidence of 1600 cases with possibly 300 deaths per year (Sims and Ostman, 1986; Haddad et al., 1987). The endemic areas of the United States include Alaska, California, Maine, and Oregon. Worldwide, the endemic areas include Canada, England, Scotland, Ireland, Norway, Germany, Belgium, France, Japan, Mexico, Malaysia, South Africa, Taiwan, and Venezuela (Sims and Ostman, 1986; Haddad et al., 1987). Recently, in a significant epidemic along the coast of Guatemala, 187 people became intoxicated and 26 died. During the initial phase of the epidemic, intravenous atropine was administered because organic phosphate poisoning was initially suspected in several patients who died. It was later discovered that saxitoxin B-1 was the cause of intoxication (Rodrigue et al., 1990). It is not known if the administration of atropine complicated the clinical presentation or treatment.

The problem of red tides and possible paralytic shellfish poisoning dates back to 1491 B.C., the time of Moses: "And all the waters that were in the river were turned to blood" (Morse, 1977). The Greeks named the Red Sea and probably derived the name from the red tide (Morse, 1977). The first clinical description of paralytic shellfish poisoning was in 1689 (Vancouver, 1798). Captain George Vancouver experienced the problem of paralytic shellfish poisoning during his exploration of the Pacific Northwest in 1793 (CDC, 1976). In 1927, a series of outbreaks and deaths in the San Francisco Bay area stimulated modern research in paralytic shellfish poisoning (Meyer et al., 1928).

Cooking shellfish contaminated with the paralytic toxins for 5 min reduces the toxin level by 30%, and only 40% when shellfish are cooked for 20 min. The toxin binds to a receptor site on the external surface of an excitable membrane and blocks transient sodium channels of the membranes in nerves and muscles with no effect on the neuromuscular synapse (Narahashi, 1972; Kao, 1972; Kao and Yeoh, 1978). Death results from respiratory failure through direct peripheral action by the toxins on the respiratory muscles. The medulla shows no evidence of impairment. The toxin can also lower mean arterial blood pressure and suppress conduction in the atrioventricular node (Evans, 1965; Acres and Gray, 1978). A dose as low as 5 mg (mouse units) of toxin can produce signs. A dose of 30 mg has been associated with death in adults, whereas ingestion of only 3 mg can be fatal to infants and young children (Hughes and Merson, 1976; Blanc et al., 1977; Zwahlen et al., 1977; Roy, 1977; Rodrigue et al., 1990).

The onset of symptoms usually occurs within 3 hr of ingestion of the toxic shellfish, although this can vary between 15 min to 10 hr depending on the quantity of ingested toxin and other factors such as age and weight of the patient, alcohol consumption, and source of contamination (broth, meat, etc.). Paresthesia of the gums, tongue, lips, and face with the sensation of constriction of the throat are the first presenting signs. Incoherent speech and aphonia along with paresthesia are seen in all of the cases reported and are pathognomonic. The paresthesia progresses to the neck and extremities in most patients. This is accompanied by dizziness, ataxia, dysmetria, and a floating sensation (cerebellar syndrome). Paresis or paralysis follows. With the onset of respiratory paralysis, cyanosis ensues. Abdominal distention with urinary retention is seen on physical examination. In half of the patients who survive the intoxication, asthenia and moderate memory loss occur for up to 3 weeks. Other signs include weakness, malaise, prostration, headache, hypersalivation, intense thirst, perspiration, dysphagia, myalgia, tachycardia, abdominal cramps, nausea, vomiting, diarrhea, and anuria. Most intoxicated patients remain calm and conscious. Death occurs within 2–25 hr or the patient recovers. Survival for 12–18 hr is a good prognostic sign (McCollum et al., 1968; Rhodes et al., 1975; Hughes and Merson, 1976; Blanc et al., 1977; Zwahlen et al., 1977; Roy, 1977; CDC, 1978; Popkiss et al., 1979; McGuigan, 1981c; CDC, 1983).

Differential diagnosis includes tetrodotoxism, which produces similar symptoms; circumoral paresthesia; hypersalivation; a floating sensation; progressive numbness from face to extremities; nausea; vomiting; and diarrhea; because of tetrodotoxin's direct effect on vascular smooth muscle and the neurovascular innervation of blood vessels producing generalized vasodilation, severe hypotension (shock) is a hallmark. Severe ciguatera intoxication also needs to be considered in the differential diagnosis in patients who present atypically with gastrointestinal signs. As with the recent Guatemalan experience, organic phosphate intoxication should also be considered in the differential diagnosis (Rodrigue et al., 1990).

Treatment is supportive. The use of emetics and gastric lavage to remove residual contaminated food particles as well as alkalinization of the remaining gastric contents with sodium bicarbonate are worthwhile treatments during the first hour after ingestion. Charcoal slurries have been advocated to neutralize toxin that remains in the stomach and to prevent absorption. Although no controlled clinical trials have been conducted, the use of activated charcoal hemoperfusion may also be effective in inactivating the circulating toxin (Rand et al., 1977). Because the toxin is unstable in an alkaline environment, the use of sodium bicarbonate i.v. is recommended (Rumack, 1986). In severe intoxication, intubation and mechanical ventilation for 24–48 hr has increased survival rates (Acres and Gray, 1978; Popkiss et al., 1979). Some have advocated the uses of neostigmine to aid in artificial respiration and oxime (Paralidoxime) to reactivate acetylcholine (Roy, 1977). Monoclonal antibodies and IgG immune globulin for use in the treatment of the intoxication are still under development (Davio, 1985; Hewetson et al., 1988; Huot et al., 1989a).

IV. SCOMBROTOXIN

Scombrotoxism is a syndrome that results from ingesting spoiled fish belonging to the families Scombridae and Scombresocidae (Kahn, 1971). The most affected fish are tuna, bonito, skipjack, saury, and mackerel. Mahi-mahi, yellowtail, bluefish, amberjack, herring, sardines, and anchovies can also cause the syndrome (Kim, 1979; Pugno et al., 1983; Etkind et al., 1987). In a recent well-documented outbreak of scombrotoxism, marlin was identified as the contaminated fish (Morrow et al., 1991).

The heat-stable, histamine-like substance is formed as a result of interaction of the fish enzymes and the bacteria *Proteus, Morganella*, and *Klebsiella* when the dead fish is improperly refrigerated (Lerke et al., 1978; Murray and Hobbs, 1982). These bacterial enzymes also cause decarboxylation of histidine to histamine.

Most often diagnosed as a fish allergy, scombroid intoxication is becoming a significant form of seafood poisoning. Scombroid intoxication accounted for 4.5% of the cases of foodborne disease outbreaks reported to the CDC between

1978 and 1982 (CDC, 1985). From 1983 to 1987, 83 outbreaks and 306 cases of scombroid intoxication were reported to the CDC with no deaths (CDC, 1990). Most of the cases of poisoning reported to the CDC in the United States were from coastal areas, but outbreaks have occurred in noncoastal areas due to shipment of fish from endemic areas (CDC, 1980b, 1986b, 1989; Nosanchuk et al., 1982).

Besides histamine-like substances (saurine), histamine is commonly present in fish (Henion et al., 1981). Concentrations of histamine > 20 mg/100 mg of fish can cause the signs (CDC, 1980c). It is not clear how histamine causes these signs, as ingested histamine is usually neutralized in the intestine and produces no ill effects in humans. Saurine and histamine are heat stable; therefore, cooking does not inactivate them. A recent study demonstrated histamine and *N*-methylhistamine at high concentrations in the urine of patients intoxicated by ingesting contaminated fish. Thus, histamine, whether exogenous or endogenous, may be the cause of the intoxication (Morrow et al., 1991).

Scombroid intoxication presents within 2–16 hr after ingestion of the contaminated fish, although signs could be manifested in minutes if large quantities of toxin are present. The initial signs usually begin with skin flushing of the face and neck, headache, burning sensation of the throat, and palpations. These can be accompanied by nausea, diarrhea, abdominal pain, bronchospasm, and, less commonly, vomiting. Physical findings include a sunburn-like rash on the face and neck, rapid pulse, wheezing, and mild hypotension (CDC, 1980c; McGuigan, 1981b; Borysiewicz and Krikler, 1981; Dickerson, 1982; Russell and Maretic, 1986; Taylor et al., 1989).

Because the intoxication is not fatal, treatment is symptomatic, and if left untreated, the signs will usually resolve within 12–24 hr. To reduce signs, gastric emptying and catharsis are recommended along with intravenous administration of 300 mg of cimetidine given over 5–10 min (Blakesley, 1983). Because the toxin binds both H_1 and H_2 receptors, the use of H_1 antagonist, such as diphenhydramine (Benadryl) (50 mg i.v. along with H_2 antagonist cimetidine), should relieve signs within 30 min (Roberts et al., 1979). Epinephrine, corticosteroids, and aminophylline have been used when significant bronchospasm is present (Dickerson, 1982). Aerosolized metaproterenol sulfate (Alupent) may be more effective than aminophylline in reducing the bronchospasm.

V. BREVETOXIN

Brevetoxin is a lipid-soluble, heat-stable neurotoxin found in shellfish contaminated by the dinoflagellate *Ptychodiscus brevis*. Brevetoxin stimulates postganglionic cholinergic nerve fibers and sodium channels and inhibits neuromuscular transmission in skeletal muscle (Asai et al., 1982; Pierce, 1984). Also known as neurotoxic shellfish poisoning, epidemics have occurred along the coast of Florida, as well as along the Gulf of Mexico, the Caribbean Sea, and the coast of Spain (Steidinger and Joyce, 1973; Baden, 1983).

Since 1884, more than 35 episodes of red tide have been reported along the Florida coastline with the characteristic discolored water containing the dinoflagellate and dead or dying fish. The toxin is a human respiratory irritant when aerosolized by the surf, causing reversible rhinorrhea, conjunctivitis, and cough (Steidinger and Joyce, 1973; Asai et al., 1982; Baden, 1983). The predominant season for outbreaks of red tide and, thus, epidemics of neurotoxic shellfish poisoning, as well as irritative aerosolized dinoflagellate respiratory disease, is between January and April (Baden, 1983).

Oysters, clams, and coquina are the most common shellfish to filter the dinoflagellate and store the toxin in the hepatopancreas. The feeding shellfish can become toxic after being exposed during a red tide bloom of <5000 protozoan cells per ml of seawater.

Brevetoxin is lethal to fish and is responsible for massive fish kills. Despite the fish lethality (LD_{50} 0.2–0.5 mg/kg), there have been no human deaths reported in Florida since 1844, when the intoxication was first described (Baden, 1983). Symptoms usually begin 1–3 hr after ingestion of the contaminated shellfish, but this depends on the quantity of toxin ingested. The earliest symptom is paresthesia of the oral pharynx. Digital paresthesia may follow as well as ataxia, vomiting, and diarrhea along with hot-to-cold temperature reversal phenomena. Physical findings include mydriasis and bradycardia (Baden, 1983).

Differential diagnosis includes ciguatera intoxication and paralytic shellfish poisoning. Although ciguatera and neurotropic shellfish poisoning share hot-to-cold temperature reversal phenomena, in ciguatera poisoning, the onset is generally 2–3 days after intoxication, whereas in brevetoxin poisoning it is within the first 24 hr. In paralytic shellfish poisoning, symptoms and physical findings are similar to neurotropic shellfish poisoning but are more severe and accompanied by respiratory paralysis, which is not seen in brevetoxin intoxication. Rapid diagnosis methods to differentiate the two toxins are under development (Hewetson et al., 1988; Poli and Hewetson, 1990).

As the intoxication does not produce paralysis and respiratory failure and recovery usually occur in 2–3 days, treatment is symptomatic. Intravenous fluids are indicated for dehydration resulting from vomiting and diarrhea. Intravenous atropine is indicated to reverse symptomatic bradycardia. The patient needs to be reassured that the intoxication is self-limiting and that he or she will recover completely.

REFERENCES

Acres, J., and Gray, J. (1978). Paralytic shellfish poisoning. *Can. Med. Assoc. J. 119*: 1195–1197.

Asai, S., Krzanowski, J., Anderson, W., et al. (1982). Effects of the toxin red tide, *Ptychodiscus brevis*, on canine tracheal smooth muscle: a possible new asthma-triggering mechanism. *J. Allergy Clin. Immunol. 69*: 418–428.

Baden, D. G. (1983). Marine foodborne dinoflagellate toxins. *Int. Rev. Cyst. 82*: 99–150.

Bagnis, R., Kuberski, T., and Laugier, S. (1979). Clinical observations on 3009 cases of ciguatera fish poisoning in the South Pacific. *Am. J. Trop. Med. Hyg. 28*: 1067–1073.

Beaglehole, J. C., ed. (1961). The journals of Captain James Cook on his voyages of discovery. In *The Voyages of the Resolution and Adventure, 1772–1775*. Cambridge University Press, Cambridge, pp. 534–535.

Blakesley, M. (1983). Scombroid poisoning: Prompt resolution of symptoms with cimetidine. *Ann. Emerg. Med. 12*: 104–106.

Blanc, M. H., Zwahlen, A., and Robert, M. (1977). Symptoms of shellfish poisoning. *N. Engl. J. Med. 196*: 287–288.

Borysiewicz, L., and Krikler, D. (1981). Scombrotoxic atrial flutter. *Br. Med. J. 282*: 1434.

Bowman, P. (1984). Amitriptyline and ciguatera. *Med. J. Aust. 143*: 802.

Centers for Disease Control. (1976). Paralytic shellfish poisoning: New Brunswick, Canada. *MMWR 25*: 347–348.

Centers for Disease Control. (1978). Paralytic shellfish poisoning—Washington. *MMWR 27*: 416–417.

Centers for Disease Control. (1980a). Ciguatera fish poisoning—Maryland. *MMWR 29*: 610–611.

Centers for Disease Control. (1980b). Scombroid fish poisoning—Illlinois. *MMWR 29*: 167–168.

Centers for Disease Control. (1980c). Scombroid poisoning—New Jersey. *MMWR 29*: 106–107.

Centers for Disease Control. (1981). Ciguatera fish poisoning—St. Croix, Virgin Islands U.S. *MMWR 30*: 130–139.

Centers for Disease Control. (1982). Ciguatera fish poisoning—Bahamas, Miami. *MMWR 31*: 391–392.

Centers for Disease Control. (1983). Annual mussel quarantine—California. *MMWR 32*: 281.

Centers for Disease Control. (1985). *Food-borne Disease Outbreaks: Annual Summary 1982*. Centers for Disease Control, Atlanta, GA, 1985.

Centers for Disease Control. (1986a). Ciguatera fish poisoning—Vermont. *MMWR 35*: 263–264.

Centers for Disease Control. (1986b). Restaurant-associated scombroid fish poisoning—Alabama, Tennessee. *MMWR 35*: 264–265.

Centers for Disease Control. (1989). Scombroid fish poisoning—Illinois, South Carolina. *MMWR 38*: 140–142, 147.

Centers for Disease Control. (1990). Waterborne disease outbreaks, 1986–1988, Food-borne disease outbreaks, 5-year summary, 1983–1987. *MMWR 39*: 15–57.

Chretien, J., Fermaglich, J., and Garagusi, V. (1981). Ciguatera poisoning presentation as a neurologic disorder. *Arch. Neuro. 15*: 1225–1228.

Davio, S. R. (1985). Neutralization of saxitoxin by anti-saxitoxin rabbit serum. *Toxicon. 23*: 669–675.

Davis, R. T., and Villar, L. A. (1986). Symptomatic improvement with amitriptyline in ciguatera fish poisoning. (Let.) *N. Engl. J. Med. 315*: 65.

Dickerson, G. (1982). Scombroid fish poisoning syndrome. *Ann. Emerg. Med. 11*: 487–489.

Emerson, D., Galbraith, R., McMillan, J., and Higerd, T. (1983). Preliminary immunologic studies of ciguatera poisoning. *Arch. Intern. Med. 143*: 1931–1933.

Engleberg, N., Morris, J., Lewis, J., McMillan, J., and Pollard, R. (1983). Ciguatera fish poisoning: A major common-source outbreak in the U.S. Virgin Islands. *Ann. Intern. Med. 98*: 336–337.

Etkind, P., Wilson, M., Gallagher, K., and Cournoyer, J. (1987). Bluefish-associated scombroid poisoning. *JAMA 258*: 3409–3410.

Evans, M. H. (1965). Cause of death in experimental paralytic shellfish poisoning. *Br. J. Exp. Pathol. 46*: 245–253.

Fuhrman, F. A. (1986). Tetrodotoxin, tarichatoxin, chiriquitoxin: Historical perspectives. *Ann. NY Acad. Sci. 479*: 1–14.

Goldfrank, L., Lewin, N., and Wiesman, R. (1981). The red snapper. *Hosp. Physician 5*: 36–51.

Haddad, L., Lee, R., McConnel, O., et al. (1987). Toxic marine life. In *Clinical Management of Poisoning and Drug Overdose*, L. Haddad and B. Winchester, eds. W. B. Saunders Co., Philadelphia, pp. 303–317.

Halstead, B. W. (1965a). *Poisonous and Venomous Marine Animals of the World*, U.S. Government Printing Office, Washington, DC, vol. 1, pp. 1–155.

Halstead, B. W. (1965b). *Poisonous and Venomous Marine Animals of the World*. U.S. Government Printing Office, Washington, DC, vol. 1, pp. 157–269.

Halstead, B. W. (1967a). *Poisonous and Venomous Marine Animals of the World*. U.S. Government Printing Office, Washington, DC, vol. 2, pp. 679–901.

Halstead, B. W. (1967b). *Poisonous and Venomous Marine Animals of the World*. U.S. Government Printing Office, Washington, DC, vol. 2, pp. 1–1070.

Halstead, B. W. (1970). *Poisonous and Venomous Marine Animals of the World*. U.S. Government Printing Office, Washington, DC, vol. 3, pp. 857–884.

Halstead, B. W. (1978). *Poisonous and Venomous Marine Animals of the World*. Darwin Press, Princeton, NJ, pp. 437–548.

Halstead, B. W., and Courville, D. A. (1965). *Poisonous and Venomous Marine Animals of the World*. U.S. Government Printing Office, Washington, DC, pp. 157–270.

Hamberger, H. (1986). The neuro-ophthalmologic signs of ciguatera poisoning: A case report. *Ann. Ophthalmol. 18*: 287–288.

Heimbecker, R. O. (1979). Ciguatera poisoning—snowbirds beware [Editorial]. *Can. Med. Assoc. J. 120*: 637–638.

Henion, J., Nosanchuk, J., and Bilder, B. (1981). Capillary gas chromatographic mass-spectrum determination of histamine in tuna fish causing scombroid poisoning. *J. Chromatogr. 213*: 475–480.

Hewetson, J. F., Hall, S. E., Smith, J. I., and Beheler, J. E. (1988). Comparison of ELISA and sodium channel assay for detection of paralytic shellfish poisoning in clams and clinical specimens from intoxicated individuals. *Proc. Abst. FASEB 2*: A373.

Hill, N. J . (1982). A gourmet's gamble (tetrodon poisoning). *Oceans 15*(2): 12–14.

Holt, R., Miro, G., and DelValle, A. (1984). An analysis of poison control center reports of ciguatera toxicity in Puerto Rico for one year. *Clin. Toxicol. 22*: 177–185.

Hughes, J., and Merson, M. (1976). Fish and shellfish poisoning. *N. Engl. J. Med. 295*: 1117–1120.

Huot, R. I., Armstrong, D. L., and Chanh, T. C. (1989a). In vitro and in situ inhibition of sodium channel blocker saxitoxin by monoclonal antibodies. *J. Tox. Environ. Health 27*: 381–393.

Huot, R. I., Armstrong, D. L., and Chanh, T. C. (1989b). Protection against nerve toxicity by monoclonal antibodies to the sodium channel blocker tetrodotoxin. *J. Clin. Invest. 83*: 1821–1826.

Johnson, R., and Jong, E. (1983). Ciguatera: Caribbean and Indo-Pacific fish poisoning. *West. J. Med. 138*: 872–874.

Kahn, E. (1971). Perspective of tuna fish. *N. Engl. J. Med. 285*: 49–50.

Kao, C. Y. (1972). Pharmacology of tetrodotoxin and saxitoxin. *Fed. Proc. 31*: 1117–1213.

Kao, C. Y., and Yeoh, P. H. (1978). Different receptors for saxitoxin. *Proc. Physiol. Soc. 284*: 88P–89P.

Kim, R. (1979). Flushing syndrome to small mahimahi (scombroid fish) poisoning. *Arch. Dermatol. 115*: 963–965.

Kim, Y. H., Brown, B. G., Mosher, F. S., et al. (1975). Tetrodotoxin: Occurrence in atelopid frogs in Costa Rica. *Science 189*: 151–152.

Kodama, M., Ogata, T., and Sato, S. (1985). External secretion of tetrodotoxin from puffer fishes stimulated by electric shock. *Mar. Bio.* [Berl] *87*: 199–202.

Kuno, M., Goto, K., Oka, S., Negishi, H., Hosoyamada, A., and Inada, Y. (1988). The effect of tetrodotoxin on cardiovascular dynamics. *Jpn. J. Anesthesiol. 37*: 530–535.

Lang, W. R. (1990). Puffer fish poisoning. *Am. Fam. Physician 42*(4): 1029–1033.

Lang, W. R., Kreider, S. D., Hattwick, M., and Hobbs, J. (1988). Potential benefit of tocainide in the treatment of ciguatera: Report of 3 cases. *Am. J. Med. 84*: 1087–1088.

Lawrence, D., Enriquez, M., Lumish, R., and Maceo, A. (1980). Ciguatera fish poisoning in Miami. *JAMA 244*: 254–258.

Lee, C. (1980). Fish poisoning with particular reference to ciguatera. *J. Trop. Med. Hyg. 83*: 93–97.

Lerke, P. A., Werner, S. B., Taylor, S. L., et al. (1978). Scombroid poisoning. *West. J. Med. 129*: 381–386.

Lewis, N. (1986). Disease and development: Ciguatera fish poisoning. *Soc. Sci. Med. 23*: 983–993.

Lyn, P. C. (1985). Puffer fish poisoning: Four case reports. *Med. J. Malaysia 40*: 31–34.

McCollum, J. P. K., Pearson, R. C. M., Ingham, H. R., Wood, P. C., and Dewar, H. A. (1968). An epidemic of mussel poisoning in North-East England. *Lancet 2*: 767–770.

McGuigan, M. (1981a). Ciguatera. *Clin. Toxicol. Rev. 3*: 1–2.

McGuigan, M. (1981b). Scombroid fish poisoning. *Clin. Toxicol. Rev. 3*: 1–2.

McGuigan, M. (1981c). Shellfish poisoning. *Clin. Toxicol. Rev. 3*: 12.

Meyer, K. F., Sommer, H., and Schoenholz, P. (1928). Mussel poisoning. *J. Prev. Med. 2*: 365–394.

Mills, A. R., and Passmore, R. (1988). Pelagic paralysis. *Lancet 1* (8578): 161–164.

Morris, J. G., Lewin, P., Hargrett, N. T., Smith, C. W., Blake, P. A., and Schneider, R. (1982). Clinical features of ciguatera fish poisoning: A study of the disease in the U.S. Virgin Islands. *Arch. Intern. Med. 142*: 1990–1992.

Morse, E. V. (1977). Paralytic shellfish poisoning: A review. *JAVMA 171*(11): 1178–1180.

Morrow, J. D., Margolies, G. R., Rowland, J., and Roberts, L. J. (1991). Evidence that histamine is the causative toxin of scombroid-fish poisoning. *N. Engl. J. Med. 324*: 716–720.

Mosher, H. S., Fuhrman, F. A., Buckwald, H. D., et al. (1964). Tarichatoxin-tetrodotoxin, a potent neurotoxin. *Science 144*: 100–110.

Murray, C., and Hobbs, G. (1982). Scombrotoxin and scombrotoxin-like poisoning from canned fish. *J. Hyg. 88*: 215–219.

Narahashi, T. (1972). Mechanism of action of tetrodotoxin and saxitoxin on excitable membranes. *Fed. Proc. 31*: 1124–1132.

Noguchi, T., and Hashimoto, Y. (1973). Isolation of tetrodotoxin from a gorby, *Gobius criniger*. *Toxicon 11*: 305–307.

Nosanchuk, J., Bilder, B., and Henion, J. (1982). Scombroid fish poisoning in central New York State. *NY State J. Med. 82*: 202–203.

Palafox, N., Jain, L., Pinano, A., Gulick, T., Williams, R., and Schatz, I. (1988). Successful treatment of ciguatera fish poisoning with intravenous mannitol. *JAMA 259*: 2740–2742.

Pearce, R., Hines, C., Burns, T., and Clark, C. (1983). Ciguatera (fish poisoning). *South. Med. J. 76*: 560–561.

Pearn, J., Harvey, P., DeAmbrosis, W., Lewis, R., and McKay, R. (1982). Ciguatera and pregnancy. *Med. J. Aust. 1*: 57–58.

Pierce, R. (1984). Red tide (*Ptychodiscus brevis*) toxin aerosols: A review. *Toxicon 22*: 381–385.

Poli, M. A., and Hewetson, J. F. (1990). Antibody production and development of a radioimmunoassay for the PbTx-2-type brevetoxins. *Proceedings of Third International Conference on Ciguatera Fish Poisoning*, in press.

Popkiss, M. E. E., Horstman, D. A., and Harpur, D. (1979). Paralytic shellfish poisoning: A report of 17 cases in Cape Town. *S. Afr. Med. J. 55*: 1017–1023.

Pugno, P., Kaufman, D., and Feder, H. (1983). Bluefish: A newly discovered cause of scombroid poisoning. *J. Fam. Pract. 17*: 1071–1081.

Rand, P. W., Lawrence, F. H., Pirone, L. A., Lavigne, J. R., and LaCombe, E. (1977). The application of charcoal hemoperfusion to paralytic shellfish poisoning. *J. Maine Med. Assoc. 68*: 147–151.

Rayner, M. D. (1972). Mode of action of ciguatoxin. *Fed. Proc. 31*: 1139–1145.

Rhodes, F. A., Mills, C. G., and Popei, K. (1975). Paralytic shellfish poisoning in Papua, New Guinea. *Papua New Guinea Med. J. 18*: 197–202.

Roberts, L. J., Marney, S. R., and Oates, J. A. (1979). Blockage of the flush associated with metastatic gastric carcinoid by combined histamine H_1 and H_2 receptor antagonists. *N. Engl. J. Med. 300*: 236–238.

Rodgers, D. L., and Muench, C. (1986). Ciguatera: Scourge of seafood lovers. *Sea Frontiers / Sea Secrets 32*: 338–346.

Rodrigue, D. C., Etzel, R. A., Hall, S., De Porras, E., Velasquez, O. H., Tauxe, R. V., Kilbourne, E. M., and Blake, P. A. (1990). Lethal paralytic shellfish poisoning in Guatemala. *Am. J. Trop. Med. Hyg. 42*: 267–271.

Roy, R. N. (1977). Red tide and outbreak of paralytic shellfish poisoning in Sabah. *Med. J. Malaysia 31*: 247–251.

Rumack, B. (Ed.) (1986). Paralytic shellfish. In *Poisindex*, B. Rumack, ed. Micromedex Inc., Denver, CO, p. 50.

Russell, F., and Maretic, Z. (1986). Scombroid poisoning: Mini-review with case histories. *Toxicon 24*: 967–973.

Saito, T., Noguchi, T., Narada, T., Murata, O., and Hashimoto, K. (1985). Tetrodotoxin as a biological defence agent for puffers. *Bull. Jpn. Soc. Sci. Fish 51*: 1175–1180.

Schatz, I. J. (1989). Ciguatera fish poisoning: A jet age peril. *Hosp. Pract.*: 79–94.

Schultz, K. R. (1983). Dangerous marine organisms. In *Emergency Medicine, A Comprehensive Review*, T. C. Kravis and C. G. Warner, eds. Aspens Systems Corp., Rockville, MD, pp. 465–489.

Shantz, E. J. (1975). Poisonous red tide organisms. *Environ. Lett. 9*: 225–237.

Sheumack, D. D., Howden, M. E. H., Spence, I., et al. (1978). A neurotoxin from the venom glands of the octopus *Hapalochlaena maculosa* identified as tetrodotoxin. *Science 199*: 188–189.

Sims, J. K. (1987). A theoretical discourse on the pharmacology of toxic marine ingestions. *Ann. Emerg. Med. 16*: 1006–1015.

Sims, J. K., and Ostman, D. (1986). Puffer fish poisoning: Emergency diagnosis and management of mild human tetrodotoxication. *Ann. Emerg. Med. 15*: 1094–1098.

Steidinger, K. A., and Joyce, E. A. (1973). Florida red tides. Fla. Dept. Nat. Res., Ed. Ser.: 17.

Tahara, Y. (1910). Über das Tetrodongift. *Biochem. Z. 30*: 255–275.

Taylor, S. L., Stratton, J. E., and Nordlee, J. A. (1989). Histamine poisoning (scombroid fish poisoning): An allergy-like intoxication. *J. Toxicol. Clin. Toxicol. 27*: 225–240.

Torda, T. A., Sinclair, E., Ulyatt, D. B. (1973). Pufferfish (tetrodotoxin) poisoning: Clinical record and suggested management. *Med. J. Aust. 1*: 599–602.

Vancouver, G. (1798). *A Voyage of Discovery of the North Pacific Ocean and Round the World*. Robinson, London, vol. 2, pp. 284–286.

van der Sar, A. (1982). Ciguatera poisoning and T-wave changes. *JAMA 247*: 1345.

Vernoux, J. P., Lahlou, N., Abbad El Andaloussi, S., Riyeche, N., and Magras, L. (1985). A study of the distribution of ciguatoxin in individual Caribbean fish. *Acta Tropica* *42*: 225–233.

Withers, N. (1982). Ciguatera fish poisoning. *Ann. Rev. Med.* *33*: 97–111.

Yokoo, A. (1950). Chemical studies on tetrodotoxin: Report III, Isolation of spheroidine. *J. Chem. Soc. Japan* *71*: 591–592.

Zwahlen, A., Blanc, M. H., and Robert, M. (1977). Paralytic shellfish poisoning. *Schweiz Med. Wschr.* *107*: 226–230.

16

Analytical Methods for Marine Toxins

James M. Hungerford and Marleen M. Wekell

United States Food and Drug Administration, Bothell, Washington

I. INTRODUCTION

Problems with marine toxins are global. Toxic phytoplankton and toxin-producing bacteria are frequently implicated in seafoodborne poisonings and are of great concern to health-protection agencies around the world. Consequently, marine toxin research is a rapidly evolving field. Results of studies of phytoplankton-derived toxins, for example, are presented in ever-increasing numbers at international symposia. The number and frequency of meetings held to discuss marine toxins are also increasing.

To eliminate the public health problems posed by marine toxins requires a multidisciplinary approach. To better understand the marine toxin problem, scientists in areas as diverse as natural products chemistry, algalogy, physiology, biochemistry, and analytical chemistry have made contributions. For example, studies of the physiological effects of marine toxins on biological systems provides information to guide health agencies in establishing maximum allowable toxin levels in seafood products. Investigations of toxin production by microorganisms and of toxin movement throughout the food chain yields information useful in the design of control measures at the harvest level.

Development and validation of rugged screening methods for marine toxins is a crucial step if federal and state agencies are to protect the public health. Furthermore, since many of the toxins are quite potent even if present in shellfish and/or finfish in minute quantities, it is essential not only to develop sensitive analytical methods, but to develop reliable methods to extract toxins or to detect them within a complex sample matrix.

As investigations of the major marine intoxications gather momentum, sophisticated methods of analysis including spectroscopic and chromatographic methods provide much of our knowledge of the marine toxins. Fourier transform nuclear magnetic resonance spectrometry, mass spectrometry, and infrared spectroscopy have all played major roles in elucidating the structures of new tetrodotoxins, for example. All of these methods require submilligram to milligram quantities of relatively pure materials rather than the trace quantities of impure toxins typically available in seafood samples. Thus these methods are applied primarily in marine toxin research rather than in routine monitoring. Chromatographic methods, especially high pressure liquid chromatography (HPLC) with fluorescence detection, have the high sensitivity and specificity needed to detect trace levels of toxins in seafoods. Each year additional toxin forms are discovered within a toxin class, and occasionally an entirely new class of toxin is found. While this increases our knowledge of the marine toxins, it also creates an immediate need for increasingly diverse marine-toxin standards to support separation methods. These standards are not widely available, and so the practicality of separation-based methods as the primary means of screening seafoods for the more diverse toxin groups is called into question. There are also problems with lab-to-lab reproducibility of data, which appear to result from direct application of research analytical methods to field monitoring. These themes repeat themselves for nearly every type of marine intoxication. In the following discussion of detection and quantitation methods for the marine toxins, these and other recurring themes will become apparent.

Most marine intoxications are caused by a mixture of several structurally distinct components, often of varying toxicities. The composition or toxin profile varies considerably both within the microbes producing them and within the molluscan shellfish and finfish tainted by them. In both groups, these variations occur at the intraspecies and interspecies level. Within a given species of shellfish or finfish, toxin profiles also vary among those harvested in the same area and within an individual as a function of time. Therefore, for maximum protection of the public health, the best analytical method should detect all toxic components with *no* possibility of a false-negative result.

Mammalian bioassays are often used as part of initial efforts to manage marine toxins because their use generally does not require knowledge of the toxin chemistry. Physiological rather than structural information is obtained. For example, toxins that block conductance through the sodium channels of neurons produce similar directly observable symptoms in mice whether the toxins are of the saxitoxin group, the tetrodotoxin group, or perhaps a previously unknown family of sodium channel blockers. The same principle applies to the polyether toxins causing sodium conductance activation. Furthermore, mammalian bioassays rapidly provide information of the most fundamental nature to those protecting public health—the toxic potency of the extract; however, care should be taken to ensure that all toxins, whether lipid or water soluble, are extracted from the suspect seafood. The controversial issue of using mammals for testing in addition to the inherent problems and limitations of mammalian bioassays encourages the development of alternative bioassays, pharmacological assays, immunoassays, and chemical or separation methods to detect marine toxins in seafoods.

II. PARALYTIC SHELLFISH POISONING (SAXITOXINS)

The saxitoxins are a family of potent neurotoxins responsible for paralytic shellfish poisoning (PSP). They block the sodium channel (Catterall, 1985), which at low doses results in a tingling or burning sensation in the lips and at higher doses, paralysis of the extremities, loss of motor coordination, and even death by respiratory paralysis.

As with many of the marine toxins, it was first believed that paralytic shellfish poisoning was caused by a single compound, saxitoxin (STX). The number of known (naturally occurring) saxitoxins has grown steadily over the years. At this time 17 different saxitoxins have been found in dinoflagellates or in shellfish. This does not include decarbamoyl gonyautoxin I (dc-GTX I) and dc-GTX IV, which have been postulated but not isolated (Fig. 1). The potencies (mouse, i.p.) of the various saxitoxins vary markedly (Fig. 2). Generally, the carbamoyl toxins are most potent, the sulfocarbamoyl toxins are least potent, and the decarbamoyl toxins have intermediate potency.

It is generally believed that shellfish acquire and concentrate the saxitoxins as a result of feeding on toxic dinoflagellates. Several species of dinoflagellates are now associated with the saxitoxins, including *Alexandrium catenella* (Schantz et al., 1966; Proktor et al., 1975; Bates et al., 1978), *A. excavatum* (Desbiens et al., 1990), *A. fundyense* (Anderson et al., 1990), and *A. tamarensis* (Prakash, 1967; Anderson and Po-on-Cheng, 1988) at northern latitudes, and at more southerly latitudes, *Gymnodinium catenatum, Pyrodinium bahamense* (Taylor, 1985; Anderson et al., 1989), and *Gonyaulax polyedra* (Bruno et al., 1990). Dinoflagellate cysts deposited in bottom sediments can remain toxic for several months (Selvin et al., 1984).

While the saxitoxins are generally thought to be the products of de novo synthesis in dinoflagellates, there is evidence that some of the toxins, primarily the gonyautoxins, may also be produced by bacteria such as species of *Moraxella* (Kodama, 1990) and *Bacillus* (Ogata et al., 1990).

Toxin profiles vary widely among the various dinoflagellate species (Boyer et al., 1985; Cembella et al., 1987). There are also intraspecies variations (Maranda et al., 1985; Cembella et al., 1987); however, the toxin composition of a particular dinoflagellate strain in a given location is remarkably constant.

A. Stability

Extensive changes in toxin profile can occur within shellfish after they feed (Oshima et al., 1990). This, and considerable variations in the potency of each

R1	R2	R3	Carbamate Toxins	N-Sulfocarbamoyl Toxins	Decarbamoyl Toxins
H	H	H	STX	B1	dc-STX
OH	H	H	NEO	B2	dc-NEO
OH	H	OSO_3^-	GTX I	C3	dc-GTX I
H	H	OSO_3^-	GTX II	C1	dc-GTX II
H	OSO_3^-	H	GTX III	C2	dc-GTX III
OH	OSO_3^-	H	GTX IV	C4	dc-GTX IV

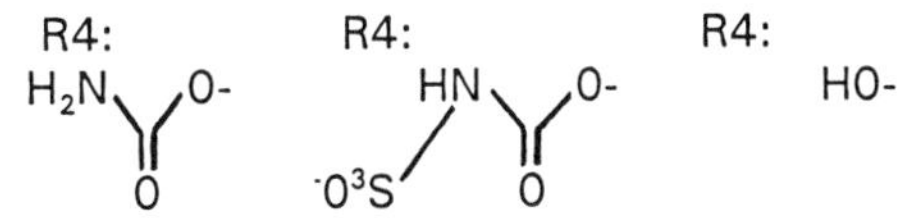

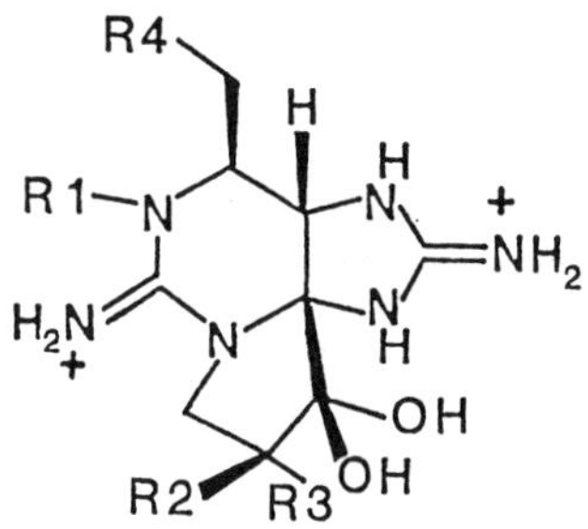

R1	R2	R3		
H	H	H	R4 = H	13-deoxycarbamoyl-saxitoxin

Figure 1 Saxitoxins. Blockers of sodium channel conductance. Abbreviations: STX, saxitoxin; NEO, neosaxitoxin; GTX, gonyautoxin.

toxin form, can lead to changes in the total potency of a shellfish sample. There is considerable interspecies variation in the ability of shellfish to interconvert and otherwise transform the various toxin forms (Kotaki et al., 1985). The littleneck clam, *Protothaca staminea*, transforms several of the saxitoxins to their decarbamoyl derivatives (Sullivan et al., 1983). Other changes in toxin profile occur due to purely nonenzymatic, physicochemical processes. Without exception, the gonyautoxins undergo epimerization, with equilibrium favoring the energetically favored alpha forms (Fix Wichmann et al., 1981; Hall, 1982). The rate of the conversion is structure and pH dependent, with more rapid epimerization occurring at neutral pH. All of the saxitoxins are readily oxidized to nontoxic products if the pH is not strictly controlled during extraction. Neutral and alkaline conditions favor oxidation; most procedures for extracting the saxitoxins recommend a pH range from 2 to 4. Under extremely acidic conditions (1 M free acid) the carbamoyl group is removed (Sullivan, 1982). Loss of the (sulfocarbamoyl) sulfate group from the sulfocarbamoyl toxins

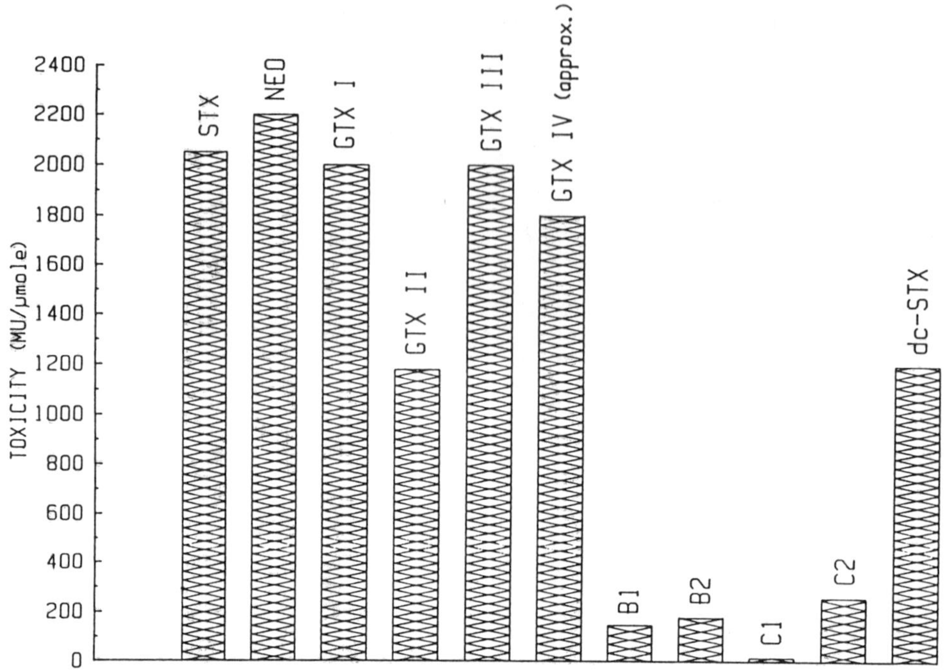

Figure 2 Toxicities (mouse intraperitoneal potencies) of the saxitoxins. One mouse unit (MU) is the amount of toxin required to kill a 20-g mouse in 15 min. Death is by respiratory paralysis (Sullivan et al., 1989).

occurs readily at pH 1 and 100°C, with conversion complete in 5 min (Hall and Reichardt, 1984). Due to the low toxicity of the sulfocarboyl toxins and the high toxicity of the carbamoyl toxins, loss of the sulfate group leads to an increase in toxicity.

In principle, "activation" of latent toxins could occur in the (acidic) mammalian stomach before the native toxins were fully absorbed. The feasibility of this gastric activation has been tested. Harada et al. (1984) found that oral administration of toxin B1 to mice and incubation of B1 with artificial and intact rat gastric juice led only to very slow conversion of B1 to STX. Additional work is needed in this area. In particular, the possibility of gastric hydrolysis of the other sulfocarbamoyl toxins should be investigated. At the present time, evaluation of human health risks by extrapolation from mouse intraperitoneal potencies is based on the assumption that there is no significant hydrolysis of the sulfocarbamoyl-toxins to more toxic carbamoyl forms following ingestion.

Since the first application of the mouse bioassay in 1937 (Sommer and Meyer, 1937), global efforts to monitor shellfish for the saxotoxins have expanded. In the United States, for example, approximately 10,000 shellfish samples were analyzed for saxitoxins in 1989 (Hungerford and Wekell, 1991). Several methods have been developed (reviewed by Sullivan, 1988) and include bioassays, pharmacological assays, immunoassays, HPLC, and continuous flow methods.

B. Bioassays

A modified version (Medcof et al., 1947) of the mouse bioassay was collaborated by McFarren (1959) in conjunction with the Association of Official Analytical Chemists (AOAC). This method remains the AOAC officially recognized procedure (Helrich, 1990) and is used extensively for PSP monitoring. It involves injection (i.p.) of a crude, aqueous shellfish extract into a mouse. Classical PSP symptoms are observed including convulsions, uncontrolled jumping, and respiratory paralysis leading to death. Initial results are expressed in mouse units, defined as the amount of saxitoxin required to kill a 20-g mouse in 15 min. Mice are calibrated with a saxitoxin standard, and the potency (i.p.) is ultimately expressed as μg saxitoxin dihydrochloride/100 g shellfish. The time elapsed from injection to death is inversely related to the overall potency. This inverse relationship restricts quantitation to death times occurring between 5 and 7 min. At longer death times the dose-response curve is nearly flat (due to low sensitivity), and at shorter death times the curve is so steep that apparent potency becomes a sensitive function of injection technique and other factors. Death times in the 5- to 7-min time period correspond to potencies (i.p.) between 0.53 and 0.73 ppm STX dihydrochloride. At levels of regulatory interest, dilutions are often required to accommodate this narrow working range, and this is one of the major disadvantages of this and many bioassays. At high levels of toxicity, interlaboratory precision is often poor (Park et al., 1986). The mouse bioassay is also subject to sample matrix effects. It has been reported that with increases in the salt level of an extract, the potency is decreased (Schantz et al., 1958). Zinc can also affect the accuracy of the bioassay (McCulloch et al., 1989).

For alternative bioassays using intact organisms, house flies (*Musca domestica*) (Siger et al., 1984; Ross et al., 1985) and brine shrimp (Betz and Blogoslawski, 1982) have been suggested.

C. Pharmacological Assays

1. *Assays at the Organ or Cell Level*

A cellular-level assay for sodium channel blockers (STX and tetrodotoxin) based on culture viability of mouse neuroblastoma cells has also been described (Kogure et al., 1989). Daigo et al. (1989) described a method for detecting saxitoxins by monitoring changes in the excitatory postsynaptic potential (EPSP) or a nerve-muscle preparation from the lobster *Panulirus japonicus*. Excitatory axons are isolated from a leg and part of the stretcher muscle is exposed by removing exoskeleton. Toxin solution is applied to the muscle surface, and after a 5-min incubation, the excitatory axons are electrically stimulated and the EPSP monitored using microelectrodes. The EPSP amplitude decreases in a dose-dependent manner, presumably due to blockage of sodium channel conductance. Several different PSP samples were prepared from toxic crabs, scallop digestive glands, oyster digestive glands, and cultures of *Gymnodinium catenatum*. The method is extremely sensitive; only 10^{-16} mol of GTX I/IV are required to completely flatten the EPSP. Nerve cell preparations, including measurements of compound action potentials (Strichartz,

1984) and voltage clamp of single neurons (Frace et al., 1986), have not been suggested for use in assays, but their use in other studies raises some interesting possibilities for future methods development.

2. Molecular Pharmacological Assays

Many of the same advantages of bioassays, from inherent selectivity for toxicity to the potential for detecting new toxin forms, may someday be realized at the molecular level by using the binding selectivity of naturally occurring proteins. In principle this could be done by constructing a detector to measure blockage of sodium ion conductance through a membrane. The feasibility of this approach is suggested by a study of blockage of single sodium channels in lipid bilayers (Moczydlowski et al., 1984). Another, perhaps more practical, approach is to detect indirectly the protein toxin binding events. Towards this goal, sodium channel receptor proteins in rat brain membranes have been used to develop a competitive displacement assay (Davio and Fontelo, 1984). Displacement of radiolabeled STX from a crude membrane preparation allows detection of as little as 0.5 ng/ml. The method has been applied to the detection only of STX (and tetrodotoxin) in human plasma, and not to a mixture of the various STXs in a shellfish tissue extract. Cross-reactivity for the STXs is an issue in the development of all methods based on "specific" protein binding, including immunoassays.

D. Immunoassays

With inherently high sensitivity and potentially high selectivity, a well-designed immunoassay kit could provide many of the desired qualities of a rapid and simple screening test for PSP toxins. In addition to the usual concerns such as cost, stability, and simplicity, a formidable challenge is posed by the need to develop a method in which the response is proportional to toxicity. Immunoassays would seem naturally well suited for this task. First, the determinant region of the antibodies is expected to have cross-reactivity to the various saxitoxin forms, since they share the common STX nucleus. Also, since the antibodies are produced as a defensive response to toxicity, the contribution of any given toxin species to the total response should be weighted in some measure by its relative toxicity. Unfortunately, the saxitoxins are small enough in size that, like all haptens, they must first be conjugated with macromolecules to elicit an immune response. Thus, it is necessary to derivatize the STX nucleus in a way that will not block those regions of the molecule which are important in both sodium channel and antibody binding.

Since antibodies were first applied to the detection of STX by Johnson and Mulberry (1966), further attempts have been made to develop immunoassays for STX and the other PSP toxins (Carlson et al., 1984; Chu and Fan, 1985; Cembella et al., 1987). Low cross-reactivity of antisera with other saxitoxins is a recurring problem, which thus far has prevented the development of an immunoassay with a response consistently proportional to the toxicity of shellfish extracts.

By far the most promising immunoassay for the saxitoxins at this date is an absorption inhibition enzyme-linked immunoassay developed in Canada

(Cembella et al., 1990), which has resulted in a commercially available kit. Briefly, the assay involves competition between immobilized STX and sample PSP toxins for limited antibody, followed by color development using an enzyme conjugate. A decrease in color compared to a negative control indicates the presence of PSP toxins. Much of the antiserum cross-reactivity pattern parallels the relative toxicities of the various saxitoxins, an important step towards the development of a practical and rapid screening method for PSP. However, while NEO is bound at a level that is initially comparable to GTX III, the binding is apparently reversible. This results in an artificially low response for NEO, and the potential exists for false-negative test results. It is also expensive. In June 1989, the cost per kit was $190 (U.S.), or about $25 per test.

Hydrogen peroxide oxidation of STX yields a fluorescent product (Bates and Rapoport, 1975). This chemistry was the basis for early attempts to develop screening methods for PSP (Shoptaugh et al., 1981). Refinements of the Bates and Rapoport reaction are widely used in many of the current instrumental methods for the saxitoxins because they are more selective for the saxitoxins than derivatizations based on other fluorescent reagents such as fluorescamine (Wright et al., 1989) or *o*-phthalaldehyde-mercaptoethanol (Onoue, 1983b; Wright et al., 1989).

E. Separation Methods

A variety of separation methods have been proposed for determining the levels of PSP toxins. Capillary electrophoresis has been proposed for the quantitation of saxitoxin. Precolumn derivatization combined with laser-induced fluorescence provided attomole detection limits. The method has not been applied to the resolution of a toxin mixture in a biological matrix (Wright et al., 1989). Conventional electrophoresis methods using gels or cellulose-acetate strips (Oshima et al., 1976; Boyer et al., 1979; Onoue et al., 1983a; Ikawa et al., 1985), thin-layer chromatography (TLC) (Mold et al., 1957; Proctor et al., 1975; Buckley et al., 1976), and HPLC have been applied extensively to the separation of the many toxin forms in biological materials.

Buckley et al. (1976) were first to detect the separated toxins by combining the Bates and Rapaport reaction with TLC. Following separation on silica gel using a pyridine, ethyl acetate, water, and acetic acid, TLC plates are sprayed with alkaline hydrogen peroxide, heated, and fluorescence is observed under a UV lamp. The *N*-hydroxy toxins give yellow-green fluorescent spots, while the other toxins fluoresce blue.

Saxitoxins have been separated by HPLC using silica (Boyer, 1980), ion-exchange (Oshima et al., 1984), aminopropyl bonded-phase (Sullivan, 1982; Luckas, 1989), cyano bonded-phase (Sullivan, 1982; Sullivan and Iwaoka, 1983), and reversed-phase columns. In all monitoring programs and in most research applications, the saxitoxins must be quantitated at sub-ppm levels in biological materials. This need for high sensitivity, and the fact that the saxitoxins are poor chromophores, plagued early efforts to develop adequate HPLC methodology. The first reported HPLC separations of the saxitoxins depended on detection of native absorbance (Boyer, 1980). While methods for separating several of the saxitoxins were described in this earliest work, all had detection limits too low for monitoring applications. In the most effective HPLC methods for the saxitoxins, fluorescence and mass spectrometric detection provide high sensitivity.

Luckas (1989) described the detection of STX and dc-STX in canned mussels by high pressure liquid chromatography–mass spectrometry (HPLC-MS). Toxins were separated on an aminopropyl bonded-phase column, and solvent was removed in a thermospray interface prior to detection in a quadrapole mass spectrometer. HPLC-MS has the potential to become one of the most powerful methods for detecting marine toxins, especially in research applications. For routine monitoring of marine toxins in seafoods, however, it is at present poorly suited due to its relatively high initial cost and lack of sufficient ruggedness. Still essentially in the development stage, interfaces and mass spectrometers for HPLC-MS are far more expensive and more delicate than fluorescence detectors.

An HPLC fluorescence method based on the *o*-phthalaldehyde-mercaptoethanol chemistry was described by Onoue et al. (1983b). Since amino acids and other materials in shellfish interfere with the *o*-phthalaldehyde-mercaptoethanol method, most researchers have opted for the specificity provided by modified versions of the Bates and Rapaport (1975) oxidation chemistry. The first postcolumn chromatography instrument for detecting saxitoxins was a low-pressure chromatography system based on a Bio-gel P-2 column and hydrogen peroxide oxidation (Buckley et al., 1978). This system did not achieve adequate resolution of the PSP toxins and did not detect any of the *N*-hydroxy toxins. However, just as the addition of modern HPLC provided the missing element to allow improved resolution of the toxins, their postcolumn oxidation and fluorescence manifold laid the groundwork for detection systems now widely used for HPLC quantitation of the saxitoxins. In his efforts to develop improved chemistries for postcolumn detection of the saxitoxins, Sullivan (1982) developed a periodate oxidation chemistry which replaced existing chemistries based on hydrogen peroxide oxidation. This was a major step in the improvement of methods for detecting saxitoxins because it allowed postcolumn detection of the *N*-hydroxy toxins with reasonable sensitivity.

The most efficient HPLC methods for determining the PSP toxins use reversed-phase columns in the ion-interaction mode. Surface-active ion-pairing agents provide a transient capacity for ion exchange by forming a charged layer at the hydrophobic surface of the column (Iskandarani and Pietrzyk, 1982). As in ion-exchange chromatography, separation of the PSP toxins by ion interaction is achieved by exploiting variations in charge arising from the uniqueness of each toxin ionization constant (pKb). The (unresolved) C group toxins are only weakly retained due to their neutral and negative charges, and they elute first; the strongly basic toxins (such as NEO and STX) are eluted last because they possess the highest positive charge. The gonyautoxins and the B toxins elute at intermediate times. The major strength of ion-interaction chromatographic methods is the ability to adjust the ion-exchange capacity by changing the concentration of ion-pairing agent and/or addition of an organic solvent.

The ion-interaction principle is used in the gradient mode with a poly(styrene,divinylbenzene) reversed-phase (SDB) column and alkylsulfonate ion-pairing agents to separate B1, B2, the four gonyautoxins (GTX I-IV), neosaxitoxin (NEO), and saxitoxin (STX) in a single run lasting about 20 min (Sullivan and Wekell, 1987). It is the authors' experience that under ideal conditions this procedure yields adequate separation of dc-GTX II and dc-GTX III, and Sullivan et al. (1985) reported that it resolved dc-NEO, but not dc-STX.

Of all the instrumental methods developed for quantitation of PSP toxins, the method of Sullivan and Wekell (1987) is the most studied. Recently it was compared with the mouse bioassay by an independent laboratory. In their study, Salter et al. (1989) report that at levels well above the regulatory limit (80 μg STX/100 g shellfish) total toxicities determined using the two methods compared well, but that at levels near this limit and lower, poor correlation was obtained. A preliminary interlaboratory study of the method was conducted recently in the authors' laboratory. The study has revealed that some commercially available SDB columns will easily resolve the above PSP toxins, while others produce unacceptable broadening of toxin peaks, especially those assigned to NEO and STX. A few of the participants in the study produced false-positive results due to overlap of toxin and sample matrix peaks even when the standard toxin mixture was well resolved. Some laboratories did not detect NEO and/or STX in an extract having a total toxicity near the 80 μg STX/100 g level (Hungerford, in Wekell, 1990).

A bonded reversed-phase (C-8) column has also been used to separate all of the above toxins and most of the decarbamoyl (dc) toxins except dc-NEO (Oshima et al., 1989), again by ion interaction with alkylsulfonates. This procedure uses two separate isocratic separations. Detection is by a periodate oxidation/fluorescence method modified from the procedure of Sullivan (1982). No interlaboratory study has been reported.

Both of the ion-interaction HPLC methods described above use simple and rapid extraction procedures which are modifications of the protocol used to prepare extracts for the AOAC mouse bioassay (Helrich, 1990). Briefly, 100 g of shellfish meat is blended with 100 ml 0.1 N HCl, and the pH is adjusted. In the procedure based on the SDB column, the extract is diluted prior to ultrafiltration through a 10-kilodalton cutoff membrane (Sullivan and Wekell, 1987). The other procedure (Oshima et al., 1989) is similar, except that the boiling step of the bioassay is retained, and the ultrafiltration step is preceded by a C18 cartridge cleanup.

The ion-interaction HPLC methods of Sullivan and Wekell (1987) and Oshima et al. (1989) have been used extensively in marine toxin research. Toxin profiles have been used in studies of the production of saxitoxins by dinoflagellates (Boyer et al., 1985) and by bacteria (Kodama et al., 1988) to aid in the discovery of a new toxin in *G. catenatum* (Oshima et al., 1990), to trace the movement of the toxins throughout the food chain (White, 1977; Haya et al., 1990), and to provide evidence for metabolic conversion of the toxins (Sullivan et al., 1983).

Increasing awareness of the dc-STXs and "C" toxins, particularly as they occur in warm water dinoflagellate species and shellfish, has spurred interest in their quantitation. Most efforts to separate and detect these toxins are modifications of the ion-pairing and postcolumn oxidation methods developed for the other known saxitoxins.

Luckas (1989) has described a modification of the above ion-pairing HPLC separations in his efforts to better separate dc-NEO, dc-STX, and the dc-GTXs in canned mussels. The method uses a more hydrophobic ion-pairing agent (octane sulfonate) than the heptane sulfonate used in the method of Oshima et al. (1989) to increase retention of the toxins to the (bonded octadecyl) reversed-phase column. Gradient elution is used to allow separation of several toxins in a single run. Thorough evaluation of the method was hampered by lack of a complete set of toxin standards.

Substitution of tetrabutyl ammonium salts (positively charged ion-pairing agenta) for alkylsulfonates in the above separations allows either the SDB (Boczar et al., 1988) or C-8 (Oshima et al., 1989) reversed-phase columns to be used to separate the negatively-charged toxins C1-C4. In separating the C-toxin group, it is the authors' view that the method of Oshima et al. (1989) using the C-8 column outperforms the SDB method of Boczar et al. (1988). The higher pH required to retain the toxins on the SDB column apparently leads to their decomposition in the course of the run, which is observed as baseline artifacts and peak tailing.

F. Continuous Flow Methods

A segmented flow analyzer has been proposed for rapid screening of shellfish samples for PSP toxins (Jonas-Davies et al., 1984). The system is considerably faster than HPLC and is simpler to set up and operate. Matrix fluorescence due to nontoxic components in the shellfish extracts interferes with quantitation. It is apparent from the data that attempts to estimate this background signal by running samples without oxidant lead to overcompensation. A pronounced, negative y-intercept is evident when segmented-flow data are plotted versus mouse bioassay results.

Flow injection analysis, in which sample is injected into an unsegmented, flowing reagent stream (Ruzicka and Hansen, 1975; Beecher et al., 1975), is being applied in the authors' laboratory to the development of an automated instrument incorporating automated background subtraction. Following injection of sample extract, the reacting sample is mixed with periodate oxidant and then split into two separate reactors. One reactor is of much lower volume than the other, resulting in a much shorter oxidation time. Recombination of the short- and long-reaction streams results in two peaks, the first of which provides an estimate of nascent sample fluorescence, while the second peak includes contributions from both nascent fluorescence and the saxitoxins. The solution conditions under which this first peak is produced are identical to those producing the second peak, except that insufficient time is provided for generation of toxin-derived fluorescence. Preliminary results suggest that subtraction of the first peak (area) from the second peak provides more accurate compensation for nascent fluorescence than is possible using a segmented stream. Due to differences in sensitivity of the periodate chemistry for the individual toxins, continuous-flow methods (flow-injection or otherwise) provide only an estimate of the total PSP toxicity of shellfish. In the case of the flow-injection method, however, the estimated signals will tend to produce false-positives rather than false-negatives. The flow-injection instrument proposed will be useful in conducting initial screening for PSP toxins with confirmation by mouse bioassay or by HPLC.

III. TETRODOTOXINS

In Japan, certain species of fish belonging to the order Tetradontiformes (pufferfish, porcupine fish, and ocean sunfish) are popular food items despite the fact that some of these fish contain potentially fatal levels of tetrodotoxin (TTX), a potent sodium channel blocker. TTX is the most toxic form of a series of structurally related compounds (Fig. 3). TTX is much more toxic than the other forms, and most of the toxicity of finfish and shellfish is due to TTX. Many other members of the TTX family of compounds have been detected as minor components in species of *Fugu* pufferfish—*F. niphobles* (Endo et al., 1988; Yasumoto et al., 1989), *F. pardalis* (Nakamura and Yasumoto, 1985; Yasumoto et al., 1989), and *F. poecilonotus* (Nakamura and Yasumoto, 1985; Yasumoto et al., 1989). These include 4-epi-TTX, 6-epi-TTX, 4,9-anhydro-TTX, 11-deoxyTTX, and 11-norTTX-6(R)-ol. Tetrodonic acid has also been reported. These compounds and a new TTX-related compound, 11-oxoTTX, have been found in the puffer *Arothron nigropunctatus* (Khora and Yasumoto, 1989). Tetrodotoxin has been released from a nontoxic, high molecular weight fraction of livers of *F. poecilonotus* by treatment with RNAase (Kodama et al., 1983). The flesh of pufferfish caught in temperate waters is believed to have low or nonexistent toxicity, but improper handling can easily result in release of the toxin from highly toxic tissues.

Symptoms of pufferfish poisoning include profuse sweating, subnormal temperature, rapid and weak pulse, tremors, and poor muscle coordination; as respiration becomes difficult (due to muscular paralysis) cyanosis appears, as does muscular twitching and tremors. In lethal episodes, death occurs by respiratory paralysis. Yotsu et al. (1989) reported that in Japan alone, pufferfish poisoning is implicated in more than 10 deaths per year. Tetrodotoxin poisonings, including deaths, have also occurred following the ingestion of certain exotic gastropods. TTX is known to occur in the ivory shell *Babylonia japonica* (Noguchi et al., 1981; Yasumoto et al., 1981), the frog shell *Tutufa lissostoma* (Noguchi et al., 1984), the trumpet shell *Charonia sauliae* (Narita et al., 1981), and the lined moon shell *Natica lineata* (Hwang et al., 1990). TTXs are also found in newts (Yotsu et al., 1989), in certain tropical and subtropical crabs (Noguchi et al., 1986), and in the eggs of the blue-ringed octopus (*Hapalochlaena maculosa*) (Sheumack et al., 1984).

Many species of bacteria are capable of producing TTX and/or anhydro-TTX (Yasumoto et al., 1986a; Simidu et al., 1987). It is now well established that these toxins accumulate in marine sediments (Kogure et al., 1989). Do et al.

	R1	R2	R3	R4
TTX	H	OH	OH	CH_2OH
4-*epi*TTX	OH	H	OH	CH_2OH
6-*epi*TTX	H	OH	CH_2OH	OH
11-deoxyTTX	H	OH	OH	CH_3
11-*nor*TTX-6(*R*)-ol	H	OH	H	OH
11-deoxy-4-*epi*TTX	OH	H	OH	CH_3
11-oxoTTX	H	OH	OH	$CH(OH)_2$

	R3	R4
4,9-anhydroTTX	OH	CH_2OH
4,9-anhydro-6-*epi*TTX	CH_2OH	OH
4,9-anhydro-11-deoxyTTX	OH	CH_3

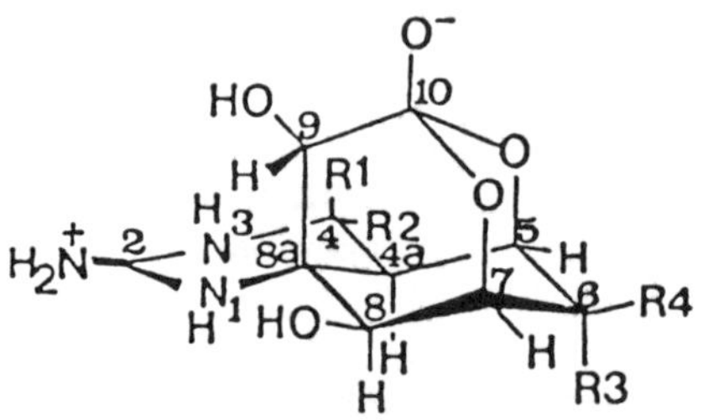

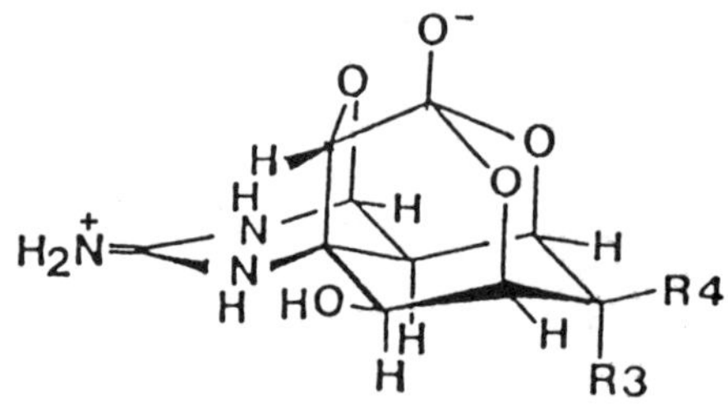

Figure 3 Tetrodotoxin (TTX) derivatives occurring in nature. Sodium channel blockers of varying potency. Alkaline oxidation affords fluorescent derivatives.

(1990) have identified TTX-producing bacteria in deep sea sediment and postulate that TTXs found in marine sediments are synthesized only by bacteria and are concentrated and deposited by benthic organisms in the food web. It appears that toxin-producing bacteria might be responsible for much of the TTX toxicity of several marine finfish and shellfish. For example, TTX-producing bacteria have been isolated from the intestines of the trumpet shell *Charonia sauliae* (Narita et al., 1989), which has been implicated in poisoning incidents (Narita et al., 1981), and from the intestines of the xanthid crab *Atergatis floridus* (Noguchi et al., 1983, 1986). One study suggests that TTX found in pufferfish is a result of their exposure to TTX-producing marine bacteria (Matsui et al., 1990). It would seem that the production of tetrodotoxins by a wide variety of bacteria, many of which are prevalent in the marine environment, could lead to TTX contamination of finfish other than pufferfish.

A. Bioassays

The mouse bioassay for TTX (Kawabata, 1978) is similar to that for the PSP toxins since both toxin groups cause blockage of the sodium channel with death by respiratory paralysis. One mouse unit is defined as the amount of TTX required to kill a (ddY strain) mouse weighing 18–21 g in 30 min after injection (i.p.).

Since bioassays provide only a composite response representing the total potency of samples, initial efforts at detecting the toxins by chemical means were predicted on an assumption that only TTX was present since the other forms had not yet been discovered.

B. Pharmacological Assays

Due to their common mechanism of intoxication (blockage of sodium conductance in neurons), many of the same pharmacological assays developed for the saxitoxins have been applied to TTX (Davio and Fontelo, 1984; Moczydlowski et al., 1984; Strichartz, 1984; Frace et al., 1986; Kogure et al., 1989; Daigo et al., 1989).

C. Immunoassay

A monoclonal antibody has been raised against a tetrodonic acid and used to develop an ELISA assay for TTX (Watabe et al., 1989). Tetrodonic acid was produced from TTX by boiling and then conjugated with bovine serum albumin. The conjugate was injected into BALB/c mice. The resulting antibody had low reactivity for TTX, but could be used to quantitate TTX in puffer livers over the range of 0.35–6 μg/well. Cross-reactivity of the antibody with other TTX forms was not reported.

D. Separation Methods

Treatment of TTX with hot alkali produces a fluorescence (excitation at 370 nm produces emission near 500 nm), which is proportional to TTX concentration (Nunez et al., 1976). The derivative responsible for the fluorescence is 2-amino-6-hydroxymethyl-8-hydroxyquinazoline (C9 base). All of the known TTX forms, including anhydro-TTX, are converted to fluorescent products following treatment with hot alkali. Conditions for maximum fluorescence vary. The optimum hydrolysis times and maximum wavelengths of fluorescence exitation and emission spectra of TTX and 6-epiTTX are comparable to 11-norTTX-6(R)-ol, whereas 11-deoxyTTX reacts with much slower kinetics to give a product with different fluorescence excitation and emission spectra. The individual maximum molar fluorescence intensities derived from each form are also different (Yotsu et al., 1989). Thus measurements of total TTX fluorescence (Nunez et al., 1976) cannot provide accurate estimates of the total toxicity of pufferfish samples because they contain a mixture of TTX forms of widely varying toxicity and fluorescence. Similarly, GC-MS methods using precolumn derivatization (alkaline hydrolysis to C9 base followed by trimethylsilation) provide only a qualitative means of confirming the presence of TTX and its isomers and congeners. More accurate methods for determining the TTX forms are based on separation prior to derivatization.

An alkaline spray reagent combined with fluorescence detection is used to provide a sensitive means of visualizing spots following electrophoresis and thin-layer separations (Kodama et al., 1983). Other derivatization chemistries have been used to generate fluorescent products from TTX. These include reaction of TTX with fluorescamine or *o*-phthalaldehyde (OPT) prior to capillary zone electrophoresis (Wright et al., 1989) and postcolumn OPT derivatization in an HPLC method (Onoue et al., 1983b). Many of the TTX separation methods, however, exploit the enhanced selectivity afforded by postcolumn alkaline derivatization after separation on cation-exchange (Yasumoto et al., 1982) or reversed-phase HPLC columns.

TTX separations using reversed-phase columns are actually ion-interaction methods in which the positively charged TTXs interact with alkylsulfonates (Nagashima et al., 1987) or heptafluorobutyrate (Yotsu et al., 1989). The ion-interaction methods have separation efficiencies superior to the ion-exchange methods, allowing the separation of all currently known TTX forms. Much of what is now known of the TTX group is due to the combined application of powerful spectroscopic techniques and these ion-interaction HPLC methods (Yotsu et al., 1989).

Other separation methods for TTX do not require derivatization but are far less sensitive than the HPLC fluorescence methods. These include TLC–fast atom bombardment mass spectrometry (Nagashima et al., 1988) and capillary isotachophoresis with potential gradient detection (Shimada, 1983). For TTX research and confirmation purposes, liquid chromatography–mass spectrometry is certainly feasible but has not been reported.

Most of the published instrumental methods for the TTXs require extensive sample workup (repeated extraction, charcoal treatment, and column chromatography) prior to the HPLC determinative step. An exception is a modification of the method of Nagashima et al. (1987), which uses C-18 and cation-exchange cartridges for rapid cleanup and has a determination limit of 0.2 ng TTX/g tissue (Fuchi et al., 1988). Of the many naturally occurring TTX forms, only the parent compound is commercially available at this time.

IV. AMNESIC SHELLFISH POISONING (DOMOIC ACID)

Domoic acid is a neurotoxic amino acid (Fig. 4). It binds to glutamate receptors in the brain, thereby causing continuous stimulation of nerve cells, and eventually lesions are formed (Teitelbaum, 1990). Victims experience headache, loss of balance, disorientation, and the usual gastrointestinal symptoms typical of most food-poisoning episodes. The most characteristic symptom, however, is persistent and apparently permanent loss of memory, thus the term amnesic shellfish poisoning (Perl et al., 1990). In December 1987, 156 individuals became ill after ingesting blue mussels (*Mytilus edulis*) cultivated and harvested at Prince Edward Island, Canada. Four elderly people died. Domoic acid (up to 900 ppm) was found in the implicated mussels (Quilliam and Wright, 1989b). It is believed that the domoic acid was produced by the diatom *Nitzschia pungens f. multiseries* and then retained by the mussels (Bates et al., 1989). As a result of these incidents, shellfish are now monitored for domoic

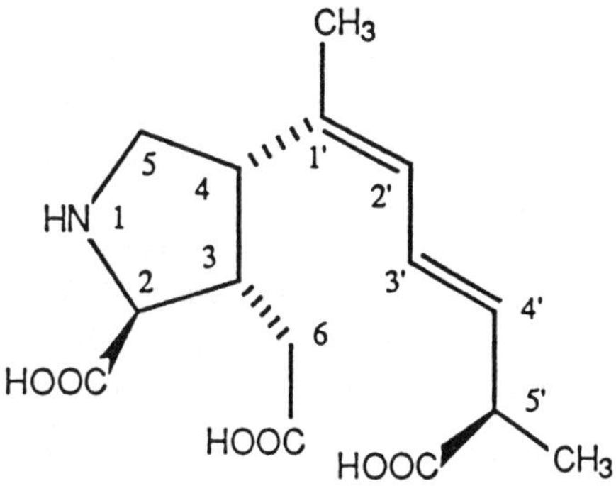

Figure 4 Domoic acid. This compound, responsible for amnesic shellfish poisoning, is a glutamate agonist. The conjugated diene (carbons 1′-4′) gives this compound a distinctive ultraviolet absorption spectrum.

acid in Canada and the United States. Examination of epidemiological data and also laboratory studies of the mammalian toxicity of domoic acid—LD_{50} (i.p.) of 3.6 mg domoic acid/kg mouse (Grimmelt et al., 1990) and lethality at 4 mg/kg in the monkey *M. fascicularis* (Tryphonas et al., 1990)—have led to the establishment of an action level of 20 ppm.

A. Stability

Domoic acid is acid labile. In spite of this, it is often extracted (for bioassay or HPLC analysis) at pH 2–4 and 100°C. A study (Lawrence et al., 1989a) has shown that the (acid) boiling step should be strictly maintained at 10 min duration to avoid excessive losses and poor recoveries. Even with these precautions, the recovery of domoic acid is low (though reproducible at about 70%) when acid extraction is used. The primary reason for using the acid extraction protocol is to produce an extract also suitable for PSP bioassay or HPLC analysis.

B. Bioassay

During initial efforts to monitor mussels for ASP toxicity, aqueous extracts were injected i.p. into mice (Iverson et al., 1989). Mice so injected show a scratching behavior, which aids in distinguishing domoic acid poisoning from PSP. Immediately following the scratching behavior, mice injected with domoic acid show uncontrolled twisting and rolling motions and loss of the righting reflex. Tremors and cyanosis occur next, followed by death. Time elapsed from injection to the onset of scratching is inversely related to dose, as is death time (Grimmelt et al., 1990). The bioassay is performed using essentially the same procedure as in the official bioassay for PSP (Helrich, 1990), except that observation times are extended. Since the mouse bioassay is not sufficiently sensitive to monitor domoic acid at the 20 ppm action level, instrumental methods were developed to provide the required sensitivity.

The presence of two conjugated double bonds in the molecule results in a strong absorbance at 242 nm, which allows for detection by monitoring absorbance at this wavelength. Acidobasic groups at the carboxylate and imino positions of domoic acid allow separation based on charge. Capillary electrophoresis (CE) has been used (Nguyen et al., 1990) to detect domoic acid in contaminated mussels. Domoic acid was readily separated from components of the mussel sample matrix in 10 min. A detection limit (signal-to-noise ratio 5:1) of 2 ppm was achieved. With excellent mass detection limits, the CE method requires only 3–15 nl sample and will find applications where sample size is severely limited. The HPLC methods described below have superior concentration detection limits.

C. Chromatographic Methods

Domoic acid is readily determined in mussels using conventional reversed-phase HPLC (Quilliam et al., 1989a). The official AOAC procedure for extracting PSP toxins from shellfish (Helrich, 1990) has been applied to a modification of the method of Quilliam et al. (1989a) for domoic acid based on reversed-phase separation with UV detection (Lawrence et al., 1989a). Recently this method was corroborated (Lawrence et al., 1990). As for the mouse bioassay (Grimmelt et al., 1990), careful timing of the acid-extraction step is crucial since domoic acid is acid-labile. Neutral aqueous extraction stabilized with methanol has been suggested as an alternative to the acid extraction (Gilgan, 1990, personal communication).

Lawrence (1989b) has proposed chemical conversion to phenylisothiocyanate derivatives and trialkyl esters as a means of confirming domoic acid in mussels. The derivatives are quantitated by reversed-phase HPLC with absorbance detection at 242 nm. Mussel tissue is extracted with HCl, as in the official HPLC method (Lawrence, 1990), except that additional sample conditioning is required. For this purpose a (strong) cation-exchange cartridge and a C-18 cartridge are used to retain and wash the extract. The detection limit was expected to be similar to the 2 ppm limit of the direct detection method of Lawrence et al. (1989a).

A precolumn-derivatization HPLC method for domoic acid has been described by Pocklington et al. (1990). Reaction of domoic acid with 9-fluorenylmethylchloroformate produces a fluorescent derivative, allowing sensitive fluorescence detection. The derivative is separated by conventional reversed-phase chromatography on a microbore (2.1 mm i.d.) column and detected at excitation and emission wavelengths of 264 nm and 313 nm, respectively. The detection limit in seawater, cultures of *N. pungens forma multiseries*, and in naturally occurring phytoplankton was 15 pg/ml (50 picomolar). The authors report that a manuscript in preparation describes a sample cleanup procedure to adapt the method to shellfish samples.

Unambiguous spectroscopic confirmation of domoic acid in shellfish tissues is achieved by GC-MS. Pleasance et al. (1990) described a method based on a two-stage extraction and production of N-trifluoroacetyl-O-silyl derivatives and capillary gas chromatography. Dihydrokainic acid is used as internal standard.

Domoic acid is commercially available, as are standard reference materials.

V. TETRAMINE POISONING (TETRAMETHYLAMMONIUM ION)

Consumption of whelks (*Neptunia arthritica, Neptunia antiqua*, and *Neptunia intersculpta*) has occasionally resulted in poisoning episodes in Japan and in Scandinavian countries (Asano and Itoh, 1960; Anthoni et al., 1989a).

The toxicity has been attributed to tetramethylammonium ion (TMA), also known as tetramine. TMA acts directly on nicotinic and muscarinic receptors, with the postsynaptic receptors expected to be the most affected in poisoning episodes (Anthoni et al., 1989b). Symptoms of TMA poisoning appear 30 min following ingestion, and recovery is complete within a few hours (Anthoni et al., 1989b). TMA is considerably less toxic than most marine toxins [estimated oral lethal dose for an adult human is 250–1000 mg TMA (Anthoni et al., 1989b)], and while TMA has been implicated in a death following ingestion of a root (Henry, 1948), there are no documented cases of whelk-derived TMA causing the death of a human (Anthoni et al., 1989b). There is evidence that other components present in the whelk salivary gland may have a synergistic effect on TMA potency (Asano and Itoh, 1959). The symptoms vary somewhat according to which of the species is consumed. *N. antiqua* and *N. arthritica* both produce headache and short periods of impaired vision (even periods of blindness), while dizziness is associated with consumption of either *N. arthritica* or *N. intersculpta* (Anthoni, 1989b).

In *N. arthritica* and *N. intersculpta* all of the tetramine is contained in the salivary gland (Asano, 1952; Asano and Itoh, 1959, 1960), while in *N. antiqua*, TMA is also found in other tissues (Anthoni et al., 1989a).

A. Bioassays

Animal bioassays based on mice (Saitoh et al., 1983; Kungsuwan et al., 1986) and killifish (Kungsuwan et al., 1986) have been proposed for quantitation of TMA, and guinea pig ileum preparations have been used in pharmacological studies of TMA toxicity (Anthoni et al., 1989a). Intraperitoneal injection of TMA into mice causes vigorous salivation, tears, convulsions, loss of balance, limp paralysis, and finally death by respiratory paralysis (Saitoh et al., 1983; Anthoni et al., 1989a).

B. Instrumental Methods

The low toxicity of TMA and its abundance in the salivary gland [0.2–7.5 parts per thousand in *N. arthritica* (Anthoni et al., 1989c)] allows the use of Fourier transform ^{1}H NMR spectroscopy to identify and even quantitate TMA in whelks (Anthoni et al., 1989c). The most time-consuming step in the NMR procedure is the freeze-drying required prior to dissolution of the residue in deuterium oxide. Other spectroscopic methods applied to the study of TMA include ^{13}C NMR (Anthoni et al., 1989a) and positive and negative ion fast-atom bombardment mass spectrometry (Larsen et al., 1988).

Separation methods for tetramine include paper chromatography (Welsh and Prock, 1958; Mathias et al., 1960; Deffner, 1961), TLC (Asano and Itoh, 1959), and ion chromatography with conductimetric detection (Saitoh et al.,

1983). Anthoni et al. have reviewed the epidemiology and pharmacology of TMA poisoning (Anthoni et al., 1989a,b) and analytical methods for determining TMA (Anthoni et al., 1989c).

The marine toxins described above are polar compounds that are readily detected well below levels where they become toxic to humans. Domoic acid and tetramine are of low potency, allowing their straightforward isolation and detection without the need for very selective and sensitive detection schemes; the potent saxitoxins and tetrodotoxins are readily converted, using selective and sensitive chemistries, to fluorescent products detectable at trace levels. In contrast, selective derivatizations are not available for the polyethers causing neurotoxic shellfish poisoning, diarrhetic shellfish poisoning, or ciguatera, and yet some of these compounds are extremely toxic and must be detected at ppb levels.

IV. NEUROTOXIC SHELLFISH POISONING (BREVETOXINS)

The marine dinoflagellate *Ptychodiscus brevis* is responsible for red tides in Florida (Davis, 1947; Steidinger, 1979). Consumption of shellfish impacted by an intense *P. brevis* bloom can be toxic to humans consuming them (Joyce, 1975). The resulting human intoxication is known as neurotoxic shellfish poisoning (NSP) (Hemmert, 1975). While there is no documented case of a human fatality (the toxic components causing NSP are far less toxic to mammals than is ciguatoxin), some of the symptoms of NSP are similar to ciguatera. Especially noteworthy is paresthesia in which sensations of hot and cold are reversed, a symptom often thought to be unique to ciguatera poisoning. The duration of NSP is, however, considerably shorter than ciguatera. NSP episodes last from 1 to 72 hr (with 17 hr most typical), while ciguatera symptoms are far more persistent.

Blooms of *P. brevis* also cause fish kills (Steidinger et al., 1973; Steidinger, 1979) with fish deaths occurring when *P. brevis* cell densities approach 5×10^5 cells/L (Steidinger et al., 1973). There is no evidence to suggest that fish exposed to *P. brevis* are toxic to humans.

The compounds responsible for the toxicity of *P. brevis* are a group of polyether lactones commonly known as the brevetoxins. So far nine (Fig. 5) have been isolated (reviewed in Baden, 1988, 1989). Six of the brevetoxins (type 1) are based on a single structural polyether backbone, and an additional three (type 2) are based on a newly described polyether backbone (see Shimizu et al., 1986). Several names for the brevetoxins have been used by various investigators. Most are based on an earlier classification of the plankton as *Gymnodinium breve* and have not been applicable since it was changed (Steidinger, 1979) to *P. brevis*. Poli et al. (1986) proposed a new notation system correlating names of toxins isolated from all laboratories. In this notation system, which has been adopted by many and will be used here, the numbering system proposed by Shimizu (1982) is used, preceded by the letters PbTx denoting *P. brevis* toxin.

The composition of the brevotoxins produced by *P. brevis* can vary according to growth phase (Roszell et al., 1990) and clone type (Baden and Thomas,

Type 1 Skeleton

	R1	R2	R3
Brevetoxin 2	H	CH_2	CHO
3	H	CH_2	CH_2OH
5	$COCH_3$	CH_2	CHO
6	H	CH_2	CHO (27,28-β-epoxide)
8	H	O	CH_2Cl

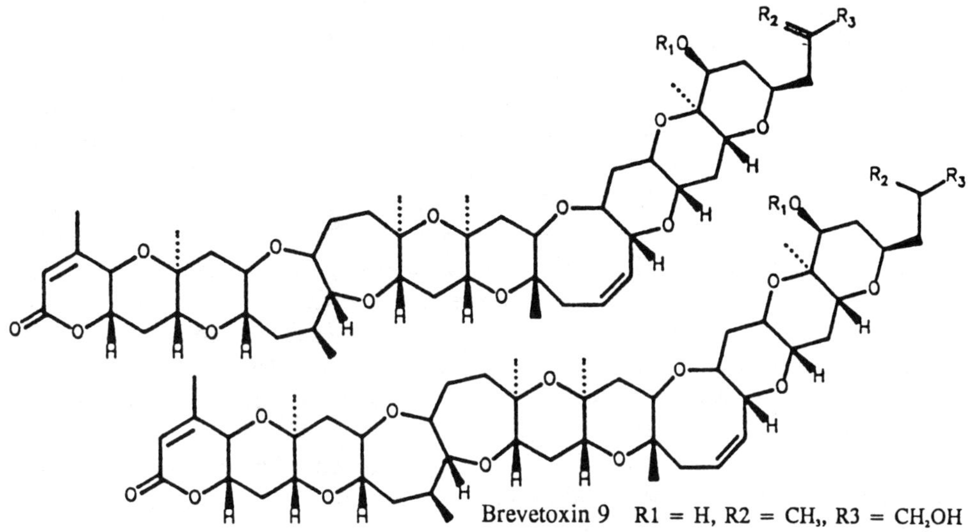

Brevetoxin 9 R1 = H, R2 = CH_2, R3 = CH_2OH

Type 2 Skeleton

	R1	R2	R3
Brevetoxin 1	H	CH_2	CHO
7	H	CH_2	CH_2OH

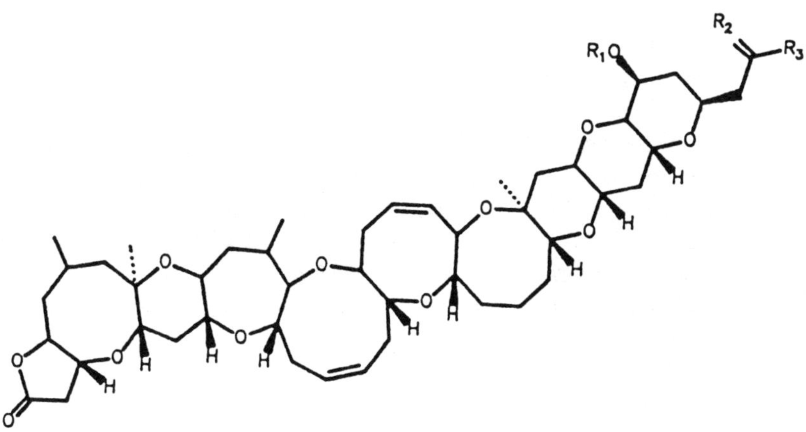

Figure 5 Brevetoxins. Enhancers of sodium-channel conductance of nerve cells. Associated with neurotoxic shellfish poisoning.

1988). In the log phase, cultures have greater levels of the aldehyde PbTx-2. As cultures progress into the stationary and declining phases, the levels of the alcohol PbTx-3 increase with a concurrent decline in PbTx-2 and other toxins such as PbTx-7 and PbTx-9 also begin to appear. The levels of PbTx-1 fluctuate during all culture phases. The findings suggest that in any new culture the aldehyde is the natural form of the toxin found and that changes in the profile can be explained by detoxification mechanisms of the dinoflagellate (Roszell et al., 1990). In other experiments using laboratory-grown cultures with growth phase controlled (log phase) and six different clone types, *P. brevis* isolates showed wide clonal variabilities in levels of PbTx-1,2 and 3 (Baden and Thomas, 1988).

In the United States, Florida has had the greatest impact from brevetoxins since most blooms of *P. brevis* occur there, although in 1987 a red tide reached North Carolina waters (Tester et al., 1988). The Florida Department of Natural Resources (FDNR), in accordance with their procedures (FDNR, 1985) and the recommendations of the National Shellfish Sanitation Program Manual of Operations (1990), closes waters to shellfish harvesting when *P. brevis* cells number 5000/L. Waters are reopened when cell densities remain below 5000/L for 2 weeks. At present, the mouse bioassay is used by the FDNR and other impacted public health agencies in official assays to detect brevetoxins. The disadvantages of this method are well known (Steidinger et al., 1973).

Several different methods for the detection or quantitation of brevetoxins are available or are under development including (1) animal bioassays (mouse, fish), (2) molecular pharmacological assays using voltage dependent sodium channel preparations, (3) immunoassays such as radioimmunoassays (RIA), ELISA, and (4) HPLC. Many of these methods have potential for application to shellfish monitoring in the management of NSP. At this time, only the mouse bioassay has been applied to the detection of the brevetoxins in shellfish.

A. Stability

Brevetoxins are stable to aqueous and organic solvents; in the dry state PbTx-2 and -3 are stable to 300°C, although in general type 2 toxins are more unstable than type 1 toxins (see Baden, 1989). The brevetoxins are affected by autoclaving for 30 minutes at 122°C (18 psi), but this is not sufficient to completely detoxify them; however, heating at 500°C is effective (Poli, 1988). They decompose at extremes of pH (<2 and >10) to the extent that Poli (1988) has recommended that laboratory glassware used in studies of PbTx-2 and -3, for example, be decontaminated by soaking in 0.1 N NaOH with exposure time dependent on toxin levels.

B. Bioassays

1. *Mouse Bioassay*

Brevetoxins are detected in shellfish meats by a standardized mouse bioassay (Delaney, 1985) based on a method originally developed by McFarren et al. (1965). Toxicity is determined by using the relationship of dose to death time of mice injected i.p. with toxic residues extracted from shellfish with diethyl ether. Since no purification is involved, relative toxicity is expressed in terms of mouse units (MU). One MU is that amount of crude toxic residue that will kill 50% of the test animals (20-g mice) in 930 min (15.5 hr). Essentially the method entails extracting acidified and boiled (5 min) shellfish homogenate with an equal volume of diethyl ether 4x (centrifuging between extractions), removing the ether under vacuum, adding cottonseed oil as a diluent, and injecting 1 ml into each of two mice. Mice are observed for 24 hours and death times are recorded. Dilutions must be made if both mice die in less than 110 min; an additional 3 mice must be injected if death occurs between 100 and 360 min. The assay can detect a minimum of 10 MU/100 g shellfish meats, which is calculated using death times, appropriate dilution factors, and correcting for mouse weight. At present, any detectable level of toxin in shellfish meats is considered as unsafe for human consumption. McFarren et al. (1965) suggest that a total of 400–500 MU of brevetoxins will produce a mild form of illness in humans and that as little as 50–80 MU can produce some symptoms of poisoning. Mice given brevetoxin i.p. exhibit an irritability immediately upon injection, followed by hindquarter paralysis, dyspnea, salivation, lacrimination, urination, defecation, and death from respiratory paralysis (Baden, 1989). Whole-body LD_{50} values for brevetoxins in mice range from 0.05 mg/kg body weight for i.v. administration to 0.5 mg/kg body weight for oral and i.p. administration (see Baden, 1989).

In 1989 the FDNR requested that the Interstate Shellfish Shippers Conference (ISSC) reduce the observation time from 24 hours to a 6 to 15.5 observation period (6 hours continuous observation). The Microbiology Committee of the ISSC recommended adoption of this request on an interim basis until publication of the new 6th edition of the American Public Health Association (APHA) Laboratory Procedures for the Examination of Seawater and Shellfish, and the change was formally proposed to the AOAC for their concurrence (Wekell, 1990). Tester and Fowler (1990) present further data and arguments to support the reduction in observation time.

2. *Fish Bioassays*

Brevetoxins are highly toxic to fin fish with lethal doses in the nanomolar concentration range; therefore, fish bioassays have been used by many investigators to assess toxicity (Baden, 1989). Symptoms of intoxication from brevetoxins in fishes include violent twisting and corkscrew swimming, defecation and regurgitation, pectoral fin paralysis, tail curvature, equilibrium loss, quiescence, vasodilation, and convulsions culminating in death due to respiratory failure (Risk et al., 1979; Baden, 1989).

A variety of fish species have been used to determine toxicities of fractions purified from culture extracts of *P. brevis* including *Lebistes reticulatus* (common guppies, Whitefleet-Smith et al., 1986), *Brachydanio rerio* (Zebra fish, Lin et al., 1981) *Gambusia affinis* (mosquito fish, Baden et al., 1988), *Oryzias latipes* (Japanese madakas, Poli, 1988), and *Cyprinadon variegatus*

(Sheepshead minnows, Pierce et al., 1985). Test fish are usually placed individually in containers of water to which toxins have been added. When levels of actual brevetoxins tested were unknown, authors have devised arbitrary fish unit (FU) values using dilution versus death time curves. Whitefleet-Smith et al. (1986), for example, defined one FU as the dilution of brevetoxin that caused death in guppies in 60 minutes. Baden et al. (1988) tested known amounts of purified toxin fractions at concentrations ranging from 1 to 64 nM and after 60 minutes of exposure determined the median lethal dose to *G. affinis* using the tables in Weil (1952).

C. Molecular Pharmacological Assays

The neurotoxins isolated from *Ptychodiscus brevis* exert their effects primarily by altering membrane properties of excitable cells by binding to Site 5 associated with the voltage-sensitivity sodium channel (VSSC) (Poli et al., 1986; Sharkey et al., 1987). In vivo binding of brevotoxin to Site 5 is believed to be the pharmacologically significant event in the onset of intoxication (Catterall, 1985; Poli et al., 1985, 1986). Specific binding leads to sodium channel activation at normal resting potential (Huang et al., 1984) and subsequent membrane depolarization. Toxic effects of dose-dependent and potency appears related to toxin hydrophobicity, so that the more hydrophobic or nonpolar brevetoxins are the most potent. Tritiated PbTx-3 binds with high affinity and specificity to rat and fish brain synaptosomes (Poli et al., 1986; Stuart and Baden, 1988). Binding is linear with increasing tissue concentration up to 0.1 mg protein/ml binding medium using fish synaptosomes (Stuart and Baden, 1988), and 0.25 mg protein/ml binding medium using rat brain synaptosomes (Poli et al., 1986). Unlabeled PbTx-3, PbTx-1, and PbTx-2 displace tritiated PbTx3 in a dose-dependent manner. The binding of brevetoxins to Site 5 of VSSC of synaptosome preparations provides the basis for a quantitative competitive assay with displacement of bound tritiated toxin by nonlabeled brevetoxins correlating directly with the potency of each toxin in whole animals (Baden et al., 1988). For example, Baden et al. (1988) showed that fewer molecules (up to 4×) of the type 2 toxins PbTx-1 and -7 were required to displace [^{3}H]-PbTx-3 (a type 1 toxin) in rat brain synaptosomes compared to levels of type 1 brevetoxins (PbTx-2,-3) with the same structural background as the ^{3}H probe. Similar results were obtained with fish (Tilapia) brain synaptosomes (Stuart and Baden, 1988), although ED_{50} values were higher (Table 1) compared to those observed in rat synaptosome preparations. The type 2 toxins PbTx-1 and PbTx-7 are also more toxic to intact fish (*G. affinis*) than are PbTx-2 and PbTx-3 in a fish bioassay (Baden et al., 1988). Therefore, results generated by the brain synaptosome assays parallel somewhat the toxicities observed in intact animals. Apparent ED_{50} (effective dose for 50% displacement of specific binding) values determined for brevetoxins in [^{3}H]-PbTx-3 displacement experiments using fish brain synaptosomes were 30 nM for PbTx-1, 70 nM for PbTx-2, and 110 nM for PbTx-3 (Stuart and Baden, 1988), and for rat brain synaptosomes corresponding values were 3.5, 17.0, and 12.0 nM, respectively (Baden et al., 1988) (Table 1).

Table 1 Correlation of Brevetoxin Potency (Fish Toxicity) with RIA, Synaptosome Assay, and Toxin Hydrophobicity

		Toxin (nM) concentration				
		Bioassay	Synaptosome		RIA	HPLC[g]
Brevetoxin type[a]	Toxin type[b]	Fish LD_{50}[c]	Fish ED_{50}[d]	Rat ED_{50}[e]	ED_{50}[f]	reversed-phase elution (min)
PbTx-1	2	4.4 (3.8–5.0)	30	3.5 (3.0–5.0)	93 (90–130)	12.5
PbTx-7	2	4.9 (2.2–10.7)		4.1 (4.0–7.0)	92 (90–120)	10.6
PbTx-2	1	21.8 (17.2–35.0)	70	17.0 (15.0–18.0)	22 (18–29)	9.6
PbTx-3	1	10.9 (7.2–22.0)	110	12.0 (10.0–15.0)	20 (16–25)	7.8

[a]Nomenclature from Poli et al., 1986.
[b]Type refers to structural backbone as shown in Fig. 1.
[c]Median lethal dose ($n = 3$), calculated according to the method of Weil (1952); *Gambusia affinis* (mosquito fish), 20 ml seawater (3.5% salinity), and 60-min assay time (Baden et al., 1981, 1988).
[d]Competitive displacement of tritiated PbTx-3 by brevetoxins in Tilapia brain synaptosomes where ED_{50} = toxin concentration at which 50% specific displacement occurs.
[e]Competitive displacement of tritiated PbTx-3 by brevetoxins in rat brain synaptosomes, average of three experiments (Baden et al., 1988).
[f]Competitive displacement of tritiated PbTx-3 from binding site in RIA, average of three experiments (Baden et al., 1988); ED_{50} defined above.
[g]C-18 reversed-phase 0.46 cm OD-5 dia × 25 cm column, 85% aqueous methanol, 1.0 ml min, 2.5 nm detection with elution time in order of increasing hydrophobicity.

D. Immunoassays

1. *Radioimmunoassay*

Specific goat antibodies directed against brevetoxins have been prepared by Baden et al. (1984, 1988). Antigen was produced by Baden et al. (1984) by reducing the aliphatic aldehyde located on the terminal portion of brevetoxin PbTx-2 (the major toxin isolated from laboratory cultures of *P. brevis*) (Baden et al., 1981) to a PbTx-3 succinate derivative and covalently coupling this to the ε amino group of lysine residues of bovine serum albumin by carbodiimide condensation in 50% of aqueous pyridine. After immunization, goat antiserum was purified by ammonium sulfate fractionation. Tritiated brevetoxin PbTx-3 probe (specific activity 10 Ci/mmol, 3H on C-42 and not exchangeable) was produced by reducing brevetoxin PbTx-2 using tritiated sodium borohydride in acetonitrile. The displacement in a dose-dependent manner of ^{3}H brevetoxin PbTx-3 probe from the antibody–antigen complex by unlabeled toxin forms the basis for a competitive RIA with a sensitivity of 600 pg and an assay linearity ranging from 1.5 to 48 ng (Baden et al., 1984). The assay detects both PbTx-2 and PbTx-3 in approximately equivalent manners because both PbTx-2 and -3 have the same structural backbone (type 1 toxins) and the only portion of the molecule (C-42) that distinguishes PbTx-2 from PbTx-3 is used as the linkage point during antigen construction. Recently, type 2 toxins, PbTx-1 and -7, were compared to PbTx-2 and -3 in their relative abilities to competitively replace tritiated brevetoxin PbTx-3 from its specific binding site in rat brain synaptosomal assays (Baden et al., 1988). Type 1 toxins, which are less toxic, were 10-fold more efficient than type 2 (more toxic) toxins at displacing tritiated PbTx-3 (a type 1 toxin) from the binding site in the RIA. Therefore, reactivity of brevetoxins in the RIA is not related to their toxicity but to their structural similarity to PbTx-3, the hapten against which antibodies were produced (Table 1). As Baden et al. (1988) have pointed out, if RIAs are to be effectively used as screening tools, antibodies must also be developed for the type 2 backbone with an appropriate mixture of the two antibody preparations (types 1 and 2) used in the assays; alternatively, if antibodies could be directed specifically at the active portion of the toxins, then binding could be more effectively correlated with toxicity. In addition, false-positive results can be obtained in the RIA with nonpotent compounds such as oxidized PbTx-2. The RIA also cross-reacts against suspected ciguatoxins (Baden et al., 1985), which may prove to be beneficial as a tool for multiple polyether marine toxin screening programs.

2. *Enzyme-Linked Immunosorbent Assay*

The RIA has been converted to a competitive ELISA using microtiter plates, with adsorbed toxin followed by either 1% gelatin in phosphate buffered saline (PBS) or specific gammaglobulin, and visualized using either PbTx-3 urease or PbTx-3 horseradish peroxidase (HRP) conjugates (Trainer and Baden, 1990). The sensitivity of the ELISA is in the pg/ml concentration range, has the potential of being more sensitive than the RIA, and requires samples of minimal size. Although ELISAs utilizing the brevetoxin-urease conjugate were successful, stability problems were encountered with loss of urease activity after 1 week. Therefore, Trainer and Baden (1990) recommended use of the HRP rather than the urease conjugate under the conditions specified. Optimization of the antibrevetoxin ELISA is necessary before it can be successfully adapted for use in field studies, however (Trainer and Baden, 1990).

E. High Pressure Liquid Chromatography

Brevetoxin content in water or culture samples has been determined by reversed-phase HPLC (Pierce et al., 1985, 1990; Poli et al., 1985; Whitefleet-Smith et al., 1986; Schulman et al., 1990). Toxic fractions have been recovered from culture samples by liquid/liquid extraction into dichloromethane and by liquid/solid adsorption onto 100- to 200-μm particles of silica bonded with octadecane (SiO_4–C-18) reverse-phase chromatography column packing described by Pierce et al. (1990). Prior to HPLC analysis, toxic extracts have also been purified by combinations of column and thin-layer chromatography on silica gel using a variety of solvents (Whitefleet-Smith et al., 1986; Schulman et al., 1990). Whitefleet-Smith et al. (1986) have used C-18 reversed-phase columns eluted with aqueous acetonitrile (72%) to separate and purify four of the brevetoxins from cell culture extracts. Separation of the nine known brevetoxins by HPLC have been achieved (Poli et al., 1986; Pierce et al., 1985; Schulman et al., 1990) using isocratic 85% aqueous methanol as the mobile phase on C-18 reversed-phase columns with UV detection (215 nm). Toxins are resolved in order of increasing hydrophobicity, which correlates to toxicity (PbTx-3, PbTx-6, PbTx-2, PbTx-7, PbTx-5, and PbTx-1) (Poli et al., 1986). The system has a detection limit of 10 ppm in the extract, corresponding to about 10 μg/L (10 ppb) in seawater (Pierce, personal communication). At this time, HPLC methods for brevetoxins have been applied only to cultures of *P. brevis* or to seawater samples. Efforts are underway at the Mote Marine Laboratory, Sarasota, Florida, to modify the extraction and cleanup procedures so that the HPLC methods can be used to monitor shellfish for brevetoxins (Pierce, personal communication). PbTx-1,2,3,7, and 9 are commercially available at this time.

VII. DIARRHETIC SHELLFISH POISONING (DSP)

In Japan, Diarrhetic Shellfish Poisoning (DSP) was first reported in 1978 as a consequence of eating mussels and scallops harvested from the Tohuku District (Yasumoto et al., 1978, 1979). Similar illnesses also occurred and were reported in Europe beginning in the 1960s (Kat, 1983, 1985). The illness, a predominantly self-limiting but severe gastroenteritis, is now well recognized as a worldwide threat to human health, affecting many thousands of consumers of molluscan shellfish and posing great economic hardships on the shellfish industry. Symptoms of individuals affected with DSP as reported by Yasumoto et al. (1978) include diarrhea (92%), nausea (80%), vomiting (79%), and abdominal pain (53%). These symptoms are not unique to DSP and therefore of limited interpretive value; it is actually the absence of symptoms, especially those of neurotoxicity (i.e., paralysis, etc.) that implicates DSP rather than other marine intoxications. DSP is easily distinguished from bacterial infection by its rapid onset time and heat stability. In a typical DSP incident, the first appearance of symptoms first occurs a few hours after ingestion. In severe cases, the onset time is as short as 30 minutes. Victims recover after 3 days regardless of medical treatment. The toxins are stable to heat, for cooked shellfish have been responsible for many causes of illness (Yasumoto et al., 1978; Kat, 1983), although prolonged boiling of hepatopancreas homogenates can decrease the concentration of one of the toxins (okadaic acid) to half of its original concentration in 163 min (Edebo et al., 1988).

Shellfish harvested in Japan and causing outbreaks of DSP contain at least 12 toxins, with structures of 9 of these determined so far (Lee et al., 1988a,b; Yasumoto, 1990; Yasumoto and Murata, 1990). The toxins can be separated into three main groups, differing in basic structures or skeletons (Lee et al., 1988a,b; Yasumoto, 1990; Yasumoto and Murata, 1990). The three groups include: (1) okadaic acid (OA) and its derivatives dinophysistoxin-1 (DTX-1) and dinophysistoxin-3 (DTX-3); (2) macrolides–pectenotoxin-1 (PTX-1), pectenotoxin-2 (PTX-2), pectenotoxin-3 (PTX-3), pectenotoxin-6 (PTX-6); and (3) a sulfated toxin–yessotoxin (YTX)—which is structurally related to the brevetoxins (contiguously transfused ether rings), but unlike brevetoxins, YTX has a terminal side chain of nine carbons and two sulfate esters and lacks carbonyl groups, and a derivative of YTX, 45 OH YTX.

The DSP toxins have varying toxicities and toxicological effects. Only OA, DTX-1, and DTX-3 are thought to be responsible for diarrhea. Only these three toxins of those tested caused fluid accumulation in ileal loop assays (Hamano et al., 1985). The toxicities (LD_{99}) of OA, DTX-1, and DTX-3 in μg/kg in mice (i.p.) are 200, 160, and 500, respectively (Yasumoto and Murata, 1990). OA may cause diarrhea by a mechanism similar to that caused by cholera toxin, by stimulating the phosphorylation of a protein that controls sodium secretion by intestinal cells (Cohen et al., 1990).

DTX-1 causes not only diarrhea, but also severe injuries to intestinal mucosa (Terao et al., 1986). PTX-1, on the other hand, is nondiarrheagenic, but does damage the liver in a way similar to that caused by fungal toxins such as cyclochlorotine (from *Penicillium islandicum*) and phalloiodine (from *Amanita phalloides*) (Terao et al., 1986). The toxicities (LD_{99}) of the PTX toxins to mice (i.p.) range from 160 to 770 μg/kg (Yasumoto and Murata, 1990).

Although YTX is also nondiarrheagenic, it can damage heart muscle (Terao et al., 1990), and kills mice (LD 99) at a dose of 100 μg/kg (IP) (Yasumoto et al., 1988).

Okadaic acid and DTX-1 were recently found to be powerful tumor promoters. This discovery raises questions as to the long-term health risks of frequent consumption of low levels of these compounds in foods. In two-stage carcinogenesis experiments on mouse skin, both toxins were of comparable potency to agents like phorbol esters (Fujiki et al., 1988; Suganuma et al., 1988). Haystead et al. (1989) suggest that tumor promotion may stem from increased phosphorylation of one or more proteins that are substrates for

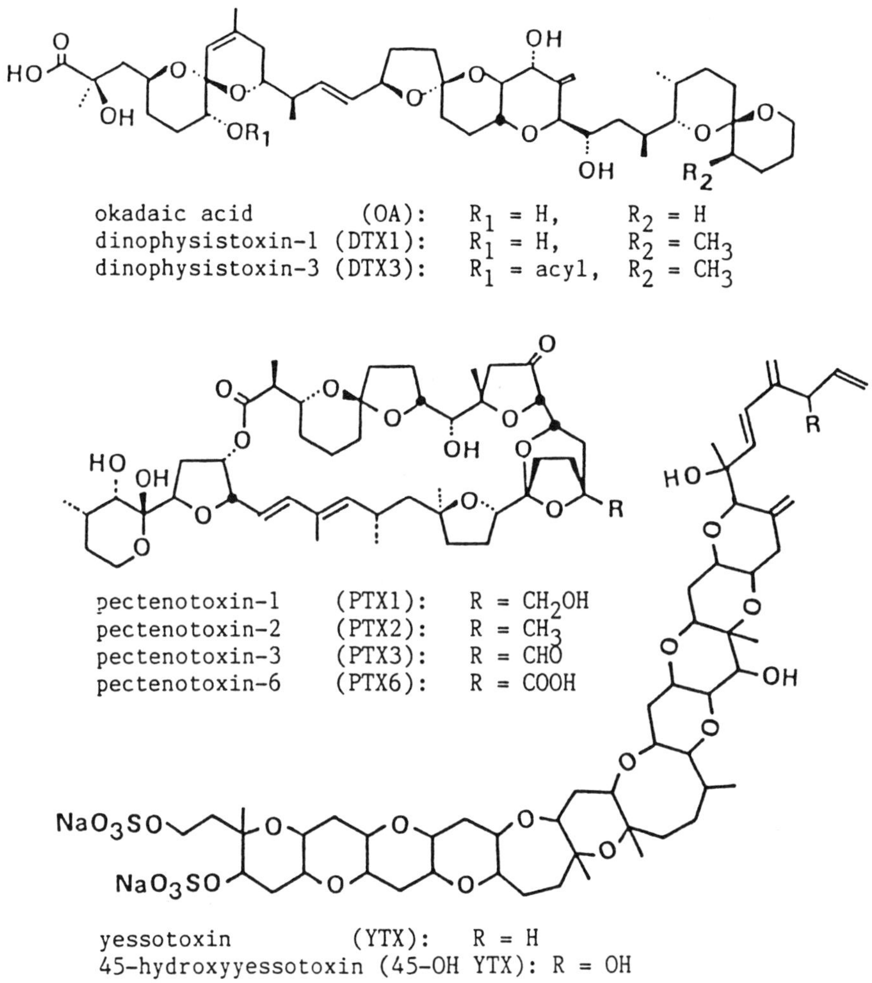

Figure 6 Diarrhetic shellfish toxins. Okadaic acid is also a potent tumor promoter.

protein kinase C and dephosphorylated by protein phosphatases 1 and 2A (which are inhibited by OA).

Mussels collected in Europe (Sweden, The Netherlands, France, and Spain) contain OA as the major toxin (Kumagai et al., 1986; Edebo et al., 1988). In Norway, mussels collected from one area (Arendal) in 1985 contained OA as the main toxic constituent, while mussels collected at another area (Sogndal) in 1986 contained DTX-1 as the major and YTX as well as a pectenotoxinlike toxin as minor toxins (Lee et al., 1988b). Mussels collected at Sogndal in 1988, however, contained DTX-1 and OA, but no YTX (Yasumoto, in Wekell, 1990). Scallops from Japan continue to show the most complicated toxin profile; for example, pectenotoxins have been detected and confirmed only in Japanese shellfish (Yasumoto and Murata, 1990).

The toxins are produced by dinoflagellates belonging to the genera *Dinophysis* and *Prorocentrum*. Difficulties in culturing *Dinophysis* sp. under laboratory conditions and their low population densities in the sea make the assignment of a species to a particular DSP outbreak challenging and somewhat controversial (Lee et al., 1989). Okadaic acid or DTX-1, and in some cases both toxins, have been found by HPLC in *Dinophysis acuminata, D. acuta, D. fortii, D. mitra, D. norvegica, D. rotundata, D. tripos*, and *Prorocentrum lima*; in addition, PTX-2 was found in *D. forti* (Lee et al., 1989). DSP toxins have also been associated with *D. sacculus* (Alvito et al., 1990; Sampayo et al., 1990). Cell densities of *D. fortii* as low as 200 cells/L have been associated with shellfish toxic to humans (Yasumoto et al., 1978).

The DSP toxin profile is diverse and dynamic, and the resulting spatial and temporal variations should be considered in designing sampling protocols. Ratios of OA to DTX-1 in *Dinophysis* cells show significant intraspecies variation (Yasumoto, 1990), and toxin profiles also vary by region, by season and even within a given area, from year to year (Yasumoto and Murata, 1990). To further complicate sampling, levels of toxins (e.g., OA) can vary in adjacent shellfish samples (e.g., mussels) at a given sampling site; shellfish at the same site but at different depths in the water column also show differences in total DSP levels (Edebo et al., 1988).

The dynamics of the toxin profile are mediated by toxin removal and possibly by toxin transformation. Since only OA, DTX-1, and PTX-2 were found in *Dinophysis* sp. cultures and other analogs found in scallops were absent in the algae (Lee et al., 1989), it is presumed (Yasumoto, 1990) that acylation of DTX-1 to DTX-3, and a series of oxidations of the 43-CH3 of PTX-2 to PTX-1 (CH20H), PTX-3 (CHO), and finally to PTX-6 (COOH) occur in the scallop hepatopancreas. The organism that produces YTX remains unknown.

The rate of removal of toxin from shellfish (depuration rate) most likely depends upon the species and may be affected by such interrelated factors as the feeding or pumping rate of the shellfish, the temperature, salinity, and the level of nontoxic algae and particulates. In Japan (using intact mouse bioassays), DSP toxins decreased from 4.4 to 2.5 MU in 1 week and then to 0.5 MU/g by the next week (Yasumoto et al., 1978). In the Netherlands, toxicity in mussels (*M. edulis*) was no longer detectable by rat bioassay after 4 weeks at water temperatures of 14–15°C (Kat, 1983). In the North Sea off the coast of Sweden (water temperatures of 1–3°C), mussels (*M. edulis*) in 1 week became toxic quite rapidly (0.4–5.4 μg OA/kg hepatopancreas). After the bloom had subsided, OA levels in mussels decreased in 1 week from 7.2 to 1.8 μg/kg as measured by HPLC with fluorescence detection (Edebo et al., 1988). These data show that in endemic areas, weekly sampling may not be sufficient for maximum protection of public health.

Most of the methods developed for the detection or quantification of DSP toxins detect the presence or the physiological action of OA toxins. Reliance on detection methods for DSP toxins specific for only OA and its derivatives, although better than no method at all, may not be adequate if resident phytoplankton in shellfish-growing areas are capable of producing the pectenotoxins and/or yessotoxins without producing the OA toxins. Hopefully, future monitoring methods can be devised that will measure all of the components of DSP toxins.

To ensure the highest sensitivities with any detection or quantitation method, it is important that recoveries of DSP toxins from shellfish are maximized. Recoveries of toxins (e.g., OA) are achieved if homogenization methods are employed that provide greatest disruption of the tissue (Edebo et al., 1988). In addition, for best results, it is important that a large number of samples be analyzed to compensate for the variation in the toxicity of shellfish at each sampling site. Methods developed to date include (1) animal bioassays; (2) suckling mouse assay; (3) intestinal loop assay; (4) cytotoxic assay; (5) immunological assays (RIA, ELISA); (6) gas chromatography (GC); and (7) HPLC (fluorescence, UV detection).

A. Bioassays

1. Mouse Bioassays

The first analytical method developed for DSP was a mouse bioassay (Yasumoto et al., 1978, 1980). An official mouse bioassay scheme published by the Ministry of Health and Welfare, Japan (1981), is cited by many investigators, and either this method or a variation of it is used for monitoring shellfish toxicity in many of the areas impacted by DSP. The assay is summarized as follows: A minimum of 200 g shellfish sample (shucked or shellstock) is transported to the laboratory on ice or, if frozen, left in the frozen state. If testing cannot be immediately completed, the samples should be frozen and transported. Samples are drained, weighed, and if possible the hepatopancreas (digestive glands or mid-gut gland) is carefully removed. Only the hepatopancreas portions are finely chopped and mixed to make the test samples. For samples for which excising only the hepatopancreas is difficult (e.g., dried samples), the entire sample is finely chopped and mixed. The sample is homogenized in 3 times the test sample volume of acetone for a minimum of 2 minutes, filtered and residue extracted two more times with 2 times test sample volume of acetone. Extracts are combined, evaporated under vacuum, taken up into 100–200 ml diethyl ether and a small volume of water. The diethyl ether layer is washed two times with distilled water, the diethyl ether removed under vacuum, and the oily residue taken up in 1% Tween 60 saline adjusting the volume of solution to equal 1.0 ml for each 20 g of shucked meats. For highly toxic samples, further dilutions may be necessary. Each of three male mice (16–20 g) is injected with either 0.5- or 1.0-ml sample. A mouse unit (MU) is defined as that amount of toxin that kills a mouse in 24 hr. The actual determination of MU is calculated using the smallest dose at which at least two of the three injected mice die within 24 hr and correcting for dilution factors and dosage given. Yasumoto et al. (1978) determined that 12 MU were sufficient to cause illness in adult humans.

The effects of i.p. injection of toxic extracts into mice are inactivation and general weakness (Yasumoto et al., 1978). Onset time ranges from 30 min to several hours, and death takes place from 100 min to 47 hr after injection depending on the dose given. Toxin in cottonseed oil and administered via stomach tube in mice elicits similar symptoms, but with a 16-fold increase in the lethal dose compared to that obtained by i.p. injection (Yasumoto et al., 1978); the toxin is also toxic to chicks (i.p.) and cats (oral). In Japan (Yasumoto and Murata, 1990), the official regulation requires toxin levels in shellfish to be below 5 MU/100 g meat. The method defines the toxicity by total lethality and toxins, and their different toxicological effects are not distinguished.

In France, the mouse bioassay method has been modified by reducing the observation period from 24 to 5 hr; less than 4 μg OA was necessary to observe a lethality time greater than 5 hr (Marcaillou-LeBaut and Masselin, 1990). A 5-hr observation time is also used for monitoring in Portugal and Spain (Alvito et al., 1990) such that a period of 5 hr after i.p. injection is the minimum survival time to allow public consumption of the corresponding shellfish. Alvito et al. (1990) found that surveillance times longer than 5 hr should be used in some instances (24–48 hr) with the mouse bioassay; some shellfish samples found positive in the suckling mouse did not cause death in intact mice until 5 hr had elapsed after injection.

2. *Rat Bioassay*

Excised hepatopancreas samples from suspect shellfish are mixed in diets fed to white rats (*Rattus norvegicus*, 100–120 g) that have been starved for 24 hr (Kat, 1983; Underdal et al., 1985). Observations are made concerning total feed intake and the consistency of the feces. Specifically the method entails mixing the hepatopancreas of 10 mussels with 6 g ground rat feed and offering this to a rat. It is noted whether rats eat or refuse the mixture. The consistency of feces produced is rated as either normal, soft diarrhea, or diarrhea. The degree of toxicity of the shellfish sample is assessed based on the observations and using a 4-point scale ranging from negative (–) to seriously toxic (+++) (Table 2). The rat bioassay has been used in The Netherlands to monitor for DSP toxins in shellfish (Kat, 1983). This method, which does not kill the animals, has been adopted for use by countries where bioassays that result in animal deaths have been made illegal. Toxicological testing methods using oral dosing are generally less sensitive than those using other routes of administration (e.g., i.v., i.p.). In addition, the rat bioassay as described here lacks quantitative precision, and it is somewhat difficult to compare data generated by this method to those using the mouse bioassay.

B. Suckling Mouse Assay

The suckling mouse test developed for assessments of bacterial virulence (Dean et al., 1972) has been adapted for detecting DSP toxins by Hamano et al., 1985, and Marcaillou-LeBaut et al., 1985. Results generated by this method are related to DSP toxicity from the effects of OA and its derivatives. The method involves intragastric administration of the shellfish extract followed by determination of fluid accumulation in the intestine, expressed as the ratio of intestinal weight to remaining body weight (R). Diarrhetic effects are estimated as follows: $R < 0.07$-negative; $R > 0.09$-positive; and $0.07 < R < 0.09$-questionably positive.

Table 2 Diarrhetic Mussel Poisoning Parameters in Relation to the Percentage Eaten of a Mussel Mixture Offered to Test Animals

Percentage eaten	Fecal consistency	Degree of toxicity	
100–90	Normal	Negative	–
90–50	Normal	Slightly toxic	+
80–50	Soft diarrhea	Moderately toxic	++
<50	Diarrhea	Seriously toxic	+++

Source: From Kat, 1983.

Marcaillou-LeBaut et al. (1985) compared the suckling mouse and intact mouse bioassays and found that both tests showed somewhat poor reproducibility. Both procedures were reported as useful in certain situations considering the lack of an alternate analytical technique. Alvito et al. (1990) in a similar comparison study found some correlations as well between the two methods.

C. Intestinal Loop Assay

The fluid accumulation in the intestine of intact rabbits and mice has been used by Hamano et al. (1985) to detect DSP. Suspensions of DSP toxins in 1% Tween 60 saline were injected into intestinal loops. A positive result was obtained when the ratio of the volume of accumulated fluid (ml) to the length of the loop (cm) was more than 1.0.

D. Cytotoxicity

1. *Rat Hepatocytes*

Underdal et al. (1985) report a testing procedure for DSP based on the measurement of lactate dehydrogenase leakage from rat hepatocytes following treatment with shellfish extracts. Preliminary results indicate the procedure may be applicable to shellfish toxicity monitoring but further work is required.

2. *Growth Inhibition L 1210 Mouse Leukemia Cells*

Yanagi et al. (1989) determined cytotoxicity of DSP toxins by measuring cell densities using a Coulter counter after incubation of 10^5 cell/ml L 1210 mouse leukemia cells in 10% fetal calf serum with DSP toxin after 48 hr at 37°C in 5% CO_2/air. Cytotoxicities of analogs of DTX-3 expressed as dose (μg/ml) causing 50% growth inhibition paralleled data generated by intact mouse bioassays, but the method was not as sensitive as the mouse bioassay and differences among the analogs was less significant.

E. Immunoassays

1. Radioimmunoassay

Development of an RIA for OA was recently reported by Levine et al. (1988b). Antibodies to OA were prepared by immunizing rabbits with OA conjugated at the carboxy function to form an amide bond with an amino group of the immunogenic carrier, bovine albumin (using carbodiimide). The RIA can detect 0.2 pmol OA. Other structurally related marine toxins such as maitotoxin, palytoxin, and brevetoxin (PbTx-2) did not inhibit binding of tritiated OA to the antibody.

2. Enzyme-Linked Immunosorbent Assay

An ELISA method was recently developed by Uda et al. (1988) and Usagawa et al. (1989). Usagawa et al. (1989) used murine monoclonal antibodies against OA prepared from hybridoma clones obtained by fusion of mouse 653 myeloma cells with mouse immune spleen cells sensitized to OA–ovalbumin conjugate. The antibody reacted with DTX-1 as well as OA, but did not react with the other toxins such as an analog of DTX-3, PTX-1, or YTX. A competitive inhibition ELISA using alkaline phosphatase as a detection system had a sensitivity of 10 μg/ml (10ppb) for OA. Organic solvents such as methanol, normally used in the extraction of DSP toxins from samples, lowers the sensitivity to OA using the ELIgw; methanol increases the background absorbance at 405 nm used in the detection system (Usagawa et al., 1989).

A commercial product is now available to measure OA using an ELISA (DSB check, Ube Industries, Ltd., Tokyo, Japan). The applicability of this kit for monitoring DTX-1 and -3 was tested recently. There was good correlation between the results obtained using an HPLC method compared to those with the kit (Kokawa et al., 1989). OA is now commercially available in the United States and Japan.

F. Gas Chromatography

GC methods have been developed to detect and separate OA toxins (Murata et al., 1982; Yasumoto et al., 1984). The toxins from diethyl ether extracts of dinoflagellate cultures were first isolated and purified using silicic acid, gel permeation chromatography, and reversed-phase partition chromatography. GC analysis of trimethylsilyl derivatives of intact toxin and methyl esters was conducted using glass columns (3 mm × 800 mm, 2% OV-101 on 60/80 mesh Uniport HP) at 315–320°C, N2 flow rate at 30 ml/min, and detection by hydrogen flame ionization.

G. High Pressure Liquid Chromatography

A method utilizing HPLC has been reported (Lee et al., 1987) and has been adopted by many investigators. This method involves extraction of shellfish with 80% methanol, purification of the extract by solvent partition and column cleanup followed by derivatization of the carboxylic acid okadaic acid toxins (OA, DTX-1, PTX-6, and PTX-7) with the fluorochrome reagent

9-anthanyldiazomethane (ADAM) to fluorescent esters. The derivatized toxins are analyzed by HPLC (Develosil ODS-5 column, 4.6 x 250 mm) using MeCN–MeOH–H_2O (8:1:1) as mobile phase with fluorescence detection (excitation 365 nm, emission 412 nm). Derivatives of OA and DTX-1 gave a linear response from 1–80 ng with recoveries (from shellfish extracts spiked with OA or DTX-1) of 95–98%.

Toxins with a primary hydroxyl group (PTX-1 and PTX-4) have been derivatized to fluorescent esters with 1-anthroyl nitrile under conditions specified by Lee et al. (1988). Analysis was carried out on a Develosil ODS column using acetonitrite–methanol (85:15) with excitation at 365 and emission at 465 nm.

The sulfated toxin YTX was chromatographed on a Develosil ODS column with methanol–sodium phosphate buffer (0.1 M, pH 5.7, 9:1) and detection at 230 nm (Lee et al., 1988a). At present this method (Lee et al., 1987) represents the nearest approach to a routine analytical technique; however, results of a recent collaborative study indicate that it is not yet sufficiently rugged for official international acceptance as a standard method (summarized by Stabel and Cembella, 1990). Most inconsistencies in this method appear to be due to the fluorescent-derivatization and sample-rinsing steps. The ADAM reagent is unstable so that resulting degradation products may yield artifact peaks on HPLC chromatograms. Deterioration of the fluorochrome reagent may also lead to incomplete derivatization of the toxin components. Therefore the reagent should be stored at low temperatures (–70°C), preferable in complete darkness in a dessicator, and should be subdivided into small aliquots to be prepared in solvent immediately before use. Since the diazo reaction involved in the derivatization procedure most likely is pH sensitive, proper pH control during the reaction is necessary. As much as half of the total toxin can be lost during the rinsing procedure during sample cleanup and is dependent on technical expertise, and the specific technique adopted. In addition, there is need for an internal standard to use in optimization of the reaction kinetics, extraction efficiency, material recovery and chromatographic stability without sacrificing precious and often unavailable toxin standards. For comparable and reproducible results, the purified fluorochrome reagent ADAM should be obtained from commercial sources rather than synthesized by each laboratory.

Two new methods for the determination of OA and its analogs have recently been introduced (Dickey and Bencsath, 1989, 1990) and are adaptions of the method introduced by Lee et al. (1987). The methods involve the derivatization of OA and its analogs with either 1-pyrenyldiazomethane (PDAM) or 1-bromoacetylpyrene (BAP). The pyrenylmethylesters (PDAM method) are generated by heating a mixture of 0.1% PDAM in ethyl acetate (w/v) and toxic extract in methanol (1:1) at 75°C for 30 min. The residue obtained after solvent removal is redissolved in hexane–chloroform (1:1) and extracted from the solid phase (Lee et al., 1987). The final eluate from SPE is dried, redissolved in acetonitrile, and analyzed by ODS reversed-phase HPLC using a mobile phase of 75% acetonitrile in water at a flow rate of 2.0 ml/min. Elution is monitored at an excitation wavelength of 340 nm and an emission wavelength of 394 nm. The pyrenylacylesters (BAP method) are generated by heating a mixture of 0.04%

(w/v) toxic extract and 0.05% diisopropylethylamine (v/v) in acetonitrile at 75°C for 30 min. The residue obtained after solvent removal is treated as described for the PDAM method. HPLC conditions are identical with the exception of excitation and emission wavelengths which are 365 and 418 nm, respectively. The lower limits of detection from spiked whole shellfish homogenates are 250 ng/g and 62 ng/gm by the PDAM and BAP methods, respectively. Recovery values from shellfish homogenates are >90% at concentrations of 1.0 μg OA/g or greater, and linearity (r values) of calibration plots are >0.998 between 62.0 ng/g and 4.0 μg/g. At present, the PDAM and BAP reagents for the determination of OA and analogs are under evaluation by independent laboratories to determine suitability of one or both methods for a collaborative study (Dickey, personal communication, 1990). At this time, only okadaic acid is commercially available.

VIII. CIGUATERA

Ciguatera is a term designating an illness caused by eating a variety of reef fishes and is most prevalent in the South Pacific and the Caribbean (see Withers, 1988; Miller, 1990a). Symptoms of the illness vary and include GI disturbances, neurological effects (e.g., paresthesia and dysesthesia-temperature reversal), and cardiovascular disorders (see Bagnis et al., 1979b; Hokama, 1988; Withers, 1988; Kodama and Hokama, 1989; Calvert, 1990). The toxic effects are cumulative and can last from several days to several months with resurgence of some symptoms after several years (Hokama, 1988; Withers, 1988). Ciguatera has been estimated to cause annually more than 20,000 illnesses worldwide (Bagnis et al., 1979a) and in the accounts for more than one-third of all finfishborne illness outbreaks (Bryan, 1988). Recent evidence indicates that levels as low as 1 ppb can cause intoxication in adults (Yasumoto and Murata, 1990).

Historically, the term ciguatera has been defined more by symptomology and by the epidemiological aspects of the illness than by the chemistry or characterization of toxin(s). Ciguatera has been one of the most difficult of the marine toxins to study due to the unpredictable and variable nature of fish toxicity, the scarcity of toxic fish to study and absence of any toxin standards, the logistics problems encountered in working in some of the endemic areas, the diversity of fish species implicated, the tedious isolation procedures required due to the extremely low toxin concentration in the fishes (ppb), and by the complex nature and multiplicity of the toxin(s).

Ciguatoxin (CTX), thought to be the main toxin in ciguateric fishes, was isolated and crystallized from Moray eel viscera in the pure form by Scheuer's group at the University of Hawaii; results of a partial chemical characterization suggested that the structure was most likely that of a polyether (Scheuer et al., 1967; Tachibana, 1980; Nukina et al., 1984; Tachibana et al., 1987). Recently, 350 μg of pure ciguatoxin was isolated (Legrand et al., 1989a,b) from viscera of over 800 moray eels, and the molecular formula of $C_{60}H_{86}NO_{19}$ was proposed on the basis of high resolution FAB mass spectral data. The structure (Figure 7a) was recently proposed (Murata et al., 1989a,b,

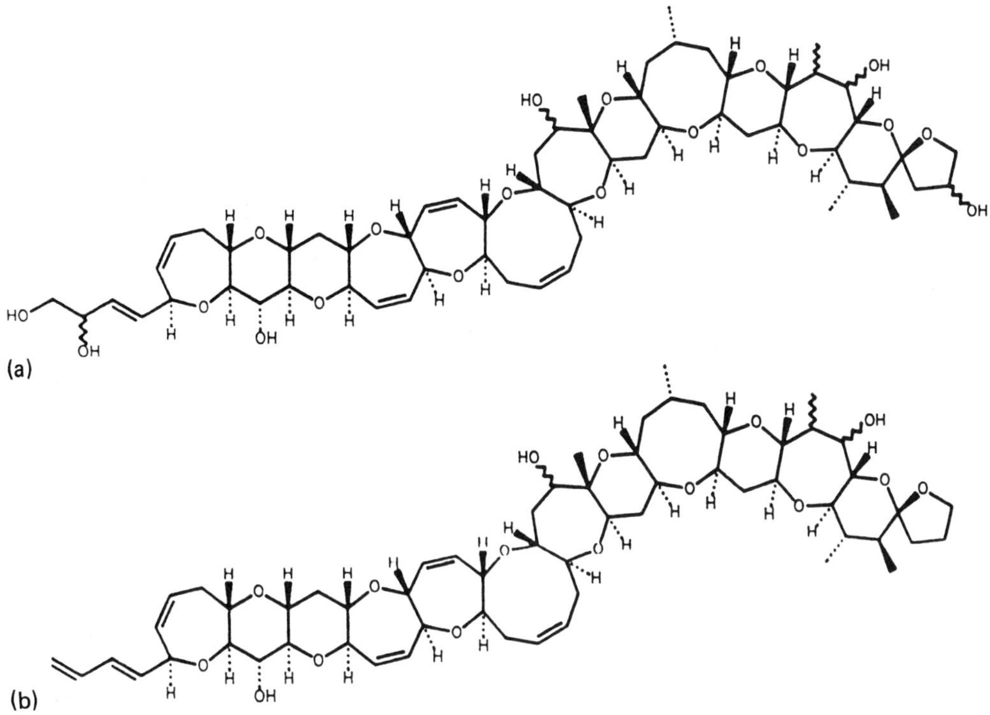

Figure 7 Ciguatoxins of known structure. Form (a) is the parent compound ciguatoxin (CTX, isolated from moray eels) and form (b) is a congener isolated from the dinoflagellate *G. toxicus*.

1990). The characteristic feature of CTX is the presence of 13 contiguously transfused ether rings of five through nine members resembling the brevetoxins and YTX (Yasumoto, 1990). In addition, several analogs of CTX have been structurally defined (Legrand et al., 1989b; Murata et al., 1989a,b, 1990; Lewis et al., 1991). Studies in French Polynesia (Yasumoto et al., 1977; Bagnis et al., 1979a) and in Hawaii (Shimizu, 1982) indicate that the toxin is first produced by an epiphytic dinoflagellate and then transmitted to various fishes through the food chain. The toxin-producing dinoflagellate *Gambierdiscus toxicus* (Yasumoto et al., 1977) produces little or variable quantities of toxin in the laboratory and shows variation in toxin production in the natural environment as well. So far *G. toxicus* has not produced CTX in culture (Yokoyama et al., 1988) but instead produces at least four less polar toxins (Legrand et al., 1990). *G. toxicus* also produces maitotoxin (MTX) (Yokoyama et al., 1988) a second important toxin in CTX, which was first detected in the surgeonfish (see Yasumoto and Murata, 1990). The structure of MTX, a polar water-soluble polyether, is still undefined. MTX is one of the most potent marine toxins known with an LD 99 of 0.13 μg/kg (i.p. mouse) (Yasumoto and Murata, 1990). At the cellular level, it induces a net influx of calcium through the plasma membrane by selectively activating or modifying voltage-dependent calcium channels (Kobayashi et al., 1986) and induces activation of single channels mainly permeable to sodium ions (Faivre et al., 1990). It is 80 times more potent than saponin in hemolytic ability and can induce severe pathomorphological changes in the stomach, heart, and lymphoid tissues in mice and rats by injection (i.p.) of as little as 200–400 ng/kg (Terao et al., 1989). Changes in lymphoid tissues are thought to be due to MTX stimulation of glands, causing release of cortisol into the blood, which produces acute involution of the thymus and other lymphoid tissues (Terao et al., 1989). MTX causes death of hepatocyte cultures by elevated intracellular calcium which inhibits mitochondrial oxidative phosphorylation causing depletion of cell ATP (Kutty et al., 1989). It causes damage and death of cultured cardiomyocytes by a similar mechanism (Santostasi et al., 1990).

Scaritoxin gives symptoms in mice similar to those of ciguatoxin and may be present in a wide variety of fish (Hashimoto, 1979). Scaritoxin has the same pharmacological properties as ciguatoxin (Yasumoto and Murata, 1990) and can be separated from ciguatoxin by silicic acid chromatography (Hashimoto, 1979), DEAE cellulose, and TLC (Yasumoto and Murata, 1990); the toxin has been mainly associated with parrotfish (scaridae).

Recent evidence has further implicated OA and its analogs (DSP toxins) as contributory agents in ciguatera (Gamboa et al., 1990; Dickey et al., 1990). Several other dinoflagellate species common to endemic areas are known to produce toxins; therefore, the full spectrum of toxins responsible for ciguatera may still be unknown. None of the ciguatera toxins are commercially available at this time.

A. Stability

Toxicity of crude ciguatoxin (both polar and less polar analogs) can be maintained in methanol solution at room temperature for at least 6 months. Crude ciguatoxin is stable in water, pyridine, acetic acid, and 1 N NaOH at 100°C for at least 10 min; under continuous air stream overnight, under sunlight exposure in methanol for 1 hr, and in metal salt solution for at least 36 hr. Toxicity was partially lost by treatment with sodium periodate in aqueous methanol at room temperatures for 75 min and by treatment with *p*-toluenesulfonic acid in methanol at 100 for 30 min. Toxicity was completely lost by treatment with 1 N HCl for 10 min and treatment with acetic anhydride in pyridine (Nukina et al., 1984).

Methods developed to detect ciguatera toxins include (1) animal bioassays; (2) varied organ and tissue assays; (3) molecular pharmacological assays; (4) immunoassays; and (5) HPLC.

B. Bioassays

Bioassays for ciguatera toxicity have involved many animal species including fish, shrimp, crayfish, frogs, mosquitos, dogs, pigs, hamsters, guinea pigs, turtles, mongoose, rabbits, chicks, cats, rats, and mice. The subject of ciguatera bioassays (and in vitro assays) has recently been thoroughly reviewed by Rakotoniaina and Miller (1990). At present, the most widely used bioassay utilizes the intact mouse.

Mice have been the animal of choice to test by injection of extracts of suspect samples for ciguatera toxicity; however, their use has been somewhat controversial due to a variable sensitivity of mice to some forms of ciguatera toxins, periodic questionable correlations of mouse toxicity to human reactions, reactions of injected mice which must be critically observed, and the form of toxic material given (Rakotoniaina and Miller, 1990).

In general, mouse bioassays involve an injection (i.p.) into mice (15–21 g) of a toxic fraction (solvent extracted from algal cultures or from flesh or viscera of fish) diluted in either saline or phosphate-buffered saline with or without Tween 60 (0.2%). The mice are observed for symptoms, which can include all or some of the following: prolonged suppression of body temperature, reduced activity, lumbar muscle contractions, unsteadiness or difficulties in walking, breathing difficulties, diarrhea, cyanosis, piloerection, reduced reflexes, and death (Kimura et al., 1982b; Hoffman et al., 1983; Sawyer et al., 1984). Toxin levels have been estimated by using rating scales such as that used by Kimura et al. (1982b) or by regression analysis of the relationship of the injected dose to the survival time (Tachibana, 1980). Mouse lethality (i.p.) estimated by Legrand et al. (1989b) for both crude and pure ciguatoxin was LD 8900 μg/kg and LD 0.4 μg/kg, respectively (where LD is the extrapolated lethal dose which would kill mice at infinite time).

C. Organ and Tissue Assays/Molecular Pharmacological Assays

Early reports on the pharmacology of ciguatoxin are conflicting due to both the variability in purity of the samples and the presence of secondary toxins (see Withers, 1988). Controversial results from in vitro and in vivo studies have surrounded the action of ciguatoxin on cholinesterase (Rakotoniaina and Miller, 1990). Early studies showed that the primary action of ciguatoxin is to increase the permeability of the excitable membranes to sodium, causing depolarization. Ciguatoxin-induced depolarization is blocked by TTX, and both this depolarization and the consequent changes in membrane excitability are antagonized by increased extracellular calcium ion concentrations (Rayner et al., 1969).

A variety of smooth muscle preparations have been utilized for testing ciguatera-type toxins, including the guinea pig vas deferens and the smooth muscle of the large intestine (see Rakotoniaina and Miller, 1990). The guinea pig ileum assay has been used by several investigators to study the effects of ciguatera-type toxins (Miller, 1990b; Rakotoniaina and Miller, 1990).

The guinea pig atrium assay has been used to detect ciguatoxin in fish tissues (Kimura et al., 1982b; Miyahara et al., 1988). The extent of inotropic effects of crude extracts on the isolated guinea pig atrium is expressed as the ratio of the amplitude of contraction occurring after addition of extract as compared to the initial amplitude of untreated atrium. In a comparison of the RIA, mouse bioassay, and guinea pig atrium assay (Kimura et al., 1982b), moderate correlation was shown between the following: RIA:mouse bioassay ($r = 0.58$); RIA:guinea pig atrium assay ($r = 0.62$); and guinea pig atrium assay:mouse bioassay ($r = 0.62$). All three assay procedures showed good correlation when ciguatoxin was at high levels in tissues. The results of these studies suggest that the three test procedures are responding to multiple toxins of similar chemical and physical properties, which may vary in toxic potency.

D. Immunoassays

Immunological methods for the analysis of polyether marine toxins (brevetoxin, palytoxin, OA, and CTX) have recently been reviewed (Hokama, 1990b).

1. *Radioimmunoassays*

An RIA procedure for the direct detection of ciguatoxin in fish tissue was developed by Hokama et al. (1977), which was successfully used in Hawaii in a mass screening of 5529 Seriola dumerili (Amberjack or Kahala) during a 2-year period. Tested fish were consumed by the public without an incidence of ciguatera (Kimura et al., 1982a,b). Although false positives were detected, these reactions have been attributed to the presence of other toxic polyethers structurally similar to CTX (Hokama, 1990b).

For the RIA, purified CTX was conjugated to human serum albumin, injected into sheep and rabbits, and antibodies were produced. The sheep antibody to CTX was used in the RIA after being purified and coupled to ^{125}I (Hokama et al., 1977).

2. *Enzyme Immunoassay (EIA)*

Hokama et al. (1983) developed an enzyme immunoassay for the detection of CTX using the same sheep serum used for the RIA. The procedure incorporating a sheep anti-CTX–horseradish peroxidase conjugate was as sensitive as the RIA but faster and less expensive. The method was further simplified by using bamboo sticks coated with correction fluid so that fish to be tested could simply be poked, the stick mixed with reagents, and the color reaction assessed by visual observation. For example, in a study (Hokama et al., 1987) using the stick test, fish were sampled by inserting the skewer end of a bamboo stick coated with liquid paper correction fluid into the dorsal anterior and ventral posterior sections of one or both sides of the fish. Each stick was inserted five times into the flesh at 1s/insertion. Each fish was examined with six sticks. The stick was air-dried and then immersed into fixative (0.3% H_2O_2 in absolute methanol) for 1 s, excess solution blotted onto tissue paper, and the stick air-dried. The stick was washed in Tris buffer (0.05 M, pH 7.5) for 10 s and excess solution blotted onto tissue paper. The stick was then immersed for 15–30 s into sheep anti-CTX-HRP (diluted just prior to use in Tris buffer + human serum albumin and 0.01% sodium azide). Excess antibody conjugate was blotted onto tissue paper. The stick was washed in two changes of Tris buffer, 10 s each, excess buffer blotted, and the stick immersed into 0.3 ml substrate (4-chloro-1-naphthol in methanol, Tris buffer, H202) for 10 min at room temperature. The intensity of the color was compared with a color scheme as follows: 0, no color; 1.0+, slightly bluish-purple; 1.5–2.0+, lightly bluish-purple; 2.0–2.5+, moderately bluish-purple; and 3.0–5.0+, moderately to intensely bluish-purple. Scoring of samples was 0–2.0+, nontoxic; 2.1–2.4+, borderline; and ≥2.5+, toxic. With this assay, 14 clinically documented toxic fishes gave a mean score of 3.1, and 60 fishes that had been consumed with no human illnesses scored 1.2 (Hokama et al., 1987, 1990).

In a competitive EIA, other polyethers such as OA, brevetoxin, MTX, and monensin cross-reacted with the CTX antibody (Hokama et al., 1984). In addition, the immunological cross-reactivity of brevetoxin to CTX has been shown using goat anti-PbTX antibody in a competitive RIA as discussed previously (Baden et al., 1984).

Most recently, monoclonal antibodies have been incorporated in the stick test procedure (Hokama et al., 1988) with the assay essentially the same except HRP was now conjugated to the anti-CTX monoclonal antibody (MAb-CTX) so that the final immersion of the stick is in the HRP substrate (4-chloronaphthol with H202). The intensity of color is read from 0 (nontoxic) to 4+ (toxic) so that scores < 1.2 are non-toxic, > 1.3–1.9 are borderline, and > 2.0 are toxic.

The latest refinement of the EIA involves a solid-phase immunobead assay (SPIA) (Hokama, 1990a). The method is similar to the stick test only in the SPIA, bamboo paddles, coated with organic base solvent correction fluid are used to insert into the flesh of test fish. The paddle is then fixed with methanol, air-dried, and immersed into an immunobead (MAb-CTX)–latex color suspension, and rinsed in saline. Any distinct coloration of the stick after 5 min is considered a positive. Appropriate positive and negative control samples are run with the test sample. The SPIA method was compared to the stick EIA using over 400 fish of various species with good agreement (Hokama, 1990a).

E. HPLC

An HPLC method was developed by Legrand et al. (1989b, 1990) for the purification of ciguatoxin from Moray eel viscera following multiple sample manipulations. The sample was subjected to extensive cleanup, with the final step involving separation of ciguatoxin from other toxins on a LiChrosorb RP 18 column (5 μm, 4.6 × 250 mm) with aqueous acetonitrile (65%) and detection at 215 nm. Previous uncertainties regarding the probable molecular formula were solved by measuring the high resolution fast atom bombardment (HRFAB) mass spectra of the ciguatoxin peak, which showed an MH + ion at m/z 1111.5770 (mean of triplicates), and the probably formula of $C_{60}H_{86}O_{19}$ (MH +, 1111.5840) was obtained. Close examination of the 1H NMR spectrum suggested the presence of a primary hydroxyl group in the toxin molecule. Legrand et al. speculated that this functional group will enable preparation of a hemisuccinate derivate, which can easily be conjugated with a protein to be used as an antigen for immunizing animals to prepare an anti-CTX for development of new immunoassay methods. They add that the hydroxyl group may also be useful for fluorescene labeling to develop a fluorometric assay.

IX. PALYTOXIN

Palytoxin originally isolated from various corals of the genus *Palythoa* is quite lethal (0.5 μg/kg, mouse, i.p.) (Yasumoto and Murata, 1990) (LD_{50}, rabbits,

0.025 μg/kg) (Fox, 1982). It has the most complicated structure (Fig. 8) of a natural product (Moore and Bartolini, 1981; Cha et al., 1982) and like okadaic acid is a potent tumor promoter (Fujiki et al., 1986). Initially, health risks due to the toxin were unclear. Recent evidence indicates that the toxin is widely distributed. It has been found in triggerfish (Fukui et al., 1987), filefish, parrotfish, and xanthid crabs from the Philippines and Singapore. Two palytoxin analogs were isolated from a red alga *Chondria armata*, a species which also produces domoic acid (see Yasumoto and Murata, 1990). Human illnesses and death have occurred after consumption of xanthid crabs (Alcala et al., 1988), mackerel (Kodama et al., 1989), and parrotfish (see Yasumoto and Murata, 1990).

The physiological action of palytoxin has been reviewed recently (Habermann, 1989). Palytoxin increases cell permeability for Na^+ and K^+ but not Ca^{2+} and at concentrations over 100 nm inhibits Na^+, K^+ATPase; because ATPase is a transmembranal protein, palytoxin can trigger a pore as soon as it has recognized the target enzyme (see Habermann, 1989). Methods to determine the presence and levels of palytoxin include (1) animal bioassays, (2) immunoassays, and (3) chromatography.

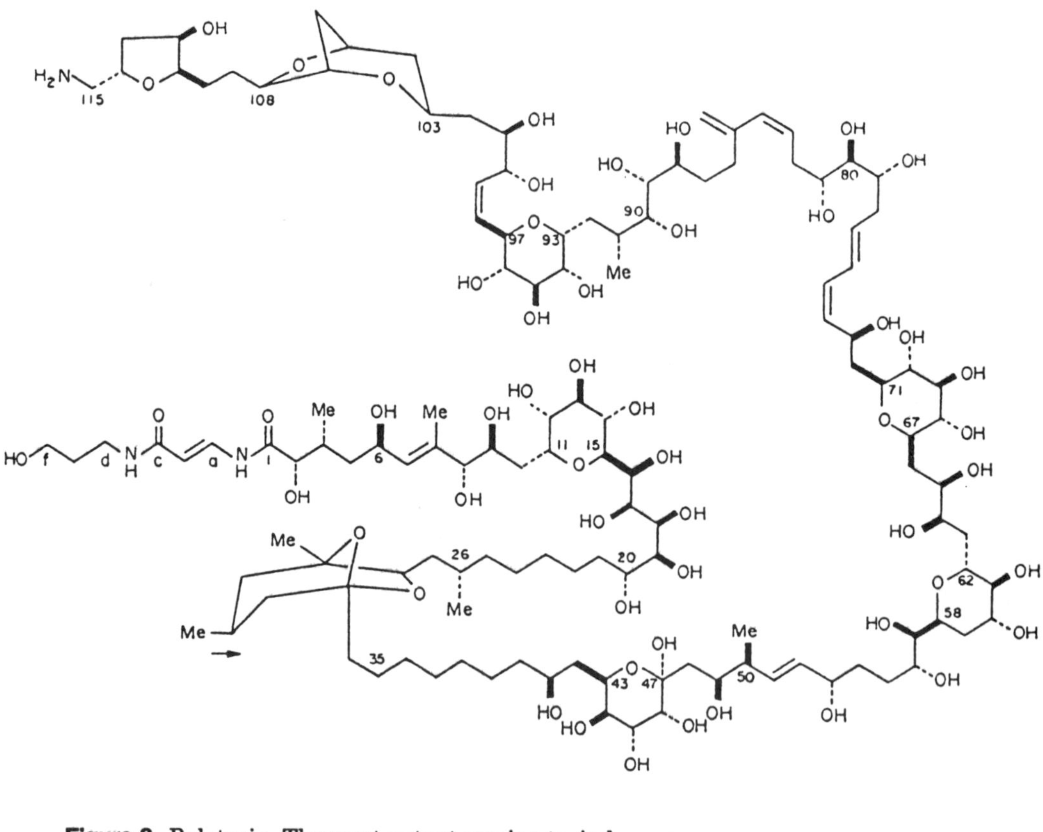

Figure 8 Palytoxin. The most potent marine toxin known.

A. Bioassays

A bioassay method (Teh and Gardiner, 1974) has been used by many investigators. Groups of three male mice (17g) are injected i.p. with suspect toxin, extracted with methanol, evaporated, resuspended in H_2O, lipids removed by diethyl ether and toxin extracted with butanol, followed by cleanup as described by Yasumoto et al. (1986b). The amount of toxin in MU is calculated from the equation $Y = 225.19\ X^{-0.99}$, where Y and X denote MU and death time in minutes, respectively.

B. Immunoassays

A radioimmunoassay was developed for palytoxin by Levine et al. (1988a). Palytoxin was labeled with ^{125}I at its terminal amine group. This labeled palytoxin bound specifically to rabbit antipalytoxin. Other toxins (MTX, OA) did not interact serologically.

C. Chromatography

1. TLC

Separation of palytoxin from other materials present in crabs was carried out by Yasumoto et al. (1986b). TLC was carried out in silica gel 60 and HN_2 F_{254} S plates with two different solvent systems: (1) pyridine–H_2O–BuOH–HOAC (10:12:15:13) and (2) 1-pentanol–pyridine–H_2O (7:7:6). The toxin on the silica gel 60 plates was detected by heating the plates after spraying with H_2SO_4, and that on $NH_2F_{254}S$ plates by exposure to UV light (254 nm).

2. HPLC

HPLC separations have been made by Yasumoto et al. (1986b) on a Develosil ODS-10/20 column (2X25 cm) with alternative use of MeOH–0.1 N HOAC (8:2) and Me CN–0.05N HOAC (5:5) and detection at 263 nm. Separations have also been conducted on an ERC ODS-1282 column (0.6 × 25 cm) with the same solvents as well as on a TSK G 3000 SW column (0.75 × 60 cm) using 0.03 N HOAC as the eluant (Yasumoto et al., 1986b) or a G 3000 SW column using as eluant 0.1 M HOAC (Fukui et al., 1987). For separation of palytoxin from triggerfish (*Melichtys vidua*), a develosil ODS column (2.0 × 25 cm) or an ERC-ODS column (0.6 × 25 cm) was eluted with acetonitrile–0.05M acetic acid (1:1) (Fukui et al., 1987).

X. SUMMARY

When protecting the public health is the objective, there is a direct relationship between the potency of a given toxin and the degree of sensitivity and selectivity required to detect it. For example, the relatively low toxicity of domoic acid allows use of simple UV detection, while the high potency of the PSP toxins demands the high sensitivity and selectivity of postcolumn derivatization or immunoassay.

At the same time, however, there are different priorities at work in the design of screening methods than in the development of determination methods for research. Research-directed methods based on sophisticated instrumentation, particularly FT-NMR, mass spectrometry, and certain HPLC separations generally yield more diverse information at the expense of speed and ruggedness.

Besides being rugged and reasonably fast, screening methods require that standards be readily available. Unfortunately, a recurring theme in the struggle to develop practical screening methods for marine toxins is the lack of primary standards. While domoic acid, and of course tetramethylammonium salts, are easily purchased, many of the most potent toxins are not. Of the extensive saxitoxin group and of all the tetrodotoxin epimers, only the parent compounds, tetrodotoxin and saxitoxin, are commercially available at the time of writing. Many of the brevetoxins can be purchased, but they are costly, as is okidaic acid. Ciguatoxin, since the structure was only recently discovered, will certainly not be available for some time. The lack of a full spectrum of analytical standards is most crippling to the success of chromatographic methods. Well-designed immunoassay kits will not suffer as much from a lack of standards as the chromatography methods, although their full characterization and refinement will be delayed, since cross-reactivity studies should include as many toxin forms as possible.

The ultimate detection method for marine toxins directly measures potency or events that mediate it. It can be argued that this is essentially what whole organism bioassays, such as the mouse bioassays, attempt. From whole organisms on down to protein binding, assays for toxicity progress from the biological to the chemical. Tissue bioassays represent one level, such as those using perfused guinea pig atria or guinea pig ileum. Cellular effects that correlate with potency can be exploited, as in the neuroblastoma cell assay for sodium channel blockers.

At the molecular level, a physicochemical event that determines the cellular response to a toxin could be used, i.e., reversible binding to a receptor, enzyme, or ion-conducting channel. This last means of detecting toxin potency has been demonstrated using competitive displacement of radiolabeled saxitoxin from nerve cell preparations.

If a reversible toxin-binding device could be refined and worked into a rugged (flow-through) geometry, it could be used to develop an automated instrument for screening and confirmation. For initial screening, sample extracts would be passed directly through the detector; positive results could then be confirmed by using a switching valve to redirect an additional portion of sample through the same detector following separation on an HPLC column. Several advantages over existing detection strategies would follow. The system would be much more rapid than whole organism bioassays, tissue bioassays, or cellular bioassays, allowing its use as a detector in automated instruments. From a public health standpoint, the most significant advantage of this approach over other chemical methods is the potential for rapid detection of new and unknown toxins.

REFERENCES

Alcala, A. C., Alcala, L. C., Garth, J. S., Yasumura, D., and Yasumoto, T. (1988). Human fatality due to ingestion of the crab *Demania reynaudii* that contained a palytoxin-like toxin. *Toxicon 26*: 105–107.

Alvito, P., Sousa, I., Franca, S., Sampayo, M. A., DeM. (1990). Diarrhetic shellfish toxins in bivalve molluscs along the coast of Portugal. In *Toxic Marine Phytoplankton*, E. Graneli, B. Sundstrom, L. Edler, and D. M. Anderson, eds. Elsevier, New York, pp. 443–448.

Anderson, D. M., and Po-on Cheng, T. (1988). Intracellular localization of saxitoxin in the dinoflagellate *Gonyaulax tamarensis. J. Phycol. 24*: 17–22.

Anderson, D. M., Sullivan, J. L., and Reguera, B. (1989). Paralytic shellfish poisoning in northwest Spain: The toxicity of the dinoflagellate *Gymnodinium catenatum. Toxicon 27*: 665–674.

Anderson, D. M., Kulis, D. M., Sullivan, J. J., and Hall, S. (1990). Toxin composition variations in one isolate of the dinoflagellate *Alexandrium-fundyense. Toxicon 28*: 885–894.

Anthoni, U., Bohline, L., Larsen, C., Nielsen, P., Neilsen, N. H., and Christophersen, C. (1989a). The toxin tetramine from the "edible" whelk *Neptunea antiqua. Toxicon 27*: 717–723.

Anthoni, U., Bohlin, L., Larsen, C., Nielsen, P., Nielsen, N. H., and Christophersen, C. (1989b). Tetramine: Occurrence in marine organisms and Pharmacology. *Toxicon 27*: 707–716.

Anthoni, U., Christophersen, C., and Nielsen, N. H. (1989c). Simultaneous identification and determination of tetramine in marine snails by proton nuclear magnetic resonance spectroscopy. *J. Agric. Food Chem. 37*: 705–707.

Asano, M. (1952). Studies of the toxic substances contained in marine animals. I. Locality of the poison of *Neptunea (Barbitonia) arthritica* Bernardi. *Jpn. Soc. Sci. Fish. 17*: 283.

Asano, M., and Itoh, M. (1959). Occurrence of tetramine and choline compounds in the salivary gland of a marine gastropod, *Neptunea arthritica* Bernardi. *Tohoku J. Agric. Res. 10*: 209.

Asano, M., and Itoh, M. (1960). Salivary poison of a marine gastropod, *Neptunea arthritica* Bernardi, and the seasonal variation of its toxicity. *Ann. N.Y. Acad. Sci. 90*: 674.

Baden, D. G. (1988). Public health problems of red tides. In *Marine Toxins and Venoms*, A. T. Tu, ed. Marcel Dekker, Inc., New York, pp. 259–277.

Baden, D. G. (1989). Brevetoxins: Unique polyether dinoflagellate toxins. *FASEB J. 3*: 1807–1817.

Baden, D. G., and Tomas, C. R. (1988). Variations in major toxin composition for six clones of *Ptychodiscus brevis. Toxicon 26*: 961–963.

Baden, D. G., Mende, T. J., Lichter, W., and Wellham, L. (1981). Crystallization and toxicology of T34: A major toxin from Florida's red tide organism, (*Ptychodiscus brevis*). *Toxicon 19*: 455.

Baden, D. G., Mende, T. J., Bikhazi, G., and Leung, I. (1982). Bronchoconstriction caused by Florida red tide toxins. *Toxicon 20*: 929–932.

Baden, D. G., Mende, T. J., Walling, J., and Schultz, D. R. (1984). Specific antibodies directed against toxins of *Ptychodiscus brevis* (Florida's red tide dinoflagellate). *Toxicon 22*: 783–789.

Baden, D. G., Mende, T. J., and Brand, L. E. (1985). Cross-reactivity in immunoassays directed against toxins isolated from *Ptychodiscus brevis*. In *Toxic Dinoflagellates*, D. M. Anderson, A. W. White, and D. G. Baden, eds. Elsevier, New York, pp. 363–368.

Baden, D. G., Mende, T. J., Szmant, A. M., Trainer, V. L., Edwards, R. A., and Roszell, L. E. (1988). Brevetoxin binding: Molecular pharmacology versus immunoassay. *Toxicon 26*: 97–103.

Bagnis, R. A., Hurtel, J. M., Chanteau, S., Chungue, E., Inoue, A., and Tasumoto, T. (1979a). Le dinoflagellate *Gambierdiscus toxicus* Adachi et Fukuyo agent causal probable de la ciguatera. *C. R. Acad. Sci. Ser. D. 289*: 671–674.

Bagnis, R. A., Kuberski, T., and Langier, S. (1979b). Clinical Observations on 3009 cases of ciguatera (fish poisoning) in the South Pacific. *Am. J. Trop. Med. Hyg. 28*: 1067–1073.

Bates, H. A., and Rapoport, H. (1975). A chemical assay for saxitoxin, the paralytic shellfish poison. *J. Agric. Food Chem. 23*: 237–239.

Bates, H. A., Kostriken, R., and Rapoport, A. (1978). The occurrence of saxitoxin and other toxins in various dinoflagellates. *Toxicon 16*: 595–601.

Bates, S. S., Bird, C. J., deFreitas, A. S. W., Foxall, R., Gilgan, M., Hanic, L. A., Johnson, G. A., McCulloch, A. W., Odense, P., Pocklington, R., Quilliam, M. A., Sim, P. G., Smith, J. C., Subba Rao, D. V., Todd, E. C. D., Walter, J. A., and Wright, J. C. L. (1989). The pennate diatom Nitzchia pungens as the primary source of domoic acid, a toxin in shellfish from Eastern Prince Edward Island, Canada. *Can. J. Fish Aquat. Sci. 46*: 1203–1215.

Beecher, G. R., Stewart, K. K., and Hare, P. E. (1975). Automated high speed analysis of discrete samples. The use of nonsegmented, continuous flow. In *Protein Nutritional Quality of Foods and Feeds*, M. Friedman, ed. Marcel Dekker, New York, Part I, p. 411.

Betz, J. M., and Blogoslawski, W. J. (1982). Toxicity of *Gonyaulax-tamaraensis-var-excavata* cells to the brine shrimp *Artemia-salina. J. Pharm. Sci. 71*: 463–465.

Boczar, B. A., Beitler, M. K., Liston, J., Sullivan, J. J., and Cattolico, R. A. (1988). Paralytic shellfish toxins in *Protogonyaulax tamarensis* and *Protogonyaulax catenella* in axenic culture. *Plant Physiol. 88*: 1285–1290.

Boyer, G. L. (1980). Chemical investigations of the toxins produced by marine dinoflagellates. Ph.D. dissertation, University of Wisconsin, Madison, Wisconsin.

Boyer, G. L., Fix-Wichmann, C., Mosser, J., Schantz, E. J., and Schnoes, H. K. (1979). Toxins isolated from Bay of Fundy scallops. In *Toxic Dinoflagellate Blooms*, D. L. Taylor and H. H. Seliger, eds. Elsevier/North-Holland, Amsterdam, pp. 373–376.

Boyer, G. L., Sullivan, J. J., Andersen, R. J., Harrison, P. J., and Taylor, F. J. R. (1985). Toxin production in three isolates of *Protogonyaulax sp.* In *Toxic Dinoflagellates*. Anderson, White, and Baden, eds. Elsevier Sci. Publ. Co., Inc., pp. 281–286.

Bruno, M., Gucci, P. M. B., Pierdominici, E., Ioppolo, A., and Volterra, L. (1990). Short Communications. Presence of saxitoxin in toxic extracts from *Gonyaulax polyedra. Toxicon. 28*: 1113–1116.

Bryan, F. L. (1988). Risks associated with vehicles of foodborne pathogens and toxins. *J. Food Protec. 51*: 498–508.

Buckley, L. J., Ikawa, M., and Sasner, J. J. (1976). Isolation of *Gonyaulax tamarensis* toxins from soft shell clams (*Mya arenaria*) and a thin-layer chromatographic-fluorometric method for their detection. *J. Agric. Food Chem. 24*: 107–111.

Buckely, L. J., Oshima, Y., and Shimizu, Y. (1978). Construction of a paralytic shellfish toxin analyzer and its application. *Anal. Biochem. 85*: 157–164.

Calvert, G. (1990). The recognition and management of ciguatera fish poisoning. In *Ciguatera Seafood Toxins*, D. M. Miller, ed. CRC Press, Boca Raton, FL, pp. 2–11.

Carlson, R. E., Lever, M. L., Lee, B. W., and Guire, P. E. (1984). Development of immunoassays for paralytic shellfish poisoning: A radioimmunoassay for saxitoxin. In *Seafood Toxins*, Ragelis, E. P., ed. American Chemical Society, Washington, DC, pp. 181–192.

Catterall, W. A. (1985). The voltage sensitive sodium channel: A receptor for multiple neurotoxins. In *Toxic Dinoflagellates*, D. M. Anderson, A. W. White, and D. G. Baden, eds. Elsevier, New York, pp. 329–342.

Cembella, A. D., Sullivan, J. J., Boyer, G. L., Taylor, F. J. R., and Anderson, R. J. (1987). Variation in paralytic shellfish toxin composition within the *Protogonyaulax tamarensis/catenalla* species complex; red tide dinoflagellates. *Biochem. System. Ecol. 15*: 171–186.

Cembella, A. D., Parent, Y., Jones, D., and Lamoureux, G. (1990). Specificity and cross-reactivity of an absorption-inhibition enzyme-linked immunoassay for the detection of paralytic shellfish toxins. In *Toxic Marine Phytoplankton*, Graneli, E., Anderson, D. M., Edler, L., and Sundstrom, B. G., eds. pp. 339–344.

Cha, J. K., Christ, W. J., Finan, J. M., Fuijoka, M., Kishi, Y., Klein, L. L., Ko, S. S., Leder, J., McWhorter, W. W., Pfaff, K. P., Yonaga, M., Uemura, D., and Hirata, Y. (1982). Stereochemistry of palytoxin 4. Complete structure. *J. Am. Chem. Soc. 104*: 7369–7341.

Chu, F. S., and Fan, T. S. L. (1985). Indirect enzyme-linked immunosorbent assay for saxitoxin in shellfish. *J. AOAC. 68*: 13–16.

Cohen, P., Holmes, C. F. B., and Tsukitani, T. (1990). Okadaic acid: A new probe for the study of cellular regulation. *Trends in Biochem. Sci. 15*: 98–102.

Daigo, K., Noguchi, T., Kawai, N., Miwa, A., and Hashimoto, K. (1989). Determination of paralytic shellfish poison by a lobster nerve-muscle preparation. In *Red Tides*, T. Okaichi, D. M. Anderson, and T. Nemoto, eds. Elsevier, New York, pp. 387–389.

Davio, S., and Fontelo, P. A. (1984). A competitive displacement assay to detect saxitoxin and tetrodotoxin. *Anal. Biochem. 141*: 199–204.

Davis, C. C. (1947). *Gymnodinium breve*: A cause of discolored water and animal mortality in the Gulf of Mexico. *Bot. Gaz. 109*: 358–360.

Dean, A. G., Ching, Y-C, Williams, R. G., and Hardan, L. B. (1972). Test for *Escherichia coli* enterotoxin using infant mice: Application in a study of diarrhea in children in Honolulu. *J. Infect. Dis. 125*: 407–411.

Deffner, G. G. J. (1961). Chemical investigations of the giant nerve fibers of the squid. V. Quaternary ammonium ions in axoplasm. *Biochim. Biophys. Acta. 50*: 555.

Delaney, J. E. (1985). In *Laboratory Procedures for the Examination of Seawater and Shellfish*. A. E. Greenberg and D. A. Hung, eds. Am. Publ. Health Assoc., Washington, DC, pp. 64–80.

Desbiens, M., Coulombe, F., Gaudreault, J., Cembella, A. D., and Larocque, R. (1990). PSP toxicity of wild and cultured blue mussels induced by Alexandrium excavatum in Gaspe Bay (Canada): Implications for aquaculture. In *Toxic Marine Phytoplankton*, E. Graneli, B. Sundstrom, L. Edler, and D. M. Anderson, eds. Elsevier, New York, pp. 459–468.

Dickey, R. W., and Bencsath, F. A. (1989). Intl. Chem. Cong. Pac. Basin Soc., Honolulu, HI, Dec. 17–22, Abst. 0630.

Dickey, R. W., and Bencsath, F. A. (1990). A comparison of methods for the HPLC fluorometric analysis of okadaic acid. In *Third Int. Cong. on Ciguatera Fish Poisoning*, Puerto Rico, April 30–May 4, 1990, Abst. pp. 6–7.

Dickey, R. W., Bobzin, S. C., Faulkner, D. J., Bencsath, F. A., and Andrzejewski, D. (1990). Identification of okadaic acid from a Caribbean dinoflagellate, *Prorocentrum concavum. Toxicon 28*: 371–377.

Do, H. K., Kogure, K., and Simidu, U. (1990). Identification of deep-sea sediment bacteria which produce tetrodotoxin. *App. Env. Microb. 56*: 1162–1163.

Edebo, L., Lange, S., Li, X. P., Allenmark, S., Lindgren, K., and Thompson, R. (1988). Seasonal, geographic, and individual variation of okadaic acid content in cultivated mussels in Sweden. *APMIS 96*: 1036–1042.

Endo, A., Khora, S. S., Murata, M., Naoki, H., and Yasumoto, T. (1988). Isolation of 11-nortetrodotoxin-6(R)-ol and other tetrodotoxin derivatives from the puffer *Fugu niphobles. Tetr. Ltrs. 29*: 4127–4128.

Faivre, J. F., Deroubaix, E., Coulombe, A., LeGrand, A. M., and Coraboeuf, E. (1990). Effect of maitotoxin on calcium current and background inward current in isolated ventricular rat myocytes. *Toxicon 28*: 925–937.

Fix Wichmann, C. F., Niemczura, W. P., Schnoes, H. K., Hall, S., Reichardt, P. B., and Darling, S. D. (1981). Structures of two novel toxins from *Protogonyaulax. J.A.C.S. 103*: 6977–6978.

Florida Department of Natural Resources (FDNR), Contingency Plan for Control of Shellfish Potentially Contaminated by Marine Biotoxins (1985). Bureau of Marine Resources, St. Petersburg, FL, pp. 1–10.

Fox, J. L. (1982). Complex structure of marine toxin unraveled. *Chem. & Eng. News 60(1)*: 19–20.

Frace, M. A., Hall, S., Brodwick, M. S., and Eaton, D. C. (1986). Effects of saxitoxin analogs in ligand competition on sodium currents of squid axons. *Am. J. Physiol. 251* (Cell. Physiol. 20): C159–C166.

Fuchi, Y., Morisaki, S., Nagata, T., Shimazaki, K., Noguchi, T., Ohtom, O. N., and Hashimoto, K. (1988). Determination of tetrodotoxin in puffer fish and shellfish by high performance liquid chromatography. *J. Food Hyg. Soc. Jpn. 29*: 306–312.

Fujiki, H., Suganuma, M., Suguri, H., Hoshizawa, S., Tanagi, K., Uda, N., Wakamatsu, K., Yamada, K., Murata, M., Yasumoto, T., and Suzimura, T. (1988). Diarrhetic shellfish toxin Dinophysistoxin is a potent tumor promoter on mouse skin. *Jpn. J. Cancer Res.* (Gann) *79*: 1089–1093.

Fujiki, H., Suganuma, M., Nakayasu, M., Hakii, H., Horiuchi, T., Takayama, S., and Sugimura, T. (1986). Palytoxin is a non-12-0-tetradecanoylphorbal-13-acetate type tumor promoter in two stage mouse skin carcinogenesis. *Carcinogenesis 7*: 707–710.

Fukui, M., Murata, M., Inoue, A., Gawel, M., and Yasumoto, T. (1987). Occurrence of palytoxin in the trigger fish, *Melichtys vidua. Toxicon 25*: 1121–1124.

Gamboa, P. M., Park, D. L., and Fremy, J. M. (1990). Extraction and purification of toxic fractions from barracuda (*Sphyraena barracuda*) implicated in ciguatera poisoning. In Third Int. Cong. on Ciguatera Fish Poisoning, Puerto Rico, April 30–May 4, 1990, Abst. pp. 3–4.

Grimmelt, B., Nijjar, M. S., Brown, J., Macnair, N., Wagner, S., Johnson, G. R., and Armend, J. F. (1990). Relationship between domoic acid levels in the blue mussel (*Mytilus edulis*) and toxicity in mice. *Toxicon 28*: 501–508.

Habermann, E. (1989). Review article: Palytoxin acts through Na^+, K^+-ATPase. *Toxicon 27*: 1171–1187.

Hall, S. (1982). Toxins and toxicity of *Protogonyaulax* from the northeast Pacific. Ph.D. dissertation, University of Alaska.

Hall, S., and Reichardt, P. B. (1984). Cryptic paralytic shellfish toxins. In *Seafood Toxins*, Ragelis, E. P., ed. American Chemical Society, Washington, DC, pp. 113–123.

Hamano, Y., Kinoshita, Y., and Yasumoto, T. (1985). Suckling mice assay for diarrhetic shellfish toxins. In *Toxic Dinoflagellates*, D. M. Anderson, A. W. White, and D. G. Baden, eds. Elsevier, New York, pp. 383–388.

Harada, T., Oshima, Y., and Yasumoto, T. (1984). Assessment of potential activation of gonyautoxin V in the stomach of mice and rats. *Toxicon 22*: 476–478.

Hashimoto, Y. (1979). *Marine Toxins and Other Bioactive Marine Metabolites*. Japanese Scientific Societies Press, Tokyo, p. 79.

Haya, K., Martin, J. L., Waiwood, B. A., Burridge, L. E., Hungerford, J. M., and Zitko, V. (1990). Identification of paralytic shellfish toxins in mackerel from Southwest Bay of Fundy, Canada. In *Toxic Marine Phytoplankton*, E. Graneli, B. Sundstrom, L. Edler, and D. M. Anderson, eds. Elsevier Science Publishing Co., Inc., pp. 350–355.

Haystead, T. A. J., Sim, A. T. R., Carling, D., Honnor, R. C., Tsukitani, Y., and Cohen, P. (1989). Effects of the tumor promoter okadaic acid on intracellular protein phosphorylation and metabolism. *Nature 337*: 78–81.

Helrich, K. (1990). Official Methods of Analysis, Assoc. Official Analytical Chemists, Arlington, VA.

Hemmert, W. H. (1975). The public health implications of Gymnodinium red tides: A review of the literature and recent events. In *First International Conference on Toxic Dinoflagellate Blooms*, V. R. Lociero, ed. MA Sci. Technol. Found., Wakefield, MA, p. 489.

Henry, A. J. (1948). The toxic principle of *Courbonia virgata*: Its isolation and identification as a tetramethylammonium salt. *Br. J. Pharmac. 3*: 187.

Hoffman, P. A., Granade, H. R., and McMillan, J. P. (1983). The mouse ciguatoxin bioassay: A dose response curve and symptomatology analysis. *Toxicon 21*: 817–824.

Hokama, Y. (1988). Ciguatera fish poisoning. *J. Clin. Lab. Anal. 2*: 44.

Hokama, Y. (1990a). Simplified solid-phase immunobead assay for detection of ciguatoxin and related polyethers. *J. Clin. Lab. Anal. 4*: 213–217.

Hokama, Y. (1990b). Immunological analysis of low molecular weight marine toxins. *J. Toxicol., Toxins Rev.* (in press).

Hokama, Y., Banner, A. H., and Boylan, D. A. (1977). A radioimmunoassay for the detection of ciguatoxin. *Toxicon 15*: 317–325.

Hokama, Y., Abad, M. A., and Kumura, L. H. (1983). A rapid enzyme immunoassay for the detection of ciguatoxin in contaminated fish tissues. *Toxicon 21*: 817–824.

Hokama, Y., Kumura, L. H., Abad, M. A., Yokochi, L., Scheurer, P. J., Nukina, M., Yasumoto, T., Baden, D. G., and Shimzu, Y. (1984). An enzyme immunoassay for the detection of ciguatoxin and competitive inhibition of related natural polyether toxins. In *Seafood Toxins*, ACS Symp. Series 262, E. Ragelis, ed. ACS, Washington, DC, pp. 307–320.

Hokama, Y., Shirai, L. K., Iwamoto, L. M., Kobayashi, M. N., Goto, C. S., and Nakawawa, L. K. (1987). Assessment of a rapid enzyme immunoassay stick test for the detection of ciguatoxin and related polyether toxins in fish tissues. *Biol. Bull. 172*: 144–153.

Hokama, Y., Honda, S. A. A., Kobayashi, M. N., Nakagawa, L. K., and Miyahara, J. T. (1988). Monoclonal antibody (MAb) in detection of ciguatoxin (CTX) and related polyethers by the stick-enzyme immunoassay (S-EIA) in fish tissues associated with ciguatera poisoning. In *Mycotoxins and Phycotoxina '88*, S. Natori, K. Hashimoto, and Y. Ueno, eds. Elsevier, Amsterdam, pp. 303–310.

Hokama, Y., Asahina, A. Y., Hong, T. W. P., Shang, E. S., and Miyahara, J. T. (1990). Evaluation of the stick enzyme immunoassay in *Caranx* sp. and *Seriola dumerili* associated with ciguatera. *J. Clin. Lab. Anal. 4*: 363–366.

Huang, J. M. C., Wu, C. H., and Baden, D. G. (1984). Depolarizing action of a red tide dinoflagellate brevetoxin on axonal membranes. *J. Pharmacol. Exp. Therapeut. 229*: 615–621.

Hungerford, J. M., and Wekell, M. M. (1991). Control measures, U.S.A. In *Toxic Algae in Food and Drinking Water*, P. Krogh and B. Hald, eds. Marcel Dekker, in press.

Hwang, D. F., Chueh, C. H., and Jeng, S. S. (1990). Occurrence of tetrodotoxin in the gastropod mollusk *Natica lineata* (lined moon shell). *Toxicon 28*: 21–27.

Ikawa, M., Auger, K., Mosley, S. P., Sasner, J. J., Noguchi, T., and Hashimoto, K. (1985). Toxin profiles of the blue-green alga *Aphanizomenon flos-aquae*. In *Toxic Dinoflagellates*, D. M. Anderson, A. W. White, and D. G. Baden, eds. Elsevier, New York, pp. 299–304.

Iskandarani, Z., and Pietrzyk, D. J. (1982). Ion interaction chromatography of organic anions on a poly(styrene-divinylbenzene) adsorbant in the presence of tetraalkylammonium salts. *Anal. Chem. 54*: 1065–1071.

Iverson, F., Truelove, J., Nera, E., Tryphonas, L., Campbell, J., and Lok, E. (1989). Domoic acid poisoning and mussel-associated intoxication: Preliminary investigations into the response of mice and rats to toxic mussel extract. *Fd. Chem. Toxic. 27*: 377–384.

Johnson, H. M., and Mulberry, G. (1966). Paralytic shellfish poison: Serological assay by passive haemagglutination and bentonite flocculations. *Nature 211*: 747–748.

Joyce, E. A. (1975). Proceedings of the Florida Red Tide Conference, 10–12 October, 1974. *Mar. Res. Publ. 8*: 3.

Jonas-Davies, J., Sullivan, J. J., Kentala, L. L., Liston, J., Iwaoka, W. T., and Wu, L. (1984). Semiautomated method for the analysis of PSP toxins in shellfish. *J. Food Sci. 49*: 1506–1516.

Kat, M. (1983). Diarrhetic mussel poisoning in the Netherlands related to the dinoflagellate Dinophysis acuminata. *Ant. van Leeuwenhoek. 49:* 417–427.

Kat, M. (1985). Dinophysis acuminata blooms, the distinct cause of Dutch mussel poisoning. In *Toxic Dinoflagellates*, D. M. Anderson, A. White, and D. Baden, eds. Elsevier, New York, pp. 73–77.

Kawabata, T. (1978). Tetrodotoxin. In *Food Hygiene Examination Manual*, Vol. II. Environmental Health Bureau, Tokyo, p. 232.

Khora, S. S., and Yasumoto, T. (1989). Isolation of 11-oxotetrodotoxin from the puffer Arothron nigropunctatus. *Tetr. Ltrs. 30*: 4393–4394.

Kimura, L. H., Abad, M. A., and Hokama, Y. (1982a). Evaluation of the radioimmunoassay (RIA) for detection of ciguatoxin (CTX) in fish tissues. *J. Fish Biol. 21*: 671–680.

Kimura, L. H., Hokama, Y., Abad, M. A., Oyama, M., and Miyahara, J. T. (1982b). Comparison of three different assays for the assessment of ciguatoxin in fish tissues: Radioimmunoassay, mouse bioassay and in vitro guinea pig atrium assay. *Toxicon 20*: 907–912.

Kobayashi, M., Kondo, S., Yasumoto, T., and Ohizumi, Y. (1986). Cardiotoxic effects of maitotoxin, a principal toxin of seafood poisoning, on guinea pig and rat cardiac muscle. *J. Pharmacol. Exp. Ther. 238*: 1077–1083.

Kodama, A. M., and Hokama, Y. (1989). Variations in symptomatology of ciguatera poisoning. *Toxicon 27*: 593–595.

Kodama, A. M., Hokama, Y., Yasumoto, T., Fukui, M., Manea, S. J., and Sutherland, N. (1989). Clinical and laboratory findings implicating palytoxin as cause of ciguatera poisoning due to *Decapterus macrosoma* (Mackerel). *Toxicon 27*: 1051–1053.

Kodama, M., Noguchi, T., Maruyama, J., Ogata, T., and Hashimoto, K. (1983). Release of tetrodotoxin and paralytic shellfish poison from puffer liver by RNAase. *J. Biochem. 93*: 243–247.

Kodama, M., Ogata, T., and Sato, S. (1988). Bacterial production of saxitoxin. Lab. Marine Biol. Chem., Sch. Fisheries Sci., Kitasato Univ., Sanriku, Iwate 022-01, Japan. *Agric. Biol. Chem. 52*: 1075–1078.

Kodama, N. (1990). Possible links between bacteria and toxin production in algal blooms. In *Toxic Marine Phytoplankton*, E. Graneli, B. Sundstrom, L. Edler, and D. M. Anderson, eds. pp. 52–61.

Kogure, K., Tamplin, M. L., Simidu, U., and Colwell, R. (1989). Tissue culture assay method for PSP and related toxins. In *Red Tides: Biology, Environmental Science, and Toxicology*, Okaichi, Anderson, and Nemoto, eds. Elsevier, Amsterdam, pp. 383–386.

Kokawa, A., Nomura, M., Murakami, J., and Kobayashi, E. (1989). *Bull. Somori Prefectural Health Institute. 26*: 45–52 (in Japanese).

Kotaki, Y., Oshima, Y., and Yasumoto, T. (1985). Bacterial transformation of paralytic shellfish toxins in coral reef crabs and a marine snail. *Bull. Jpn. Soc. Sci. Fish. 51*: 1009–1013.

Kumagai, M., Yanagi, T., Murata, M., Yasumoto, T., Kato, M., Lassus, P., and Rodriguez-Vasquez. (1986). Okadaic acid as the causative toxin of diarrhetic shellfish poisoning in Europe. *Agr. Biol. Chem. 50*: 2853–2856.

Kungsuwan, A., Noguchi, T., Kano, S., and Hashimoto, K. (1986). Assay method for tetramine in carnivorous gastropods. *Jpn. Soc. Sci. Fish. 52*: 881.

Kutty, K. F., Singh, Y., Santostasi, G., and Kirshar, G. (1989). Maitotoxin-induced liver cell death involving loss of cell ATP following influx of calcium. *Toxicol. Appl. Pharmacol. 101*: 1–10.

Larsen, C., Anthoni, U., Christophersen, C., Nielen, P. H. (1988). Diagnostic positive and negative ion fast atom bombardment mass spectrometry of low molecular weight ammonium compounds of marine origin. *Biomed. Envir. Mass. Spectr. 17*: 187.

Lawrence, J. F., Charbonneau, C. F., Menard, C., Quilliam, M. A., and Sim, P. G. (1989a). Liquid chromatographic determination of domoic acid in shellfish products using the paralytic shellfish poison extraction procedure of the Association of Official Analytical Chemists. *J. Chromatog. 462*: 349–356.

Lawrence, J. F., Charbonneau, C. F., Page, B. D., and LaCroix, M. A. (1989b). Confirmation of domoic acid in molluscan shellfish by chemical derivatization and reversed-phase liquid chromatography. *J. Chrom. 462*: 419–425.

Lawrence, J. F., Charbonneau, C. F., and Menard, C. (1990). Collaborative study of the liquid chromatographic determination of domoic acid in mussels using the paralytic shellfish poison extraction procedure of the Association of Official Analytical Chemists. *J. AOAC* (in press).

Lee, J. S., Yanagi, T., Kanna, R., and Yasumoto, T. (1987). Fluorometric determination of diarrhetic shellfish toxins by high performance liquid chromatography. *Agric. Biol. Chem. 51*: 877.

Lee, J. S., Murata, M., and Yasumoto, T. (1988a). Analytical methods for determination of diarrhetic shellfish toxins. In *Mycotoxins and Phycotoxins '88*, S. Natori, K. Hashimoto, and Y. Ueno, eds. Elsevier, Amsterdam, pp. 327–334.

Lee, J. S., Tangen, K., Dahl, E., Hovgaard, P., and Yasumoto, T. (1988b). Diarrhetic shellfish toxins in Norwegian mussels. *Nippon Suisan Gakkaishi. 54*: 1953–1957.

Lee, J. S., Igarashi, T., Fraga, S., Dahl, E., Hovgaard, P., and Yasumoto, T. (1989). Determination of diarrhetic shellfish toxins in various dinoflagellate species. *J. Appl. Phycol. 1*: 147–152.

Legrand, A. M., Fukui, M., and Yasumoto, T. (1989a). Characterization of ciguatoxins at different stages of the food chain. Intl. Chem. Cong. Pac. Basin Soc., Honolulu, HI, Dec. 17–22, 1989, Abst. 0626.

Legrand, A. M., Litaudon, M., Genthon, J. N., Bagnis, R., and Yasumoto, T. (1989b). Isolation and some properties of ciguatoxin. *J. Appl. Phycol. 1*: 183–188.

Legrand, A. M., Cruchet, P., Bagnis, R., Murata, M., Ishibashi, Y., and Yasumoto, T. (1990). Chromatographic and spectral evidence for the presence of multiple ciguatera toxins. In *Toxic Marine Phytoplankton*, E. Graneli, ed. pp. 374–378.

Levine, L., Fukiki, H., Gjika, H. B., and van Vunakis, H. (1988a). A radioimmunoassay for palytoxin. *Toxicon 26*: 1115–1121.

Levine, L., Fujiki, H., Kiyoyuki, Y., Ojika, M., Gjirka, H., and Van Vanakis, H. (1988b). Production of antibodies and development of a radioimmunoassay for okadaic acid. *Toxicon 26*: 1123–1128.

Lin, Y., Risk, M., Ray, S. M., Van Engen, D., Clardy, J., Golik, J., James, J. C., and Nakanishi, K. (1981). Isolation and structure of brevetoxin B from the "red tide" dinoflagellate *Ptychodiscus brevis* (*Gymnodinium breve*). *J. Am. Chem. Soc. 103*: 6773.

Luckas, B. (1989). The occurrence of decarbamoyl-saxitoxin in canned mussels. Presentation at WHO consultation on public health aspects of seafood-borne zoonotic diseases. Hannover, Germany.

Maranda, L., Anderson, and Shimizu, Y. (1985). Comparison of toxicity between populations of *Gonyaulax tamarensis* of Eastern North American waters. *Estuarine, Coastal and Shelf Science. 21*: 401–410.

Marcaillou-LeBaut, C., and Masselin, P. (1990). Recent data on diarrhetic shellfish poisoning in France. In *Toxic Marine Phytoplankton*. E. Graneli, B. Sundstrom, L. Edler, and D. M. Anderson, eds. Elsevier, New York, pp. 487–492.

Marcaillou-LeBaut, C., Lucas, D., and LeDean, L. (1985). Dinophysis acuminata toxin: Status of toxicity bioassays in France. In *Toxic Dinoflagellates*, D. M. Anderson, A. W. White, and D. G. Baden, eds. Elsevier, New York, pp. 485–488.

Mathias, A. P., Ross, D. M., and Schachter, M. (1960). The distribution of 5-hydroxytryptamine, tetramethylammonium, homarine, and other substances in sea anemones. *J. Physiol. 142*: 56P.

Matsui, T., Taketsugu, S., Sata, H., Yamamori, K., Kodama, K., Ishii, A., Hirose, H., and Shimizu, C. (1990). Toxification of cultured puffer fish by the administration of tetrodotoxin producing bacteria. *Nippon Suisan Gakkaishi. 56*: 705.

McCulloch, A. W., Boyd, R. K., DeFreitas, A. S. W., Foxall, R. A., Jamieson, W. D., Laycock, M. V., Quilliam, M. A., Wright, J. L. C., Boyko, V. J., McLaren, J. W., Miedema, M. R., Pocklington, R., Arsenault, E., and Richard, D. J. A. (1989). Zinc from oyster tissue as causative factor in mouse deaths in official bioassay for paralytic shellfish poison. *J. AOAC 72*: 384–386.

McFarren, E. F. (1959). Report on collaborative studies of the bioassay for paralytic shellfish poison. *J. AOAC 42*: 263–271.

McFarren, E. F., Tanabe, H., Silva, F. J., Wilson, W. B., Campbell, J. E., and Lewis, K. H. (1965). The occurrence of a ciguatera-like poison in oysters, clams, and *Gymnodinium breve* cultures. *Toxicon 3*: 111–123.

Medcof, J. C., Leim, A. H., Neeler, A. B., Neeler, A. W. H., Gibbard, J., and Naubert, J. (1947). Paralytic shellfish poisoning on the Canadian Atlantic coast. *Bull. Fish Res. Board Canada. 75*: 1–32.

Miller, D. M., ed. (1990a). *Ciguatera Seafood Toxins*, CRC Press, Boca Raton, FL.

Miller, D. M. (1990b). The guinea-pig ileum: An assay system for ciguatera-type toxins. In *Ciguatera Seafood Toxins*, D. M. Miller, ed. CRC Press, Boca Raton, FL, pp. 103–116.

Ministry of Health and Welfare, Japan (1981). *Food Sanitation Research 7(31)*: 60–65. Translated from the Japanese by L. Mottet and M. Mottet, for Bigelow Laboratory for Ocean Sciences, West Boothbay Harbor, ME, 1987.

Miyahara, J. T., Kamibayashi, C. K., and Hokama, Y. (1988). Pharmacological characterization of the toxins in ciguateric fishes. In *Mycotoxins and Phycotoxins '88*, S. Natori, K. Hashimoto, and Y. Ueno, eds. Elsevier, Amsterdam, pp. 399–406.

Moczydlowski, E., Hall, S., Garber, S., Strichartz, G., and Miller, C. (1984). Voltage-dependent blockade of muscle Na+ channels by guanidinium toxins. *J. Gen. Physiol. 84*: 687–704.

Mold, J. D., Bowden, J. P., Stanger, D. W., Maurer, J. E., Lynch, J. M., Wyler, R. S., Schantz, E. J., and Riegal, B. (1957). Paralytic shellfish poison. VII. Evidence for the purity of the poison isolated from toxic clams and mussels. *J. Am. Chem. Soc. 79*: 5235–5238.

Moore, R. E., and Bartolini, G. (1981). Structure of palytoxin. *J. Am. Chem. Soc. 103*: 2491–2494.

Murata, M., Shimatani, M., Sugitani, H., Oshima, Y., and Yasumoto, T. (1982). Isolation and structural elucidation of the causative toxin of the diarrhetic shellfish poisoning. *Bull. Jpn. Soc. Sci. Fish. 48*: 549–552.

Murata, M., Legrand, A., Ishibashi, Y., and Yasumoto, T. (1989a). Structures of ciguatoxin and its congener. *J. Am. Chem. Soc. 111*: 8929–8931.

Murata, M., Legrand, A. M., and Yasumoto, T. (1989b). A probable partial structure of ciguatoxin isolated from the moray eel *Gymnothorax javanicus*. *Tet. Lett. 30*: 3793–3796.

Murata, M., Legrand, A. M., Ishibashi, Y., Fukui, M., and Yasumoto, T. (1990). Structures and configurations of ciguatoxin from the moray eel *Gymnothorax javanicus* and its likely precursor from the dinoflagellate *Gambierdiscus toxicus*. *J. Am. Chem. Soc. 112*: 4380–4386.

Nagashima, Y., Maruyama, J., Noguchi, T., and Hashimoto, K. (1987). Analysis of paralytic shellfish poison and tetrodotoxin by ion-pairing high performance liquid chromatography. *Bull. Jpn. Soc. Sci. Fish. 53*: 819–823.

Nagashima, Y., Nishio, S., Noguchi, T., Arakawa, O., Kanoh, S., and Hashimoto, K. (1988). Detection of tetrodotoxin by thin-layer chromatography/fast atom bombardment mass spectrometry. *Anal. Biochem. 175*: 258–262.

Nakamura, M., and Yasumoto, T. (1985). Tetrodotoxin derivatives in puffer fish. *Toxicon. 23*: 271–276.

Narita, H., Miwa, N., Akahane, S., Masumoti, H., Mizuno, S., Noguchi, T., Shida, Y., and Hashimoto, K. (1989). Tetrodotoxin productivity of bacteria isolated from trumpet shell *Charonia sauliae* intestine. *J. Food Hyg. Soc. Japan. 30*: 518–521.

Narita, H., Noguchi, T., Maruyama, J., Ueda, Y., Hashimoto, K., Watanabe, Y., and Hida, K. (1981). Occurrence of tetrodotoxin in a trumpet shell, Boshubora: *Charonia sauliae*. *Bull. Jpn. Soc. Fish. 47*: 935–941.

National Shellfish Sanitation Program. (1990). In *Manual of Operations*, U.S. Food and Drug Administration, Washington, DC.

Nguyen, A.-L., Luong, J. H. T., and Masson, C. (1990). Capillary electrophoresis for detection and quantitation of domoic acid in mussels. *Anal. Ltrs. 23*: 1621–1634.

Noguchi, T., Maruyama, J., Ueda, Y., Hashimoto, K., and Harada, T. (1981). Occurrence of tetrodotoxin in the Japanese ivory shell *Babylonia japonica*. *Bull. Jpn. Soc. Sci. Fish 47*: 909–913.

Noguchi, T., Uzu, A., Koyama, K., Maruyama, J., Nagashima, Y., and Hashimoto, K. (1983). Occurrence of tetrodotoxin as the major toxin in a xanthid crab *Atergatis floridus*. *Bull. Jpn. Soc. Sci. Fish. 49*: 1887–1892.

Noguchi, T., Maruyama, J., Narita, H., and Hashimoto, K. (1984). Occurrence of tetrodotoxin in the gastropod mollusk *Tutufa lissostoma* (frog shell). *Toxicon 22*: 219–226.

Noguchi, T., Jeon, J.-K., Arakawa, O., Sugita, H., Deguchi, Y., Shida, Y., and Hashimoto, K. (1986). Occurrence of tetrodotoxin and anhydrotetrodotoxin in *Vibrio* sp. isolated from the intestines of a xanthid crab. *Atergatis floridus*. *J. Biochem. 99*: 311–314.

Nukina, M., Koyanagi, L. M., and Scheuer, P. J. (1984). Two interchangeable forms of ciguatoxin. *Toxicon 22*: 169–176.

Nunez, M. T., Fischer, S., and Jaimovich, E. (1976). A fluorimetric method to determine tetrodotoxin. *Anal. Biochem. 72*: 320–325.

Ogata, T., Kodama, M., Komaru, K., Sakamoto, S., Sato, S., and Simidu, S. (1990). Production of paralytic shellfish toxins by bacteria isolated from toxic dinoflagellates. In *Toxic Marine Phytoplankton*, E. Graneli, B. Sundstrom, L. Edler, and D. M. Anderson, eds. Elsevier, pp. 311–315.

Onoue, Y., Noguchi, T., Maruyama, J., Hashimoto, K., and Seto, H. (1983a). Properties of two toxins newly isolated from oysters. *J. Agric. Food Chem. 31*: 420–423.

Onoue, Y., Noguchi, T., Nagashima, and Hashimoto, K. (1983b). Separation of tetrodotoxin and paralytic shellfish poisons by high-performance liquid chromatography with a fluorometric detection using o-phthalaldehyde. *J. Chromatog. 257*: 373–379.

Oshima, Y., Fallon, W. E., Shimzu, Y., Noguchi, T., and Hashimoto, Y. (1976). Toxins of the *Gonyaulax* sp. and infested bivalves in Owase Bay. *Bull. Jpn. Soc. Sci. Fish. 42*: 851–856.

Oshima, Y., Machida, M., Sasaki, K., Tamaoki, Y., and Yasumoto, T. (1984). Liquid chromatographic-fluorometric analysis of paralytic shellfish toxins. *Agric. Biol. Chem. 48*: 1707–1711.

Oshima, Y., Sugino, K., and Yasumoto, T. (1989). Latest advances in HPLC analysis of paralytic shellfish toxins. In *Mycotoxins and Phycotoxins 88*, S. Natori, K. Hashimoto, and Y. Ueno, eds. Elsevier, Amsterdam, pp. 319–326.

Oshima, Y., Sugino, K., Itakura, H., Hirota, M., and Yasumoto, T. (1990). Comparative studies on paralytic shellfish profile of dinoflagellates and bivalves. In *Toxic Marine Phytoplankton*, E. Graneli, B. Sundstrom, L. Edler, and D. M. Anderson, eds. Elsevier, New York, pp. 391–396.

Park, D. L., Adams, W. N., Graham, S. L., and Jackson, R. C. (1986). Variability of mouse bioassay for determination of paralytic shellfish poisoning toxins. *J. Assoc. Offic. Anal. Chem. 69*: 547–550.

Perl, Trish, M., Bedard, M. S. M., Kosatsky, T., Hockin, J. C., Todd, E. C. D., and Remis, R. S. (1990). An outbreak of toxic encephalopathy caused by eating mussels contaminated with domoic acid. *N. Engl. J. Med. 322*: 1775–1780.

Pierce, R., Brown, R. C., and Kucklick, J. R. (1985). Analysis of *Ptychodiscus brevis* toxins by Reverse Phase HPLC. In *Toxic Dinoflagellates*, D. M. Anderson, A. W. White, and D. G. Baden, eds. Elsevier, New York, pp. 309–314.

Pocklington, R., Milley, J. E., Bates, S. S., Bird, C. J., DeFreitas, A. S. W., and Quilliam, M. A. (1990). Trace determination of domoic acid in seawater and phytoplankton by high-performance liquid chromatography of the fluorenylmethoxycarbonyl (FMOC) derivative. *Intern. J. Environ. Anal. Chem. 38*: 351–368.

Poli, M. A. (1988). Laboratory procedures for detoxification of equipment and waste contaminated with brevetoxins PbTx-2 and PbTx-3. *J. Assoc. Off. Anal. Chem. 71*: 1000–1002.

Poli, M. A., Mende, T. J., and Baden, D. G. (1985). Characterization of the *Ptychodiscus brevis* polyether binding component in excitable membranes. In *Toxic Dinoflagellates*, D. M. Anderson, A. W. White, and D. G. Baden, eds. Elsevier, New York, pp. 357–362.

Poli, M. A., Mende, T. J., and Baden, D. G. (1986). Brevetoxins, unique activators of voltage-sensitive sodium channels, bind to specific sites in rat brain synaptosomes. *Mol. Pharmacol. 30*: 129–135.

Prakash, A. (1967). Growth and toxicity of a marine dinoflagellate, *Gonyaulax tamarensis. J. Fish. Res. Bd. Canada. 24*: 1589–1600.

Proctor, N. H., Chan, S. L., and Trevor, A. J. (1975). Production of saxitoxin by cultures of *Gonyaulax catanella. Toxicon. 13*: 1–9.

Quilliam, M. A., Sim, P. G., McCulloch, A. W., and MacInnes, A. G. (1989a). High performances liquid chromatography of domoic acid, a marine neurotoxin. *J. Environ. Anal. Chem. 36*: 139–154.

Quilliam, M. A., and Wright, J. L. C. (1989b). The amnesiac shellfish poisoning mystery. *Anal. Chem. 61*: 1053A–1059A.

Rakotoniaina, C. A., and Miller, D. M. (1990). Assays for ciguatera-type toxins. In *Ciguatera Seafood Toxins*, D. M. Miller, ed. CRC Press, Boca Raton, FL, pp. 73–86.

Raynor, M. D., Baslow, M. H., and Kosaki, T. I. (1969). Marine toxins from the Pacific. Ciguatoxin: Not an in vivo anticholinesterase. *J. Fish. Res. Bd. Can. 26*: 2208–2222.

Risk, M., Lin, Y. Y., McFarlane, R. D., Ramanujam, U. M. S., Smith, L. L., and Trieff, L. (1979). Purification and chemical studies on a major toxin from *Gymnodium breve*. In *Toxic Dinoflagellate Blooms*, D. L. Taylor and H. H. Selizer, eds. Elsevier, New York, pp. 335–344.

Ross, M. R., Siger, A., and Abbott, B. C. (1985). The house fly: An acceptable subject for paralytic shellfish toxin bioassay. In *Toxic Dinoflagellates*, D. M. Anderson, A. W. White, and D. G. Baden, eds. Elsevier, New York, pp. 433–438.

Roszell, L. E., Schulman, L. S., and Baden, D. G. (1990). Toxin profiles are dependent on growth stages in cultured *Ptychodiscus brevis*. In *Toxic Dinoflagellates*, E. Graneli, B. Sundstrom, L. Edler, and D. M. Anderson, eds. Elsevier, New York, pp. 403–406.

Ruzicka, J., and Hansen, E. H. (1975). Flow injection analysis. Part I. A new concept of fast continuous flow analysis. *Anal. Chim. Acta, 78* 145. Danish Pat. Appl. No. 4846/74, September 1974; subsequent U.S. Pat. No. 4,022,575.

Saitoh, H., Oikawa, K., Takano, T., Kamimura, K. (1983). Determination of tetramethylammonium ion in shellfish by ion chromatography. *J. Chromatogr. 281*: 397.

Salter, J. E., Timperi, R. J., Hennigan, L. J., Sefton, L., and Reece, H. (1989). Comparison evaluation of liquid chromatographic and bioassay methods of analysis for determination of paralytic shellfish poisons in shellfish tissues. *J. Assoc. Off. Anal. Chem. 72*: 670–673.

Sampayo, M. A., Alvito, P., Franca, S., and Spusa, I. (1990). Dinophysis spp. toxicity and relation to accompanying species. In *Toxic Marine Phytoplankton*, E. Graneli, B. Sundstrom, L. Edler, and D. M. Anderson, eds. Elsevier, New York, pp. 215–220.

Santostasi, G., Kutty, R. K., Bartorelli, A. L., Yasumoto, T., and Krisna, G. (1990). Maitotoxin-induced myocardial cell injury: Calcium accumulation followed by ATP depletion precedes cell death. *Toxicol. and Appl. Pharmacol. 102*: 164–173.

Sawyer, P., Jollow, D., Scheuer, P., York, R., McMillan, J., Withers, N., Fudenberg, H., and Higer, T. (1984). The effect of ciguatera-associated toxins in mice. In *Seafood Toxins*, American Chemical Society Symposium Series No. 262, Ragelis, E., ed. ACS, Washington, DC, pp. 322–329.

Schantz, E. J., McFarren, E. F., Schafer, M. L., and Lewis, K. H. (1958). Purified poison for bioassay standardization. *J. Assoc. Offic. Anal. Chem. 41*: 160–168.

Schantz, E. J., Lynch, J. M., Vayada, G., Masumoto, K., and Rapoport, H. (1966). The purification and characterization of the poison produced by *Gonyaulax catenella* in axenic culture. *Biochemistry 5*: 1191–1195.

Scheuer, P. J., Takahashi, W., Tsutsumi, J., and Yoshida, T. (1967). Ciguatoxin: Isolation and chemical nature. *Science 155*: 1267–1268.

Schulman, L. S., Roszell, L. E., Mende, T. J., King, R. W., and Baden, D. G. (1990). A new polyether toxin from Florida's red tide dinoflagellate *Ptychodiscus brevis*. In *Toxic Marine Phytoplankton*, E. Graneli, B. Sundstrom, L. Edler, and D. M. Anderson, eds. Elsevier, New York, pp. 407–412.

Selvin, R. C., Lewis, C. M., Yentsch, C. M., and Hurst, J. W. (1984). Seasonal persistence of resting cyst toxicity in the dinoflagellate *Gonyaulax tamarensis* var. excavata. *Toxicon 22*: 817–820.

Sharkey, R. G., Joner, E., Couraud, F., Baden, D. G., and Catterall, W. A. (1987). Allosteric Modulation of Neurotoxin Binding to Voltage-Sensitive Voltage Channels by *Ptychodiscus brevis* Toxin 2. *Mol. Pharm. 31*: 270–27x.

Sheumack, D. D., Howden, M. E. H., and Spence, I. (1984). Occurrence of a tetrodotoxin-like compound in the eggs of the venomous blue-ringed octopus (*Hapalochlaena maculosa*). *Toxicon 22*: 811–812.

Shimada, K., Ohtsuru, M., Yamaguchi, T., and Nigota, K. (1983). Determination of tetrodotoxin by capillary isotachophoresis. *J. Food Sci. 48*: 665–680.

Shimizu, Y. (1982). Recent progress in marine toxin research. *Pure Appl. Chem. 54*: 1973–1980.

Shimizu, Y., Chou, H. N., Bando, G., VanDuyne, G., and Clarddy, J. (1986). Structure of Brevetoxin-A (GB-1 toxin), the most potent toxin in the Florida red tide organism *Gymnodinium breve* (*Ptychodiscus brevis*). *J. Am. Chem. Soc. 108*: 514–515.

Shoptaugh, N. H., Carter, P. W., Foxall, T. L., Sasner, J. J., and Ikawa, M. (1981). Use of fluorometry for the determination of *Gonyaulax tamarensis* var. excavata toxins in New England shellfish. *J. Agric. Food Chem. 29*: 198–200.

Siger, A., Abbott, B. C., and Ross, M. (1984). Response of the house fly to saxitoxins and contaminated shellfish. In *Seafood Toxins*, E. P. Ragelis, ed. ACS, Washington, D.C., pp. 193–196.

Simidu, U., Noguchi, T., Hwang, D.-F., Shida, Y., and Hashimoto, K. (1987). Marine bacteria which produce tetrodoxin. *Appl. Env. Micro. 53*: 1714–1715.

Sommer, H., and Meyer, K. F. (1937). Paralytic shellfish poisoning. *Arch. Pathol. 24*: 560–598.

Stabell, O. B., and Cembella, A. D. (1990). Standardizing extraction and analysis techniques for marine phytoplankton toxins. In *Toxic Marine Phytoplankton*, E. Graneli, B. Sundstrom, L. Edler, and E. M. Anderson, eds. Elsevier, New York, pp. 518–521.

Steidinger, K. A. (1979). Collection, enumeration, and identification of free living marine dinoflagellates. In *Toxic Dinoflagellate Blooms*, D. L. Taylor and H. H. Seliger, eds. Elsevier/North-Holland, Amsterdam, pp. 435–442.

Steidinger, K. A., Burklew, M. A., and Ingle, R. M. (1973). The Effects of *Gymnodinium breve* toxin on estuarine animals. In *Marine Pharmacognosy*, D. F. Martin and G. M. Padella, eds. Academic Press, New York, pp. 179–202.

Steidinger, K. A., Burklew, M. A., and Ingle, R. M. (1973). Effects of *Gymnodinium breve* toxin on estuarine animals. In *Marine Pharmacognosy*, D. F. Martin and G. M. Padilla, eds. Academic Press, New York, p. 127.

Strichartz, G. (1984). Structural determinants of the affinity of saxitoxin for neuronal sodium channels: Electrophysiological studies on frog peripheral nerve. *J. Gen. Physiol. 84*: 281–305.

Stuart, A. M., and Baden, D. G. (1988). Florida red tide brevetoxins and binding in fish brain synaptosomes. *Aquat. Toxicol. 13*: 271–280.

Suganuma, M., Fujiki, H., Suguri, H., Yoshizawa, S., Hirota, M., Nakayasu, M., Ojuuka, M., Wakamatsu, K., Yamado, K., and Sugimura, T. (1988). Okadaic acid. An additional non-phorbol-12 tetradecanoaate-13-acetate type tumor promoter. *Proc. Natl. Acad. Sci. USA 85*: 1768–1771.

Sullivan, J. J. (1982). Paralytic shellfish poisoning—analytical and biochemical investigations. Doctoral dissertation, University of Washington, Seattle.

Sullivan, J. J. (1988). Methods of analysis for DSP and PSP toxins in shellfish: A review. *J. Shellfish Res. 7*: 587–595.

Sullivan, J. J., and Iwaoka, W. T. (1963). High pressure liquid chromatographic determination of toxins associated with paralytic shellfish poisoning. *J. Assoc. Off. Anal. Chem. 66*: 297–303.

Sullivan, J. J., and Wekell, M. M. (1987). The application of high performance liquid chromatography in a paralytic shellfish poisoning monitoring program. In *Seafood Quality Determination*, D. E. Kramer and J. Liston, eds. pp. 357–371.

Sullivan, J. J., Iwaoka, W. T., and Liston, J. (1983). Enzymatic transformation of PSP toxins in the littleneck clam (*Protochaca staminea*). *Biochem. and Biophys. Res. Commun. 114*: 465–472.

Sullivan, J. J., Wekell, M. M., and Kentala, L. L. (1985). Application of HPLC for the determination of PSP toxins in shellfish. *J. Food Sci. 50*: 26–29.

Sullivan, J. J., Wekell, M. M., and Hall, S. (1988). Detection of paralytic shellfish toxins. In *Marine Toxins*, A. Tu, ed. Marcel Dekker, New York, pp. 87–106.

Tachibana, K. (1980). Structural studies on marine toxins. Ph.D. thesis, University of Hawaii, Honolulu, as cited by Legrand et al., 1989.

Tachibana, K., Nukina, M., Joh, Y. G., and Scheuer, P. J. (1987). Recent developments in the molecular structure of ciguatoxin. *Biol. Bull. 172*: 122–127.

Taylor, F. J. R. (1985). The taxonomy and relationships of red tide flagellates. In *Toxic Dinoflagellates*, D. M. Anderson, A. W. White, and E. G. Baden, eds. Elsevier Science Publishing, New York, pp. 11–26.

Teh, Y. F., and Gardiner, J. E. (1974). Partial purification of *Lophozozymus pictor* toxin. *Toxicon 12*: 601–603.

Teitelbaum, J. S., Zatorre, R. J., Carpenter, S., Gendron, D., Evans, A. C., Gjedde, A., and Cashman, N. R. (1990). Neurologic sequelae of domoic acid intoxication due to the ingestion of contaminated mussels. *N. Engl. J. Med. 322*: 1781–1787.

Terao, K., Ito, E., Yanagi, T., and Yasumoto, T. (1986). Histopathological studies on experimental marine toxin poisoning. I. Ultrastructural changes in the small intestine and liver of suckling mice induced by dinophysistoxin-1 and pectenotoxin-1. *Toxicon 24*: 1141–1151.

Terao, K., Ito, E., Kakinuma, Y., Igarashi, K., Kobayashi, M., Ohizumi, Y., and Yasumoto, T. (1989). Histopathological studies on experimental marine toxin poisoning. Pathogenesis of experimental maitotoxin poisoning. *Toxicon 27*: 979–988.

Terao, K., Ito, E., Orada, M., Murata, M., and Yasumoto, T. (1990). Histopathological studies on experimental marine toxin poisoning. 5. The effects in mice of yessotoxin isolated from pactinopectin-yessoensis and of a sulfated derivative. *Toxicon 28*: 1095–1104.

Tester, P. A., and Fowler, P. K. (1990). Brevetoxin contamination of *Mercenaria mercenaria* and *Crassostrea virginica*: A management issue. In *Toxic Marine Phytoplankton*, E. Graneli, B. Sundstrom, L. Edler, and D. M. Anderson, eds. Elsevier, New York, pp. 499–503.

Tester, P. A., Stumpf, R. P., and Fowler, P. K. (1988). Red tide, the first occurrence in North Carolina waters: An overview. *Proc. Oceans 88 Conf.*, Baltimore, MD, October 31–November 2, 1988, pp. 808–811.

Trainer, V. L., and Baden, D. G. (1990). Enzyme immunoassay of brevetoxins. In *Toxic Marine Phytoplankton*, E. Graneli, B. Dundstrom, L. Edler, and D. M. Anderson, eds. Elsevier, New York, pp. 430–435.

Tryphonas, L., Truelove, J., and Iverson, F. (1990). Acute parenteral neurotoxicity of domoic acid in *Cynomolgus* monkeys *Macaca fascicularis*. *Toxicol. Pathol. 18*: 297–303.

Uda, T., Itoh, Y., Nishimuri, M., Usagawa, T., and Yasumoto, T. (1988). Enzyme immunoassay using monoclonal antibody specific for diarrhetic shellfish poisons. In *Mycotoxins and Phycotoxins*, S. Natori, K. Hashimoto, and Y. Ueno, eds. Elsevier, New York, pp. 335–342.

Underal, B., Yndestad, M., and Aune, T. (1985). DSP intoxication in Norway and Sweden, Autumn 1984–Spring 1985. In *Toxic Dinoflagellates*, D. M. Anderson, A. W. White, and D. G. Baden, eds. Elsevier, New York, pp. 489–494.

Usagawa, T., Nishimuri, M., Itoh, Y., Uda, T., and Yasumoto, T. (1989). Preparation of monoclonal antibodies against okadaic acid prepared from the sponge *Halichondria okadai*. *Toxicon 27*: 1323–1330.

Watabe, S., Sato, Y., Nakaya, M., Hashimoto, K., Atsushi, E., Kaminogawa, S., and Yamauchi, K. (1989). Monoclonal antibody raised against tetrodonic acid, a derivative of tetrodotoxin. *Toxicon 27*: 265–268.

Weil, C. S. (1952). Tables for the convenient calculation of media-effective dose (LD_{50} or ED_{50}) and instructions in their use. *Biometrics 1*: 249.

Wekell, M. M. (1990). Seafood toxins. *J. Assoc. Off. Anal. Chem. 73*: 113–117.

Welsh, J. H., and Prock, P. B. (1958). Quaternary ammonium bases in the coelenterates. *Biol. Bull. 115*: 551.

White, A. W. (1977). Dinoflagellate toxins as probable cause of an Atlantic Herring (*Clupea harengus harengus*) kill, and pteropods as apparent vector. *J. Fish. Res. Board Can. 34*: 2421–2424.

Whitefleet-Smith, J., Boyer, G. L., and Schnoes, H. K. (1986). Isolation and spectral characteristics of four toxins from the dinoflagellate *Ptychodiscus brevis*. *Toxicon 24*: 1075–1090.

Withers, N. W. (1988). Ciguatera fish toxins and poisoning. In *Handbook of Natural Toxins*, Vol. 3, *Marine Toxins and Venoms*, A. T. Tu, ed. Marcel Dekker, Inc., New York, pp. 31–61.

Wright, B. W., Ross, G. A., and Smith, R. D. (1989). Capillary zone electrophoresis with laser fluorescence detection of marine toxins. *J. Microcolumn Separations 1*(2): 85–89.

Yanagi, T., Murata, M., Torigoe, K., and Yasumoto, T. (1989). Biological activities of semi synthetic analogs of dinophysistoxin-3, the major diarrhetic shellfish toxin. *Agric. Biol. Chem. 53*: 525–529.

Yasumoto, T. (1990). Marine microorganisms toxins—a review. In *Toxic Marine Phytoplankton*, E. Graneli, B. Sundstrom, L. Edler, and D. M. Anderson, eds. Elsevier, New York, pp. 3–8.

Yasumoto, T., and Murata, M. (1990). Polyether toxins involved in seafood poisoning. In *Marine Toxins, Origin, Structure, and Molecular Pharmacology*. ACS Symposium Series 418, S. Hall and G. Strichartz, eds. pp. 120–132.

Yasumoto, T., Nakajima, L., Bagnis, R., and Adachi, R. (1977). Finding of a dinoflagellate as a likely culprit of ciguatera. *Nippon Suisan Gakkaishi 43*: 1021–1026.

Yasumoto, T., Oshima, Y., and Yamaguchi, M. (1978). Occurrence of a new type of shellfish poisoning in the Tohoku District. *Bull. Jpn. Soc. Sci. Fish. 44*: 1249–1255.

Yasumoto, T., Oshima, Y., and Yamaguchi, M. (1979). Occurrence of new type of toxic shellfish in Japan and chemical properties of toxin. In *Toxic Dinoflagellate Blooms*, D. T. Taylor and H. H. Seeliger, eds. Elsevier, New York, pp. 395–398.

Yasumoto, T., Oshima, Y., Sugawara, W., Fuguyo, Y., Oguri, H., Igarashi, T., and Fujita, N. (1980). Identification of *Dinophysis fortii* as the causative organism of diarrhetic shellfish poisoning. *Bull. Jpn. Soc. Sci. Fish. 46*: 1405–1411.

Yasumoto, T., Oshima, Y., Hosaka, M., and Miyakoshi, S. (1981). Occurrence of tetrodotoxin in the ivory shell *Babylonia japonica* from Wakasa Bay. *Bull. Jpn. Soc. Sci. Fish. 47*: 929–934.

Yasumoto, T., Nakamuar, M., Oshima, Y., and Takahata, J. (1982). Construction of a continuous tetrodotoxin analyzer. *Bull. Jpn. Soc. Sci. Fish. 48*: 1481–1483.

Yasumoto, T., Murata, M., Oshima, Y., Matsumoto, G. K., and Clardy, J. (1984). Diarrhetic shellfish poisoning. In *Seafood Toxins*, E. Ragelis, eds. American Chemical Society, Washington, DC, pp. 207–214.

Yasumoto, T., Nagai, H., Yasumura, D., Michishita, T., Endo, A., Yotsu, M., and Kotaki, Y. (1986a). Interspecies distribution and possible origin of tetrodotoxin. *Ann. N.Y. Acad. Sci. 479*: 44–51.

Yasumoto, T., Yasumura, D., Ohizumi, Y., Takahashi, M., Alcala, A., and Alcalo, L. C. (1986b). Palytoxin in two species of xanthid crab from the Philippines. *Agric. Biol. Chem. 50*: 163–167.

Yasumoto, T., Murata, M., Lee, J. S., and Torigae, K. (1988). Polyether toxins produced by dinoflagellates. In *Mycotoxins and Phycotoxins*, S. Natori, K. Hashimoto, and Y. Ueno, eds. Elsevier, Amsterdam, pp. 375–382.

Yasumoto, T., Yotsu, M., Endo, A., Murata, M., and Naoki, H.(1989). Interspecies distribution and biogenetic origin of tetrodotoxin and its derivatives. *Pure and Appl. Chem. 61*: 505–508.

Yokoyama, A., Murata, M., Oshima, Y., Iwashita, T., and Yasumoto, T. (1988). Some chemical properties of maitotoxin, a putative calcium channel agonist isolated from a marine dinoflagellate. *J. Biochem. 104*: 184–187.

Yotsu, M., Endo, A., and Yasumoto, T. (1989). An improved tetrodotoxin analyzer. *Agric. Biol. Chem. 53*: 893–895.

VI

GOITER

17

Naturally Occurring Goitrogens

Pavel Langer and Nikolaj Michajlovskij

Slovak Academy of Sciences, Bratislava, Czech and Slovak Federal Republic

I. INTRODUCTION

Several extensive reviews have been published describing mostly recent advances in phytochemistry of naturally occurring substances with goitrogenic activity (Fenwick et al., 1983; Van Etten and Tookey, 1983), their effects on the development of experimental and human goiter (Langer and Greer, 1977; Gaitan, 1980, 1983, 1986a, 1990; Langer, 1983), or analyzing the possibilities of the use of plant material containing some toxic compounds in feeding domestic animals (Fenwick and Curtis, 1980; Clandinin and Robbles, 1981; Thomke, 1981). However, for a complex evaluation of possible effects of a variety of environmental goitrogens on human thyroid, it seems to be reasonable to also report some advances in thyroid pathophysiology, genetic and hereditary bases of thyroid disorders, and their molecular mechanisms. It is our intention not to repeat basic information published by others, but rather to present a synthetic comprehensive view on present medical and chemical problems of environmental goitrogens.

II. DEFINITION OF GOITROGENS AND GENERAL MECHANISMS OF THEIR ACTION

Goitrogens are compounds of various chemical structures, the administration of which to humans or animals for a certain time results in an increase of thyroid size, which is called goiter.

A. Normal Thyroid Size and Goiter

By classical definition, goiter means an enlarged thyroid. However, before defining goiter we should define the normal thyroid. According to the prevailing view, the normal thyroid should not be prominent over the neck surface and should be undetectable by palpation. However, this definition has recently been seriously challenged (Langer, 1989) by findings with ultrasonographic volumetry showing that even among unpalpable thyroids a great variety of sizes may actually exist. Thus, the upper limit of normal thyroid size is currently shifting down to the category of unpalpable thyroids. It appears that a normal or "minimum size" thyroid may exist perhaps only in some countries with abundant iodine intake such as Iceland, Norway, Sweden, Japan, the United States, Canada, and some others. In several other countries even unpalpable thyroids may finally appear to be enlarged if examined by ultrasonography, which means that even the effect of environmental goitrogens should be traced in such terms. The normal thyroid may therefore be defined as a gland with a normal (i.e., euthryoid) function in which the growth mechanisms were not stimulated to overcome any deteriorating influences.

B. Endemic Goiter and Iodine Deficiency Disease

Previously, if the prevalence of palpable goiters in a certain area was greater than 10%, it was considered to be affected by endemic goiter. However, since goiter is only one of several serious signs of iodine deficiency resulting in several degrees of neural and mental deficiency, cretinism being the most severe, the term endemic goiter has recently been replaced by iodine deficiency disease (IDD), and three levels of severity of IDD have been defined (Hetzel, 1987).

C. General View on the Mechanism of Thyroid Growth

Under steady-state conditions, there exists a certain equilibrium between the production of thyroid hormone by the thyroid and its disposal by peripheral tissues, which results in more or less stable levels of thyroxine (T_4) and triiodothyronine (T_3) in blood plasma and in more or less stable and regular release of thyroid stimulating hormone (TSH) from the pituitary. Any interfering influence that results in a decrease of thyroid hormone supply to the periphery (including the pituitary, which is the site of the feedback effect of thyroid hormone) will finally result in an increased release of TSH and subsequently in thyroid growth.

Several exogenous agents (among them iodine deficiency and environmental goitrogens) or endogenous influences may interfere with steady state at the level of biosynthesis of thyroid hormones, of their binding to plasma carrier proteins, and thus of their transport to peripheral tissues and disposal rate and, finally, of their peripheral metabolism. All such effects may disturb the steady state of the pituitary-thyroid axis and, if severe and long-lasting enough, they may result in a development of goiter. However, a variety of less severe disorders may result from less severe or transient effects as well.

TSH is recognized as the main factor regulating thyroid growth. Its blood level increases in response to either a decrease of biosynthesis and production or peripheral metabolism of thyroid hormone due to the factors mentioned above. Recently, however, the participation of several other growth factors has been demonstrated such as insulinlike growth factor (IGF), epidermal growth factor (EGF), transforming growth factor (TGF), and endothelial cell growth factor (Greil et al., 1989).

Several biochemical pathways may be involved in the regulation of thyroid cell proliferation, such as (1) activated adenylate cyclase–cAMP system via TSH receptor, (2) cAMP-independent EGF mechanism, and (3) phosphatidylinositol-Ca^{2+} cascade. Some factors may even activate thyroid growth without activating hormone biosynthesis.

The final result of the action of growth factors may be either a hypertrophy of cells without increasing their number or hyperplasia resulting from an increased total number of cells. Recently, a polyclonal or heterogenous nature of thyroid follicular cells was demonstrated, which means that there exist several families of thyroid cells differing in their metabolic properties and responses to growth factors. This also means that they actually show highly individual growth programs (Huber et al., 1990).

D. Basal Views on Iodine Requirement and Metabolism

It has been established that a plasma iodine level of 1 μg/L is essential to prevent iodine-deficiency goiter (Beckers and Delange, 1980). To maintain such a level, a minimum daily intake between 40 and 120 μg iodine is necessary depending mainly on the individual variations in the absorption from the gastrointestinal tract, which may thus be considered an important factor determining whether some inhabitants of an iodine-deficient area will develop goiter or not. The other factor regulating plasma iodide level, i.e., renal iodide clearance, appears to be relatively constant. Though 160 μg iodine daily for adults and 200 μg daily for adolescents and pregnant or lactating women was proposed as a safe level, some authors recently recommended the range 200–300 μg daily, while the actual intake in about 30% of the examined population in the United States and Canada was between 200 and 500 μg daily, values up to 1000 μg still being considered safe from the view of possible side effects (Matovinovic, 1983). In contrast, in most areas of endemic goiter the intake of iodine was found to be less than 50 μg daily. This was evaluated from the urinary excretion of iodine, which satisfactorily reflects dietary iodine intake (Hetzel, 1987).

Worldwide monitoring of hundreds of millions of people shows that iodine deficiency is the principal etiological factor of endemic goiter and that the increase of iodine intake will result in a decrease of goiter prevalence (Hetzel, 1987). Similarly, it is well known and repeatedly confirmed that, in general, iodine intake will counteract the effect of various goitrogenic compounds (Greer, 1957; Langer and Greer, 1977). In contrast, several reports show that increasing intake of iodine may result in an increased incidence of Hashimoto's autoimmune thyroiditis, presumably in genetically predisposed individuals, and, in addition, some environmental goitrogens may apparently increase the incidence of such thyroiditis with concomitant goitrous enlargement of the thyroid despite high iodine intake (Gaitan, 1986b; Fort et al., 1990).

E. Possible Approaches to Evaluation of Goitrogen Participation in Human Thyroid Disorders

Though the participation of goitrogens in the etiology of endemic goiter in some areas has been repeatedly postulated, several reports have been poorly documented and apparently overestimate the data obtained in animal experiments by extrapolating them to human population. This problem has been repeatedly reviewed (Greer, 1962; Langer and Greer, 1977; Langer, 1983; Gaitan, 1980, 1983). However, as mentioned above, manifested goiter should be considered a maximum result of several endogenous (genetic, hereditary, metabolic, etc.) and exogenous influences (nutrition, environment, etc.), and the possible role of goitrogens should also be evaluated at the level of subclinical disorders by keeping in mind molecular events, which may be a field of further research (Thomas and Williams, 1988).

In addition, it should be recalled that any goitrogenic effects increase with a decreasing intake of iodine. Second, several groups of normal individuals have a temporarily increased demand for iodine (adolescents, pregnant and lactating women, etc.), which, if not met, results in a relative iodine deficiency. Third, groups of people with inborn errors of thyroid hormone biosynthesis (Stanbury, 1983) or with hereditary predisposition to develop autoimmune thyroiditis may be more sensitive to the effect of goitrogens than a normal population, even with a rich iodine intake (Gaitan, 1986b). Finally, a different functional spectrum of several families of thyroid follicular cells should be taken into account (Huber et al., 1990).

It appears a rather difficult task to demonstrate a role for goitrogens in the etiology of endemic goiter in certain areas. Perhaps detailed and long-term metabolic studies in a large number of individuals would serve this purpose. A statistical approach should be considered as reasonable and economical. In general, there are two situations in which the active role of goitrogens in goiter epidemiology may be suggested: (1) when two or more neighboring and in several points (socioeconomical, nutritional, genetic, environmental, etc.) closely related and comparable areas have about the same iodine intake but strikingly different goiter prevalence, such as described for two parts of Idjwi Island in Zaire (Delange and Ermans, 1976; Ermans et al., 1983) or for some areas of Vietnam (Hershman et al., 1983), or (2) when a high percentage of goiter exists in some areas with evidently sufficient iodine intake, as recently demonstrated for some areas of Colombia and Kentucky (Gaitan, 1986b).

III. DISTRIBUTION OF ENVIRONMENTAL GOITROGENS

The term "naturally occurring goitrogens" has recently been replaced by "environmental goitrogens" (Gaitan, 1983), since they may occur either as natural constituents or as anthropogenic contaminants in foodstuffs, water supplies, and air.

A. Goitrogens of Natural Origin

This group consists mainly of organic compounds in a wide variety of plants, several of them representing essential components of human or animal nutrition, from which they may be transferred to milk and meat products. Their common property is that they are breakdown products of their parent glucosides (see Sec. V.A).

Recently the formation of some goitrogenic compounds of polyphenolic structure was detected in decaying organic matter by microbial activity during the humidification process. In this way they became present in coals, shales and soils, from which they are transferred to water sources (Gaitan, 1980, 1986a,b,c; Thomas and Williams, 1988).

Finally, the antithyroid effect of T-2 mycotoxin, originating in fungi that contaminate corn and other products, has been reported (Van Middlesworth, 1986).

1. Sulfur-Containing Glucosides

Some aglucones of glucosinolates belong to the first natural goitrogens discovered, such as L-5-vinyl-oxazolidine-2-thione or goitrin (Fig. 1) (Astwood et al., 1949), thiocyanate (Silink and Marsikova, 1951; Michajlovskij and Langer, 1958; Langer and Michajlovskij, 1958), or isothiocyanates (Fig. 2) (Langer and Stolc, 1965; Langer, 1966a,b). Nowadays more than 100 glucosinolates are known, which occur predominantly in crucifers and in several other

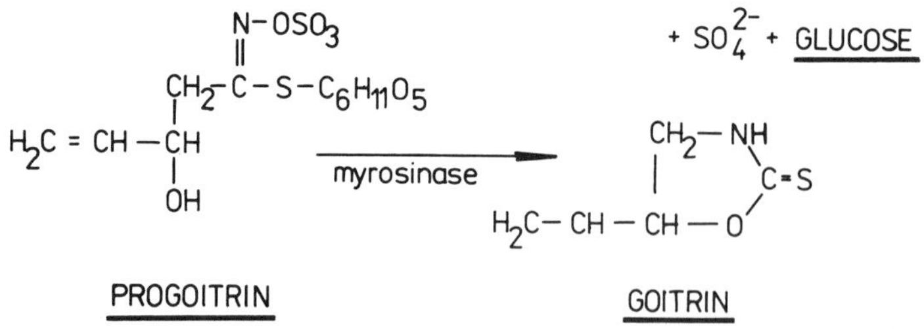

Figure 1 Enzymic splitting of progoitrin to goitrin (L-5-vinyl-oxazolidine-2-thione) by the action of myrosinase. The same reaction takes place in the intestine by the action of bacterial thioglucosidases.

plant families. Their chemical structures and natural distribution in plants have been repeatedly reviewed (Ettlinger and Kjaer, 1968; Kjaer, 1973; Langer and Greer, 1977; Gaitan, 1980; Fenwick et al., 1983; Van Etten and Tookey, 1983; Langer, 1983; Sones et al., 1984; Fenwick et al., 1986). The seeds contain much higher concentrations of glucosinolates than the green parts. Various authors found 5–200 mg/kg goitrin, 5–500 mg/kg thiocyanate, and 4–200 mg/kg total glucosinolates in green parts of various crucifers, while 10–30 g/kg of these compounds were detected in seeds. The world production of rapeseed in 1970–1973 was about 8 million tons, which means about 250,000 tons of glucosinolates.

2. *Cyanogenic Glucosides*

Several cyanogenic glucosides are present in at least 2000 species of higher plants (including cassava, maize, bamboo shoots, sweet potatoes, lima beans,

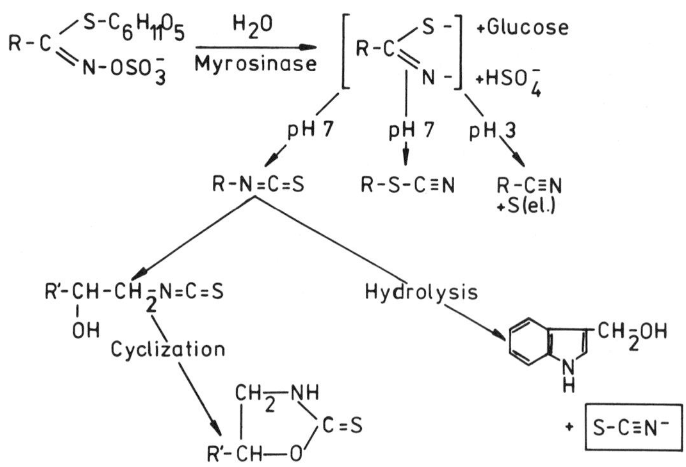

Figure 2 Scheme of enzymic splitting of glucosinolates by the action of myrosinase at various pHs (for R groups see Table 1).

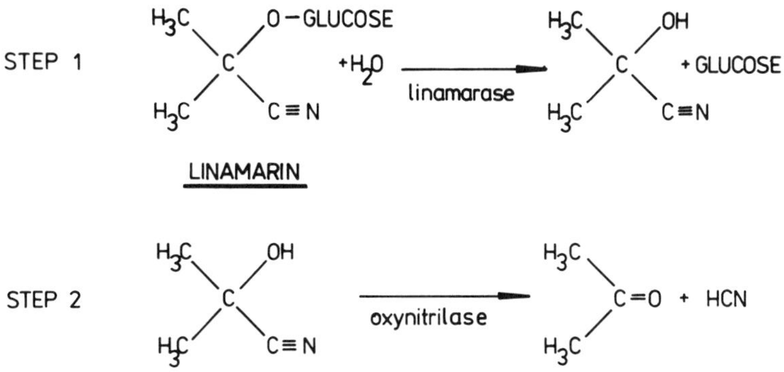

Figure 3 Two steps of enzymic splitting of cyanogenic glucoside Linamarin with a final liberation of hydrocyanic acid, which in the organism is detoxicated to thiocyanate.

and millets) among approximately 110 families as repeatedly reviewed (Siegler, 1975). Perhaps the most important of them appears to be cassava, furnishing the basic food for several hundred million inhabitants in tropical countries, the global production of its root in 1977 being 110 million tons (Cooke and Coursey, 1981). It contains the cyanogenic glucosides linamarin and lotaustralin yielding 15–400 mg cyanide/kg fresh food (Fig. 3). The same or similar glucosides are present in white clover, line seeds, beans, almonds, bamboo shoots, apricots, prunes, cherries, yam, cicad, maize, peas, etc.

3. *Flavonoid Glucosides and Humid Substances*

Bioflavonoids are polyhydroxyphenols with C_6-C_3-C_6 structures (Fig. 4) that exert thiourealike effect, being several times more potent than the widely used antithyroid drug propylthiouracil (Gaitan, 1984, 1986a, 1990; Gaitan et al., 1989). They are present in polymeric (tannins) or oligomeric (pigments) forms of flavonoid glucosides in a wide variety of plants, some of them representing staple foods or fodders (millet, sorghum, beans, ground nuts, etc.). The most important source of flavonoids appears to be pearl millet (*Penisetum americanum Lecke*), which, because of its perennial growth, constitutes a main source of food energy in semiarid tropics. Flavonoid glucosides are hydrolyzed by intestinal bacteria to flavonoid glucosides, and such bacterial hydroxylation of β ring together with a middle ring fission results in a formation of phenolic acid, gallic acid, and highly potent goitrogenic monomers such as resorcinol, phloroglucinol, and orcinol (Gaitan, 1986a, 1990; Thomas and Williams, 1988). Recently, a goitrogenic effect of millet, extracts of millet, and purified glycosylflavones has been demonstrated in rats (Gaitan et al., 1989).

Furthermore, flavonoid-type humic compounds are principal organic substances of soils and waters, and bioflavonoid structures may represent a link between plant goitrogens and those present in coal, soils, and water. For instance, as much as 8% of shale bitumen is constituted of phenols, which are also major organic pollutants in aqueous effluents from coal-conversion processes (Gaitan, 1986a,c, 1990).

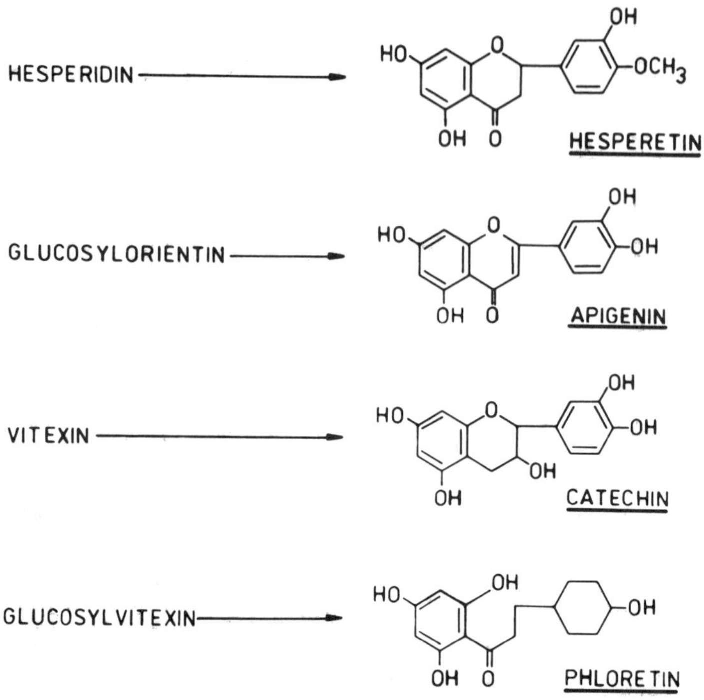

Figure 4 Aglucones of the most widespread glycosylflavonoids.

B. Goitrogenic Contaminants of Anthropogenic Origin

Several groups of organic compounds are introduced into food chains and other natural cycles by human activities.

1. *Industrial Waste-Water Effluents*

One of the richest sources of industrial contaminants is aqueous effluents from coal-conversion processes which contain resorcinol, substituted resorcinols, and other phenolic compounds (≤4 g/L), thiocyanate (~1 g/L) (Gaitan, 1986a), hydroxypyrimidines and phthalate esters (which undergo biodegradation by bacteria, resulting in a production of goitrogenic dihydroxybenzoic acid), and polycyclic aromatic hydrocarbons, the most potent of which are 3,4-benzpyrene and 3-methylcholantrene. All compounds mentioned have been found to possess potent antithyroid activity.

2. *Polyhalogenated Biphenyls*

Polychlorinated biphenyls (PCBs) have a great and growing variety of industrial applications. Though their use in the United States was restricted to closed systems in 1971 and totally banned in 1978, they widely contaminated the ecosystems, and they are expected to exert long-term effects due to their very long biological half-lives. Until 1978 an estimated 69,000 tons of PCBs contaminated the air, water, and water sediments in the United States and, further, 390,000 tons of PCBs are still in service. Though banned in the United States, the contamination of other parts of the world goes on, resulting in such disasters as happened in the Italian town Soveso with 2,3,7,8-tetrachlorodibenzo-*p*-dioxin (Bastomsky, 1977).

Apparently the primary mode of environmental distribution is atmospheric transport from sites of use and disposal. From atmospheric sources, PCBs are accumulated by plant foliage and flushed to surface waters. The most important exposures are that of industrial workers, which may result in increased mortality from cancer (Brown, 1987) and increased incidence of hypothyroidism (Bahn et al., 1980), and that of individuals consuming freshwater fish from contaminated streams or lakes (e.g., fish from the Great Lakes contained about 5 mg PCBs/kg). In 1972 the estimated content of PCBs in 45% of the American population was about 1 μg/g body fat (Sonstegard and Leatherland, 1976), while in seriously contaminated areas of the river Krupa in Yugoslavia, the concentration of PCBs was as high as 117 μg/g fish and 320 μg/g human skin fat (Jan and Tratnik, 1988).

Polybrominated biphenyls (PBBs) are used exclusively as fire retardants, but their accidental introduction into the food chain occurred in Michigan in 1973 when they were added by mistake to the mineral mixture feed for cattle and poultry instead of calcium chloride. A goitrogenic effect of PCBs (Bastomsky, 1977; Collins and Capen, 1980) and PBBs (Allen-Rowlands et al., 1981; Akoso et al., 1982) in rats was repeatedly observed.

3. *Organochlorine Insecticides*

Some pesticides used worldwide either in malaria control or in agriculture, such as DDT (2,2-bis-[*p*-chlorophenyl]-1,1,1-trichloromethane), DDE (2,2-bis-[*p*]chlorophenyl]-1,1-dichloroethylene), and Dieldrin, are ubiquitous contaminants of water and food products. Human milk is among the especially contaminated ones. These compounds are insoluble in water and resistant to destruction by light and oxidation, so they are almost biologically and environmentally undegradable (Gaitan, 1988). Their goitrogenic effect has been demonstrated in homing pigeons (Jefferies and French, 1969).

4. *Fungicides*

Ethylene bisdithiocarbamates are widely used in agriculture as fungicides. Their residues on the surface of treated objects may be degraded by heat to ethylenethiourea, which has been repeatedly shown to be goitrogenic (O'Neill and Marshall, 1984) as well as carcinogenic and teratogenic in animals.

5. *Bacteriostatics (Sulfonamides and Antibiotics)*

Various sulfonamide compounds and antibiotics are widely used in animal husbandry as feed additives and medications. In the United States almost 1.5 million kg of antibiotics were given to pigs in 1978 alone (Matovinovic, 1983). The goitrogenic effect of several antibiotics (Saito et al., 1972) or sulfonamides (Fullerton and Kushmaul, 1987) in rats have been repeatedly demonstrated.

IV. METABOLISM OF PLANT GOITROGENS IN THE ORGANISM AND THEIR MECHANISM OF ACTION

A. Glucosinolates and Their Aglucones

As a first step, the glucosinolates are subjected to enzymatic splitting by the enzyme myrosinase, which is present in the plant tissue and released from special cells after the destruction by culinary preparation or chewing. In addition, similar thioglucosidases are present in intestinal bacteria and may also contribute to enzymatic splitting, even in such cases when the plant enzyme has been inactivated by cooking. Individual aglucones are then easily absorbed from the gastrointestinal tract (see Sec. V.A).

1. *Thiocyanate*

In addition to exogenous thiocyanate originating from foods, another fraction called endogenous thiocyanate is formed from cyanide and sulfur donors through the enzymatic action of rhodanese (see Langer and Greer, 1977). The most important cyanide donor and thus a source of endogenously formed thiocyanate is hydrocyanic acid originating from cyanogenic glucosides (see below), while the sulfur for endogenous formation of thiocyanate is mostly contributed from endogenous sources (thiosulfate, sulfur-containing amino acids, etc.). Among the most important sources of exogenous (or preformed) thiocyanate is glucobrassicin and related glucosinolates (Fenwick et al., 1983).

Thiocyanate distribution in the organism, except in the brain, resembles that of iodide or chloride. There are several anion-concentrating tissues (thyroid, salivary glands, gastric mucosa, mammary glands, etc.) in which iodide, thiocyanate, and some other anions compete for the same binding sites.

In various organs the conversion of thiocyanate sulfur to sulfate has been demonstrated (Maloof and Soodak, 1963), and about 4.5% of labeled sulfur of ^{35}S-thiocyanate was found in the urine of rats (Funderbunk and van Middlesworth, 1971). There exists a common pool of thiocyanate carbons, and apparently cyanide originating from other sources may also enter this cycle (Wood, 1975). However, the oxidation of thiocyanate sulfur to sulfate removes it irreversibly from thiocyanate pool.

After a single dose there is a rapid distribution of thiocyanate in the extracellular fluid. Its subsequent decrease apparently depends on the extracellular fluid turnover rate related to numerous factors such as water balance, kidney function, hormonal regulation of electrolyte and water metabolism, etc. Like some univalent anions, thiocyanate may inhibit the active transport of iodide both in the thyroid and in extrathyroidal iodide-concentrating tissues. This effect finally results in an increase of iodide supply to the kidneys (van Middlesworth, 1960). Another effect of thiocyanate consists of displacement of thyroxine from plasma protein carriers, which results in an increase of thyroxine flux to the tissues. Under experimental conditions a single dose of thiocyanate may inhibit the pituitary-thyroid axis; this axis may later be stimulated due to the increased activity of thyrotropic hormone (Langer, 1968). Recently, a considerable accumulation of unusual iodinated protein in the thyroid has been found in mice fed thiocyanate (Van Middlesworth, 1985). The inhibition of thyroid peroxidase—an enzyme essential for thyroid hormone biosynthesis—and of thyroid hormone synthesis by thiocyanate (Langer and Michajlovskij, 1972) and other antithyroid compounds (Taurog et al., 1989) has been repeatedly reported.

2. *Isothiocyanates*

Possible oxidation of isothiocyanate sulfur to sulfate was demonstrated by findings of labeled sulfate in the urine after administration of ^{35}S-*p*-bromophenylisothiocyanate (Langer, 1966c). In addition, the formation of goitrogenic thiohydantoins from isothiocyanates and amino acids by the well-known Edman's reaction, which might spontaneously proceed under slightly alkaline pH in the upper intestine, cannot be excluded (Langer et al., 1964). After the administration of naturally occurring methyl-, ethyl-, butyl-, and allylisothiocyanate, their mercapturic acids were found in the urine (Mennicke et al., 1988). Finally, after the ingestion of rapeseed meal, 1-cyano-2-hydroxy-3-butene and hydroxynitrile were found in milk (Papas et al., 1979). It should be added that isothiocyanates exert teratogenic, toxic, fungistatic, bacteriostatic, and other effects and were found to inhibit carcinogenic effects of several chemical carcinogens (reviewed by Wattenberg et al., 1986) (see also Sec. V.A). It has been reported that a decreased somatomedin synthesis resulting from the administration of plant goitrogens may be responsible for peripheral hypothyroidism (Jahreis et al., 1985) and that the treatment of rapeseed meal with Cu^{2+} resulted in normal growth in pigs (Schone et al., 1990).

Goitrogenic effect of allylisothicyanate (Langer and Stolc, 1965) and some other isothiocyanates (Bachelard et al., 1963) has been demonstrated in rats and also in vitro, which apparently means that this type of compound may directly affect the thyroid without first being metabolized (Langer and Greer, 1968). It also appeared that the three main groups of goitrogenic aglucones from various plant species such as thiocyanate, isothiocyanates, and oxazolidinethiones apparently act together on the thyroid after ingestion of natural plant material and thus may be considered as the so-called "Brassica-factor" (Langer, 1966a,b).

B. Glucosylflavonoids and Their Aglucones

The problems of chemistry and metabolism of this widespread group of compounds have been extensively reviewed by Gaitan (1986a,b,c; 1990) and are briefly summarized in Sec. III.A.1.

V. CHEMISTRY OF NATURALLY OCCURRING GOITROGENS

A. Glucosinolates and Their Breakdown Products

The first two glucosinolates—Sinigrin from black mustard (*Sinapis nigra*) and Sinalbin from white mustard (*Sinapis alba*)—were discovered 150 years ago. Their names were first derived from the Latin name of the plant from which they were also isolated (e.g., Glucocheirolin from Cheiranthus), but later with the growing number of such compounds they were replaced by semisystematic names in which all members of this class are called glucosinolates (GSs) and a prefix is added identifying the variable part of the molecule (R) (see Fig. 2). Thus, Sinigrin becomes 2-propenyl-GS or allyl-GS, Sinalbin becomes *p*-hydroxy-benzyl-GS, etc. All glucosinolates possess the same basic skeleton with a sulfonated oxime moiety and thioglucoside moiety. They differ only in the chemical structure of the side chain R.

It should be kept in mind that from the point of goitrogenic activity, glucosinolates are only inactive parent compounds of several active aglucones, which are breakdown products liberated from glucosinolates by the action of thioglucoside glucohydrolase, still commonly called by its original name "myrosinase." So far, this enzyme has been found in all plants containing glucosinolates, but in the intact plant it is localized separately from GSs in special cells called idioblasts (Kjaer, 1960) or myrosin cells (Iversen et al., 1979; Pocock et al., 1987). The damage of plant tissue (homogenization, milling, grinding, preparing food, etc.) brings the enzyme and substrate (GS) into contact, and thus the hydrolysis may be started, strongly activated by L-ascorbic acid (Ettlinger et al., 1961; Schwimmer, 1961; Henderson and McEwen, 1972). The spectrum of active breakdown products is determined by the nature of the glucosinolate side chain, reaction conditions, and the presence of some cofactors (pH, ferrous ions, protein cofactors, etc.). Since several excellent reviews were published on the chemistry of glucosinolates (Kjaer, 1960; Fenwick et al., 1983; McGregor et al., 1983), we present here only fundamental information.

The main products of glucosinolate hydrolysis are shown in Figure 2. By the action of this enzyme, first glucose is released and an unstable intermediate is formed (not shown), which breaks down at weakly acidic pH or in the presence of ferrous ions to nitrile (R-CN), elementary sulfur, and bisulfate. At neutral pH, however, the intermediate undergoes a Lossen rearrangement to produce isothiocyanate (R-NCS) and bisulfate. In rare instances organic isothiocyanates (R-SCN) may be formed under the action of a cofactor in seeds of *Thlaspi arvense* and *Lepidium sativum* (Gmelin and Virtanen, 1959). According to a side chain (R) of GS, isothiocyanates of alkyl, alkanyl, methylthioalkyl, methylsulfinylalkyl, methylsulfonylalkyl or aromatic configuration are formed. They may be separated into volatile and nonvolatile isothiocyanates. The most widespread natural isothiocyanate is allylisothiocyanate (from Sinigrin) with known goitrogenic effect (Langer and Stolc, 1965; Langer, 1966a,b). All such isothiocyanates are stable in aqueous solutions with the exception of the following two groups.

1. GSs with a hydroxyl group on the second carbon of the side chain, such as Progoitrin (2-hydroxybutenyl-GS), give rise to an isothiocyanate which forms oxazolidinethione (5-vinyl-oxazolidine-2-thione or goitrin) by spontaneous cyclization. Progoitrin is frequently present in Brassica foodstuffs (Fenwick et al., 1983; Sones et al., 1984), and its aglucone goitrin is one of the most active naturally occurring goitrogens (Langer and Greer, 1977).
2. Indole-containing GSs (Glucobrassicin and its congeners) and *p*-hydroxybenzyl-GS (Sinalbin) also give rise to unstable isothiocyanates, which are

promptly hydrolyzed to form corresponding hydroxyproducts (alcohols, R-OH) and thiocyanate ion (SCN^-) (Gmelin and Virtanen, 1961, 1962; Kawakishi et al., 1967). Figure 2 shows the hydrolysis of 3-methyl-indolyl-isothiocyanate liberated from Glucobrassicin. The appropriate 3-hydroxy-methylindole (indolyl-3-carbinol, I3C) is also unstable and polymerizes to the 3,3′-diindolylmethan; in the presence of ascorbic acid it forms ascorbigen—the bound form of ascorbic acid (Prochazka and Sanda, 1960). The other GSs of this group are subjected to similar reactions. Thus, Glucobrassicin as a regular component of Brassicia vegetables may be the source not only of goitrogenic thiocyanate, but also of physiologically active indoles, i.e., indolylacetonitrile as a plant growth stimulator (auxin) (Kutacek et al., 1966) or the I3C and other indoles as effective anticarcinogenic compounds in Brassica plants (Wattenberg et al., 1986; Bradfield and Bjeldanes, 1987; McDanell et al., 1987, 1988; Dashwood et al., 1988).

From Figure 2 it is clear that several physiologically active compounds are formed from glucosinolates in the presence of myrosinase. They are responsible for the pungent taste of important condiments (horseradish, mustard, etc.) and also contribute to the characteristic flavors of brassica and other vegetables. However, the presence of about 4–8% of glucosinolates in Brassica plants used for feeding animals remains a serious economical problem, since several of them are used as pasture, forage, or silage (kale, turnip, etc.) or as fodder flour following the extraction of oils from seeds (*Brassica napus, Brassica campestris, Brassica juncea, Crambe abyssinica*, etc.). Animals are fed predominantly with such products in a raw form, which means that the toxic aglucones may be entirely released (see Langer and Greer, 1977; Fenwick and Curtis, 1980).

Although a large number (up to 100) of GSs occur mainly in the Crucifers, about 30 of these are present in the Brassica in which about 3–6 different glucosinolates were found in individual species. The differences in the presence and content of individual GSs were also found between individual parts of the same plant (e.g., green parts vs. seeds).

Since several reviews have appeared about the occurrence and content of glucosinolates in the plant kingdom (Kjaer, 1960; Langer and Greer, 1977; Fenwick et al., 1983; Langer, 1983; Sones et al., 1984; McDanell et al., 1988), only some of the most widespread glucosinolates and their breakdown products are listed in Table 1.

B. Hydrolysis of Glucosinolates Under Different Conditions

The above-presented breakdown of glucosinolates by the action of myrosinase takes place in pure systems only with the use of an enzyme of known quality under controlled pH. However, during the cooking of vegetables and the preparation of animal feed, various steps of autolysis take place due to the action of myrosinase after the disintegration of plant tissues. Under such uncontrolled conditions the structure of some final products may be somewhat different from that described above. First, even the myrosinase itself occurs in several isoenzyme forms (Bjorkman, 1976; Kjaer and Larsen, 1977; MacLeod

Table 1 Glucosinolates[a] and Their Breakdown Products Occurring in Brassica Plants

Glucosinolate (original name)	R Group	Isothiocyanates (ITC)[b]
		Stable isothiocyanates:
Glucocapparin	CH_3-	Methyl-ITC
Sinigrin	CH_2=CH-CH_2-	2-Propenyl-ITC (Allyl-ITC)
Gluconapin	CH_2=CH-$(CH_2)_2$-	3-Butenyl-ITC
Glucobrassicanapin	CH_2=CH-$(CH_2)_3$-	4-Pentenyl-ITC
Glucoibervirin	CH_3-S-$(CH_2)_3$-	3-Methyl-thio-propyl-ITC
Glucoerucin	CH_3-S-$(CH_2)_4$-	4-Methyl-thio-butyl-ITC
Glucoberteroin	CH_3-S-$(CH_2)_5$-	5-Methyl-thio-pentyl-ITC
Glucoiberin	CH_3-SO-$(CH_2)_3$-	3-Methyl-sulfinyl-propyl-ITC
Glucoraphanin	CH_3-SO-$(CH_2)_4$-	4-Methyl-sulfinyl-butyl-ITC
Glucoalyssin	CH_3-SO-$(CH_2)_5$-	5-Methyl-sulfinyl-pentyl-ITC
Glucocheirolin	CH_3-SO_2-$(CH_2)_3$-	3-Methyl-sulfonyl-propyl-ITC
Glucotropaeolin	C_6H_5-CH_2-	Benzyl-ITC
Gluconasturtiin	C_6H_5-$(CH_2)_2$-	2-Phenyl-ethyl-ITC
		Unstable isothiocyanates:
Progoitrin	CH_2=CH-CH(OH)-CH_2-	(2-Hydroxy-3-butenyl-ITC)[c]
Glucobrassicin	Indolyl-3-CH_2-	(3-Indolyl-methyl-ITC)[d]
Neoglucobrassicin	1-Methoxy-indolyl-3-CH_2-	(1-Methoxy-3-indolyl-methyl-ITC)[d]
Sinalbin	*p*-HO-C_6H_4-CH_2-	(*p*-Hydroxy-benzyl-ITC)[d]

[a]See Figure 2 for generalized structure.
[b]R-N=C=S.
[c]Cyclization to the goitrin (5-vinyl-oxazolidin-2-thione).
[d]Hydrolyzed to the SCN^- + corresponding hydroxy-derivatives (alcohols).

and Rossiter, 1986), which show different sensitivities to activation with ascorbic acid or inactivation by heating. In addition, a number of factors shift the process of hydrolysis in favor of the formation of nitriles rather than of isothiocyanates, and thus it is generally accepted that nitriles are major products of such autolysis (Fenwick et al., 1983). From a practical viewpoint, the formation of nitriles under acidic conditions appears to be important, since it may take place in processed vegetables such as sauerkraut, pickled cabbage, cole slaw, etc. (Daxenbichler et al., 1980). Moreover, the formation of some nitriles would presumably occur when the ingested vegetables reach the acidic pH of the stomach, unless the myrosinase has not been destroyed by cooking. Nevertheless, it has been shown that the autolysis of previously cooked cauliflower (10 min in boiling water) yielded 80% of autolytic products as compared with the appropriate raw vegetables (Bradfield and Bjeldanes, 1987). This apparently shows that either common cooking practices do not inactivate the myrosinase to any significant extent or that some other thermostable factors may be involved in this process (unfortunately, the latter authors did not estimate the activity of myrosinase in their cooked cauliflower).

The cooking of glucosinolates or heating of seeds of Crucifers at 125°C for various periods was reported to result in nitrile formation (Hasapis and MacLeod, 1982). In some plants (*Crambe abyssinica, Brassica napus*) an epithiospecifier protein was found which is heat unstable and favors the formation of nitrile and epithionitrile (Tookey, 1973). At pH 4.5–5.5 the formation of isothiocyanate by myrosinase was strongly inhibited by ferrous ion, while such effect was notably depressed at pH 6.5 and disappeared at pH 7.5 (Uda et al., 1986a). However, under the simultaneous presence of thiol compounds (cysteine, glutathione) and Fe^{2+}, strong acceleration of nitrile formation was found even at pH 6.5 (Uda et al., 1986b). A nonenzymatic breakdown of glucosinolates to nitriles was also observed in the presence of ferrous ions (Youngs and Perlin, 1967; Austin et al., 1968).

The hydrolysis of indole glucosinolates in the above conditions gives rise to some different products. Thus, by autolysis of the Brassica plant material the indolyl-3-carbinol (I3C) is the major metabolite generated within the first 20 min, but it is not stable under the autolytic conditions, more than 80% being converted to other products within 24 h (Bradfield and Bjeldanes, 1987). In the presence of Fe^{2+} without myrosinase a red-violet complex of Glucobrassicin is formed, and only 2% of indolylacetonitrile (auxin) is liberated. Of the other ions tested (Mg^{2+}, Ni^{2+}, Zn^{2+}, Cd^{2+}, Mn^{2+}, Co^{2+}, Cr^{3+}, Fe^{3+}), only Cu^{2+} was active, and after the incubation of a solution of 2 mM Cu^{2+} per 1 mM Glucobrassicin for 24 h, up to 1% of indolylacetonitrile was formed (Michajlovskij, 1974). Following UV irradiation of aqueous solution of Glucobrassicin, the same products of enzymatic cleavage were found as after autolysis (i.e., sulfate, glucose, thiocyanate, and indolyl-3-carbinol), while the UV photolysis of other glucosinolates (Sinigrin, Sinalbin, Progoitrin, Glucoiberin) was not so rapid, and only the formation of glucose and bisulfate, but not that of isothiocyanate, goitrin, or nitriles, was observed (Michajlovskij, 1968).

The isothiocyanates (ITCs) liberated show a high reactivity. Thus, in the presence of ammonia, aniline, and other amino compounds (amino acids, proteins) or thiol compounds, they form mono- and disubstituted thiourea derivatives (Kjaer et al., 1953; Kawakishi and Kaneko, 1987). Such reactions occur even spontaneously under alkaline conditions. In acidic conditions these thioureas may easily cyclize to form thiohydantoins (Edman's reaction) via intermediate carbamyl derivatives. Several of the latter groups of compounds may be goitrogenic and toxic (Langer et al., 1964; Macholz et al., 1986).

The above-described myrosinaselike hydrolysis, especially that of Progoitrin, by gastrointestinal bacteria was recently reexamined in rats (Oginsky et al., 1965). During the incubation of Progoitrin with feces or with the content of cecum or colon of germ-free animals in vitro, no degradation could be detected, but the incubation with microflora of conventional rats resulted in considerable hydrolysis of that glucosinolate. Simultaneously it was found that the cyclization of hydroxybutenyl ITC to goitrin and the formation of corresponding thioureas and thiohydantoins with proteins, amino acids, etc. are competitive reaction steps (Macholz et al., 1986). Thus, it was suggested that the goitrogenic and toxic effects of Progoitrin cannot be attributed to the effect of goitrin only. For instance, the possible etiological role in the pathogenesis of Spanish toxic oil syndrome in May 1981 was the consumption of insufficiently purified technical rapeseed oil which contained 2-hydroxy-3-butenyl-ITC and aniline as denaturating agent. They formed the toxic 2-hydroxy-3-butenyl-phenylthiourea and the more toxic cyclic compound 1-phenyl-5-vinyl-2-imidazolidine-thione, though a recent work suggests that these conclusions should be reevaluated (Verhaar et al., 1989).

Crucifers and especially Brassica vegetables may be consumed either raw or cooked—steamed, dried, or otherwise processed including initial cutting, blanching, freezing, pickling, or fermenting. The cooking results in various biochemical processes such as thermal hydrolysis of glucosinolates, evaporation of volatile ITCs, decomposition of ITCs, etc. There are several studies on the effect of cooking and other kinds of processing of these vegetables on the content of glucosinolates and their breakdown products (Michajlovskij et al., 1970; Srinivasa Kumar and Chandrasekhara, 1973; Mullin and Sahasrabudhe, 1978; Maheshwari et al., 1980; Srisangnam et al., 1980; Daxenbichler et al., 1980; Sones et al., 1984; Slominski and Campbell, 1989), which were reviewed by Fenwick et al. (1983). In most cases it was shown that about one third to one half of glucosinolate content is decreased by cooking (Michajlovskij et al., 1970; Sones et al., 1984). After cooking, volatile ITCs disappeared completely, and some others (goitrin, iberin) were partly or completely decomposed, but all thiocyanate liberated is stable enough to remain in the boiled material. So far, only a few reports exist on the influence of thermal processes on the goitrogenic activity of vegetables. Thus, a decrease of goitrogenic activity of steamed vegetables by about 30–50% was found in rabbits as compared with that of raw material (Podoba et al., 1957). Similarly, a decrease of thiocyanate content and a proportional decrease of goitrogenic activity in cooked vegetables were found (Michajlovskij, 1964).

C. Isolation, Identification, and Analysis of Glucosinolates and Their Breakdown Products

The methods of isolation, identification, and quantification of glucosinolates and their breakdown products were developed in parallel with the new analytical techniques and instrumentation, which led to significant advances in methodology for analysis of glucosinolates over the pasts three decades. All other and newer methods of sample preparation, GS identification, and both the direct and indirect methods for determining GS content are summarized in some reviews (Kjaer, 1960; Gmelin, 1964; Langer and Greer, 1977; Langer, 1983; Fenwick et al., 1983; McDanell et al., 1988) and completely treated in a special review (McGregor et al., 1983). In the latter review consideration is given to the suitability of direct or indirect methods for a rapid screening or precise discriminating measurements and also to the standardization of methods for regulatory and quality control. Only general principles of procedures and newer methods of GS estimation will be given here, with particular attention to the estimation of goitrogenic GSs in Brassica vegetables, while some other problems, like the estimation of GSs in rapeseed meal, will be mentioned only briefly.

1. Sample Preparation, Inactivation of Myrosinase and Cofactors

Crucial step for the isolation and estimation of GSs is the inactivation of myrosinase and cofactors by boiling of the entire and intact plant segments (or defatted seeds) in methanol followed by the reextraction of the material in boiling 70% methanol. After homogenization of boiled material and filtration of combined methanol extracts, the methanol is evaporated under vacuum, and the residue (aqueous GS concentrate) is stored at –20°C until required for analysis. Alternatively, the vegetable samples are quickly frozen at –40°C, ground in a frozen state, and then extracted with boiling methanol (Heaney and Fenwick, 1980a). Freeze-drying has also been used to reduce moisture content (Mullin and Sahasrabudhe, 1977). Freezing may facilitate the handling of a large number of samples, since these may be accumulated and stored in the frozen or freeze-dried state over 6 months without any decomposition of GSs. However, any occasional thawing should be avoided, since the myrosinase during such storage is still active. For analysis, the frozen samples are weighed and then extracted with boiling methanol as indicated above.

The concentrated aqueous extracts of GS can be directly used for the identification of GS by paper chromatography (PC) (Kjaer, 1960; Olsen and Sorensen, 1981) or thin-layer chromatography (TLC) (Wagner et al., 1965; Underhill and Kirkland, 1971) or subjected to further purification before subsequent analytical steps. Previously the aqueous extracts were preextracted with solvents (ethylenechloride, chlorophorm), and the remaining water phase containing GS was then used for the extraction of isothiocyanates and goitrin after their liberation by myrosinase (Appelquist and Josefsson, 1967; Langer and Gschwendtova, 1969; Wetter and Youngs, 1976). Recent purification methods are based on the trapping of anionic GS with a suitable ionex (Sephadex A-25, DEAE-Sephadex A-25, etc.) and, after washing with water, eluted with pyridine acetate (Thies, 1977).

2. Indirect Methods

All products of enzymatic hydrolysis of GSs including sulfate and glucose are useful for GS identification and quantitation. For such purpose the aqueous extracts are incubated under optimal conditions (neutral pH, 30 min at 30°C), which give rise only to ITC and other aglucones such as oxazolidinethiones and thiocyanate. For the hydrolysis either crude preparation of myrosinase from seeds (Schwimmer, 1961; Appelquist and Josefsson, 1967) or purified commercial enzyme (Heaney et al., 1988) may be used.

Total Content of Glucosinolates. The most convenient method for the rapid and screening estimation of total content of GS, especially in breeding programs of Brassica crops and seeds, is that based on colorimetric estimation of glucose released from GS by myrosinase (Lein, 1970; van Etten and Daxenbichler, 1977; Thies, 1985; Saini and Wratten, 1987; Heaney et al., 1988). For instance, in a purified extract corresponding to 4 g of wet Brassica plants, the total GS content was reliably estimated with the aid of a diagnostic glucose kit (Heaney and Fenwick, 1980a). Recently an improved method used the separation of GS from final aqueous solution on a mini-column of DEAE-Sephadex A-25 (Heaney et al., 1988). After washing, the glucose is liberated from the GS by the action of myrosinase directly on the column (incubation for 2 h at 25°C) and estimated in the eluate using a glucose kit. The method is suitable for rapid determination of total GS in rapeseed without any defatting step.

The total GS content may also be estimated by direct spectrophotometry in unhydrolyzed extracts as colored complex of GS with tetrachloropalladate. This method (Thies, 1982) is suitable for a rapid screening of rapeseed (only a few seeds are required) and is apparently more sensitive than the glucose oxidase/hexokinase test paper method (Lein, 1970).

Total Content of Indole Glucosinolates. This may be simply measured in aqueous homogenates of Brassica vegetables after autolysis of GS with endogenous myrosinase (30 min at room temperature) or in enzymatically hydrolyzed GS extracts. The liberated thiocyanate is then estimated in the deproteinized filtrate photometrically with Fe^{3+}. Of several modifications of this method (see Langer and Greer, 1977; Langer, 1983; Fenwick et al., 1983; McGregor et al., 1983), the most precise is that in which, after the addition of $HgCl_2$ solution to destroy $Fe(SCN)_2$–complex, the background is also measured and subtracted from the original value (Johnston and Jones, 1966). However, the methods based on the oxidation of thiocyanate ion such as the photometric method by Aldridge as adopted to plant material (Michajlovskij and Langer, 1958; Jurges and Thies, 1980) are about 10 times more sensitive and also very simple. Recently, a gas chromatographic method for direct estimation of thiocyanate in vegetables (only 1 g of desiccated sample is required) was elaborated (Serrano et al., 1988). The difference between total GS content and indole GS content (i.e., thiocyanate content multiplied by 7.7) corresponds to the partial content of other ITCs and goitrin-producing GSs in plant material. This process, however, was not yet frequently used.

Isothiocyanates and Goitrin. Several methods for the separation, identification, and estimation of ITCs and goitrin were described. Originally, important progress was reached by ITC transformation to thiourea derivatives. After that the thioureas may be easily separated by PC or TLC and estimated with subsequent UV-spectrophotometry at 240 nm (Kjaer, 1960; VanEtten and Daxenbichler, 1977). For the separation of goitrin from ITC, some combined extractions with organic solvents (ethylene chloride, chloroform, ether, iso-octaine-ether, etc.) from myrosinase hydrolyzate were used, and goitrin was also estimated spectrophotometrically (Appelquist and Josefsson, 1967; Langer and Gschwendtova, 1969; Wetter and Youngs, 1976).

ITCs and goitrin are also easily estimated with advanced methods such as gas-liquid chromatography (GLC) (Daxenbichler and VanEtten, 1977; Daxenbichler et al., 1980), GLC/mass spectrometry (Spencer and Daxenbichler, 1980), or HPLC (Maheshwari et al., 1979; Josefsson and Akerstrom, 1979). The estimation of indole products of Glucobrassicin (i.e., indolylmethyl-GS) in Brassica vegetables after autolysis using reverse-phase HPLC is also possible (Bradfield and Bjeldanes, 1987).

Direct Estimation of Glucosinolates. A direct estimation of GSs in purified plant extracts after inactivation of myrosinase is frequently utilized using GC (Olsen and Sorensen, 1980) or HPLC (Helboe et al., 1980). Such methods were further improved by the introduction of glucosinolate desulfation with sulfatase isolated from edible snail (*Helix pomatia*) followed by liquid chromatography (LC) (Sang and Truscott, 1984), HPLC (Minchinton et al., 1982; Spinks et al., 1984), and GC including the determination of indole-desulfo-GC (Heaney and Fenwick, 1980b). For the separation and identification of GSs, GC/mass spectrometry (Eagles et al., 1981a,b) or NMR spectra of $^3H,^{13}C$-GC (Cox et al., 1984) were satisfactorily utilized. Recently a new and highly sensitive enzyme-linked immunosorbent assay (ELISA) for alkenyl-GS has been developed (Hassan et al., 1988).

Isolation and Identification of Glucosinolates. Essentially similar procedures are used for the isolation of GSs, but higher quantities of most suitable material are used for extraction. Thus, Sinigrin is extracted from seeds of *B. juncea*, Progoitrin from seeds of *B. napus* or Glucobrassicin from the leaves of *B. oleracea*, var *gemmifera*. Compared with the tedious and time-consuming previous methods (Kjaer, 1960; Gmelin, 1964), the new methods are simple and rapid (Hanley et al., 1983): the frozen ground plant material (1 kg) is extracted with boiling methanol (2 L), the extract evaporated to dryness, taken up in water (500 ml), filtered through Celite, applied to the column of acidic alumina, washed with water, and then GSs were finally eluted with 1% potassium sulfate. After evaporation to dryness the eluate is extracted with hot methanol (desalting), which is then evaporated to dryness. The residue is taken up in a little water and freeze-dried to obtain a partially purified product, which may be further purified with DEAE-Sephadex A-25 column, and GSs may be eluted with ammonium bicarbonate. The combined fractions of GSs are evaporated and desalted by freeze-drying (e.g., Glucobrassicin is converted to the tetramethylammonium salt and recrystallized from aqueous propan-2-ol). A still more rapid method was developed using flash chromatography for the isolation and purification of GSs (Peterka and Fenwick, 1988). In this procedure only 40 min are needed for the separation, and the column scan may be run in parallel. Both methods give yields in gram quantities of highly purified products as checked by GC (Heaney and Fenwick, 1980b), mass spectrometry (Fenwick et al., 1980), melting point and NMR spectroscopy (Cox et al., 1984), HPLC (Spinks et al., 1984), and glucose release method (Heaney et al., 1988). The most recent methods of identification of desulfoglucosinolates using thermospray liquid chromatography/mass spectrometry can also be used (Hogge et al., 1988).

REFERENCES

Akoso, B. T., Sleight, S. D., Nachreiner, R. F., and Aust, S. D. (1982). Effects of purified polyborominated biphenyl congeners on the thyroid and pituitary gland in rats. *J. Am. Coll. Toxicol. 1*: 23–36.

Allen-Rowlands, C. F., Castracena, V. D., Hamilton, M. G., and Seifter, J. (1981). Effect of polybrominated biphenyls (PBB) on the pituitary-thyroid axis of the rat. *Proc. Soc. Exp. Biol. Med. 166*: 506–514.

Appelquist, L. A., and Josefsson, E. (1967). Method for quantitative determination of isothiocyanates and oxazolidinethiones in digests of seed meals of rape and turnip rape. *J. Sci. Food Agric, 18*: 510–519.

Astwood, E. B., Greer, M. A., and Ettlinger, M. G. (1949). L-5-vinyl-2-thiooxzolidone, an antithyroid compound from yellow turnip and from Brassica seeds. *J. Biol. Chem.* *181*: 121–130.

Austin, F. J., Gent, C. A., and Wolff, J. A. (1968). Degradation of natural thioglucosides with ferrous salts. *J. Agric. Food. Chem.* *16*: 752–755.

Bachelard, H. S., McQuillan, M. T., and Trikojus, V. M. (1963). An investigation of antithyroid activities of isothiocyanates and derivatives. *Aust. J. Biol. Sci.* *16*: 177–191.

Bahn, A., Mills, J. L., Snyder, P. J., Gann, P. H., Houten, L., Bialik, O., Hollman, L., and Utiger, R. (1980). Hypothyroidism in workers exposed to polybrominated biphenyls. *N. Engl. J. Med.* *302*: 31–33.

Bastomsky, C. H. (1977). Goitres in rats fed polychlorinated biphenyls. *Canad. J. Physiol. Pharmacol.* *55*: 288–292.

Beckers, C., and Delange, F. (1980). Iodine deficiency. In *Endemic Goiter and Endemic Cretinism*, J. B. Stanbury and B. S. Hetzel, eds. John Wiley, New York, pp. 199–217.

Bjorkman, R. (1976). Properties and function of plant myrosinases. In *The Biology and Chemistry of the Cruciferae*, J. G. Vaughan, A. J. MacLeod, B. M. G. Jones, eds. Academic Press, New York, pp. 191–205.

Bradfield, C. A., and Bjeldanes, L. F. (1987). High-performance liquid chromatographic analysis of anticarcinogenic indoles in *Brassica oleracea*. *J. Agric. Food Chem.* *35*: 46–49.

Brown, D. P. (1987). Mortality of workers exposed to polychlorinated biphenyls—an update. *Arch. Environm. Health* *42*: 333–339.

Clandinin, D. R., and Robbles, A. R. (1981). Rapeseed meal in animal nutrition: Non-ruminant animals. *J. Am. Oil Chem. Soc.* *58*: 682–694.

Collins, W. T., and Capen, C. C. (1980). Ultrastructural and functional alterations of the rat thyroid gland produced by polychlorinated biphenyls compared with iodide excess and deficiency, and thyrotropin and thyroxine administration. *Virchow's Arch. Cell Path.* *33*: 213–231.

Cooke, R. D., and Coursey, D. G. (1981). Cassava: A major cyanide-containing food crop. In *Cyanide in Biology*, B. Vanesland, ed. Academic Press, New York, pp. 93–114.

Cox, I. J., Hanley, A. B., Belton, P. S., and Fenwick, G. R. (1984). N.M.R. spectra (^{3}H, ^{13}C) of glucosinolates. *Carbohydrate Res.* *132*: 323–329.

Dashwood, R. H., Arbogast, D. N., Fong, A. T., Hendricks, J. D., and Bailey, G. S. (1988). Mechanisms of anti-carcinogenesis by indole-3-carbinol: detailed in vivo DNA binding dose-response studies after dietary administration with aflatoxin B_1. *Carcinogenesis* *9*: 427–432.

Daxenbichler, M. E., and VanEtten, C. H. (1977). Glucosinolates and derived products in cruciferous vegetables: Gas-liquid chromatographic determination of the aglucon derivatives from cabbage. *J. AOAC* *60*: 950–953.

Daxenbichler, M. E., VanEtten, C. H., and Williams, P. H. (1980). Glucosinolate products in commercial sauerkraut. *J. Agric. Food Chem.* *28*: 809–814.

Delange, F. M., and Ermans, A. M. (1976). Endemic goiter and creatinism, naturally occurring goitrogens. In *Pharmacological Therapy*, Vol. 1, J. N. Hershman and G. A. Bray, eds. Pergamon Press, New York, pp. 57–93.

Eagles, J., Fenwick, G. R., and Heaney, R. K. (1981a). Gas chromatography chemical ionization mass spectrometry of glucosinolate derivatives. *Biomed. Mass Spectrom.* *8*: 278–282.

Eagles, J., Fenwick, G. R., Gmelin, R., and Rakow, D. (1981b). The chemical ionization mass spectra of glucosinolates (mustard oil glucosides) and desulphoglucosinolates. *Biomed. Mass Spectrom.* *8*: 265–269.

Ermans, A. M., Bourdoux, P., Kinthaert, J., Lagasse, R., Luvivila, K., Mafuta, M., Thilly, C. H., and Delange, F. (1983). Role of cassava in the etiology of endemic goitre and cretinism. In *Cassava Toxicity and Thyroid: Research and Public Health Issues*, F. Delange and R. Ahluwalia, eds. Agricultural Development Research Center, Ottawa, Canada, pp. 9–26.

Ettlinger, M. G., and Kjaer, A. (1968). Sulfur compounds in plants. *Recent Advances in Phytochemistry*, Vol. 1, T. J. Masbry, ed. Appleton-Century-Crofts, pp. 60–144.

Ettlinger, M. G., Dateo, G. P., Harrison, B. W., Mabry, T. J., and Thompson, C. P. (1961). *Proc. Natl. Acad. Sci. USA 47*: 1875–1880.

Fenwick, G. R., and Curtis, R. F. (1980). Rapeseed meal and its use in poultry diets. *Anim. Feed Sci. Technol. 5*: 255–263.

Fenwick, G. R., Eagles, J., Gmelin, R., and Rakow, D. (1980). The mass spectra of glucosinolates and desulphoglucosinolates. *Biomed. Mass Spectrom. 7*: 410–412.

Fenwick, G. G., Heaney, R. K., and Mullin, W. J. (1983). Glucosinolates and their breakdown products in food and food plants. *CRC Crit. Rev. in Food Sci. and Nutrit. 18*: 123–201.

Fenwick, G. R., Heaney, R. K., Hanley, A. B., and Spinks, E. A. (1986). Special report No. 14: Glucosinolates in food plants. AFRC Food Research Institute, Norwich, Biennal Report 1983–1984, pp. 31–36.

Fort, P., Moses, N., Fasano, M., Goldberg, T., and Lifshitz, F. (1990). Breast and soy-formula feedings in early infancy and the prevalence of autoimmune thyroid disease in children. *J. Am. Coll. Nutrit. 9*: 164–167.

Fullerton, F. R., Kushmaul, R. J., Suber, R. L., and Littlefield, N. A. (1987). Influence of oral administration of sulfamethazine on thyroid hormone levels in Fisher 344 rats. *J. Toxicol. Environm. Health 22*: 175–185.

Funderburk, C. F., and van Middlesworth, L. (1971). The effect of thiocyanate concentration on thiocyanate distribution and excretion. *Proc. Soc. Exp. Biol. Med. 136*: 1249–1252.

Gaitan, E. (1980). Goitrogens in the etiology of endemic goiter. In *Endemic Goiter and Endemic Cretinism*, J. B. Stanbury and B. S. Hetzel, eds. John Wiley, New York, pp. 219–236.

Gaitan, E. (1983). Role of naturally occurring goitrogens in the etiology of endemic goiter. In *Cassava Toxicity and Thyroid: Research and Public Health Issues*, F. Delange and R. Ahluwalia, eds. International Development Research Center, Ottawa, Canada, pp. 27–34.

Gaitan, E. (1984). Endemic goiter in Western Colombia. *Ecology of Disease 2*: 295–308.

Gaitan, E. (1986a). Environmental goitrogens other than iodine deficiency. *IDD Newsletter 2*: 11–13.

Gaitan, E. (1986b). Iodine sufficient goiter and autoimmune thyroiditis: The Kentucky and Colombian experience. In *Frontiers in Thyroidology*, G. Medeiros-Neto and E. Gaitan, eds. Plenum Press, New York, pp. 19–26.

Gaitan, E. (1986c). Environmental goitrogens. In *The Thyroid Gland: Practical Clinical Treatise*, L. Van Middlesworth, ed. Year Book Medical Publishers, Chicago, pp. 263–280.

Gaitan, E. (1988). Goitrogens. *Bailliere's Clin. Endocrin. Metab. 2*: 683–702.

Gaitan, E. (1990). Goitrogens in food and water. *Annu. Rev. Nutr. 10*: 21–39.

Gaitan, E., Lindsay, R. H., Reichert, R. D., Ingbar, S. H., Cooksey, R. C., Legan, J., Meydrech, E. F., Hill, J., and Kubota, K. (1989). Antithyroid and goitrogenic effects of millet: Role of C-glycosylflavones. *J. Clin. Endocrin. Metab. 68*: 707–714.

Gmelin, R. (1964). Chemie der S-haltigen Brassica-Inhaltstoffe und ihre Beziehungen in der Brassica-Faktoren. In *Naturally Occurring Goitrogens and Thyroid Function*, J. Podoba and P. Langer, eds. Veda, Bratislava, pp. 17–33.

Gmelin, R., and Virtanen, A. I. (1959). A new type of enzymatic cleavage of mustard oil glucosides. *Acta Chem. Scand. 13*: 1474–1475.

Gmelin, R., and Virtanen, A. I. (1961). Glucobrassicin, der Precursor von SCN^-, 3-Indolylacetonitril und Ascorbigen in Brassica Oleracea spezies. *Ann. Acad. Sci. Fenn., Ser. A, II. Chemica 107*: 1–25.

Gmelin, R., and Virtanen, A. I. (1962). Neoglucobrassicin, ein zweiter SCN^- Precursor vom Indoltyp in Brassica-Arten. *Acta Chem. Scand. 14*: 507–510.

Greer, M. A. (1957). Goitrogenic substances in food. *Am. J. Clin. Nutr. 5*: 440–444.

Greer, M. A. (1962). The natural occurrence of goitrogenic agents. *Rec. Progr. Horm. Res. 18*: 187–219.

Greil, W., Rafferzeder, M., Bechtner, G., and Gartner, R. (1989). Release of an endothelial cell growth factor from cultured porcine thyroid follicles. *Molec. Endocrin. 3*: 858–867.

Hanley, A. B., Heaney, R. K., and Fenwick, G. R. (1983). Improved isolation of glucobrassicin and other glucosinolates. *J. Sci. Food Agric. 34*: 869–873.

Hasapis, X., and MacLeod, A. J. (1982). Benzylglucosinolate degradation in heat-treated *Lepidium sativum* seeds and detection of a thiocyanate-forming factor. *Phytochemistry 21*: 1009–1013.

Hassan, F., Rothnie, N. E., Yeung, S. P., and Palmer, M. V. (1988). Enzyme-linked immunosorbens assays for alkenyl glucosinolates. *J. Agric. Food Chem. 36*: 398–403.

Heaney, R. K., and Fenwick, G. R. (1980a). Glucosinolates in Brassica vegetables. *J. Sci. Food Agric. 31*: 775–793.

Heaney, R. K., and Fenwick, G. R. (1980b). The analysis of glucosinolates in Brassica species using gas chromatography. *J. Sci. Food. Agric. 31*: 593–599.

Heaney, R. K., Spinks, E. A., and Fenwick, G. R. (1988). Improved method for the determination of the total glucosinolate content of rapeseed by determination of enzymatically released glucose. *The Analyst 113*: 1515–1518.

Helboe, P., Olsen, O., and Sorensen, H. (1980). Separation of glucosinolates by high-performance liquid chromatography. *J. Chromatogr. 197*: 199–205.

Henderson, H. M., and McEwen, T. J. (1972). Effect of ascorbic acid on thioglucosidases from different crucifers. *Phytochemistry 11*: 3127–3133.

Hershman, J. H., Dang Tran Due, Sharp, B., Le My, Kent, J. R., Le Ngoc Binh, Reed, A. W., Lam Dinh Phuc, van Herle, A. J., Nguyen Anh Thai, Tran Xuang Troung, Nguyen Van Van, Sugawara, M., and Pekary, A. E. (1983). Endemic goiter in Vietnam. *J. Clin. Endocrin. Metab. 57*: 243–253.

Hetzel, B. (1987). An overview of the prevention and control of iodine deficiency disorders. In *The Prevention and Control of Iodine Deficiency Disorders*, B. S. Hetzel, J. T. Dunn, and J. B. Stanbury, eds. Elsevier, Amsterdam, pp. 7–31.

Hogge, L. R., Reed, D. W., and Underhill, E. W. (1988). The identification of desulfoglucosinolates using thermospray liquid chromatography-mass spectrophotometry. *J. Chromatogr. 26*: 348–351.

Huber, G., Derwahl, M., Kaempf, J., Peter, H.-J., Gerber, H., and Studer, H. (1990). Generation of intercellular heterogeneity of growth and function in cloned rat thyroid cells (FRTL-5). *Endocrinology 126*: 1639–1645.

Iversen, T. H., Baggerud, C., and Beisvaag, T. (1979). Myrosin cells in Brassicacae roots. *Z. Pflanzenphysiol. 94*: 143–155.

Jahreis, G., Hesse, V., Plenert, W., Hennig, A., Schone, F., and Ludke, H. (1985). Influence of phytogenic substances with thyreostatic effect in combination with iodine on the thyroid hormones and somatomedin level in pigs. *Exp. Clin. Endocrinol. 85*: 183–190.

Jan, J., and Tratnik, M. (1988). Polychlorinated biphenyls in residents around the river Krupa, Slovenia, Yugoslavia. *Bull. Environ. Contam. Toxicol. 41*: 809–814.

Jefferies, D. J., and French, M. C. (1969). Avian thyroid: Effect of pp, DDT on size and activity. *Science 166*: 1278–1280.

Johnston, T. D., and Jones, D. I. H. (1966). Variations in the thiocyanate content of kale varieties. *J. Sci. Food Agric. 17*: 70–71.

Josefsson, E., and Akerstrom, L. (1979). High performance liquid chromatographic method for the determination of 5-vinyl-2-oxazolidinethione in milk. *J. Chromatogr. 174*: 465–468.

Jurges, K., and Thies, W. (1980). Quantitative Analyse des Indolglucosinolatgehaltes in Samen und Blättern von *Brassica napus* und *B. campestris*. *Z. Pflanzenzucht. 84*: 168–178.

Kawakishi, S., and Kaneko, T. (1987). Interaction of proteins with allyl isothiocyanate. *J. Agric. Food Chem. 35*: 85–88.

Kawakishi, S., Namiki, M., Watanabe, H., anad Muramatsu, K. (1967). Studies on the decomposition of Sinalbin. *Agricult. Biol. Chem. 31*: 823–830.

Kjaer, A. (1960). Naturally derived isothiocyanates (mustard oils) and their parent glucosides. In *Progress in the Chemistry of Organic Natural Products*, L. Zechmeister, ed. Springer, Berlin, pp. 122–176.

Kjaer, A. (1973). The natural distribution of glucosinolates: A uniform group of sulfur-containing glucosides. *Nobel 25, Chemistry in Botanical Classification*, pp. 229–234.

Kjaer, A., and Larsen, P. O. (1977). Non-protein amino acids, cyanogenic glucosides and glucosinolates. In *Biosynthesis, a Specialist Periodical Report*, The Chemical Society, London, pp. 120–135.

Kjaer, A., Rubinstein, K., and Jensen, K. A. (1953). Unsaturated 5-carbon isothiocyanates. *Acta Chem. Scand. 7*: 518–527.

Kutacek, M., Bulgakov, R., and Oplistilova, K. (1966). On the auxin activity of glucobrassicin in biological tests. *Biologia Plantarum 8*: 252–255.

Langer, P. (1966a). Synergic effect of naturally occurring goitrogens on the thyroid gland of rats. *Physiol. Bohemoslov. 15*: 162–166.

Langer, P. (1966b). Antithyroid action of small doses of some naturally occurring compounds. *Endocrinology 79*: 1117–1122.

Langer, P. (1966c). Some basic observations on the metabolism of naturally occurring goitrogenic compounds. In *Endemic Goiter and Allied Diseases*, K. Silink and K. Cerny, eds. Veda, Bratislava, pp. 197–206.

Langer, P. (1968). Fluctuation of thyroid function following a single and repeated administration of antithyroid drugs. *Endocrinology 83*: 1268–1272.

Langer, P. (1983). Naturally occurring food toxicants: Goitrogens. In *CRC Handbook of Naturally Occurring Food Toxicants*, M. Rechcigl, Jr., ed. CRC Press, Boca Raton, FL, pp. 101–129.

Langer, P. (1989). Normal thyroid size versus goiter—postmortem thyroid weight and ultrasonographic volumetry versus physical examination. *Endocrin. Exper. 23*: 67–76.

Langer, P., and Greer, M. A. (1968). Antithyroid action of some naturally occurring isothiocyanates in vitro. *Metabolism 17*: 596–605.

Langer, P., and Greer, M. A. (1977). *Antithyroid Substances and Naturally Occurring Goitrogens*. Karger, Basel.

Langer, P., and Gschwendtova, K. (1969). Micro-estimation of major mustard oil and oxazolidinethione in small amounts of plant material. *J. Sci. Food. Agric. 20*: 535–539.

Langer, P., and Michajlovskij, N. (1958). Präformiertes Rhodanid in Nahrungsmitteln als Hauptursache der Rhodanausscheidung im Harn. *Hoppe-Seyler's Z. Physiol. Chem. 312*: 31–36.

Langer, P., and Michajlovskij, N. (1972). Effect of naturally occurring goitrogens on thyroid peroxidase and influence of some compounds on iodide formation during the estimation. *Endocrin. Exper.* *6*: 97–103.

Langer, P., and Stolc, V. (1965). Goitrogenic activity of allyl-isothiocyanate—a widespread natural mustard oil. *Endocrinology 76*: 151–155.

Langer, P., Drobnica, L., and Augustin, J. (1964). On the possible mechanism of the antithyroid activity of isothiocyanates. *Physiol. Bohemoslov. 13*: 450–456.

Lein, K. A. (1970). Quantitative Bestimmungsmethoden für Samenglucosinolate in Brassica-Arten und ihre Anwendung in die Zuchtung von glucosinolatarmen Raps. *Z. Pflanzenzucht. 63*: 137–154.

Macholz, R., Ackermann, H., Biedrich, M., Henschel, K. P., Kujawa, M., Lewerenz, H.-J., Przybilski, H., Schnaak, W., Schulze, J., and Woggon, H. (1986). Studies on the degradation of glucotropaeolin and progoitrin toxicity and reactivity of splitting products. In *Proc. of Euro Food Tox. II*, Institute of Toxicology, Zurich, pp. 40–45.

MacLeod, A. J., and Rossiter, J. T. (1986). Isolation and examination of thioglucosinolate glucohydrolase from seeds of *Brassica napus. Phytochemistry 25*: 1047–1051.

Maheshwari, P. N., Stanley, D. W., Gray, J. I., and Van der Voort, F. R. (1979). An HPLC method for simultaneous quantitation of individual isothiocyanates and oxazolidinethione in myrosinase digests of rapeseed meal. *J. Am. Oil Chem. Soc. 56*: 837–841.

Maheshwari, P. N., Stanley, D. V., Van der Voort, F. R., and Gray, J. I. (1980). The heat stability of allyl glucosinolate (sinigrin) in aqueous and model systems. *Can. Inst. Food Sci. Technol. J. 13*: 28–35.

Maloof, F., and Soodak, M. (1963). Intermediary metabolism of thyroid tissue and the action of drugs. *Pharm. Rev. 15*: 45–95.

Matovinovic, J. (1983). Endemic goiter and cretinism at the dawn of the third millenium. *Ann. Rev. Nutr. 3*: 341–412.

McDanell, R., McLean, A. E. M., Hanley, A. B., Heaney, R. K., and Fenwick, G. R. (1987). Differential induction of mixed-function oxidase (MFO) activity in rat liver and intestine by diet containing processed cabbage: Correlation with cabbage levels of glucosinolates and glucosinolate hydrolysis products. *Food Chem. Toxicol. 25*: 363–368.

McDanell, R., McLean, A. E. M., Hanely, A. B., Heaney, R. K., and Fenwick, G. R. (1988). Chemical and biological properties of indole glucosinolates (glucobrassicins): A review. *Food Chem. Toxicol. 26*: 59–70.

McGregor, D. I., Mullin, W. J., and Fenwick, G. R. (1983). Review of analysis of glucosinolates. *J. AOAC 66*: 825–850.

Mennicke, W. H., Gorler, K., Krumbiegel, G., Lorenz, D., and Rittmann, N. (1988). Studies on the metabolism and excretion of benzyl isothiocyanate in man. *Xenobiotica 18*: 441–447.

Michajlovskij, N. (1964). Nahrungsmittel als Rhodanidtrager. In *Naturally Occurring Goitrogens and Thyroid Function*, J. Podoba and P. Langer, eds. Veda, Bratislava, pp. 39–48.

Michajlovskij, N. (1968). The effect of UV-irradiation on glucobrassicin and other glucosinolates (mustard oil glucosides). *Experientia 24*: 223–224.

Michajlovskij, N. (1974). Degradation of glucobrassicin and formation of auxine in the presence of ferrous and cuprous ions (in Russian). In *Biological Role of Microelements and their Use in Agriculture and Medicine*, J. V. Peive and G. F. Khailova, eds. Nauka, Moscow, pp. 283–289.

Michajlovskij, N., and Langer, P. (1958). Gehalt einiger Nahrungsmittel an präformiertes Rhodanid. *Hoppe-Seyler's Z. Physiol. Chem. 312*: 26–30.

Michajlovskij, N., Sedlak, J., and Kostekova, O. (1970). Content of naturally occurring goitrogens in boiled plants of Brassica family. *Endocrin. Exper. 4*: 51–62.

Minchinton, I., Sang, J., Burke, D., and Truscott, J. W. (1982). Separation of desulphoglucosinolates by reversed-phase high performance liquid chromatography. *J. Chromatogr. 247*: 141–148.

Mullin, W. J., and Sahasrabudhe, M. R. (1977). Glucosinolate content of cruciferous vegetable crops. *Can. J. Plant Sci. 57*: 1227–1230.

Mullin, W. J., and Sahasrabudhe, M. R. (1978). Effect of cooking on the glucosinolates in cruciferous vegetables. *Can. Inst. Food Sci. Technol. J. 11*: 50–59.

Oginsky, E. L., Stein, A. E., and Greer, M. A. (1965). Myrosinase activity in bacteria as demonstrated by the conversion of progoitrin to goitrin. *Proc. Soc. Exp. Biol. Med. 119*: 360–364.

Olsen, O., and Sorensen, H. (1980). Sinalbin and other glucosinolates in seeds of double low rape species and *Brassica napus* v. *Bronowski*. *J. Agr. Food Chem. 28*: 43–48.

Olsen, O., and Sorensen, H. (1981). Recent advances in the analysis of glucosinolates. *J. Am. Oil Chem. Soc. 58*: 857–865.

O'Neill, W. M., and Marshall, W. D. (1984). Goitrogenic effect of ethylenethiourea on rat thyroid. *Pesticide Biochem. Physiol. 21*: 92–101.

Papas, A., Ingalls, J. R., and Campbell, L. D. (1979). Studies on the effects of rapeseed meal on thyroid status of cattle. *J. Nutrit. 109*: 1129–1135.

Peterka, S., and Fenwick, G. R. (1988). The use of flash chromatography for the isolation and purification of glucosinolates (mustard oil glucosides). *Fat Sci. Technol. 90*: 61–64.

Pocock, K., Heaney, R. K., Wilkinson, A. P., Beaumont, J. E., Vaughan, J. G., Fenwick, G. R. (1987). Changes in myrosinase activity and isoenzyme pattern, glucosinolate content and the cytology of myrosin cells in the leaves of heads of three cultivars of English white cabbage. *J. Sci. Food Agric. 41*: 245–257.

Podoba, J., Samel, M., Stukovsky, R., and Michajlovskij, N. (1957). Studies on goitrogenic effect of vegetables from endemic area of Island Schutt (in Slovak). *Bratisl. Lek. Listy 37*: 67–74.

Prochazka, Z., and Sanda, V. (1960). Isolation of pure ascorbigen and some other indole derivatives from Savoy cabbage. *Coll. Czechoslov. Chem. Commun. 25*: 270–280.

Saini, H. S., and Wratten, N. (1987). Quantitative determination of total glucosinolates in rapeseed and meal digests. *J. AOAC 70*: 141–145.

Saito, K., Jujio, T., Hashizume, I., Yamada, T., Onaya, T., Uehara, T., Kajihara, A., Kojima, A., and Takemura, Y. (1972). Studies on goitrogenic action of mimocycline and related compounds. *Endocrinology 90*: 1192–1201.

Sang, J. P., and Truscott, R. J. W. (1984). Liquid chromatographic determination of glucosinolates in rapeseed as desulfoglucosinolates. *J. of the AOAC 67*: 829–837.

Schone, P., Jahreis, G., Lang, R., Seffner, W., Groppel, B., Henning, A., and Ludke, H. (1990). Effect of varying glucosinolate and iodine intake via rapeseed meal diets on serum thyroid hormone level and total iodine in the thyroid in growing pigs. *Endocrin. Exper. 24*: (in press).

Schwimmer, S. (1961). Spectral changes during the action of myrosinase on sinigrin. *Acta Chem. Scand. 15*: 535–544.

Serrano, M. R. F. O., Lopez, M. D. R., and Palomares, H. (1988). Determination of SCN^- in vegetables by gas chromatography in relation to endemic goiter. *J. Analyt. Toxicol. 12*: 307–309.

Siegler, D. S. (1975). Isolation and characterization of naturally occurring cyanogenic compounds. *Phytochemistry 14*: 9–29.

Silink, K., and Marsikova, L. (1951). Thiocyanate and endemic goiter. *Nature* (London) *167*: 528–529.

Slominski, B. A., and Campbell, L. D. (1989). Formation of indole glucosinolate breakdown products in autolyzed, steamed and cooked Brassica vegetables. *J. Agric. Food Chem.* *37*: 1297–1302.

Sones, K., Heaney, R. K., and Fenwick, G. R. (1984). An estimate of the mean daily intake of glucosinolates from cruciferous vegetables in the UK. *J. Sci. Food Agric.* *35*: 712–720.

Sonstegard, R. A., and Leatherland, J. F. (1976). The epizootiology and pathogenesis of thyroid hyperplasia in Coho salmon (*Oncorhynchus kisutch*) in Lake Ontario. *Cancer Res.* *36*: 4467–4473.

Spencer, G. F., and Daxenbichler, M. E. (1980). Gas chromatography-mass spectrophotometry of nitriles, isothiocyanates and oxazolidinethiones derived from cruciferous glucosinolates. *J. Sci. Food Agric.* *31*: 359–367.

Spinks, E. A., Sones, K., and Fenwick, G. R. (1984). The quantitative analysis of glucosinolates in cruciferous vegetables, oilseeds and forage crops using high performance liquid chromatography. *Fette, Seifen, Anstrichmmittel* *86*: 228–231.

Srisangnam, C., Salunke, D. K., Reddy, N. R., and Dull, G. G. (1980). Quality of cabbage. II. *J. Food Qual.* *3*: 233–241.

Srinivasa Kumar, C. V., and Chandrasekhara, N. (1973). Effect of processing on ascorbigen in cabbage (*Brassica oleracea*). *J. Food Sci. Technol. (Mysore)* *10*: 42–50.

Stanbury, J. B. (1983). Inherited metabolic disorders of the thyroid system. In *Werner's The Thyroid*, 5th ed., S. H. Ingbar and L. E. Braverman, eds. J. B. Lippincott, New York, pp. 687–695.

Taurog, A., Dorris, M. L., and Guziec, F. S. (1989). Metabolism of ^{35}S and ^{14}C-labeled 1-methyl-2-mercaptoimidazole in vitro and in vivo. *Endocrinology* *124*: 30–39.

Thies, W. (1977). Analysis of glucosinolates in seed of rapeseed (*Brassica napus* L.): Concentration of glucosinolates by ion exchange. *Z. Pflanzenzucht.* *79*: 331–335.

Thies, W. (1982). Complex formation between glucosinolates and tetrachloropalladate and its utilization in plant breeding. *Fette, Seifen, Anstrichmittel* *84*: 338–342.

Thies, W. (1985). Determination of glucosinolate content in commercial rapeseed loads with a pocket reflectometer. *Fette, Seifen, Anstrichmitt.* *87*: 347–350.

Thomas, G. A., and Williams, E. D. (1988). Aetiology of simple goitre. *Bailliere's Clin. Endocrin. Metab.* *2*: 703–718.

Thomke, S. (1981). Review of rapeseed meal in animal nutrition: Ruminant animals. *J. Am. Oil Chem. Soc.* *58*: 805–824.

Tookey, H. L. (1973). Crambe thioglucoside glucohydrolase (E.C.3.2.3.1.1): Separation of a protein required for epithiobutane formation. *Can. J. Biochem.* *51*: 1654–1660.

Uda, Y., Kurata, T., and Arakawa, N. (1986a). Effects of pH and ferrous ion on the degradation of glucosinolates by myrosinase. *Agric. Biol. Chem.* *11*: 2735–2740.

Uda, Y., Kurata, T., and Arakawa, N. (1986b). Effects of thiol compounds on the formation of nitriles from glucosinolates. *Agric. Biol. Chem.* *11*: 2741–2746.

Underhill, E. W., and Kirkland, D. F. (1971). Gas chromatography of trimiethylsilyl derivatives of glucosinolates. *J. Chromatogr.* *57*: 47–54.

Van Etten, C. H., and Daxenbichler, M. E. (1977). Glucosinolates and derived products in cruciferous vegetables: Total glucosinolates by retention on anion exchange resin and enzymatic hydrolysis to measure released glucose. *J. AOAC* *60*: 946–949.

Van Etten, C. H., and Tookey, H. L. (1983). Glucosinolates. In *CRC Handbook of Naturally Occurring Food Toxicants*, M. Rechcigl, Jr., ed. CRC Press, Boca Raton, FL, pp. 15–30.

Van Middlesworth, L. (1960). Re-evaluation of certain aspects of iodine metabolism. *Recent Progr. Horm. Res.* *16*: 405–438.

Van Middlesworth, L. (1985). Thiocyanate feeding with low iodine diet causes chronic iodine retention in thyroids of mice. *Endocrinology 116*: 665–670.

Van Middlesworth, L. (1986). T-23 mycotoxin intensifies iodine deficiency in mice fed low iodine diet. *Endocrinology 118*: 583–586.

Verhaar, H. J. M., Kammuler, M. E., Terlouw, J. K., Brandsma, L., and Seinen, W. (1989). Spanish toxic oil syndrome: An isothiocyanate-derived compound cannot be substantiated as a causative agent. *Fd. Chem. Toxic. 27*: 205–206.

Wagner, H., Horhammer, L., and Nufer, H. (1965). Zur Dünnschichtchromatografie von Senfolen und Senfolgukosiden. *Arzneimitt.-Forsch. 15*: 453–457.

Wattenberg, L. W., Hanley, A. B., Barany, G., Sparnins, V. L., Lam, L. K. T., and Fenwick, G. R. (1986). Inhibition of carcinogenesis by some minor dietary constitutents. In *Diet, Nutrition and Cancer*, Y. Hayashi, ed. Japan Sci. Soc. Press and Tokyo/VNU Sci. Press, Utrecht, pp. 193–203.

Wetter, L. R., and Youngs, C. G. (1976). A thiourea-UV assay for total glucosinolate content in rapeseed meals. *J. Am. Oil Chem. Soc. 53*: 162–164.

Wood, J. L. (1975). Biochemistry. In *Chemistry and Biochemistry of Thiocyanic Acid and its Derivatives*, A. A. Newman, ed. Academic Press, New York, pp. 156–221.

Youngs, C. G., and Perlin, A. S. (1967). Fe(2)-catalyzed decomposition of sinigrin and related thioglucosides. *Can. J. Chem. 45*: 1801–1803.

VII

TERATOGENY

18

Natural Teratogens in Foods and Drugs

James L. Schardein

International Research and Development Corporation, Mattawan, Michigan

I. INTRODUCTION

Naturally occurring foods are generally assumed to be pure and free of toxicity. Indeed, "natural" is defined as existing or formed by nature. Attitudes bordering on deification of "naturalness" by the public are responsible for this misconception. Actually, there are naturally occurring toxins in food, for instance, alkaloids in potato and caffeine in tea and coffee, to name but two. In addition, hundreds of different chemicals are intentionally added to foods during processing, in the way of preservatives, flavors, coloring agents, etc., to make them more palatable, keep longer, or facilitate their preparation. This process is not a new one: salt, for instance, was used to preserve meat over 3000 years ago (Buist, 1986). Foods are also contaminated through pesticide spraying, whose residues then enter our food chain indirectly, adding further adulteration. As so well stated by another writer, "food is only a mixture of chemicals and not all of them are dietarily beneficial" (Crosby, 1969).

It is not the same with drugs having a natural origin. For the most part, they are derived from plants and generally do not share the adulteration processes that were described for food. Like all chemicals, however, they demonstrate toxicity when consumed in excessive quantities. Teratogenesis is one of these toxicities.

It is these "natural" toxins, or more specifically, teratogens, in food and drugs that are of interest in this presentation: those that occur under natural conditions in the foods we eat (the basic "foodstuffs") and in the drugs we are medicated with. Naturally occurring teratogens in plants have been covered in an earlier volume in this series (Keeler, 1983), as have the mycotoxins affecting food supplies and fungal-produced antibiotics (Hood and Szczech, 1983). Thus, the myriad of additives, pollutants, and contaminants found in food, drugs used to increase animal production, and other intentional or unintentional additives are not included here.

By strict lexicon, "teratogens" are those substances that induce congenital structural malformations. Placed in contemporary context, however, this process is but one of four classes of adverse outcome, the others being fetal growth retardation, embryo/fetal mortality, and functional impairment, the sum representing developmental toxicity. All are possible and equivalent outcomes of disruptive development, and as such will be discussed as appropriate in this text. Although much more data exist for laboratory species than for humans in this science, both are considered here, especially since it is the human that we are trying to protect from such endeavors. In some cases, no clear distinction exists with respect to whether a given chemical is a drug or food; caffeine is a good example. In these cases classification is determined solely on the basis of the former having pharmacological activity and, therefore, therapeutic utility in the usual context.

II. NATURAL TERATOGENS IN FOODS

A. Nutrients (General)

Good reviews on nutrients obtained from food sources and their effect on abnormal development have been published on animals (Giroud, 1968; Hurley, 1980, 1985; Moghissi, 1981; Pfeiffer and Barnes, 1981; Renwick, 1982; Warren, 1983; Brent, 1985; Pieters, 1985).

B. Macronutrients

Several interesting associations have been published relating to the complex molecules known as macronutrients that comprise the three food groups: carbohydrates, fats, and proteins.

In the case of the *carbohydrates*, one group of investigators reported that 10–45% of 152 cases of human malformation had abnormal blood glucose values indicative of carbohydrate disorder (Navarette et al., 1967). No animal studies with carbohydrates proper have been published to my knowledge.

With *fats* proper, dietary fat during gestation to rabbits was said to result in eye defects in their offspring, but the study lacks sufficient detail to interpret and is of historic interest only (Maeda, 1937). A more recent experiment in rats fed a cyclic monomer isolated from fried fat was said not to result in teratogenic activity (Artman, 1969).

Studies involving *protein* proper are not available. One experimental study has indicated that pregnancy maintenance is impaired by diets containing less than 6% protein, at least in the rat (Nelson and Evans, 1953).

C. Micronutrients

A number of micronutrients existing naturally in food have been examined for teratogenic properties when ingested or dosed orally to animals. Lactose or milk sugar is a disaccharide found in milk. Given orally at doses as high as 4000 mg/kg/day during organogenesis to mice, rats, and rabbits produced no teratogenic effects, but increased resorption in all three species (Beltrame and Cantone, 1973).

A number of amino acids essential to human nutrition have been investigated for their effects on mammalian development. Leucine and lysine, when fed in excess quantities (up to 25%) during gestation days 5 to 15 to rats, had no teratogenic effects, but both resulted in reduced offspring survival (Cohlan and Stone, 1961). Methionine, another essential amino acid, was given in dietary concentrations of 4% to rats throughout gestation (Viau and Leathem,

1973). No terata were produced, but like leucine and lysine, the agent caused increased fetal mortality. Still another amino acid, phenylalanine, has shown marked effects on development of the conceptus. Feeding in the diet to guinea pigs, rats, and primates resulted, respectively, in malformation; cataracts, stunting, and death; and significant learning deficits (Kerr et al., 1968; Luse et al., 1970; Kronick et al., 1987). Quantities required to elicit these toxicities were on the order of 3.5–7.0% in the diet. Several forms of yet another amino acid have been investigated, and produced variable results in animals. L-Tyrosine given orally to rats and mice by gavage on gestation days 1–10 resulted in microscopic vertebral and adjacent soft tissue abnormalities in one report (Schlack et al., 1970). Lower doses of D,L-m-, or L-tyrosine had no such effect in rats treated orally by gavage on selected days of or throughout pregnancy in another study (Kitchin and DiStefano, 1976).

Linoleic acid is an essential fatty acid. In the 10% oxidized form in the diet during pregnancy, it gave variable results. In mice, no teratogenesis was observed, but in rats, 9% of the offspring had urogenital abnormalities when the nutrient was given at a twofold higher dose than in mice (Cutter and Schneider, 1973).

Calcium is the only mineral reported to be associated with congenital malformation following excess. This was reported in the large collaborative study published by Heinonen et al. (1977). They found a suggestive association among a series of over 1000 women taking calcium in the first 4 months of pregnancy, and the frequency of central nervous system malformations in their issue. Further associations have not appeared, nor have animal studies been done to confirm this finding. Essential fatty acids fed to rats in a reproduction study was said to have produced adverse effects on fertility in the second generation, but no specific teratogenicity (Hafiez, 1974).

D. Sugars

Sucrose is processed from sugar cane or sugar beets for use as a sweetening agent for food. Older studies with this chemical implicated it in disrupted development. In one study in the guinea pig, huge doses of 5–10 g/kg/day in the last one half of gestation were said to result in skeletal alterations (Seta, 1931). In another study, these same high doses given in the diet to rabbits prior to conception and continuing in gestation resulted in hydrocephaly (Sumi, 1960). These studies have not been replicated, and more recent studies at similar oral dosages to mice, rats, and rabbits have not recorded any adverse developmental effects (Fritz and Hess, 1968; Klotzsche, 1969; Lorke, 1969).

Glucose, also known as dextrose, blood sugar, grape sugar, and corn sugar, occurs naturally in the free state in fruits and other plant parts. It had no teratogenic activity in rats when fed as 30% of diet (Telford et al., 1962).

E. Cooking Oils

Several processed oils derived from plants and used in food preparation have been studied with respect to effects on mammalian development. Fortunately, they have demonstrated little or no potential for developmental toxicity, including teratogenicity, in animal models. Hence they are considered safe for human consumption in the context of reproduction and development.

Corn (maize) oil has been thoroughly studied on two counts: first, because it has often been used in the laboratory as a suspending vehicle for a wide variety of drugs and chemicals during testing; second, because early studies with corn oil in laboratory animals reported toxicity.

Of these studies anomalous development was described in rats (Khera and McKinley, 1972), cats (Khera, 1973), and hamsters (Ottolenghi et al., 1974); a rabbit study was negative under the regimen used (Keeler, 1971). Studies in rodents reported by Kimmel et al. (1985) also confirmed an increased number of fetuses in rats and mice per litter with malformations, and more recent studies in mice and rats at dosages up to 10 ml/kg during major organogenesis caused reduced food and water consumption of the dams, but no developmental toxicity (Price et al., 1989). This ambiguity of results in a number of studies in a variety of species conducted over a period of almost 20 years remains unresolved, and it remains to be seen whether future studies will clarify the reported results.

Rapeseed oil had no reported teratogenicity from oral administration to mice and rats, but fewer and smaller offspring were reported in one study (Beare et al., 1961; Neubert and Dillmann, 1972).

F. Egg Albumen

A large quantity of egg white or albumen hydrolysate fed in the diet to pregnant rats did not result in malformed offspring (Yangimoto et al., 1983).

G. Vitamins

Vitamins can be defined as substances essential for the maintenance of normal metabolic functions of the body, which are supplied exogenously, because they are not synthesized in the body. Well-balanced diets normally provide adequate amounts of vitamins.

There are many situations when the concentration of one or more vitamins in the body is suboptimal, culminating in deficiency states characterized by a variety of manifestations. To alleviate these manifestations may require administration of the vitamin in chemical form. Large doses of a vitamin may also be employed for disorders unrelated to vitamin deficiency. As such, they can be considered drugs, and it is these situations rather than deficiency states that are of interest in this presentation, since excessive administration of vitamins, notably lipid-soluble vitamins, can have toxic manifestations. A chemical described as "fat soluble factor," now known to be a complex of vitamins A and D, was reported almost 70 years ago to produce rudimentary limbs in piglets in what is considered to be the first report of a teratogenic response in a mammal (Zilva et al., 1921).

1. Retinol

This is a fat-soluble vitamin present naturally as beta-carotene in fruits and vegetables: the body converts it to vitamin A or retinol. The structural

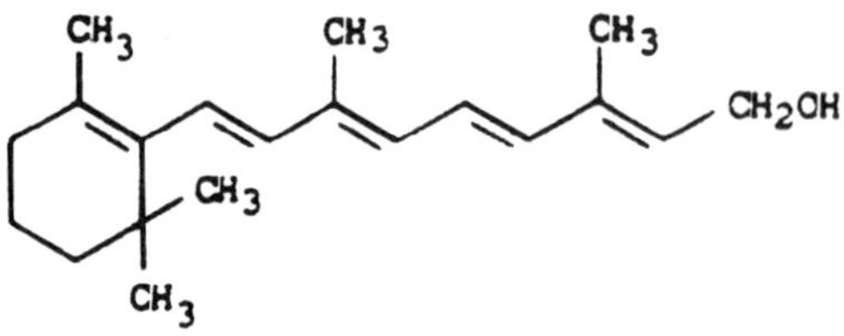

Figure 1 Chemical structure of retinol.

formula of retinol is shown in Figure 1. The recommended daily allowance has been set at 2000 IU (infants) to 5000 IU (adults).

In excessive amounts, retinol is a universal teratogen, producing a wide variety of malformations in seven species of mammals (Table 1). Based on the minimum dosage required to elicit effects, the mouse is the most sensitive species, but even subteratogenic doses have been reported to result in behavioral disturbances in rat offspring (Malakhovsky, 1969). It has been suggested that the vitamin acts directly on the embryo by interfering with migrating mesodermal cells (Morriss, 1976).

Over the years, occasional case reports have appeared associating intake of retinol by mothers with congenital malformations in their offspring. Five such cases are known (Stange et al., 1978; Von Lennep et al., 1985; Schardein, 1985), but recent faddish practices of megadosing with vitamins have raised additional concerns, and the U.S. Food and Drug Administration has now on file a total of 17 cases of human malformation from excess retinol intake during pregnancy (Rosa et al., 1986). Central nervous defects have predominated, but cardiovascular defects, microtia, facial clefts, and urinary defects have been described. This association has been strengthened with publication of a recent

Table 1 Representative Laboratory Teratologic Studies: Retinol

Species	Oral dosage (IU)	Treatment interval (in gestation)	Malformations observed	Ref.
Rat	35,000	4–16	Multiple, esp. CNS	Cohlan, 1953a,b
Mouse	10,000	8–13	Multiple head	Kalter and Warkany, 1959
Guinea pig	50,000	10–13	Jaw and tongue	Giroud and Martinet, 1959a,b
Hamster	20,000	7–10	Multiple	Marin-Padilla and Ferm, 1965
Pig	3–10,000,000	12–42	Eye	Palludan, 1966
Dog	125,000	17–22	Cleft palate, ear, tail	Wiersig and Swenson, 1967
Rabbit	41,000	5–14	Face and digit	Giroud and Martinet, 1958

case-control study indicating risk and the suggestion that congenital birth defects from the vitamin may be underestimated (Werler et al., 1989). The California State Public Health Department has also issued a pregnancy hazard alert on excessive vitamin A intake during pregnancy (Kizer et al., 1990). Concerned about this trend, the U.S. Teratology Society has taken the public position that human dosages of retinol should not exceed 8000 IU without risk to the fetus (Teratology Society Position Paper, 1987).

2. *B-Complex Vitamins*

In contrast to retinol, the B-complex vitamins are water soluble and are found in a wide variety of foods. None of the five tested by the oral route has been teratogenic in laboratory animals (Table 2). Several other B vitamins have been tested by parenteral routes, and they too with one exception (B_4: adenine) have not reacted positively, at least in the dosages and regimens employed, and are not included here since parenteral administration of natural teratogens is outside the scope of this presentation.

No human cases of congenital malformation have been reported for vitamin B intake during pregnancy.

3. *Ascorbic Acid*

Ascorbic acid or vitamin C is a water-soluble vitamin found naturally in fruit and vegetables. The recommended dietary allowance is 35–60 mg daily.

The vitamin had no teratogenic activity in any of four species tested in the laboratory (Table 3). Serum levels of ascorbic acid in humans were reported not to have any relationship to the presence or absence of malformations (Martin et al., 1957).

Table 2 Laboratory Teratologic Studies: B-Complex Vitamins

B vitamin	Species	Oral dosage (mg/kg)	Treatment interval (in gestation)	Malformations observed	Ref.
B_{12}, Cyanocobalamin	Rat	3,000	whole gestation	None	Newberne, 1963
B_6, Pyridoxine	Rat	80	6–15	None	Khera, 1975
B_5, Pantethine	Mouse	600	6–12	None	Oshima et al., 1966
	Rat	600	6–12	None	Oshima et al., 1966
B_{15}, Pangamic acid	Rat	c. 40	1-term	None	Telford et al., 1962
B_1, Thiamine	Rat	c. 330	1-term	None	Telford et al., 1962

Table 3 Laboratory Teratologic Studies: Ascorbic Acid

Species	Oral dosage (mg/kg)	Treatment interval (in gestation)	Malformations observed	Ref.
Mouse	1000	6–15	None	Frohberg et al., 1973
Rat	1000	6–15 or 0–21	None	Frohberg et al., 1973
Guinea pig	c. 1000	Whole gestation	None	Nandi et al., 1973
Rabbit	500	?	None	Carpi and Scarinci, 1974

4. *Vitamin D*

Vitamin D or cholecalciferol is a fat-soluble vitamin freely available naturally in fish. The recommended dietary allowance of the vitamin ranges from 5 to 10 mg/day; it is essential for normal growth and development. High oral doses of vitamin D are teratogenic in the mouse and rat (Table 4), and other classes of developmental toxicity including growth retardation, embryolethality, and impairment of ossification have been reported in animal studies.

Vitamin D has been implicated circumstantially as a cause of the syndrome of supravalvular aortic stenosis and idiopathic hypercalcemia in humans (Garcia et al., 1964; Friedman, 1968), a charge denied by other investigators (Antia et al., 1967). Difficulties in proving this association exist, but the syndrome has been produced experimentally in the rabbit (Friedman and Roberts, 1966; Chan et al., 1979), lending further support for the role played by vitamin D in this malformation.

Other forms of the vitamin are also teratogenic (see Table 4). Calcitriol administration had no effect in rats from the proscribed regimen, but at the same dosage was associated with a few malformations in several litters in rabbits. Hydroxycholecalciferol was associated with gall bladder agenesis and

Table 4 Laboratory Teratologic Studies: Vitamin D

D vitamin	Species	Oral dosage (mg/kg)	Treatment interval (in gestation)	Malformations observed	Ref.
Cholecalciferol	Mouse	50000 (IU)	5–7	CNS & skeletal	Zane, 1976
	Rat	40000 (IU)	10–21	Skeletal	Ornoy et al., 1972
Calcitriol	Rat	0.3	7–15	None	McClain et al., 1978
	Rabbit	0.3	7–18	Multiple	McClain et al., 1978
Ergocalciferol	Rat	c. 30	1–5	None	Sharma et al., 1972
Hydroxy-cholecalciferol	Rabbit	0.02–0.5	6–18	Cleft palate, gall bladder	Makita et al., 1977

Table 5 Laboratory Teratologic Studies: Vitamin E

Species	Oral dosage (mg/kg)	Treatment interval (in gestation)	Malformations observed	Ref.
Rat	c. 650	1-term	None	Telford et al., 1962
Mouse	591 (IU)	10 or 7–11	None	Hook et al., 1974

cleft palate in a few rabbit bunnies. Ergocalciferol given in the preimplantation period of pregnancy was not associated with malformations in the rat.

5. Vitamin E

Vitamin E or alpha-tocopherol is another fat-soluble vitamin present naturally in some fruits, seeds, nuts, and oils. The recommended daily intake is 3–10 mg, and it has as one important function the promotion of normal growth and development.

Vitamin E given orally was not teratogenic in rodents (Table 5). One experiment in which the vitamin was given subcutaneously at doses as high as 300 mg/kg/day on 3 days during organogenesis to mice resulted in cleft palate and growth retardation (Momose et al., 1972).

There have been no positive case reports in humans for hypervitaminosis E. One group of investigators associated blood serum tocopherol levels to pregnancy outcome, specifically stillbirth and malformation (Vobecky et al., 1974), but this association has not been strengthened since the initial report.

H. Fruits

1. Ackee

A plant called Ackee (Akee), scientifically known as *Blighia sapida*, is a food source in the West Indies. An old anecdotal report described six cases in which babies with macroglossia and exomphalos were born following ingestion by their mothers of unripe fruit of the plant during early pregnancy (Persaud and Kaplan, 1970). This finding remains unconfirmed, but extracts of the plant have proved to be developmentally toxic to rats in the laboratory (Persaud, 1971). Two dipeptides isolated from the plant, hypoglycin A and hypoglycin B, were reported to be teratogenic in the rat (Persaud, 1967, 1972).

2. Black Cherry

The wild black cherry plant, *Prunus serotina*, has been associated with the production of malformations in swine. Selby et al. (1971) reported an outbreak of tail, anal, and hindlimb deformities in 13 of 184 piglets born to 13 sows bred and maintained in a pasture in which the plant was growing in Missouri. Sows bred by the same boar in an adjacent pasture free of *Prunus* delivered normal piglets. The investigators speculated that a cyanogenic glycoside was the responsible teratogen. Additional field or experimental studies on the plant have not been published since this report.

3. Betel

Betel, a name applied to areca nut (*Areca catechu*) or betel leaf or bean (*Piper betel*), is commonly chewed, being a custom indulged in by some 200 million people throughout East Africa, India, Southeast Asia, and Melanesia (DeCosta and Griew, 1982). Because betel chewing has been linked to oral and esophageal cancer, it has also been suspect as inducing adverse pregnancy outcome in the human.

Only one study on this assumption exists in the published literature. Antenatal records of 400 women from Papua, New Guinea, who had chewed betel throughout pregnancy were examined (DeCosta and Griew, 1982). These were matched with control women who had never chewed betel. There were no significant differences between the two groups with respect to congenital malformations, perinatal mortality, or other parameters of offspring characteristics or outcome except for birth weights. Babies born to betel-chewing mothers were significantly smaller than their control counterparts (mean 2999 g vs. 3080 g). The babies were otherwise healthy, and the author considered the clinical significance of this finding doubtful.

Apparently no laboratory animal studies have been done on betel.

4. Rosaceae (Amygdalin)

Amygdalin is a glycoside occurring in the seeds of *Rosaceae* genera, principally bitter almonds, but also peaches and apricots. Amygdalin given intravenously on gestation day 8 to pregnant hamsters resulted in multiple abnormalities in a high proportion of the offspring (Willhite, 1982). The metabolite cyanide was considered the teratogenic moiety. No human studies with amygdalin have occurred to my knowledge.

I. Cassava

Cassava (gari) is the tuberous root of a shrublike plant (*Manihot esculenta* Crantz) cultivated in tropical rain forests. The plant is an important staple source of carbohydrate for 450–500 million people in 26 countries (Cock, 1982). The edible portions of the tubers contain cyanide, about 90% of which is found in the form of the substance linamarin (Gomez and Valdivieso, 1983). Through metabolism, ingestion of cassava results in the release and absorption of cyanide, the quantity dependent on a number of factors. Acute poisoning, ataxic neuropathy, endemic goiter, and cretinism have been associated with cassava diets in humans (Montgomery, 1965). Because of these facts, it has been suspected, by local clinicians in Africa at least, that the plant is a cause of congenital anomalies as well, but the reports are strictly anecdotal and lack scientific foundation at this time.

The plant has been teratogenic in animals under certain conditions. In the rat, cassava supplied as 80% of the diet on gestational days 1–15 resulted in a low incidence of limb defects, ablepharia, and microcephaly (Singh, 1981). Diets containing the same concentration fed to hamsters did not induce malformations, but did result in maternal toxicity and other developmental toxicity, including reduced fetal weight and retardation of skeletal ossification (Frakes et al., 1984). Cassava meals containing high concentrations of cyanide were more toxic developmentally than lower concentrations (Frakes et al., 1986).

In contrast to dietary administration, oral doses of the linamarin form by intubation was a teratogenic regimen in the hamster (Frakes et al., 1985). Doses of 120 or 140 mg linamarin/kg on day 8 of gestation were associated with maternal toxicity and an increased incidence of vertebral and rib anomalies and encephalocele in the offspring, but had no effect on other developmental parameters as had been seen earlier. The signs of toxicity in both mothers and offspring were consistent with the toxicity pattern of cyanide.

The potential of cassava being teratogenic in the human seems unlikely based on dosage considerations (Frakes et al., 1985). A woman would have to consume about 2.7 kg of cassava flour containing 200 mg/kg cyanide to achieve the teratogenic doses shown in the animal studies.

J. Potato

The potato, *Solanum tuberosum*, is a common high-carbohydrate food source. It contains 150 distinct chemicals (Rhodes, 1979). A number of years ago, a British scientist published a brief note suggesting that specific but unidentified substances in winter-stored potatoes, presumably blighted by *Phytophthora infestans*, were responsible for induction of neural tube defects like anencephaly and spina bifida in individuals in the British Isles and elsewhere where similar dietary customs prevailed (Renwick, 1972). The publication of this ominous note elicited a flurry of experimental studies to confirm or deny the hypothesis in both animal studies and the epidemiological evidence in humans in a number of countries. The subject of blighted potatoes has been reviewed (Schardein, 1985).

In short, initial studies in rats fed potato concentrates were negative, but some marmosets fed concentrates of blighted potatoes reportedly developed cranial defects (Poswillo et al., 1972). The latter study could not be replicated (Poswillo et al., 1973), and the remainder of the animal studies in hamsters, swine, and rabbits fed blighted potatoes were either negative or gave contradictory results. A similar lack of association was apparent from human populations examined from a number of countries including Taiwan, Canada, the United States, Australia, Scotland, and Britain.

Of 10 or so specific chemicals extracted from potato and tested for teratogenic potential, the results were equally ambivalent. A number were outright negative, including caffeic acid, chlorogenic acid, scopoletin, terpenoid phytolexin, and tomatidine, and several others provided both positive and negative results: chaconine, cytochalasin B, and solanine. Only two chemicals, potato glycoalkoloid and solasodine, appeared to possess unequivocal teratogenic properties (in rats and hamsters). The results thus laid to rest the hypothesis that blighted potatoes are an etiological factor in the induction of central nervous system defects in the human population; no interest has been shown in published reports since 1978.

K. Lupine

Lupine is a field plant of several *Lupinus* genera. It possesses many alkaloids, especially of the quinolizidine group. While it is not normally ingested by humans, it may have indirect adverse health consequences through the food chain.

It was reported a number of years ago that consumption of the plant by grazing heifers during days 40–70 of gestation could result in arthrogryposis, torticollis, scoliosis, and cleft palate in about one quarter of the calves produced (Shupe et al., 1967). The abnormalities observed provoked the term "crooked calf disease" for their manifestation. More specifically, it was subsequently shown that the quantity required by intubation to demonstrate this effect was 0.57–0.68 kg of the plant (Keeler, 1973a,b). The same investigator went on to show that a specific chemical constituent of the plant, anagyrine, was the responsible teratogen (Keeler, 1976).

More recently, a report appeared suggesting that anagyrine was also suspect as a human teratogen. In the case described, a severely anemic child with bilateral forelimb and digital defects was born to a woman who reportedly drank goat's milk contaminated with the chemical as the primary source of milk during her pregnancy. The family's goat herd and puppies born to their pet dog on the same farm with similar limb defects were offered as additional evidence that the chemical was responsible for the birth defects (Kilgore et al., 1981). A further description of the case was published later providing additional circumstantial evidence for the validity of the case (Ortega and Lazerson, 1987).

L. Caffeine

Three methylxanthines commonly found in foods are pharmacologically active: caffeine, theobromine, and theophylline. A review of their toxicology has been published (Tarka, 1982). Theobromine and theophylline are more appropriately considered in Section III.

Caffeine is a purine alkaloid flavoring agent, chemically known as 1,3,7-trimethylxanthine (Fig. 2), and occurs naturally in more than 60 species of plants. Principal sources are of the Angiosperm genera *Ilex, Miconia, Coffea, Paullinia, Cola, Theobroma,* and *Camellia*. The chemical is of great societal importance due to its ubiquitous usage and the fact that it has been listed until recently as "generally recognized as safe" (GRAS) for its multiple uses.

Foods and beverages containing caffeine have a history of human usage dating back several thousand years. The most notable of these are, of course, coffee, tea, cocoa, and chocolate. Caffeine comprises 1–2% (dry weight) of roasted coffee beans, 3.5% of fresh tea leaves, and about 2% of mate leaves (Spiller, 1984; Graham, 1984a,b). As a hot beverage, coffee came into use by the Arabians c. 1000 A.D., while tea was first mentioned as early as 2737 B.C. (Roberts and Barone, 1983). Worldwide, tea is the most popular caffeine-containing beverage, followed by coffee. In this country, however, about 75% of the per capita consumption of caffeine is in coffee (Graham, 1978). Caffeine also has uses other than as a flavoring agent in beverages: as a flavor in baking

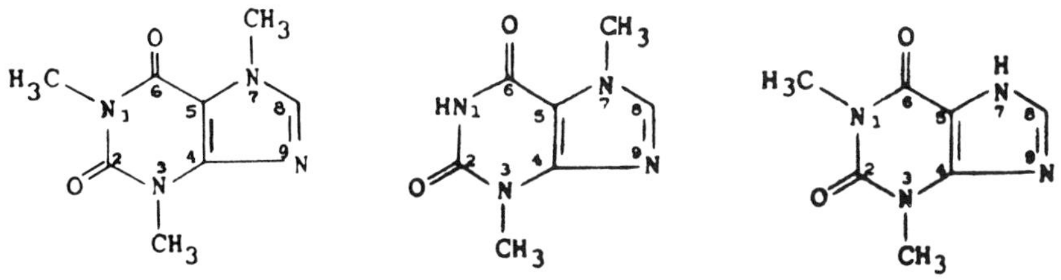

(a) (b) (c)

Figure 2 Chemical structures of some xanthines: (a) caffeine, (b) theobromine, (c) theophylline.

goods and desserts as cocoa and chocolate, and as a stimulant therapeutically in both prescription drugs and over-the-counter (OTC) preparations. However, the latter lead to relatively inconsequential intakes (FDA, 1980).

The quantity of caffeine in various foods and drugs can be quite variable; values generally accepted for caffeine intake are as shown in Table 6. The per capita consumption of caffeine from all sources is estimated to be about 200 mg/day, or about 3–7 mg/kg/day (Barone and Roberts, 1984). For the population of greatest concern from our perspective—the pregnant woman—approximately 43% consume coffee and 75% consume tea during pregnancy (Hill et al., 1977); a reliable estimate for caffeine consumption from all sources would appear to average about 2.1 mg/kg/day (Select Committee, 1978).

The developmental toxicity profile of caffeine has been reviewed in detail recently by Nolen (1989). It was initially established as a teratogen by

Table 6 Caffeine Content of Representative Products

Product	Measure	Avg. content (mg)	Ref.
Coffee			
Ground roasted	5 oz. cup	83	Burg, 1975
Instant	5 oz. cup	66	Gilbert, 1981
Decaffeinated	5 oz. cup	3	Burg, 1975
Tea			
Leaf or bag	5 oz. cup	42	Burg, 1975
Instant	5 oz. cup	28	Burg, 1975
Hot chocolate (cocoa)	5 oz. cup	4	Zoumas et al., 1980
Cola beverages			
Regular	12 oz. serving	35	Gilbert, 1984
Decaffeinated	6 oz. serving	trace	NSDA, 1982
Chocolate			
Milk	1 oz.	6	Zoumas et al., 1980
Sweet	1 oz.	20	Zoumas et al., 1980
Baking	1 oz.	60	Zoumas et al., 1980
Drugs	Capsule/tablet	15–200	Select Committee, 1978

Nishimura and Nakai (1960) some 30 years ago. The chemical has been tested in three species by a variety of routes, as shown by selected representative studies in Table 7. As can be seen, the teratogenic response varies somewhat with the dosage, route, and species, but digital defects (ectrodactyly) are common to all treatments. Other classes of developmental toxicity, i.e., reduction in fetal body weight, embryolethality, with or without observable maternal toxicity, have been variably recorded.

Perhaps the experiment best typifying the developmental toxicity outcome from caffeine exposure in laboratory animals is that reported as a quasi-official study designed for the purpose of establishing safe levels of caffeine in cola beverages (Collins et al., 1981). This study, too, meets presentday experimental standards, and except for the strain of animal used (Osborne-Mendel) cannot be criticized for study design or reporting of results. In this study, groups of 61 rats each were intubated orally with 0, 6, 12, 40, 80, or 125 mg caffeine/kg on days 0–19 of gestation; a concurrent control group received distilled water to serve as controls.

Maternal toxicity culminated in death of six animals at the 125 mg/kg dosage. Weight gain was significantly decreased in dams at all doses, as was food intake. Developmentally, there was increased embryonic resorption at doses of 80 and 125 mg/kg, reduced fetal body weight at 40 mg/kg/day and above, and malformations of the digits at levels of 80 and 125 mg/kg/day. The type of malformation described was ectrodactyly and ranged in severity from hypoplastic development of a nail to the absence of one or more digits. The NOEL for frank teratogenesis was thus 40 mg/kg.

The malformation occurred mostly in the hind appendages and was observed in approximately 4% of limbs at 80 mg/kg and in 11% at 125 mg/kg. Hemorrhage of the limbs was an accompanying feature. Developmental toxicity was also manifested by reduced ossification of various sorts of the sternum at all dose levels. The average number of fetuses with at least one sternebral variation per litter increased significantly from 6 to 125 mg/kg, and

Table 7 Laboratory Teratologic Studies: Caffeine

Species	Route	Threshold teratogenic dose (mg/kg)	Treatment interval (in gestation)	Malformations observed	Ref.
Mouse	ip	100 × 2	12	Cleft palate, limb, digit	Fujii et al., 1969
	sc	200	12	Cleft palate, limb, digit	Fujii et al., 1969
	po	50	6–18	Digit	Bertrand et al., 1966
	dw	250	5–18	Cleft palate, limb	Elmazar et al., 1982
Rat	po	25	2–15	Digit	Bertrand et al., 1970
Rabbit	po	100	1–15	Digit	Bertrand et al., 1970

the number of litters containing fetuses with at least one sternebral variation increased significantly at doses of 40, 80, and 125 mg/kg. Additionally, skeletal variations of sites other than sternum were increased significantly at these latter dose levels, affecting vertebral centra and arches, long bones and skull bones. Interestingly, the skeletal effects were shown to be reversible in later experiments (Collins et al., 1987).

In sum, a clear NOEL was not established for either the mother or fetus from this study, there being maternal and developmental effects, however minor, at 6 mg/kg. More importantly, however, no unique toxicity to the fetus occurred, there thus being no hazard to development at doses at least threefold greater than the average daily intake in the human.

The route of administration appears to play a crucial role in the response in the laboratory studies. Bolus oral doses by intubation, for example, as in the study detailed above, elicited toxicity patterns not evident when the chemical was given orally via the drinking water. Nolen (1981) gave the equivalent of 20–80 mg/kg caffeine as instant or brewed coffees in the drinking water to rats through two pregnancies and observed as the only overt sign of toxicity in either mother or fetus a delay in fetal sternal ossification at the highest dose.

There have been other interesting reports of the effects of caffeine on mammalian development. The results of studies assessing postnatal behavior following oral prenatal caffeine administration to rats have not clearly demonstrated treatment-related effects. Positive effects, usually indicative of increased activity, and often associated with retarded growth, have been reported in some studies (Sobotka et al., 1979; Holloway, 1982; Groisser et al., 1982; Peruzzi et al., 1985), but were countered by negative or equivocal results in others (Butcher et al., 1984; Gullberg et al., 1986). An interesting finding was recently reported in a two-generation reproduction study in mice given caffeine via their drinking water (Sinton, 1989). This investigator found functional effects expressed in the second-generation offspring, although ingestion occurred only in the first generation. Further studies are clearly warranted to clarify the developmental toxicity of caffeine.

The almost universal use of foods and beverages containing caffeine, the teratogenic activity of caffeine in laboratory animals, and the high daily intake of caffeine during pregnancy as cited earlier, has led to concern of major proportions over the hazard the chemical presents to humans. The published associations between caffeine consumption and developmental toxicity in the human to date have been reviewed recently (Schardein and Keller, 1989; Al-Hachim, 1989). Of a dozen studies published between 1974 and 1986 reporting associations to low birth weights, stillbirth, spontaneous abortion, or congenital malformations as pregnancy outcomes among caffeine users, there was no convincing evidence for association between caffeine consumption of usual amounts and the occurrence of any class of developmental toxicity. It has been stated, however, by recent reports of animal and human data relating to caffeine, that "it might be prudent to limit intake to approximately 300 mg/day during pregnancy in view of decreases in birth weight which might occur at or about this level of consumption" (Berger, 1988; Caan and Goldhaber, 1989). Further, recent studies suggest that women who consume more than the equivalent of one cup of coffee per day were half as likely to become pregnant, per cycle, as women who drank less; a dose-response effect on fertility was present (Wilcox et al., 1988; Wilcox, 1989; Christianson et al., 1989).

III. NATURAL TERATOGENS IN DRUGS

A. Theobromine

Theobromine is known chemically as 3,7-dimethylxanthine (Fig. 2), and occurs naturally as 1.5–3% of the base in the bean of *Theobroma cacao*, the same plant source (cacao tree) for cocoa and chocolate. The chemical has therapeutic properties as a diuretic, smooth muscle relaxant, vasodilator, and cardiac stimulant.

In the laboratory, theobromine has given variable results in teratologic studies. In the mouse, high doses (500–600 mg/kg) injected intraperitoneally on gestation day 12 induced fetal malformations (Fujii and Nishimura, 1969). The chemical was also teratogenic in the rabbit (Tarka et al., 1986a). Oral doses of 25–200 mg/kg administered by intubation resulted in vascular and digital malformations, increased death and resorption, and reduced fetal body weight and increased developmental variations characterized by reduced ossification at doses of 75 mg/kg and higher. These developmental effects were accompanied by excessive maternal toxicity at the highest dosage level (200 mg/kg). However, oral doses of 21–63 mg/kg admixed in the diet resulted only in delayed skeletal ossification of sternebrae and metacarpal bones at doses of 41 mg/kg and higher.

Teratologic studies in rats have been limited to a dietary study and the chemical was not teratogenic (Tarka et al., 1986b). In this study, theobromine was admixed in the diet in concentrations of 0.0675 and 0.135% (approximately 49 and 97 mg/kg, respectively) and fed to rats on gestation days 6–19. There was no maternal or developmental toxicity elicited with the exception of delayed ossification of sternebrae and pubic bones at the 0.135% level. It is not known whether the difference in teratogenic response in rats and rabbits is due to species reaction or to route of administration. It is known that unchanged theobromine is found in sera of both species following administration of the chemical (Tarka et al., 1986a,b).

No reports of the drug affecting human pregnancy have appeared. It should be of some comfort too, that the highest doses of theobromine administered orally in the cited studies in laboratory animals correspond to a consumption greater than 7.5–10 lb of milk chocolate per day.

B. Theophylline

The third xanthine considered here, theophylline, chemically designated 1,3-dimethylxanthine (Fig. 2), occurs naturally in small quantities in several species of the *Camellia* genus. It has important therapeutic utility as a diuretic, vasodilator, cardiac stimulant, smooth muscle relaxant, and bronchodilator. It is of particular interest in this presentation, since it is the bronchodilator of choice for asthma and chronic obstructive pulmonary disease in the pregnant patient (Briggs et al., 1983).

Theophylline is teratogenic in mice by several routes of administration. By the intraperitoneal route, single doses of 100 mg/kg and higher on gestation day 10, 11, 12, or 13 induced cleft palate, digit, and predominant left-sided limb defects; embryolethality was also increased at the 150 and 200 mg/kg dosages (Tucci and Skalko, 1978). When administered via drinking water in concentrations of 0.075–0.2% on gestational days 6–15, malformations accompanied by increased resorptions and reduced fetal body weight were observed in the presence of maternal toxicity as well (George et al., 1986).

In contrast, theophylline was not teratogenic in the rat by either parenteral or dietary administration at dosages comparable to those utilized in mice. Doses of 200 mg/kg subcutaneously to rats on day 10 or 11 of organogenesis did not result in malformations (Maren and Ellison, 1972). Dietary admixtures containing 0.15–0.4% theophylline on gestation days 6–15 to rats resulted in maternal toxicity, increased fetal resorption and reduced fetal body weight, but no malformations (George et al., 1986). No adverse effects have been reported from human pregnancies. Given the maximum human therapeutic dose of 18 mg/kg/day, it would appear to be sufficiently less than levels affecting development in animals as to be of little or no concern.

C. Tobacco

Tobacco is an important field crop in several parts of the world. Scientifically, tobacco as utilized is the dried leaf of *Nicotiana tabacum*, but at least seven other plant genera are used as substitutes for this species throughout the world. It is indulged in by many millions of people through smoking, chewing, or snuffing.

While over 500 chemicals have been isolated from the particulate and gaseous phases of tobacco smoke, the principal chemical present in tobacco is the alkaloid nicotine. Chemically, it is 3-(1 methyl-2-pyrrolidinyl)pyridine (Fig. 3). Tobacco leaves contain nicotine in amounts ranging from 0.6 to 9%, as well as lesser amounts of nornicotine and tobacco camphor. The roots of tobacco also contain the major pyridine alkaloid anabasine as well as anatabine. Anabasine is known chemically as 3(2-piperidinyl)pyridine (see Fig. 3). Nicotine no longer has therapeutic application; taken in tobacco, it can act as a stimulant, depressant, or tranquilizer.

For our purposes, the common tobacco plant *Nicotiana tabacum* and wild tree tobacco *N. glauca* are the species of greatest interest. There are a number of issues associated with tobacco in the context of "natural teratogens." First, the tobacco plant itself has teratogenic properties in range animals when ingested. Second, chemicals extracted from tobacco are teratogenic under certain experimental conditions. Finally, tobacco has marked effects on development when smoked. We will consider these conditions separately.

Ingestion of *N. tabacum* stalks by swine was observed to cause leg deformities in several hundred piglets (Crowe, 1969). The induction of limb malformations, i.e., arthrogryposis, was subsequently confirmed in swine fed tobacco

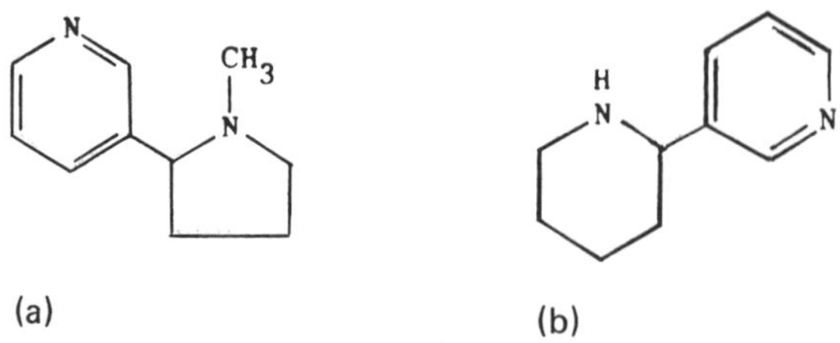

Figure 3 Chemical structure of principal alkaloids in tobacco: (a) nicotine and (b) anabasine.

stalks or leaf filtrates of this plant species as one source of diet (Crowe and Swerczek, 1974) and in swine fed *N. glauca* parts (Keeler et al., 1981; Keeler and Crowe, 1983). In addition, palate closure defects were observed in the latter study.

Arthrogryposis and cleft palate were also shown to be induced in calves in which cattle were fed *N. glauca* (Keeler, 1980; Keeler et al., 1981; Keeler and Crowe, 1981, 1983).

The teratogenic properties of nicotine, the primary alkaloid in the tobacco plant, are weak. The injection of 0.008–0.025 mg nicotine/g body weight to mice either subcutaneously or intraperitoneally during organogenesis induced limb and digit skeletal defects and resorption (Nishimura and Nakai, 1958). Higher doses injected subcutaneously in rats had the effect of reducing fetal body weight and viable litters, but not of inducing malformations (Hudson and Timiras, 1972). Effects on postnatal behavior have also been reported in the rat (Martin and Becker, 1970; Fung, 1988). There were no reported teratogenic effects in rabbits (Vara and Kinnunen, 1951) or in cattle or swine (Keeler, 1980).

The smoking of tobacco is, of course, one of the major threats to public health existent. It presents particular dangers to women of childbearing age (Greenwood, 1979). This is of widespread concern, since estimates are that 20–50% of women in the United States smoke during pregnancy (Abel, 1980). In fact, smoking is the most important single preventable determinant of low birth weight and perinatal mortality in this country (Longo, 1982).

The premise that exposure to tobacco smoke could be hazardous to fetal development date back to early in the present century (Guillian and Gy, 1907; Fleig, 1908). Since that time, literally hundreds of publications have addressed the toxicity in mother and child resultant from cigarette smoking during pregnancy. All studies considered, maternal smoking does not appear to be a major factor in the induction of congenital malformations (Schardein, 1985). As noted earlier, however, other developmental toxicity of major proportions results from this habit. The profile of this toxicity can be summarized as follows.

Birth weight deficits of up to 250 g for full-term newborns are clearly associated with smoking (Stein and Susser, 1984). There is a dose-response relationship between this deficit and the number of cigarettes smoked (Meyer et al., 1976). The reduction in birth weight appears to be a direct effect on fetal growth, since affected infants display symmetrical fetal growth retardation, deficits in crown-heel length, chest circumference, and head circumference, as well as birth weight (Miller et al., 1976; Report of the Surgeon General, 1983).

Direct relationships to other adverse pregnancy outcomes from cigarette smoking have also been demonstrated. These include increased incidences of abruptio placentae, bleeding during pregnancy, premature rupture of membranes, fetal deaths, neonatal mortality, and sudden infant death syndrome (Rush and Kass, 1972; Meyer et al., 1975; Meyer and Tonascia, 1977; Report of the Surgeon General, 1983).

A growing body of data indicates there may also be functional effects on infants of smoking mothers. Several controlled studies have shown deficits in growth, intellectual and emotional development, and behavior (Butler and Goldstein, 1973; Dunn et al., 1976; Report of the Surgeon General, 1983; Naeye and Peters, 1984).

Because of this wide range of adverse effects related to cigarette smoking during pregnancy, it has been suggested that a descriptive diagnostic term, such as "fetal tobacco syndrome" be applied to infants relating to this maternal behavior under certain conditions (Neiburg et al., 1985). Omitting other causes of adverse pregnancy outcome, i.e., hypertension, congenital infection or anomaly, the term can be applied when the mother smoked five or more cigarettes a day throughout pregnancy, and the newborn has symmetrical growth retardation at term defined as a birth weight < 2500 g and a ponderal index > 2.32. Whether such labeling of this pattern of toxicity is necessary, no one would argue about the need to recognize cigarette smoking as a serious threat to public health.

Nicotine in the stalks was implicated as the causative chemical teratogen to limb defects in the animal studies with *N. tabacum*, it being found in high content (1058 ppm) in the stalk in one study (Menges et al., 1970). In contrast, the principal alkaloid of *N. glauca* is anabasine, and oral doses of 2.6–1066 mg/kg of the chemical given to swine induced cleft palate and arthrogryposis in the piglets as had been observed earlier in the tobacco-feeding studies (Keeler et al., 1984). This suggests that anabasine may be the active teratogenic molecule. However, the chemical was reported to be not teratogenic in rats and rabbits (Ryabchenko, 1982). In humans, the precise mechanism for the reported effects following smoking is not known; the available data support the view for the effect on birth weight that nicotine and/or carbon monoxide can cause intrauterine hypoxia. Further definition of causative factors of tobacco toxicity must await further experimentation.

D. Podophyllum and Derivatives

The mayapple or mandrake plant (*Podophyllum peltatum*) has medicinal use in the topical treatment of warts of several types, and also has utility as a cathartic and has been used experimentally as an antitumor agent. The active compound of the plant is believed to be podophyllotoxin, a highly liquid-soluble β-D-glucoside (Fig. 4).

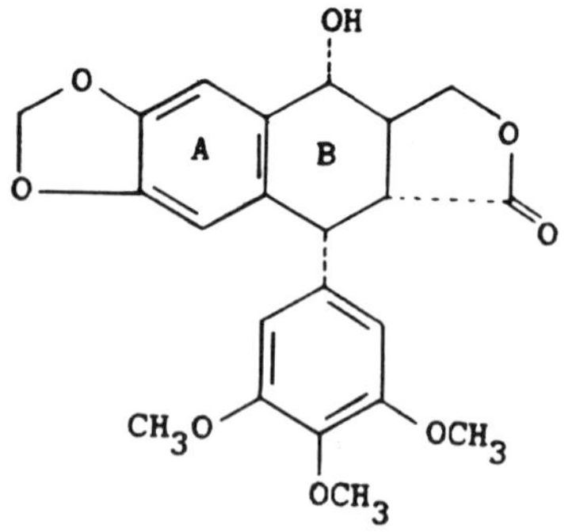

Figure 4 Chemical structure of podophyllotoxin.

Podophyllotoxin showed no teratogenic activity in mice, rats, or rabbits treated parenterally during pregnancy (Didcock et al., 1952). It did cause resorption in the rat (Thiersch, 1963), however, as evidence of developmental toxicity potential.

Three semisynthetic podophyllotoxin derivatives have also shown teratogenic activity. The first two, etoposide (VP-16-213) and teniposide (VM-26), both induced multiple malformations in mice when injected intraperitoneally with 0.5–2 mg/kg/day on one day in gestation (Sieber et al., 1978). The third, mitopodozide or Proresid®, produced multiple malformations in rats when injected intraperitoneally with doses of 100–120 mg/kg/day on gestation days 8–14 (Tanase and Suzuki, 1967).

Podophyllum resin, the dried alcoholic extract of the rhizome roots of the plant, not only was embryotoxic in the mouse when given intraperitoneally (Joneja and LeLiever, 1974), but was teratogenic in the rat when given orally on gestation days 8–12 as evidenced by minor skeletal alterations in the fetuses (Dwornik and Moore, 1967). Peltatin (α and β forms) glucosides also found in rhizomes of the plant were embryotoxic in mice, as evidenced by increased resorption following oral dosing of c. 40–160 mg/kg/day on one or two days in early gestation (Wiesner et al., 1958).

Several reports have also appeared concerning podophyllum and human usage in pregnancy. In the first case reported, a woman took six herbal "slimming" tablets containing 30 mg each podophyllum plus other natural extracts per day for about 3.5 weeks during the fifth to ninth weeks of her pregnancy (Cullis, 1962). At birth, her infant had several skin tags, polyneuritis, growth retardation, limb malformations, and heart defects, which were suspected to have been caused by podophyllum. In the second case, podophyllum resin was applied topically to vulval warts during the 32nd week of pregnancy and resulted in intrauterine death of the conceptus (Chamberlain et al., 1972). In the last reported case, podophyllum was applied topically in 25% concentration five times at the end of the second trimester of pregnancy (weeks 23–29); she also was administered several antimalarial medications (Karol et al., 1980). The patient gave birth to an infant with preauricular skin tags and a simian crease on one hand. The authors suggested that podophyllum

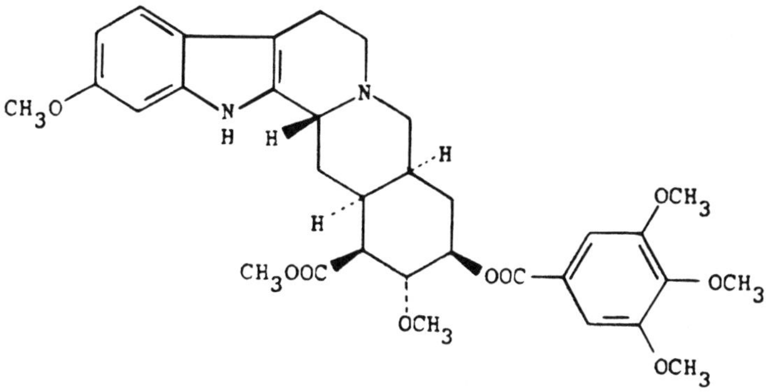

Figure 5 Chemical structure of reserpine.

be avoided during pregnancy, and this advice appears to be warranted based on the cases presented to date.

E. Reserpine

Reserpine (Serpasil®), a therapeutically useful antihypertensive drug, is obtained from the roots of the *Rauwolfia serpentina* plant. It has utility in veterinary practice as well. Its chemical structure is shown in Figure 5.

The drug is not a potent teratogen (Table 8). In laboratory models, it was teratogenic upon parenteral administration at dosages of 0.1/mg/kg/day and higher to rats. In addition to structural abnormalities, postnatal functional alterations have been induced (Buelke-Sam et al., 1989). Studies in other species, including guinea pigs, hamsters, and rabbits were not teratogenic, although other developmental toxicity was mentioned in the latter species.

Over the many years the drug has been marketed, about 300 normal babies have been reported following treatment of the mother (Schardein, 1985; Czeizel, 1988), and only one case report describing malformation has appeared (Pauli and Pettersen, 1986). This was a child with multiple malformations whose mother was treated with 0.5 mg/day on days 13–41 of her pregnancy.

Table 8 Laboratory Teratologic Studies: Reserpine

Species	Dosage and route (mg/kg/day)	Treatment interval (in gestation)	Malformations observed	Ref.
Rat	0.1–2 im	9 or 10	Multiple	Goldman and Yakovac, 1965
Guinea pig	c. 0.3–7 im	Preimplantation	None	Deanesly, 1966
Hamster	0.5–1 sc	1–3	None	Harper, 1972
Rabbit	0.125–0.5 im	2–11	None	Kehl et al., 1956

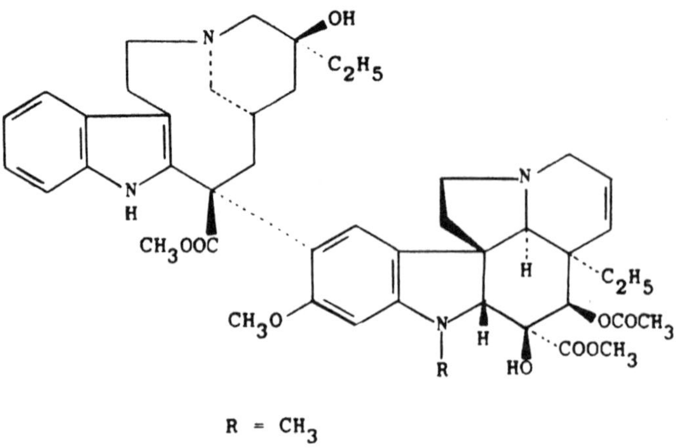

Figure 6 Chemical structure of a representative *Vinca* alkaloid: vinblastine.

F. *Vinca* Alkaloids

Two important anticancer drugs have been obtained from the periwinkle plant (*Vinca rosea*). Both are potent teratogens in multiple laboratory species. The first of these, called vinblastine (Fig. 6) or Velban®, induced polymorphic malformations in rats (Cohlan et al., 1964; DeMyer, 1964), mice (Joneja and LeLiever, 1974), hamsters (Ferm, 1963b), and rabbits (Morris, 1970) following very low parenteral doses.

Reports of two normal babies have appeared with the drug (Rosenweig et al., 1964; Armstrong et al., 1964), but it also probably is developmentally toxic in the human as well. The other drug obtained from this plant, vincristine or Oncovin®, also is a potent teratogen in rats (DeMyer, 1965), hamsters (Ferm, 1963b), mice (Sieber et al., 1978), and rabbits (Szabo and Kang, 1969). The drug also induced abortion and several malformations in primates (Courtney and Valerio, 1968; Wilson, 1971). Like vinblastine, the drug probably has the potential for inducing developmental toxicity in the human species, although some 11 normal babies are known from treatment (Schardein, 1985).

G. Maytansine

Maytansine has, like the *Vinca*-derived anticancer alkaloidal agents vinblastine and vincristine, an origin from a plant, *Maytensus* sp. in this case. Intraperitoneal doses of only 0.1 mg/kg produced multiple malformations in mice when injected on a single day of gestation (Sieber et al., 1978). No reports in humans have been published.

H. Colchicine

Colchicine is an alkaloid having therapeutic utility as a uricosuric agent or gout suppressant. It is obtained from the *Colchicum autumnale* plant, better known as the autumn crocus. It is depicted chemically in Figure 7.

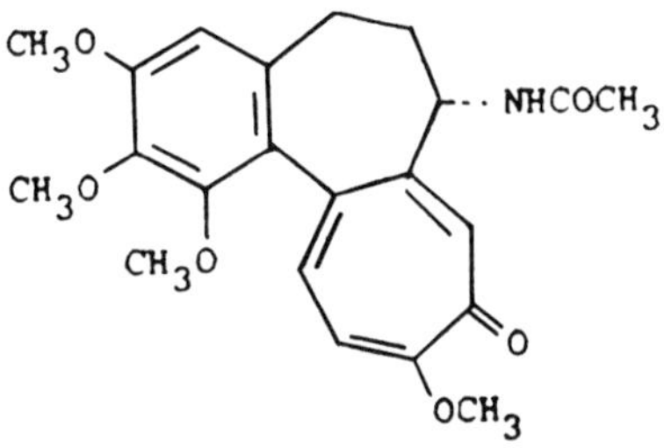

Figure 7 Chemical structure of colchicine.

The drug is teratogenic in a number of laboratory species (Table 9). In addition to the three species listed, the drug is also apparently teratogenic in the rabbit, but experimental details were lacking (Szabo et al., 1971). Another publication alluded to 34 pregnant cattle treated in the absence of abortion and malformations (Katsilambros, 1963). The developmental toxicity profile of colchicine demonstrates the drug has some hazard potential. In a well-conducted study in mice, multiple malformations and increased resorption occurred at dosages in the absence of maternal toxicity (Sieber et al., 1978). This situation is a unique one, even though there are a large number of human cases known in which the resulting offspring were normal (Schardein, 1985).

I. Solanaceae Anticholinergics

Several therapeutically useful agents have their origins in plant genera of the Solanaceae family, which include belladonna, mandrake, and jimson weed species. The three drugs considered here are atropine, hyoscyamine, and scopolamine. They are similar chemically (Fig. 8) and are used medicinally in a variety of indications affected by their anticholinergic pharmacological activity.

Atropine has been studied with respect to its effect on development in laboratory animals, and the results have been largely negative with respect to teratogenic potential (Table 10). Two studies in mice provided disparate results

Table 9 Laboratory Teratologic Studies: Colchicine

Species	Dosage and route (mg/kg/day)	Treatment interval (in gestation)	Malformations observed	Ref.
Mouse	0.5–2.5 sc	2–14 (single)	Multiple	Shoji and Makino, 1966
Rat	c. 0.2 ip	10–14	Multiple	Van Dyke and Ritchey, 1947
Hamster	10–20 iv	8	Eye, skeletal, closure defects	Ferm, 1963a

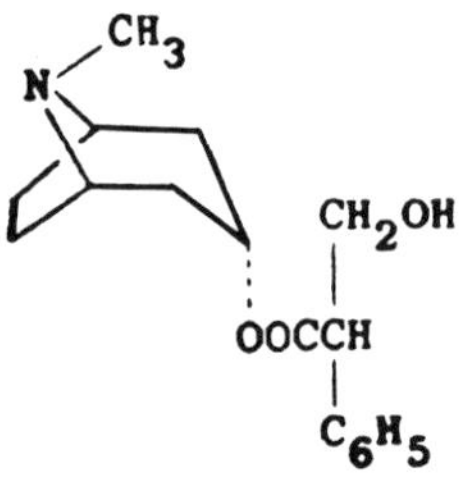

Figure 8 Chemical structure of atropine.

under almost an identical experimental regimen: no terata were observed in one study, while the other recorded 5.2% offspring with skeletal abnormalities. Rats and dogs were not reactive under the experimental conditions tested, although in the dog, atropine sulfate given bitches in gestation caused dystocia and resultant death of the puppies. Human studies have not implicated the drug as toxic developmentally.

No published laboratory teratologic studies exist on either scopolamine or hyoscyamine. A few reports have alluded to absence of congenital malformations in humans with both drugs (Schardein, 1985; Yu et al., 1988).

J. Tubocurarine

Tubocurarine (Fig. 9) is a curare component having therapeutic utility as a skeletal muscle relaxant. It is derived from the *Chondodendron* plant genus.

The drug has given ambiguous results in animals. In mice, intramuscular dosages of 0.6–5 mg/kg on the 13th gestational day were not developmentally toxic (Jacobs, 1971). In rats, a smaller dose (about 0.5 mg/kg) given by injection on single days late in gestation caused intrauterine growth retardation and clubfoot (Shoro, 1977). A single case report in the human 20 years ago that has remained unsubstantiated described arthrogryposis in a child treated the 10th to 12th gestational weeks (Jago, 1970).

Table 10 Laboratory Teratologic Studies: Atropine

Species	Dose and route (mg/kg/day)	Treatment interval (in gestation)	Malformations observed	Ref.
Mouse	50 sc	9	Skeletal	Arcuri and Gautieri, 1973
	50 sc	8, 9, or 10	None	Zellers, 1979
Rat	c. 80 sc	11–17 (2-day intervals)	None	Maeda and Yasuda, 1979
Dog	1–50 oral	?	None	Back et al., 1961

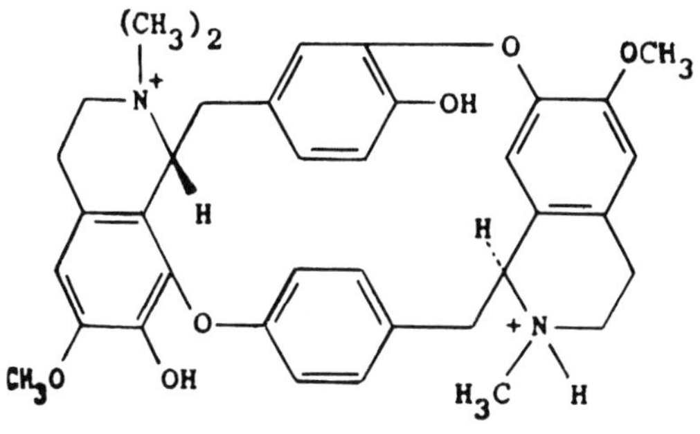

Figure 9 Chemical structure of tubocurarine.

K. Ergot Derivatives

Two drugs obtained from ergot (*Claviceps purpurea*), ergonovine and ergotamine, have therapeutic utility as oxytocic agents. The former is also used specifically as a vasoconstrictor in migraine headache.

The first, ergonovine (Fig. 10), has had limited testing. In the only reported study of which I am aware, pregnant rats injected intravenously with 10 mg/kg of the drug on gestation day 14 elicited no teratogenicity (Leist and Grauwiler, 1974). A single case report in the human some time ago described Poland anomaly resulting from treatment with a large dose of the drug in the first trimester (David, 1972). The case remains unconfirmed.

The other drug, ergotamine (Fig. 10), has been studied experimentally in mice, rats, and rabbits by the oral route but did not induce malformation at doses as high as 300 mg/kg/day when given during the period of major organogenesis (Grauwiler and Schon, 1973). The drug induced other developmental toxicity in both mice and rats, however. A single human case report described prune perineum in the infant of a woman treated with the drug several times

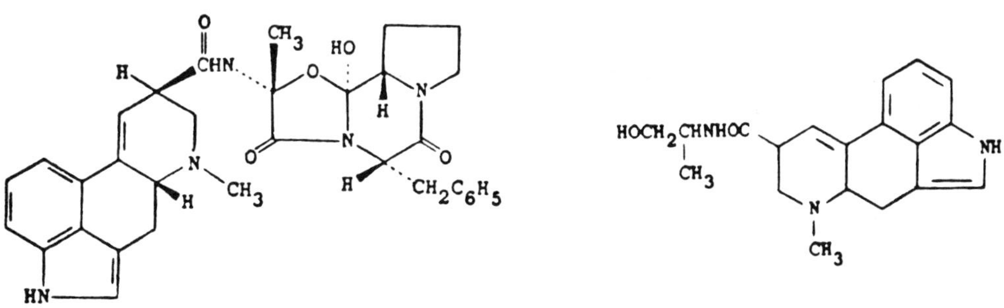

(a) (b)

Figure 10 Chemical structure of several ergot-derived drugs: (a) ergotamine and (b) ergonovine.

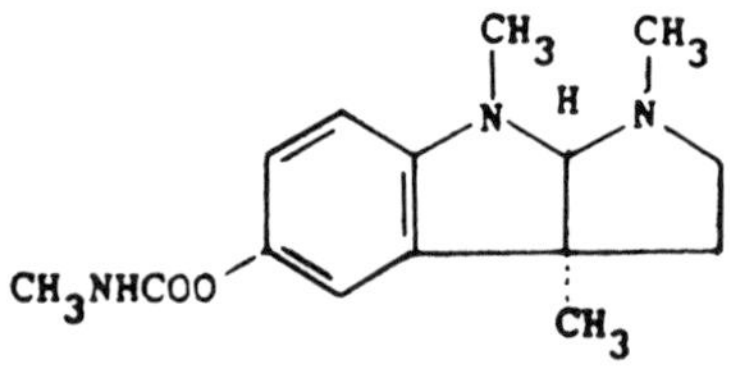

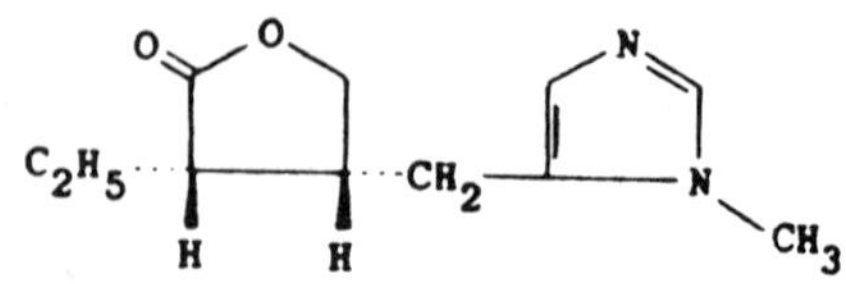

Figure 11 Chemical structures of several cholinergic drugs: (a) physostigmine and (b) pilocarpine.

during the first 8 weeks of pregnancy (Peeden et al., 1979), but further cases have not appeared.

L. Cholinergics

Several useful cholinergic drugs obtained from different plant genera are represented here—physostigmine and pilocarpine.

Physostigmine or eserine is a parasympathomimetic drug that is obtained from the calabar bean, also known scientifically as *Physostigma venenosum*. It has a number of therapeutic indications relating to its cholinergic, miotic pharmacological action. Chemically it is a pyrol methylcarbamate ester (Fig. 11).

The drug has been tested for teratogenic potential in only a single study. In that experiment, pregnant mice injected subcutaneously on gestation day 8 or 9 with 0.005 mg resulted in skeletal defects in about 10% of the offspring (Arcuri and Gautieri, 1973).

Pilocarpine (Fig. 11) is obtained from *Pilocarpus jaborandi* and is used in treating glaucoma. The only report describing the drug's effect on development was published by Kropp and Forward (1963). They gave 100 mg/kg of the drug to rats subcutaneously through pregnancy, and reported effects on dentition.

M. Ephedrine

Ephedrine (Fig. 12) is a widely used adrenergic drug and is obtained from several species of the *Ephedra* genus. The drug has only been studied in a

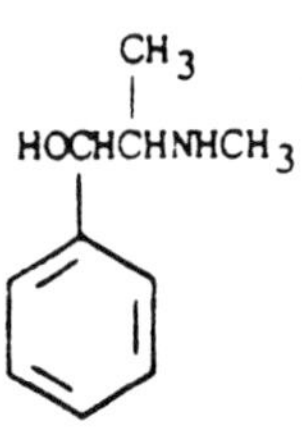

Figure 12 Chemical structure of ephedrine.

single species. In the reported study, pregnant rats were treated intraperitoneally on gestation days 9, 10, and 11 at doses ranging from 0.1 to 50 mg/kg/day (Kanai et al., 1986). Ventricular septal defects were reported in some offspring. With respect to hazard to humans, the large collaborative study reported a suggestive association between its use during the first 4 months of pregnancy and the incidence of minor malformations (Heinonen et al., 1977). No further reports have appeared, to my knowledge, to confirm or deny this association.

N. Opium Derivatives

Two very useful medicines are derived from the opium poppy, known scientifically as *Papaver somniferum*. Having strong narcotic properties, both codeine and morphine (Fig. 13) are used therapeutically as potent analgesics.

With respect to codeine, oral doses at the tested levels did not induce terata in rabbits and rats when administered during major organogenesis (Table 11). When injected subcutaneously, however, malformations were observed in both mice and hamsters. These latter dosages were higher, however, than the oral dosages used in the other two species. No case report or other associations to congenital malformations in humans have been published, but the large collaborative study reported a suggestive association between the use of codeine in the first four months of pregnancy and respiratory malformations in the subsequent issue (Heinonen et al., 1977), although this has not been corroborated since.

Similar results have been obtained in animal studies with morphine (Table 11). Central nervous system malformations were induced in mouse and hamster fetuses, while no malformations were observed in rats and rabbits, although the dosages were smaller in the latter. Two older reports listed limb defects in single human cases following morphine administration in pregnancy, but a number of other published reports found no relationship to treatment (Schardein, 1985).

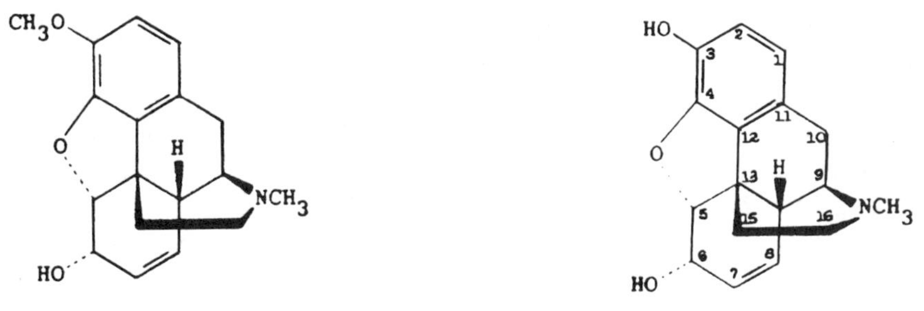

(a) (b)

Figure 13 Chemical structure of several narcotic analgesics: (a) codeine and (b) morphine.

Table 11 Laboratory Teratologic Studies: Codeine, Morphine

Drug	Species	Dosage and route (mg/kg/day)	Treatment interval (in gestation)	Malformations observed	Ref.
Codeine	Mouse	100 sc	7–11 (single) or 8 & 9	Skeletal	Zellers and Gautieri, 1977
	Rat	10–120 oral	6–15	None	Lehmann, 1976
	Hamster	73–360 sc	8	Skull	Geber and Schramm, 1975
	Rabbit	5–30 oral	6–18	None	Lehmann, 1976
Morphine	Mouse	100–500 sc	8 or 9	CNS	Harpel and Gautieri, 1968
	Rat	20 sc	2–5, 7–9 or 11–13	None	Becker and Johannesson, 1973
	Hamster	300 sc	8	CNS	Geber, 1970
	Rabbit	50 or 100 sc	?	None	Raye et al., 1977

O. Hallucinogenic Alkaloids

There are three illicit drugs obtained from plants that have had medicinal uses over many years, but are known contemporaneously as street drugs of abuse due to having mind-altering effects, i.e., euphoria, hallucinations, deliria, when ingested or smoked. They all have addictive properties as well. At least one third of the population of the United States over the age of 12 reports using marijuana, cocaine, or psychotherapeutic drugs according to an official government survey (Dattel, 1990). The drugs to be discussed are mescaline, marijuana, and cocaine.

The first of these, mescaline, is isolated from peyote, the flowering heads of *Lophophora williamsii*. Chemically it is trimethoxybenzeneethanamine (Fig. 14). The drug has been studied developmentally only in the hamster. In the reported study, dosages ranging from 0.45 to 3.25 mg/kg administered subcutaneously on day 8 of gestation produced runted fetuses, increased resorption, and defects of the central nervous system (Geber, 1967).

The second drug of this group, marijuana, also known as hemp, hashish, ganja, pot, cannabis, etc., comes from the dried flowering tops of *Cannabis sativa L.* The active constituents of the plant are isomeric tetrahydrocannabinols (Fig. 14). The plant is ubiquitous, and while cultivation of *Cannabis* is illegal in the United States, it remains one of the biggest cash crops in several states.

The chemical is teratogenic in a number of species (Table 12). Injection of marijuana resin or extract induced malformations in rats, rabbits, and hamsters. A conventional teratology type study in the mouse with resin was negative, but cleft palate was reported in F_2 generation offspring in another study in which marijuana smoke was inhaled on gestation day 10 (Nishimura

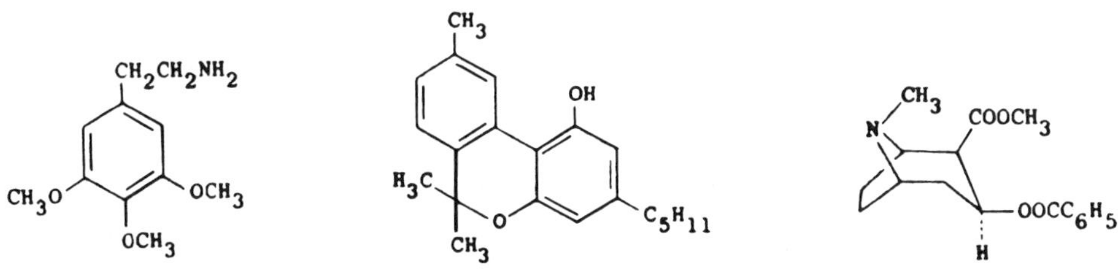

(a) (b) (c)

Figure 14 Chemical structures of several hallucinogenic alkaloids: (a) mescaline, (b) cannabinol, and (c) cocaine.

and Tanimura, 1976). A single oral study with marijuana was negative in primates.

Human studies are difficult to interpret because doses used of illicit drugs and pattern of use are unknown variables, and multiple drug use of street drugs is common. A few case reports describing several types of malformations occurring in the offspring of users have been published (Schardein, 1985), but a recent study found no association with congenital anomalies (Witter and Niebyl, 1990). Low birth weight and short gestation have also been reported in several studies (Hingson et al., 1982; Linn et al., 1983; Zuckerman et al., 1989). However, it seems unlikely due to the nature of exposure with marijuana that it will be known with certainty whether there are real effects relating to drug use.

The last drug of the group, cocaine (ecgonine) (Fig. 14), is obtained from the leaves of the cocaine plant (*Erythroxylum coca*) of South America and is at present one of the most important drugs known to man. It has been used as a topical anesthetic, but its use today as a recreational drug of abuse far transcends its therapeutic utility. A recent estimate was that up to 2 million

Table 12 Laboratory Teratologic Studies: Marijuana

Species	Dosage form and route (mg/kg/day)	Treatment interval (in gestation)	Malformations observed	Ref.
Mouse	16 resin ip	6 or 1–6	None	Persaud and Ellington, 1967
Rat	4.2 resin ip	1–6	Limb, digit, closure	Persaud and Ellington, 1968
Rabbit	250–500 extract sc	7–10	Multiple	Geber and Schramm, 1969
Hamster	100–300 extract sc	6–8	Multiple	Geber and Schramm, 1969
Primate	1.4–2.1 resin oral	?	None	Grilly et al., 1974

American women over age 18 use the drug (Dattel, 1990). It is colloquially known as "snow," "coke," "gold dust," "lady," and a smokable form called "crack."

In spite of the known effects on human development of cocaine, as will be described below, only a few studies have been done with respect to the effects of the drug in the laboratory. It is known that doses of 20–60 mg/kg/day by parenteral routes during 3 or 6 days of the organogenesis period cause congenital malformations in the mouse (Mahalik et al., 1980; Finnell et al., 1990). A similar regimen in the rat instead of malformation caused increased resorption and reduced fetal body weight (Fantel and Macphail, 1982). Given later in gestation to rats, doses of 60 mg/kg/day cocaine produced changes in startle reaction and exploratory behavior, increased locomotor activity and other postnatal functional effects (Foss and Riley, 1988; Hutchings et al., 1989; Smith et al., 1989). Based on these findings, cocaine is an active developmental toxicant in the laboratory, producing the full spectrum of developmental toxicity.

Cocaine has adverse effects on human development as well. According to a large series of studies, cocaine use in pregnancy significantly reduces fetal birth weight, increases the rates of spontaneous abortion, stillbirth, preterm labor and delivery, perinatal morbidity and mortality, and is associated with higher malformation rates (Bingol et al., 1987; Chasnoff et al., 1987; MacGregor et al., 1987; Frank et al., 1988; Landy and Hinson, 1988; Hadeed and Siegel, 1989; Keith et al., 1989; Little et al., 1989; Neerhof et al., 1989; Zuckerman et al., 1989). Among the malformations reported, central nervous system, eye, vascular, genitourinary tract, and cardiac have been cited specifically, but it is too early to characterize a syndrome attributable to the drug (Chasnoff et al., 1988; Ferriero et al., 1988; Fulroth, 1989; Greenland et al., 1989; Little et al., 1989). In addition to the developmental toxicity described above, infants of cocaine users, in addition to marked addiction withdrawal symptoms, suffer from functional impairments (Chasnoff et al., 1989; Hume et al., 1989). This chemical is clearly a societal problem of major proportions).

P. Quinine

Quinine, chemically known as 6′-methoxycinchonan-9-ol (Fig. 15) is an alkaloid derived in 1–8% concentration from the bark of *Cinchona* trees, cultivated in South America and Java. It has been widely used to treat malaria over many years. Another drug derivative from the bark in 0.25–3% concentration is quinidine, commonly used as a cardiac depressant in antiarrhythmic states. Of the two, only quinine has been studied with respect to effects on development.

A wide variety of species have been investigated for teratogenic potential (Table 13). Of these, only the guinea pig and chinchilla have been reported to be subject to teratogenic insult. The drug is of greater concern as it relates to the human species. The subject has been reviewed (Schardein, 1985). The large number of published studies over the past 50 years indicate a wide variety of congenital malformations supposedly induced by the drug, especially at high, even abortifacient dose levels. The cause for concern is with the defects

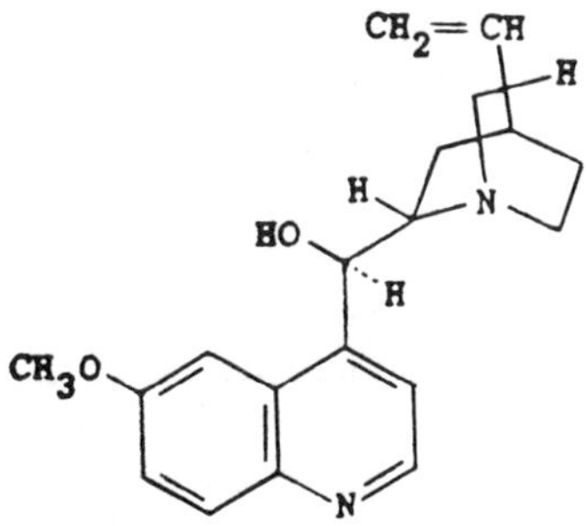

Figure 15 Chemical structure of quinine.

associated with auditory nerve hypoplasia, resulting in clinical descriptions of varying degrees of hearing loss. This finding is strengthened by the presence of similar lesions in guinea pigs treated experimentally throughout gestation.

IV. DISCUSSION AND SUMMARY

This survey of "natural teratogens" in foods and drugs has disclosed a rather limited number of such agents. And of this number, few have demonstrated hazard potential to humans. While it is true that the majority of agents discussed herein have evidenced developmental toxicity potential, including teratogenesis, in laboratory animal models, this is to be expected, in line with the principle that virtually all agents at some dose to a given species of animal under proper conditions will elicit adverse developmental effects on the conceptus (Karnofsky, 1965).

Table 13 Laboratory Teratologic Studies: Quinine

Species	Dosage and route (mg/kg/day)	Treatment interval (in gestation)	Malformations observed	Ref.
Mouse	125–500 oral	6,10,6–10, or 0–17	None	Tanimura and Lee, 1972
Rat	50 various	7–14	None	Neuweiler and Richter, 1964
Rabbit	100 oral	18–28	None	Savini et al., 1971
Guinea pig	200 sc	throughout	Inner ear	Covell, 1936
Dog	15–50 im	18–48	None	Savini, et al., 1971
Primate	20–200 oral	24–26 or 27–29	None	Tanimura and Lee, 1972
Chinchilla	90–150 oral	4–14	Central nervous system	Klosovskii, 1963

A small number of these agents, however, have teratogenic or other adverse effects in the human species, and judicious use during pregnancy is warranted. In the first group of these agents of concern are quinine and vitamins A and D. Under normal use, these probably present little hazard, the adverse effects attributed to them manifested only at high doses—abortifacient ones with quinine, and megadoses in the case of the vitamins. At any rate, in the case of quinine, the drug labeling should serve as sufficient warning to avoid use of the drug during pregnancy. With vitamin A hypervitaminosis, hazard alerts to the public with the recommendation that daily doses not exceed 8000 IU have appeared in print (Teratology Society Position Paper, 1987; Werler et al., 1989; Kizer et al., 1990) and should serve at least in part to alert the public to limit dosage of this OTC product to the recommended level. The situation with respect to hypervitaminosis D is less clear, but the available evidence with respect to supravalvular aortic stenosis in humans is sufficient to restrict use to recommended daily allowances of this vitamin during pregnancy.

A second small group of agents of concern are the chemotherapeutic agents discussed, including the *Vinca* alkaloids and maytansine. Risk-benefit considerations apply in their use and, by this process, are of less immediate concern.

Caffeine is the third agent or groups of agents of concern. This concern stems not from the aspect of induction of congenital malformations in offspring of consumers ingesting the chemical in beverages, because the net result of epidemiological studies conducted appears to indicate they are unable to make such an association. Rather, it is the recent publications attesting to lowered birth weights (Hogue, 1981; Berger, 1988; Caan and Goldhaber, 1989) and impaired fertility rates (Wilcox et al., 1988; Wilcox, 1989; Christianson et al., 1989; Wyngaard, 1989) among users of even seemingly moderate quantities of caffeine that give rise to this concern, especially in light of the universal consumption of the chemical. Further studies are clearly in order to better establish the effect of caffeine on human pregnancy.

The final two "natural" agents of concern with respect to potential for induction of adverse developmental effects in human pregnancy are tobacco (smoking) and cocaine. Both represent societal issues of major proportions. As noted earlier, smoking is the most important single preventable determinant of low birth weight and perinatal mortality in the United States (Longo, 1982). Clearly the habit confers no benefit to the fetus whatsoever (Abel, 1980). In addition to increased mortality and decreased birth weight, increased spontaneous abortion, and adverse functional effects in offspring, among other toxicity are common sequelae, although the habit does not appear to be a major factor on teratogenesis. Tobacco smoking is clearly dangerous to reproductive health (Greenwood, 1979).

The other "natural" teratogen, cocaine, has assumed tremendous interest recently due to its predominant place as an addictive drug of abuse. Five million Americans are thought to be using the drug regularly (MacGregor et al., 1987), and in one urban area (Detroit), an estimated 10% of pregnant women use it (Anon., 1986). Widespread availability, the selective euphoria induced by its use, and use other than by intravenous injection are the main reasons for this popularity. Unfortunately, however, the drug is teratogenic and is associated with increased spontaneous abortion, reduced fetal birth weight, preterm delivery, increased perinatal morbidity and mortality, and disrupts central nervous system development. Exposure to cocaine clearly is detrimental to the human fetus. Educational programs aimed at prevention of the initiation of cocaine use would be highly desirable to alert the general public to the damages of cocaine use. It among all "natural teratogens" surveyed in this review is the most hazardous developmental toxicant at present.

REFERENCES

Abel, E. L. (1980). Smoking during pregnancy: a review of effects on growth and development of offspring. *Human Biol. 52*: 593–626.

Al-Hachim, G. M. (1989). Teratogenicity of caffeine (review). *Europ. J. Obstet. Gynecol. Repro. Biol. 31*: 237–247.

Anon., *Pediatric News*, February, 1986, p. 64.

Antia, A. U., Wiltse, H. E., Rowe, R. D., Pitt, E. L., Levin, S., Ottesen, O. E., and Cooke, R. E. (1967). Pathogenesis of the supravalvular aortic stenosis syndrome. *J. Pediatr. 71*: 431–441.

Acuri, P. A., and Gautieri, R. F. (1973). Morphine-induced fetal malformations 3: Possible mechanisms of action. *J. Pharm. Sci. 62*: 1626–1634.

Armstrong, J. G., Dyke, R. W., and Fouts, P. J. (1964). Vinblastine sulfate treatment of Hodgkin's disease during a pregnancy. *Science 143*: 703.

Artman, N. R. (1969). The chemical and biological properties of heated and oxidized fats. In *Advances in Lipid Research*, vol. 7. Pooletti, R., Kritchevsky, D., eds. Academic Press, New York, p. 245.

Back, K. C., Newberne, J. W., and Weaver, L. C. (1961). A toxicopathologic study of endobenzyline bromide, a new cholinergic blocking agent. *Toxicol. Appl. Pharmacol. 3*: 422–430.

Barone, J. J., and Roberts, H. (1984). Human consumption of caffeine. In *Caffeine*, P. B. Dews, ed. Springer, New York, pp. 59–73.

Beare, J. L., Gregory, E. R., Smith, D. M., and Campbell, J. A. (1961). The effect of rapeseed oil on reproduction and on the composition of rat milk fat. *Can. J. Biochem. 39*: 195–201.

Becker, B. A., and Johannesson, T. (1973). Persistent effects of transplacentally administered morphine in the Sprague-Dawley rat. *Teratology 8*: 215.

Beltrame, D., and Cantone, A. (1973). Maternal and foetal toxicity induced by lactose. *Teratology 8*: 215.

Berger, A. (1988). Effects of caffeine consumption on pregnancy outcome—a review. *J. Repro. Med. 33*: 945–956.

Bertrand, M., Schwam, E., Frandon, A., Vagne, A., and Alary, J. (1966). Sur un effet teratogene systematique et specifique de la cafeine chez les rongeurs. *C. R. Soc. Biol. 159*: 2199–2201.

Bertrand, M., Girod, J., and Rigaud, M. F. (1970). Ectrodactylie provoquee par la cafeine chez les rongeurs: role des facteurs specifiques at genetiques. *C. R. Soc. Biol. 164*: 1488–1489.

Bingol, N., Fuchs, M., Diaz, V., Stone, R. K., and Gromisch, D. S. (1987). Teratogenicity of cocaine in humans. *J. Pediat. 110*: 93–96.

Brent, R. L. (1985). Maternal nutrition and congenital malformations. *Birth Defects 21*: 1–8.

Briggs, G. G., Bodendorfer, T. W., Freeman, R. K., and Yaffe, S. J. (1983). *Drugs in Pregnancy and Lactation. A Reference Guide to Fetal and Neonatal Risk*. Williams and Wilkins, Baltimore.

Buelke-Sam, J., Ali, S. F., Kimmel, G. L., Slikker, W., Newport, G. D., and Harmon, J. R. (1989). Postnatal function following prenatal reserpine exposure in rats-neurobehavioral toxicity. *Neurotox. T. 11*: 515–522.

Buist, R. (1986). *Food Chemical Sensitivity. What It Is and How to Cope with It*. Avery Publ. Group, Inc., Garden City, New York.

Burg, A. W. (1975). How much caffeine in the cup. *Tea Coffee Trade 147*: 40–42.

Butcher, R. E., Vorhees, C. V., and Wootten, V. (1984). Behavioral and physical development of rats chronically exposed to caffeinated fluids. *Fund. Appl. Toxicol. 4*: 1–13.

Butler, N. R., and Goldstein, H. (1973). Smoking in pregnancy and subsequent child development. *Br. Med. J. 4*: 573–575.

Caan, B. J., and Goldhaber, M. K. (1989). Caffeinated beverages and low birth-weight: A case-control study. *Am. J. Publ. Health 79*: 1299–1300.

Carpi, C., and Scarinci, V. (1974). Effects of ascorbic acid on embryonic and fetal development in rats and rabbits. *Studi Urbinati, Fac. Farm. 47*: 107–116.

Chamberlain, M. J., Reynolds, A. L., and Yeoman, W. B. (1972). Toxic effect of podophyllum application in pregnancy. *Br. Med. J. 3*: 391–392.

Chan, G. M., Bachino, J. J., Mehlhorn, D., Bove, K. E., Steichen, J. J., and Trang, R. C. (1979). The effect of vitamin D on pregnant rabbits and their offspring. *Pediatr. Res. 13*: 121–126.

Chasnoff, I. J., Burns, K. A., and Burns, W. J. (1987). Cocaine use in pregnancy: Perinatal morbidity and mortality. *Neurobehav. Toxicol. Teratol. 9*: 291–293.

Chasnoff, I. J., Chisum, G. M., and Kaplan, W. E. (1988). Maternal cocaine use and genitourinary tract malformations. *Teratology 37*: 201–204.

Chasnoff, I. J., Griffith, D. R., MacGregor, S., Dirkes, K., and Burns, K. A. (1989). Temporal patterns of cocaine use in pregnancy. Perinatal outcome. JAMA 261: 1741–1744.

Christianson, R. E., Oechsli, F. W., and Vandenberg, B. J. (1989). Caffeinated beverages and decreased fertility. *Lancet 1*: 378.

Cock, J. H. (1982). Cassava: A basic energy source in the tropics. *Science 218*: 755–762.

Cohlan, S. Q. (1953a). Excessive intake of vitamin A during pregnancy as a cause of congenital anomalies in the rat. *Am. J. Dis. Child. 86*: 348–349.

Cohlan, S. Q. (1953b). Excessive intake of vitamin A as a cause of congenital anomalies in the rat. *Science 117*: 535–536.

Cohlan, S. Q., and Stone, S. M. (1961). Effects of dietary and intraperitoneal excess of L-lysine and L-leucine on rat pregnancy and offspring. *J. Nutr. 74*: 93–95.

Cohlan, S. Q., Dancis, J., and Kitay, D. (1964). Vinblastine. *Lancet 1*: 1390.

Collins, T. F. X., Welsh, J. J., Black, T. N., and Collins, E. (1981). A comprehensive study of the teratogenic potential of caffeine given by oral intubation to rats. *Regulat. Toxic. Pharmacol. 1*: 355–378.

Collins, T., Welsh, J., Black, T., Whitby, K., and O'Donnell, M. (1987). Potential reversibility of skeletal effects in rats exposed *in utero* to caffeine. *Food Chem. Tox. 25*: 647–663.

Courtney, K. D., and Valerio, D. A. (1968). Teratology in the *Macaca mulatta*. *Teratology 1*: 163–172.

Covell, W. P. (1936). Cytologic study of effects of drugs on cochlea. *Arch. Otolaryngol. 23*: 633–641.

Crosby, D. G. (1969). Natural toxic background in the food of man and his animals. *J. Agric. Food Chem. 17*: 532–538.

Crowe, M. W. (1969). Skeletal anomalies in pigs associated with tobacco. *Mod. Vet. Pract. 50*: 54–55.

Crowe, M. W., and Swerczek, T. W. (1974). Congenital arthrogryposis in offspring of sows fed tobacco (*Nicotiana tabacum*). *Am. J. Vet. Res. 35*: 1071–1073.

Cullis, J. E. (1962). Congenital deformities and herbal "slimming tablets." *Lancet 2*: 511–512.

Cutter, M. G., and Schneider, R. (1973). Malformations produced in mice and rats by oxidized linoleate. *Food Cosmet. Toxicol. 11*: 935–942.

Czeizel, A. (1988). Reserpine is not a human teratogen. *J. Med. Genet. 25*: 787.

Dattel, B. J. (1990). Substance abuse in pregnancy. *Sem. Perinat. 14*: 179–187.

David, T. J. (1972). Nature and etiology of the Poland anomaly. *N. Engl. J. Med. 287*: 487–489.

Deanesly, R. (1966). The effects of reserpine on ovulation and on the corpus luteum of the guinea-pig. *J. Reprod. Fertil. 11*: 429–438.

DeCosta, C., and Griew, A. R. (1982). Effects of betel chewing on pregnancy outcome. *Aust. NZ. J. Obstet. Gynaecol. 22*: 22–24.

DeMyer, W. (1964). Vinblastine-induced malformations of face and nervous system in two rat strains. *Neurology* (Minneap.) *14*: 806–808.

DeMyer, W. (1965). Cleft lip and jaw induced in fetal rats by vincristine. *Arch. Anat. Pathol.* (Paris) *48*: 181–186.

Didcock, K. A., Picard, C. W., and Robson, J. M. (1952). The action of podophyllotoxin on pregnancy. *J. Physiol.* (London) *117*: 65–66P.

Dunn, H. G., McBurney, A. K., and Ingram, S. (1976). Maternal cigarette smoking during pregnancy and the child's subsequent development: I. Physical growth to age 6-1/2 years. *Can. J. Public Health 67*: 499–505.

Dwornik, J. J., and Moore, K. L. (1967). Congenital anomalies produced in the rat by podophyllin. *Anat. Rec. 157*: 237.

Elmazar, M. M. A., McElhatton, P. R., and Sullivan, F. M. (1982). Studies on the teratogenic effects of different oral preparations of caffeine in mice. *Toxicology 23*: 57–71.

Fantel, A. G., and Macphail, B. J. (1982). The teratogenicity of cocaine. *Teratology 26*: 17–19.

FDA. (1980). Caffeine content of various products. *FDA Talk Paper TX80-45*. FDA, Washington, DC.

Ferm, V. H. (1963a). Colchicine teratogenesis in hamster embryos. *Proc. Soc. Exp. Biol. Med. 112*: 775–778.

Ferm, V. H. (1963b). Congenital malformations in hamster embryos after treatment with vinblastine and vincristine. *Science 141*: 426.

Ferriero, D. M., Partridge, J. C., and Wong, D. F. (1988). Congenital-defects and stroke in cocaine-exposed neonates. *Ann. Neurol. 24*: 348–349.

Finnell, R. H., Toloyan, S., Van Waes, M., and Kolivas, P. W. (1990). Preliminary evidence for a cocaine-induced embryopathy in mice. *Toxicol. Appl. Pharmacol. 103*: 228–237.

Fleig, C. (1908). Influence de la fumee de tabac et de la nicotine sous la developpement de l'organisme. *Compt. Rend. Soc. Biol.* (Paris) *64*: 683–685.

Foss, J. A., and Riley, E. P. (1988). Behavioral evaluation of animals exposed prenatally to cocaine. *Teratology 37*: 517.

Frakes, R. A., Willhite, C. C., and Sharma, R. P. (1984). Teratogenic potential of dietary cassava in the golden hamster. *Toxicologist 4*: 87.

Frakes, R. A., Sharma, R. P., and Willhite, C. C. (1985). Developmental toxicity of the cyanogenic glycoside linamarin in the golden hamster. *Teratology 31*: 241–246.

Frakes, R. A., Sharma, R. P., Willhite, C. C., and Gomez, G. (1986). Effect of cyanogenic glycosides and protein content in cassava diets on hamster prenatal development. *Fund. Appl. Toxicol.* 7: 191–198.

Frank, D. A., Zuckerman, B. S., Amaro, H., Aboagye, K., Bauchner, H., Cabral, H., Fried, L., Hingson, R., Kayne, H., and Levenson, S. M. (1988). Cocaine use during pregnancy—prevalence and correlates. *Pediatrics 82*: 888–895.

Friedman, W. F. (1968). Vitamin D and the supravalvular aortic stenosis syndrome. *Adv. Teratol. 3*: 85–96.

Friedman, W. F., and Roberts, W. C. (1966). Vitamin D and the supravalvar aortic stenosis syndrome. *Circulation 34*: 77–86.

Fritz, H., and Hess, R. (1968). Prenatal development in the rat following administration of cyclamate, saccharin and sucrose. *Experientia 24*: 1140–1141.

Frohberg, H., Gleich, J., and Kieser, H. (1973). Reproduction-toxicologic studies on ascorbic acid in mice and rats. *Arzneim. Forsch. 23*: 1081–1082.

Fujii, T., and Nishimura, H. (1969). Teratogenic actions of some methylated xanthines in mice. *Okajimas Fol. Anat. Jap. 46*: 167–175.

Fujii, T., Sasaki, H., and Nishimura, H. (1969). Teratogenicity of caffeine in mice related to its mode of administration. *Jap. J. Pharmac. 19*: 134–138.

Fulroth, R., Phillips, B., and Durand, D. J. (1989). Perinatal outcome of infants exposed to cocaine and/or heroin *in utero*. *Am. J. Dis. Child. 143*: 905–910.

Fung, Y. K. (1988). Postnatal behavioral-effects of maternal nicotine exposure in rats (technical note). *J. Pharm. Pha. 40*: 870–872.

Garcia, R. E., Friedman, W. F., Kabock, M. M., and Rowe, R. D. (1964). Idiopathic hypercalcemia and supravalvular aortic stenosis: Documentation of a new syndrome. *N. Engl. J. Med. 271*: 117–120.

Geber, W. F. (1967). Congenital malformations induced by mescaline, lysergic acid diethylamide, and bromolysergic acid in the hamster. *Science 158*: 265–267.

Geber, W. F. (1970). Blockade of teratogenic effect of morphine and dihydromorphinone by nalorphine and cyclazocine. *Pharmacologist 12*: 296.

Geber, W. F., and Schramm, L. C. (1969). Teratogenicity of marihuana extract as influenced by plant origin and seasonal variation. *Arch. Int. Pharmacodyn. Ther. 177*: 224–230.

Geber, W. F., and Schramm, L. C. (1975). Congenital malformations of the central nervous system produced by narcotic analgesics in the hamster. *Am. J. Obstet. Gynecol. 123*: 705–713.

George, J. D., Price, C. J., Marr, M. C., and Kimmel, C. A. (1986). Developmental toxicity of theophylline (THEO) in mice and rats. *Teratology 33*: 70–71.

Gilbert, R. M. (1981). Caffeine: Overview and anthology. In *Nutrition and Behavior*, S. A. Miller, ed. Franklin Institute, Philadelphia, pp. 145–166.

Gilbert, R. M. (1984). Caffeine consumption. In *Progress in Clinical and Biological Research*, Vol. 159, *The Methylxanthine Beverages and Foods: Chemistry, Consumption and Health Effects*, G. A. Spiller, ed. Liss, New York, pp. 185–213.

Giroud, A. (1968). Nutrition of the embryo. *Fed. Proc. 27*: 163–184.

Giroud, A., and Martinet, M. (1958). Repercussions de l'hypervitaminose A chez l'embryon de lapin. *C. R. Soc. Biol.* (Paris) *152*: 931–932.

Giroud, A., and Martinet, M. (1959a). Extension a plusieurs especes de mammiferes des malformations embryonnaires par hypervitaminose A. *C. R. Soc. Biol.* (Paris) *153*: 201–202.

Giroud, A., and Martinet, M. (1959b). Teratogenese par hypervitaminose A chez le rat, la souris, le cobaye, et le lapin. *Arch. Fr. Pediatr. 16*: 971–975.

Goldman, A. S., and Yakovac, W. C. (1965). Teratogenic action in rats of reserpine alone and in combination with salicylate and immobilization. *Proc. Soc. Exp. Biol. Med. 118*: 857–862.

Gomez, G., and Valdivieso, M. (1983). The effect of variety and plant age on cyanide content, chemical composition and quality of cassava roots. *Nutr. Rep. Int. 27*: 857–865.

Graham, D. M. (1978). Caffeine: Its identity, dietary sources, intake and biological effects. *Nutr. Rev. 36*: 97–102.

Graham, H. N. (1984a). Tea: The plant and its manufacture; chemistry and consumption of the beverage. In *Progress in Clinical and Biological Research*, Vol. 159, *The Methylxanthine Beverages and Foods: Chemistry, Consumption, and Health Effects*, G. A. Spiller, ed. Liss, New York, pp. 29–74.

Graham, H. N. (1984b). Mate in: *Progress in Clinical and Biological Research*, Vol. 158, *The Methylxanthine Beverages and Foods: Chemistry, Consumption, and Health Effects*, G. A. Spiller, ed. Liss, New York, pp. 179–183.

Grauwiler, J., and Schon, H. (1973). Teratological experiments with ergotamine in mice, rats, and rabbits. *Teratology* 7: 227–236.

Greenland, V. C., Delke, I., and Minkoff, H. L. (1989). Vaginally administered cocaine overdose in a pregnant woman. *Obstet. Gynecol. 74*: 476–477.

Greenwood, S. G. (1979). Warning: cigarette smoking is dangerous to reproductive health. *Fam. Plan. Perspect. 11*: 168–172.

Grilly, D. M., Ferraro, D. P., and Braude, M. C. (1974). Observations on the reproductive activity of chimpanzees following long-term exposure to marihuana. *Pharmacology 11*: 304–307.

Groisser, D. S., Rosso, P., and Winick, M. (1982). Coffee consumption during pregnancy: Subsequent behavioral abnormalities of the offspring. *J. Nutr. 112*: 829–832.

Guillian, G., and Gy, A. (1907). Recherches experimentales sur l'influence de l'intoxication tabagique sur la gestation. *Compt. Rend. Soc. Biol.* (Paris) *63*: 583–584.

Gullberg, E. I., Ferrell, F., and Christensen, H. D. (1986). Effects of postnatal caffeine exposure through dam's milk upon weanling rats. *Pharmacol. Biochem. Behav. 24*: 1695–1701.

Hadeed, A. J., and Siegel, S. R. (1989). Maternal cocaine use during pregnancy—effect on the newborn infant. *Pediat. 84*: 205–210.

Hafiez, A. A. (1974). Prostaglandin E_2 prevents impairment of fertility in rats fed a diet deficient in essential fatty acids. *J. Reprod. Fertil. 38*: 273–286.

Harpel, H. S., and Gautieri, R. F. (1968). Morphine-induced fetal malformations I. Exencephaly and axial skeletal fusions. *J. Pharm. Sci. 57*: 1590–1597.

Harper, M. J. K. (1972). Agents with antifertility effects during preimplantation stages of pregnancy. In *Biology of Mammalian Fertilization and Implantation*, K. S. Moghissi and E. S. E. Hafez, eds. Charles C. Thomas, Springfield, IL, pp. 431–492.

Heinonen, O. P., Slone, D., and Shapiro, S. (1977). *Birth Defects and Drugs in Pregnancy*, Publishing Sciences Group, Littletown, MA.

Hill, R. M., Craig, J. P., Chaney, M. D., Tennyson, L. M., and McCulley, L. B. (1977). Utilization of over-the-counter drugs during pregnancy. *Clin. Obstet. Gynecol. 20*: 381–394.

Hingson, R., Alpert, J. J., Day, N., Dooling, E., Kayne, H., Morelock, S., Oppenheimer, A., and Zuckerman, B. (1982). Effects of maternal drinking and marijuana. *Pediatrics 70*: 539–545.

Hogue, C. J. (1981). Coffee in pregnancy. *Lancet 1*: 554.

Holloway, W. R. (1982). Caffeine: Effects of acute and chronic exposure on the behavior of neonatal rats. *Neurobehav. Toxic. Terat. 4*: 21–32.

Hood, R. D., and Szczech, G. M. (1983). Teratogenicity of fungal toxins and fungal-produced antimicrobial agents. In *Handbook of Natural Toxins*, Vol. 1, A. T. Tu, ed. Marcel Dekker, New York.

Hook, E. B., Healy, K. M., Niles, A. M., and Skalko, R. G. (1974). Vitamin E: Teratogen or anti-teratogen? *Lancet 1*: 809.

Hudson, D. B., and Timiras, P. S. (1972). Nicotine injection during gestation; impairment of reproduction, fetal viability, and development. *Biol. Reprod.* 7: 247–253.

Hume, R. F., O'Donnell, K. J., Stanger, C. L., Killam, A. P., and Gingras, J. L. (1989). *In utero* exposure-observations of fetal behavioral state may predict neonatal outcome. *Am. J. Obstet. Gynecol. 161*: 685–690.

Hurley, L. S. (1980). *Developmental Nutrition*. Prentice Hall, Englewood Cliffs, NJ.

Hurley, L. S. (1985). Report of the workshop on nutrition. *Prog. Clin. Biol. Res. 163b*: 365–368.

Hutchings, D. E., Fico, T. A., and Dow-Edwards, D. L. (1989). Prenatal cocaine-maternal toxicity, fetal effects and locomotor-activity in rat offspring. *Neurotox. Teratol. 11*: 65–69.

Jacobs, R. M. (1971). Failure of muscle relaxants to produce cleft palate in mice. *Teratology 4*: 25–30.

Jago, R. H. (1970). Arthrogryposis following treatment of maternal tetanus with muscle relaxants. *Arch. Dis. Child. 45*: 277–279.

Joneja, M. G., and LeLiever, W. C. (1974). Effects of vinblastine and podophyllin on DBA mouse fetuses. *Toxicol. Appl. Pharmacol. 27*: 408–414.

Kalter, H., and Warkany, J. (1959). Teratogenic action of hypervitaminosis A in strains of inbred mice. *Anat. Rec. 133*: 396–397.

Kanai, T., Nishikawa, T., Satoh, A., and Kajita, A. (1986). Cardiovascular teratogenicity of ephedrine in rats. *Cong. Anom. 26*: 246.

Karnofsky, D. A. (1965). Drugs as teratogens in animals and man. *Ann. Rev. Pharmacol. 5*: 447–472.

Karol, M. D., Conner, C. S., Watanabe, A. S., and Murphrey, K. J. (1980). Podophyllum: Suspected teratogenicity from topical application. *Clin. Toxicol. 16*: 283–286.

Katsilambros, L. (1963). Colchicine in the preventive treatment of the rubella embryopathy. *Arch. Inst. Pasteur Hellen. 9*: 97–99.

Keeler, R. F. (1971). Teratogenic compounds of *Veratrum californicum* (Durand). II. Gestational chronology and compound specificity in rabbits. *Proc. Soc. Exp. Biol. Med. 136*: 1174–1179.

Keeler, R. F. (1973a). Lupin alkaloids from teratogenic and nonteratogenic lupins. I. Correlation of crooked calf disease incidence with alkaloid distribution determined by gas chromatography. *Teratology 7*: 23–30.

Keeler, R. F. (1973b). Lupin alkaloids from teratogenic and nonteratogenic lupins. II. Identification of the major alkaloids by tandem gas chromatography-mass spectrometry in plants producing crooked calf disease. *Teratology 7*: 31–36.

Keeler, R. F. (1976). Lupin alkaloids from teratogenic and nonteratogenic lupins. III. Identification of anagyrine as the probable teratogen by feeding trials. *J. Toxicol. Environ. Health 1*: 887–898.

Keeler, R. F. (1980). Congenital defects in calves from maternal ingestion of *Nicotiana glauca* of high anabasine content. *Clin. Toxicol. 15*: 417–426.

Keeler, R. F. (1983). Naturally occurring teratogens from plants. In *Handbook of Natural Toxins*, Vol. 1, A. T. Tu, ed. Marcel Dekker, New York.

Keeler, R. F., and Crowe, M. W. (1981). Congenital deformities in livestock induced by maternal *Nicotiana* ingestion. *Teratology 23*: 44A.

Keeler, R. F., and Crowe, M. W. (1983). Congenital deformities in swine induced by wild tree tobacco, *Nicotiana glauca. Toxicology 20*: 47–58.

Keeler, R. F., Balls, L. D., and Ponter, K. (1981). Teratogenic effects of *Nicotiana glauca* and concentration of anabasine, the suspect teratogen in plant parts. *Cornell Vet. 71*: 47–53.

Keeler, R. F., Crowe, M. W., and Lambert, E. A. (1984). Teratogenicity in swine of the tobacco alkaloid anabasine isolated from *Nicotiana glauca. Teratology 30*: 61–69.

Kehl, R., Audibert, A., Gage, G., and Amarger, J. (1956). Action de la reserpine a differentes periodes de la gestation chez la lapine. *C. R. Soc. Biol.* (Paris) *150*: 2196–2199.

Keith, L. G., MacGregor, S., Friedell, S., Rosner, M., Chasnoff, I. J., and Sciarra, J. J. (1989). Substance abuse in pregnant women—recent experience at the Perinatal Center for Chemical-Dependence of Northwestern Memorial Hospital. *Obstet. Gynecol. 73*: 715–720.

Kerr, G. R., Chamove, A. S., Harlow, H. F., and Waisman, H. A. (1968). "Fetal PKU": The effect of maternal hyperphenylalaninemia during pregnancy in the rhesus monkey (*Macaca mulatta*). *Pediatrics 42*: 27–36.

Khera, K. S. (1973). Teratogenic effects of methylmercury in the cat; note on the use of this species as a model for teratogenicity studies. *Teratology 8*: 293–304.

Khera, K. S. (1975). Teratogenicity studies in rats given high doses of pyridoxine (vitamin B6) during organogenesis. *Experientia 31*: 469–470.

Khera, K. S., and McKinley, W. P. (1972). Pre- and postnatal studies on 2,4,5-trichlorophenoxyacetic acid, 2,4-dichlorophenoxyacetic acid, and their derivatives in rats. *Toxicol. Appl. Pharmacol. 22*: 14–28.

Kilgore, W. W., Crosby, D. G., Craigmill, A. L., and Poppen, N. K. (1981). Toxic plants as possible human teratogens. *Calf. Agric. 35*: 11–12.

Kimmel, C. A., Price, C. J., Sadler, B. M., Tyle, R. W., and Gerling, F. S. (1985). Comparison of distilled water and corn oil vehicle controls from historical teratology study data. *Toxicologist 5*: 185.

Kitchin, K. T., and Di Stefano, V. (1976). L-dopa and brown fat hemorrhage in the rat pup. *Toxicol. Appl. Pharmacol. 38*: 251–263.

Kizer, K. W., Fan, A. M., Bankowaska, J., Jackson, R. J., and Lyman, D. O. (1990). Vitamin A—a pregnancy hazard alert. *West. J. Med. 152*: 78–81.

Klosovskii, B. N. (1963). *The Development of the Brain and Its Disturbance by Harmful Factors*. MacMillan, New York.

Klotzsche, C. (1969). Teratogenic and embryotoxic effects of cyclamate, saccharin, and saccharose. *Arzneim. Forsch. 19*: 925–928.

Kronick, J. B., Whelan, D. T., and McCallion, D. T. (1987). Experimental hyperphenylalaninemia in the pregnant guinea pig, possible phenylalanine teratogenesis and p-chlophenylalanine embryotoxicity. *Teratology 36*: 245–258.

Kropp, B. N., and Forward, R. B. (1963). The effect of pilocarpine on teeth and salivary glands in the rat embryo. *Anat. Rec. 145*: 250–251.

Landy, H. J., and Hinson, J. (1988). Placental absorption associated with cocaine use: Case report. *Reprod. Toxicol. 1*: 203–205.

Lehmann, V. H. (1976). Teratologic studies in rabbits and rats with the morphine derivative codeine. *Arneim. Forsch. 26*: 551–554.

Leist, K. H., and Grauwiler, J. (1974). Ergometrine and uteroplacental blood supply in pregnant rats. *Teratology 10*: 316.

Linn, S., Schoenbaum, S. C., Monson, R. R., Rosner, R., Stubblefield, P. C., and Ryan, K. J. (1983). The association of marijuana use with outcome of pregnancy. *Am. J. Public Health 73*: 1161–1164.

Little, B. B., Snell, L. M., Klein, V. R., and Gilstrap, L. C. (1989). Cocaine abuse during pregnancy—maternal and fetal implications. *Obstet. Gynecol. 73*: 157–160.

Longo, L. D. (1982). Some health consequences of maternal smoking: Issues without answers. *Birth Defects 18*: 13–31.

Lorke, D. (1969). Investigations into the embryotoxic and teratogenic action of cyclamate and saccharin in the mouse. *Arzneim. Forsch. 19*: 920–922.

Luse, S. A., Rhys, A., and Lessey, R. (1970). Effects of maternal phenylketonuria on the rat fetus. *Am. J. Obstet. Gynecol. 108*: 387–390.

MacGregor, S., Keith, L., Chasnoff, I., Rosner, M., Chisum, G., Shaw, P., and Minogue, J. (1987). Cocaine use during pregnancy: Adverse perinatal outcome. *Am. J. Obstet. Gynecol. 157*: 686–697.

Maeda, T. (1937). Experimental studies on the malformation of eye by administration of fat. *Nisson Igaku 26*: 1935–1958.

Maeda, H., and Yasuda, M. (1979). Induction of digital malformations in rat fetuses by combined administration of papaverine hydrochloride and atropine sulfate. *Teratology 20*: 157.

Mahalik, M. P., Gautieri, R. F., and Mann, D. E (1980). Teratogenic potential of cocaine hydrochloride in CF-1 mice. *J. Pharm. Sci. 69*: 703–706.

Makita, T., Kato, M., Matuzawa, K., Ojima, N., Hasimoto, Y., and Noguchi, T. (1977). Safety evaluation studies on the hormonal form of vitamin D3. III. Teratogenicity in rabbits by oral administration. *Iyakuhin Kenkyu 8*: 615–624.

Malakhovsky, V. G. (1969). Behavioral disturbances in rats receiving teratogenic agents antenatally. *Biull. Eksp. Biol. Med. 68*: 1230–1232.

Maren, T. H., and Ellison, A. C. (1972). The teratological effect of benzolamide, a new carbonic anhydrase inhibitor. *Johns Hopkins Med. J. 130*: 116–123.

Marin-Padilla, M., and Ferm, V. H. (1965). Somite necrosis and developmental malformations induced by vitamin A in the golden hamster. *J. Embryol. Exp. Morphol. 13*: 1–8.

Martin, J. C., and Becker, R. F. (1970). The effects of nicotine administration *in utero* upon activity in the rat. *Psychon. Sci. 19*: 59–60.

Martin, M. P., Bridgforth, E., McGanity, W. J., and Darby, W. J. (1957). The Vanderbilt cooperative study of maternal and infant nutrition X. Ascorbic acid. *J. Nutr. 62*: 201–224.

McClain, R. M., Hoar, R. M., and Pfitzer, E. A. (1978). Reproduction studies with calcitrol (dihydroxyvitamin D3). *Toxicol. Appl. Pharmacol. 45*: 242.

Menges, R. W., Selby, L. A., Marienfeld, C. J., Aue, W. A., and Greer, D. L. (1970). A tobacco related epidemic of congenital limb deformities in swine. *Environ. Res. 3*: 285–302.

Meyer, J., Jonas, B. S., and Tonascia, J. A. (1976). Perinatal events associated with maternal smoking during pregnancy. *Am. J. Epidemiol. 103*: 464–476.

Meyer, M. B., and Tonascia, J. A. (1977). Maternal smoking, pregnancy complications, and perinatal mortality. *Am. J. Obstet. Gynecol. 128*: 494–592.

Meyer, M. B., Tonascia, J. A., and Buck, C. (1975). The interrelationship of maternal smoking and increased perinatal mortality with other risk factors; further analysis of the Ontario perinatal mortality study, 1960–1961. *Am. J. Epid. 100*: 443–451.

Miller, H. C., Hasseinein, K., and Hensleigh, P. A. (1976). Fetal growth retardation in relation to maternal smoking and weight gain in pregnancy. *Am. J. Obstet. Gynecol. 125*: 55–60.

Moghissi, K. S. (1981). Risks and benefits of nutritional supplements during pregnancy. *Obstet. Gynecol. 58*: 68–78S.

Momose, Y., Akiyoski, S., Mori, K., Nishimura, N., Fujishima, H., Imaizumi, S., and Agata, I. (1972). On teratogenicity of vitamin E. Reports from the Dept. of Anatomy. *Mie Perfectual Univ. School of Medicine 20*: 27–35.

Montgomery, R. D. (1965). The medical significance of cyanogen in plant foodstuffs. *Am. J. Clin. Nutr. 17*: 103–113.

Morris, J. M. (1970). Postcoital antifertility agents and their teratogenic effect. *Contraception 2*: 85–97.

Morriss, G. M. (1976). Vitamin A and congenital malformations. *Int. J. Vitam. Nutr. Res. 46*: 220–222.

Naeye, R. L., and Peters, E. C. (1984). Mental development of children whose mothers smoked during pregnancy. *Obstet. Gynecol. 64*: 60–107.

Nandi, B. K., Majumder, A. K., Subramanian, N., and Chatterjee, I. B. (1973). Effects of large doses of vitamin C in guinea pigs and rats. *J. Nutr. 103*: 1688–1695.

Navarrete, V. N., Torres, I. H., Rivera, I. R., Shor, V. P., and Gracia, P. M. (1967). Maternal carbohydrate disorder and congenital malformations. *Diabetes 16*: 127–130.

Neerhof, M. G., MacGregor, S. N., Retzky, S. S., and Sullivan, T. P. (1989). Cocaine abuse during pregnancy—peripartum prevalence and perinatal outcome. *Am. J. Obst. Gynecol. 161*: 633–638.

Neiburg, P., Marks, J. S., McLaren, N. M., and Remington, P. L. (1985). The fetal tobacco syndrome. *JAMA 253*: 2998–2999.

Nelson, M. M., and Evans, H. M. (1953). Relation of dietary protein levels to reproduction in the rat. *J. Nutr. 51*: 71–84.

Neubert, D., and Dillmann, I. (1972). Embryotoxic effects of mice treated with 2,4,5-trichlorophenoxyacetic acid and 2,3,7,8-tetrachlorodibenzo-p-dioxin. *Naunyn Schmiedebergs Arch. Pharmakol. 272*: 243–264.

Neuweiler, W., and Richter, R. H. H. (1964). In *Medikamentose Pathogenese fetaler Missbildungen*, T. Koller, H. Erv, eds. Karger, Basel, pp. 47–79.

Newberne, P. M. (1963). Effect of vitamin B12 deficiency and excess on the embryonic development of the rat. *Am. J. Vet. Res. 24*: 1304–1312.

Nishimura, H., and Nakai, K. (1958). Developmental anomalies in offspring of pregnant mice treated with nicotine. *Science 127*: 877–878.

Nishimura, H., and Nakai, K. (1960). Congenital malformations in offspring of mice treated with caffeine. *Proc. Soc. Exp. Biol. Med 104*: 140–142.

Nishimura, H., and Tanimura, T. (1976). *Clinical Aspects of the Teratogenicity of Drugs*. Excerpta Medica, American Elsevier Publishing Co., New York.

Nolen, G. A. (1981). The effect of brewed and instant coffee on reproduction and teratogenesis in the rat. *Toxic. Appl. Pharmac. 58*: 171–183.

Nolen, G. A. (1989). The developmental toxicology of caffeine. In *Issues and Reviews in Teratology*, Vol. 4. H. Kalter, ed. Plenum, New York, pp. 305–350.

NSDA (National Soft Drink Association). (1982). *What's in Soft Drinks*, 2nd ed., Washington, DC.

Ornoy, A., Kaspi, T., and Nebel, L. (1972). Persistent defects of bone formation in young rats following maternal hypervitaminosis D. *Israel J. Med. Sci. 8*: 943–949.

Ortega, J. A., and Lazerson, J. (1987). Anagyrine-induced red cell aplasia, vascular anomaly, and skeletal dysplasia. *J. Pediatr. 111*: 87–89.

Oshima, Y., Morita, H., Kanno, Y., and Tachizawa, H. (1966). Biological studies on pantethine. III. Teratogenic effects of pantethine in the experimental animal. *Bitamin. 34*: 32–36.

Ottolenghi, A. D., Haseman, J. K., and Suggs, F. (1974). Teratogenic effects of aldrin, dieldlrin, and endrin in hamsters and mice. *Teratology 9*: 11–16.

Palludan, B. (1966). Swine in teratological research. In *Swine in Biomedical Research*. L. K. Bustad and R. O. McClellan, eds. Battelle Mem. Inst., Columbus, OH, pp. 51–78.

Pauli, R. M., and Pettersen, B. J. (1986). Is reserpine a human teratogen? *J. Med. Genet. 23*: 267–268.

Peeden, J. N., Wilroy, R. S., and Soper, R. G. (1979). Prune perineum. *Teratology 20*: 233–236.

Persaud, T. V. N. (1967). Foetal abnormalities caused by the active principle of the fruit of *Blighia sapida* (Ackee). *W. Indian Med. J. 16*: 193–197.

Persaud, T. V. N. (1971). Mechanism of teratogenic action of hypoglycin-A. *Experientia 27*: 414.

Persaud, T. V. (1972). Effects of intra-amniotic administration of hypoglycin B on fetal development in the rat. *Exp. Pathol.* (Jena) *6*: 55–58.

Persaud, T. V. N., and Ellington, A. C. (1967). Cannabis in early pregnancy. *Lancet 2*: 1306.

Persaud, T. V. N., and Ellington, A. C. (1968). The effects of *Cannabis sativa L.* (Ganja) on developing rat embryos. Preliminary observations. *W. Indian Med. J. 17*: 232–234.

Persaud, T. V. N., and Kaplan, S. (1970). The effects of hypoglycin A, a leucine analog, on the development of rat and chick embryos. *Life Sci. 9*: 1305–1313.

Peruzzi, G., Lombardelli, G., Abbracchio, M. P., Coen, E., and Cattabeni, F. (1985). Perinatal caffeine treatment: Behavioral and biochemical effects in rats before weaning. *Neurobehav. Toxic. Terat. 7*: 453–460.

Pfeiffer, C. C., and Barnes, B. (1981). Role of zinc, manganese, chromium, and vitamin deficiencies in birth defects. *Int. J. Environ. Stud. 17*: 43–56.

Pieters, J. J. (1985). Nutritional teratogens: a survey of epidemiological literature. *Prog. Clin. Biol. Res. 163b*: 419–429.

Poswillo, D. E., Sopher, D., and Mitchell, S. (1972). Experimental induction of foetal malformation with "blighted" potato: a preliminary report. *Nature 239*: 462–464.

Poswillo, D. E., Sopher, D., Mitchell, S. J., Coxon, D. T., Curtis, R. F., and Price, K. R. (1973). Further investigations into the teratogenic potential of imperfect potatoes. *Nature 244*: 367–368.

Price, C. J., George, J. D., Sadler, B. M., Marr, M. C., Kimmel, C. A., Schwetz, B. A., and Morrissey, R. E. (1989). Teratologic evaluation of corn oil (CO) or distilled water (DW) in CD-1 mice and CD rats. *Toxicologist 9*: 269.

Raye, J. R., Dubin, J. W., and Blechner, J. N. (1977). Fetal growth retardation following maternal morphine administratoin: Nutritional or drug effect? *Biol. Neonate 32*: 222–228.

Renwick, J. H. (1972). Spina bifida, anencephaly, and potato blight. *Lancet 2*: 967–968.

Renwick, J. J. (1982). Food and malformation. *Practitioner 226*: 1947–1953.

Report of the Surgeon General, Dept. of Health and Human Services (1983). *The Health Consequences of Smoking for Women*. Publication 410-889/1284, Washington, D.C., pp. 191–249.

Rhodes, M. E. (1979). The "natural" food myth. *The Sciences*, May/June 1979.

Roberts, H. R., and Barone, J. J. (1983). Caffeine: History and use. *Food Tech. 37*: 32–39.

Rosa, F. W., Wilk, A. L., and Kelsey, F. O. (1986). Teratogen update: Vitamin A congeners. *Teratology 33*: 355–364.

Rosenweig, A. I., Crews, Q. E., and Hopwood, H. G. (1964). Vinblastine sulfate in Hodgkins disease in pregnancy. *Ann. Intern. Med. 61*: 108–112.

Rush, D., and Kass, E. H. (1972). Maternal smoking: A reassessment of the association with perinatal mortality. *Am. J. Epidemiol. 96*: 183–196.

Ryabchenko, V. P. (1982). Effect of anabasine hydrochloride on the embryogenesis of white rats and rabbits. *Farmakol. Toksikol. 45*: 87–90.

Savini, E. C., Moulin, M. A., and Herrou, M. F. (1971). Experimental study of the effects of quinine on the fetus of rats, rabbits, and dogs. *Therapie 26*: 563–574.

Schardein, J. L. (1985). *Chemically Induced Birth Defects*. Marcel Dekker, New York.

Schardein, J. L., and Keller, K. A. (1989). Potential human developmental toxicants and the role of animal testing in their identification and characterization. *CRC Crit. Rev. Toxicol. 19*: 251–339.

Schlack, L., Salinas, A., Lopez, A., and Trabucco, E. (1970). Effects of high levels of l-tyrosine upon neural tube closure. *J. Pediat. 77*: 716.

Selby, L. A., Menges, R. W., Houser, E. C., Flatt, R. E., and Case, A. A. (1971). Outbreak of swine malformations associated with the wild black cherry, *Prunus serotina. Arch Environ. Health 22*: 496–501.

Select Committee on GRAS Substances (1978). *Evaluation of the Health Aspects of Caffeine as a Food Ingredient*, SCOGS-89, FASEB, Bethesda, NTIS NO. PB 283-441/AS.

Seta, S. (1931). Effect of maternal nutrition during pregnancy on the skeletal development of the fetus. *Nisshin Igahu 21*: 486–504.

Sharma, S. N., Kamboj, V. P., and Kar, A. B. (1972). Anti-implantation effect of dihydrotachysterol and calciferol in rats. *Curr. Sci. 41*: 181–182.

Shoji, R., and Makino, S. (1966). Preliminary notes on the teratogenic and embryocidal effects of colchicine on mouse embryos. *Proc. Jap. Acad. 42*: 822–827.

Shoro, A. A. (1977). Intra-uterine growth retardation and limb deformities produced by neuromuscular blocking agents in the rat fetus. *J. Anat. 123*: 341–350.

Shupe, J. L., Binns, W., James, L. F., and Keeler, R. F. (1967). Lupine, a cause of crooked calf disease. *J. Am. Vet. Med. Assoc. 151*: 198–203.

Sieber, S. M., Whang-Peng, J., Botkin, C., and Knutsen, T. (1978). Teratogenic and cytogenic effects of some plant derived antitumor agents (vincristine, colchicine, maytansine, VP-16-213 and VM-26) in mice. *Teratology 18*: 31–48.

Singh, J. D. (1981). The teratogenic effects of dietary cassava on the pregnant albino rat: A preliminary report. *Teratology 24*: 289–291.

Sinton, C. M. (1989). Preliminary indications that functional effects of fetal caffeine exposure can be expressed in a second generation. *Neurotoxicol. Teratol. 11*: 357–362.

Smith, R. F., Mattran, K. M., Kurkjian, M. F., and Kurtz, S. L. (1989). Alterations in offspring behavior induced by chronic prenatal cocaine dosing. *Neurotox. Teratol. 11*: 35–38.

Sobotka, T. J., Spaid, S. L., and Brodie, R. E. (1979). Neurobehavioral teratology of caffeine exposure in rats. *Neurotoxicology 1*: 403–416.

Spiller, M. A. (1984). The chemical components of coffee. In *Progress in Clinical and Biological Research*, Vol. 158, *The Methylxanthine Beverage and Foods: Chemistry, Consumption and Health Effects*, G. A. Spiller, ed. Liss, New York, pp. 91–147.

Stange, L., Carlstrom, K., and Erikkson, M. (1978). Hypervitaminosis A in early human pregnancy and malformations of the central nervous system. *Acta Obstet. Gynecol. Scand. 57*: 289-291.

Stein, Z. A., and Susser, M. (1984). Intrauterine growth retardation: Epidemiological issues and public health significance. *Semin. Perinatol. 8*: 5–14.

Sumi, T. (1960). Experimental studies on the congenital hydrocephalus due to excessive sugar. *J. Osaka City Med. Cent. 9*: 351–359.

Szabo, K. T., and Kang, Y. J. (1969). Comparative teratogenic studies with various therapeutic agents in mice and rabbits. *Teratology 2*: 270.

Szabo, K. T., Free, S. M., Birkhead, H. A., Kang, Y. J., Alston, E., and Henry, M. (1971). The embryotoxic and teratogenic effects of various agents in the fetal mouse and rabbit. *Toxicol. Appl. Pharmacol. 19*: 371–372.

Tanase, H., and Suzuki, Y. (1967). Teratogenic effect of podophyllotoxin derivate (SP-1). Report 1. Effects upon rat embryos. *Congenital Anomalies 7*: 61.

Tanimura, T., and Lee, S. (1972). Discussions on the suspected teratogenicity of quinine to humans. *Teratology 6*: 122.

Tarka, S. M. (1982). The toxicology of cocoa and methylxanthines: A review of the literature. *CRC Crit. Rev. Toxic. 9*: 275–312.

Tarka, S., Applebaum, R., and Borzelleca, J. (1986a). Evaluation of the teratogenic potential of cocoa and theobromine in New Zealand White rabbits. *Food Chem. Toxicol. 24*: 363–374.

Tarka, S., Applebaum, R., and Borzelleca, J. (1986b). Evaluation of the perinatal, postnatal and teratogenic effects of cocoa powder and theobromine in Sprague-Dawley/CD rats. *Food Chem. Toxicol. 24*: 375–382.

Telford, I. R., Woodruff, C. S., and Linford, R. H. (1962). Fetal resorption in the rat as influenced by certain antioxidants. *Am. J. Anat. 110*: 29–36.

Teratology Society Position Paper (1987). Guest editorial: Vitamin A during pregnancy. *Teratology 35*: 267–268.

Thiersch, J.B. (1963). Effect of podophyllin (P) and podophyllotoxin (PT) on the rat litter *in utero*. *Proc. Soc. Exp. Biol. Med. 113*: 124–127.

Tucci, S. M., and Skalko, R. G. (1978). The teratogenic effects of theophylline in mice. *Toxicol. Lett. 1*: 337–341.

VanDyke, J. H., and Ritchey, M. G. (1947). Colchicine influence during embryonic development in rats. *Anat. Rec. 97*: 375.

Vara, P., and Kinnunen, O. (1951). Effect of nicotine on the female rabbit and developing fetus. *Ann. Med. Exp. Biol. Fenn. 29*: 202–213.

Viau, A. T., and Leathem, J. H. (1973). Excess dietary methionine and pregnancy in the rat. *J. Reprod. Fertil. 33*: 109–111.

Vobecky, J. S., Vobecky, J., Shapcott, D., Blanchard, R., Lafond, R., Cloutier, D., and Munan, L. (1974). Serum alpha-tocopherol in pregnancies with normal or pathological outcomes. *Can. J. Physiol. Pharmacol. 52*: 384–388.

Von Lennep, E., El Khazen, N., DePierreau, A., Rodesh, F., and Van Regemorter, N. (1985). A case of partial sirenomelia and possible vitamin A teratogenesis. *Prenatal Diag. 5*: 35–40.

Warren, M. P. (1983). Effects of undernutrition on reproductive function in the human. *Endocr. Rev. 4*: 363–377.

Werler, M. M., Rosenberg, L., and Mitchell, A. A. (1989). First trimester vitamin A use in relation to birth defects. *Teratology 39*: 489.

Wiersig, D. O., and Swenson, M. J. (1967). Teratogenicity of vitamin A in the canine. *Fed. Proc. 26*: 486.

Wiesner, B. P., Wolfe, M., and Yudkin, J. (1958). The effects of some antimitotic compounds on pregnancy in the mouse. *Stud. Fertil. 9*: 129–136.

Wilcox, A. (1989). Caffeinated beverages and decreased fertility. *Lancet 1*: 840.

Wilcox, A., Weinberg, C., and Baird, D. (1988). Caffeinated beverages and decreased fertility. *Lancet 2*: 1453–1456.

Willhite, C. C. (1982). Congenital malformations induced by Laetrile. *Science 215*: 1513–1515.

Wilson, J. G. (1971). Use of rhesus monkeys in teratological studies. *Fed. Proc. 30*: 104–109.

Witter, F. R., and Niebyl, J. R. (1990). Marijuana use in pregnancy and pregnancy outcome. *Am. J. Perinatol. 7*: 36–38.

Wyngaard, J. B. (1989). Caffeine may be associated with reduced fertility. *JAMA 261*: 1864.

Yanagimoto, Y., Niii, N., Fujii, Y., Murakami, H., Matsuda, M., Yamamoto, E., Sano, Y., Yamazaki, K., Takao, S., Hara, H., and Watanabe, M. (1983). Effects of egg white hydrolysate on reproduction. *Clin. Rep. 17*: 3894–3903.

Yu, J. F., Yang, Y. S., Wang, W. Y., Xiong, G. X., and Chen, M. S. (1988). Mutagenicity and teratogenicity of chlorpromazine and scopolamine. *Chin. Med. J. 101*: 339–345.

Zane, C. E. (1976). Assessment of hypervitaminosis D during the first trimester of pregnancy on the mouse embryo. Preliminary report. *Arzneim. Forsch. 26*: 1589–1590.

Zellers, J. E. (1979). Influence of atropine and diphenhydramine on the teratogenic capability of codeine in CF-1 mice. *Dissert. Abst. Int. B. 39*: 870.

Zellers, J. E., and Gautieri, R. F. (1977). Evaluation of teratogenic potential of codeine sulfate in CF-1 mice. *J. Pharm. Sci. 66*: 1727–1731.

Zilva, S. S., Golding, J., Drummond, J. C., and Coward, K. H. (1921). The relation of the fat-soluble factor to rickets and growth in pigs. *Biochem. J. 15*: 427–437.

Zoumas, B. L., Kreiser, W. R., and Martin, R. A. (1980). Theobromine and caffeine content of chocolate products. *J. Food Sci. 45*: 314–316.

Zuckerman, B., Frank, D. A., Hingson, R., Amaro, H., Levenson, S. M., Kayne, H., Parker, S., Vinci, R., Aboagye, K., Fried, L. E., Cabral, H., Trimperi, R., and Bauchner, H. (1989). Effects of maternal marijuana and cocaine use on fetal growth. *N. Engl. J. Med. 320*: 762–768.

VIII

ANTIBIOTICS

19

Antibiotic Residues in Foods

Irtaza H. Siddique

Tuskegee University, Tuskegee, Alabama

I. INTRODUCTION

Many sulfonamides and antibiotics have had profound effects and impacts on the life and health of human beings as well as animals. The use of sulfonamides and antibiotics over the years has made it possible to successfully treat and alleviate the effects of many diseases. Their development, wide use in the treatment and prevention of disease, growth promotion and feed efficiency in livestock, pig, veal, fish, and poultry production during the past 50 or more years has been described extensively in the scientific literature (Anderson et al., 1952; Weinstein et al., 1960; Siddique, 1983; Nichols and Keys, 1984). The challenges of population growth have led to increased efforts to find resources to enhance animal food production to its maximum by employing all available means known to scientists. It has been claimed by the Council for Agricultural Science and Technology that without the use of antibiotics in food animals, the efficiency of weight gains will be reduced and the methods of raising animals would become less efficient.

In recent years, public health concern over different aspects of drug use in veterinary medicine and the presence of drug residues in foods of animal origin has grown rapidly. In addition to antibiotics, many other chemicals are used in animal husbandry that may be transferred to food products of animal origin (Huber, 1971). This chapter shall focus on a discussion of the use and effects of important sulfonamides and antibiotics as they relate to medical and veterinary practice.

II. THERAPEUTIC USE OF ANTIMICROBIAL DRUGS IN ANIMALS

In a report by a joint Food and Agriculture Organization/World Health Organization (FAO/WHO, 1984) expert consultation committee, the term "veterinary drug" was defined as any substance applied or administered to any food-producing animal, such as meat- or milk-producing animals, poultry, fish, or bees, whether used for therapeutic, prophylactic, or diagnostic purposes or for modification of physiological functions, and for prevention and treatment of diseases in food-producing animals. Sulfonamides and modern antibiotics are widely used for the treatment of many localized and generalized infections in animals. However, the search for newer and better drugs for use on entire herds or flocks of animals that can be administered through feedstuffs or drinking water is a continuous process. It is estimated that over 100 million kg of these drugs are being used worldwide annually (Steele and Beran, 1984). The impact of these vast amounts of drugs on human and on animal health, agriculture, ecology, and the environment are exceedingly important as they often lead to potential drug residues in foods and the environment.

III. SUBTHERAPEUTIC USE OF ANTIMICROBIAL DRUGS IN ANIMALS

The administration of sulfonamides, principally sulfamethazine and sulfathiozole, and antibiotics such as tetracyclines, penicillin, virginiamycin, and tylosin, in subtherapeutic doses to livestock through feed and/or water is well described in the literature (Nichols and Keys, 1984). These drugs exert their effects on animals in at least four different ways: (1) direct growth promotion, (2) metabolic activity, (3) nutrient sparing effect, and (4) disease control. The antibiotics thus not only help increase the rate of weight gain and improve feed efficiency, but also prevent many potential diseases in animals.

A. Growth Promotion

Antibiotics, e.g., penicillin, inhibit the growth of many gram-positive organisms, which consequently leads to development of increased numbers of *Escherichia coli* and other intestinal bacterial flora that play an important role in the synthesis of essential vitamins and amino acids. As animals are given antimicrobial drugs in feeds on a continuous basis, their intestinal wall structures become thinner and more absorptive. Because of this, these drugs are employed mainly to improve and contribute to the production of beef, lamb, poultry, and pork (Steele and Beran, 1984).

B. Metabolic Effect

There is evidence to suggest that antibiotics contribute to modification of metabolic reactions. For example, tetracyclines have been shown to affect water and nitrogen excretion (Steele and Beran, 1984). Detailed information on metabolic activity has been evaluated and documented by other workers (Huber, 1971; Mandell and Sande, 1985a).

C. Nutrient-Sparing Effect

Antimicrobial drugs have nutrient-sparing effects and act by depressing microorganisms in the intestinal flora which compete with the host animals for essential nutrients, thereby increasing the availability of nutrients through chelation and/or by increasing absorption from the digestive tract (Steele and Beran, 1984).

D. Disease Prevention

The effects of subtherapeutic feeding of antimicrobial drugs are very pronounced. This response is greater in animals in contaminated environments or in those previously used in live-stock production. Tetracyclines in feedlot cattle have been shown to reduce the incidence of liver abscesses from over 50% to about 18% with an increase in marketing weight. Similar studies have indicated increase in weight gains and feed efficiency in other species of food animals. In the United States, nearly 100% of chickens and turkeys, 90% of swine and veal calves, and 60% of beef cattle receive rations containing antimicrobial drugs during at least some part of their growth periods (Steele and Beran, 1984).

IV. ADVERSE REACTIONS TO SULFONAMIDES

The sulfonamide drugs were the first effective chemotherapeutic agents to be employed systemically for the prevention and cure of bacterial infections in people. Later, the sulfonamides were used therapeutically in veterinary practice and subsequently used extensively at subtherapeutic levels in feed in the practice of animal husbandry (FAO/WHO, 1984). The adverse reactions of people following consumption of meat and poultry with sulfa residues are numerous and varied, and the overall incidence of such reactions is about 5%.

A. Hypersensitivity Reactions

Sensitivity reactions may involve the skin and mucous membrane in the form of and including urticaria, petechial rashes, exfoliative dermatitis, and photosensitivity. The dermal effects was about 1.5% with sulfadiazine therapy and about 2% with sulfisoxazole. In previously sensitized persons, immediate reactions of the anaphylactoid type have been observed. Serum sickness, which sometimes appears following sulfonamide therapy, may be accompanied by fever, joint pain, conjunctivitis, bronchospasm, and urticarial eruptions. In previously sensitized individuals particularly, the drug fever occurs in about 3% of cases with sulfisoxazole (Weinstein et al., 1960; Mandell and Sande, 1985).

B. Development of Bacterial Resistance to Sulfonamides

It is reported that bacteria develop resistance to sulfonamides in vitro and in vivo by random mutation and selection or by transfer of resistance by plasmids. Studies performed to date indicate that the resistance so developed is usually irreversible and thus limits the full effectiveness of sulfonamides as therapeutic agents.

C. Effects of Sulfonamides on the Hematopoietic System

Sulfonamide therapy has occasionally resulted in acute hemolytic anemia. Also, there is a marked decrease in erythrocyte and hemoglobin levels, leukocytosis, reticulocytosis, bilirubinemia, and hemoglobinuria, which may be followed by acute renal tubular necrosis (Weinstein et al., 1960).

D. Other Effects of Sulfonamides

Other reactions to sulfonamides include goiter and hypothyroidism, arthritis, and various neuro-psychiatric disturbances. Focal or diffuse necrosis of the liver due to direct toxicity or sensitization also occurs in less than 0.1% of patients. Experimentally, sulfamethazine has reportedly produced follicular cell adenomas of the thyroid glands in rats and mice (Mandell and Sande, 1985a).

V. ADVERSE EFFECTS OF ANTIBIOTICS

Following the use of antibiotics, their residues will, at some level, be present in edible products of treated animals. Such products, when consumed, may be hazardous to human health (Caldwell and Cliff, 1974) (Figs. 1 and 2, Table 1). These hazardous manifestations can be classified into the following categories.

A. Development of Resistance by Microorganisms

The resistance of pathogenic microorganisms to antimicrobial agents and their transmission to humans is one of the most important issues and concerns of contemporary drug therapy, which merits our serious attention. Venkateswaran isolated antibiotic-resistant salmonella from raw meat and other food samples that had multiple drug resistance (Venkateswaran et al., 1988). In another outbreak of salmonella in 1985, the isolated strain was found to be resistant to tetracycline, erythromycin, clindamycin, sulfisoxazole, sulfadiazine, triple sulfa, cefoperazone, streptomycin, mezlocillin, piperacillin, carbenicillin, penicillin, ampicillin, and kanamycin (Schuman et al., 1989).

In a similar study (Vecht et al., 1989) the antibiotic-resistant *Staphylococcus aureus* was isolated from milk and meat of slaughtered animals and wounds of slaughterhouse workers. It has been suggested that these highly resistant organisms can be transmitted to humans directly or through food prepared under unsanitary conditions. Experimental studies conducted by Corpet (1987) showed that continuous administration of small doses of ampicillin and chlortetracycline in gnotobiotic mice resulted in resistant *E. coli*.

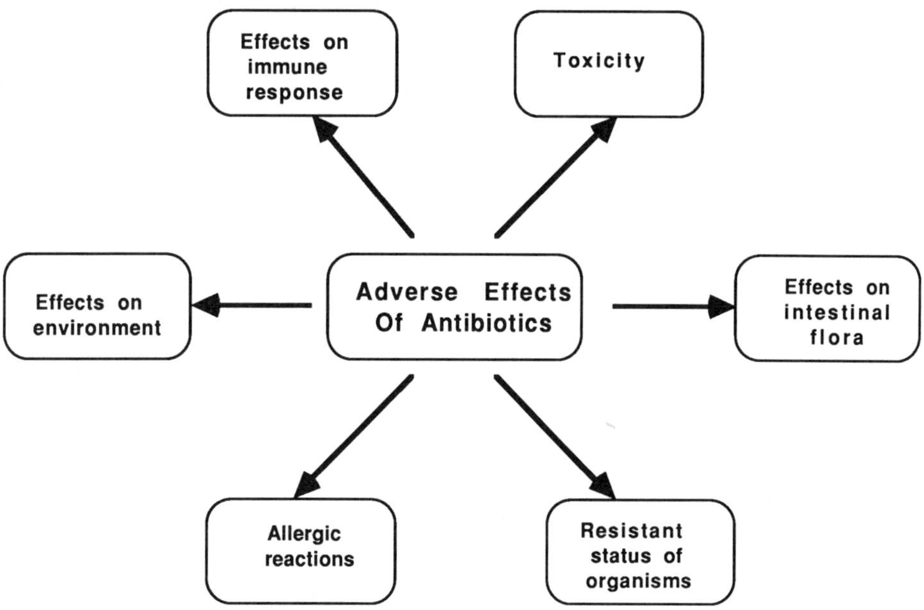

Figure 1 Adverse effects of antibiotics.

Table 1 Adverse Reactions in Humans Suspected to Be Caused by Consumption of Foods Containing Penicillin Residues

Year (sex, age)	Symptoms	Comments	Penicillin source	Total consumed
1958 (male, 54 yr)	Generalized exfoliative dermatitis	Victim had prior history of penicillin allergy. No assay of milk to confirm penicillin residues.	Milk	Unknown
1958 (female, 55 yr)	Acute dermatitis with erythema and exudation of skin on the face, neck, hands, and forearms	Victim had prior history of skin disease unrelated to penicillin allergy. No assay of milk to confirm penicillin.	Milk	Unknown
1958 (male, 44 yr)	Generalized rash, edema of the skin, swollen, painful lymph nodes	Victim had prior history of skin rashes unrelated to penicillin allergy. Victim was a farmer who had treated a cow with intramammary penicillin and subsequently drank the milk.	Milk	Unknown
1961 (female, 25 yr)	Eczematous eruptions on the face, arms, and trunk	Victim had history of penicillin allergy. Following admission to a hospital, victim was given uncontaminated milk—no reaction. Milk was spiked with 40 IU penicillin—adverse reaction. Milk was spiked with penicillin + penicillinase—no reaction.	Milk, butter, goat's milk	40 IU

1969 (female, 42 yr)	Pruritus, erythema, rash, severe headaches	Victim had history of extreme penicillin allergy.	Milk, ice cream	2480 IU
1972 (male)	Pruritus on face and fingers, generalized rash	Victim previously had been treated with penicillin. A pig was slaughtered 3 days after an injection of penicillin. Victim (a butcher) consumed one bite of meat from the pig and suffered the reaction.	Meat	12 IU
1980 (female, 52 yr)	Urticaria, pruritus, itchy sensations on eyes and palms	Victim had previous history of penicillin allergy. One prior reaction traced to milk. Victim consumed fruit drink ("Wink") and reaction occurred within 5 minutes. Bioassay of fruit drink detected a "penicillin-like" substance.	Fruit drink	26 IU
1981 (female, 37 and 42 yr)	Pruritus, anesthesia of the oral mucosa	Victims had prior history of penicillin allergy. Experimental study in which nine persons with allergies to penicillin were fed raw pork from a pig injected with 3 million units of penicillin b.i.d. for 3 days, then slaughtered. Two of nine volunteers reacted.	Raw meat	6–10 IU

Source: Sundlof, 1989. Reprinted with permission.

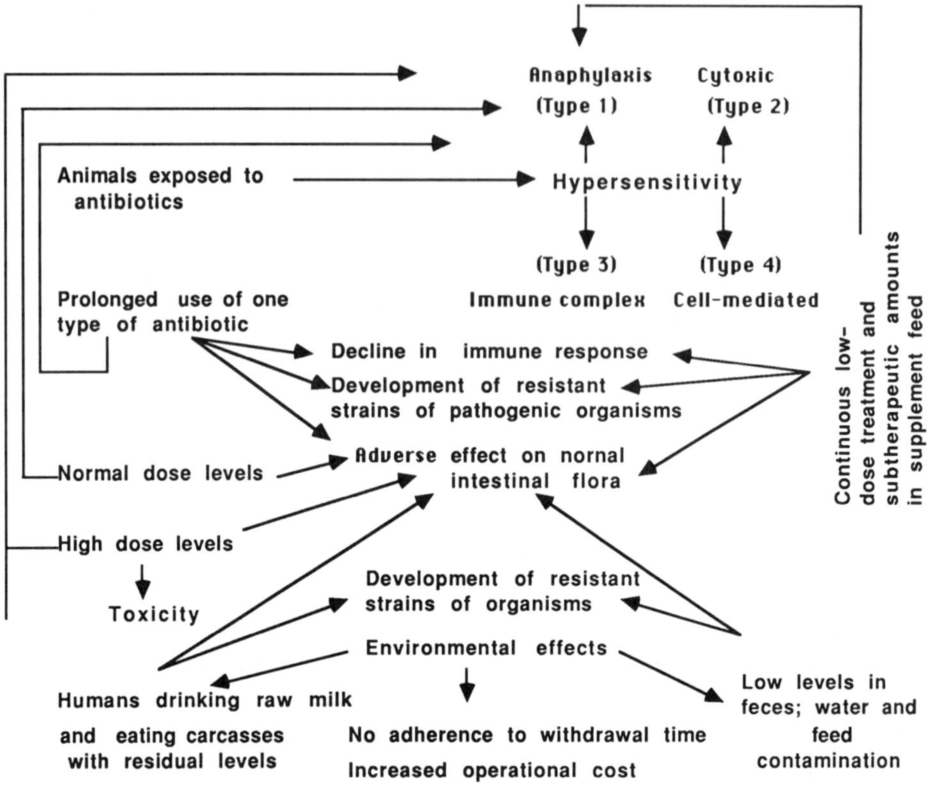

Figure 2 Detailed adverse effects of antibiotics.

Bacteria acquire drug resistance by mutation, conjugation, and transduction. According to these authors, fecal contamination of meat during slaughter may result in the transfer of antibiotic-resistant *E. coli* to the meat. As suggested by Okolo (1986), in the human gut *E. coli* could transfer resistance to other organisms present in the gut. It is believed that the ingestion of residues of antimicrobial agents may either exert a selective pressure on the intestinal flora of consumers and favor the growth of the microorganisms with natural or acquired resistance or give rise, directly or indirectly, the development of acquired resistance in pathogenic enteric bacteria. However, this issue has not been resolved with any measurable satisfaction (FAO/WHO, 1984). Several workers (Anderson et al., 1952; Loken et al., 1971; Levy et al., 1974; Evangelisti et al., 1975; Neu et al., 1975; Hinton et al., 1987) have reported on the transmission of drug resistance by several intestinal bacteria following their exposure to antibiotics in the gut of animals and their transmission to humans.

B. Economic Impacts of Antibiotics

According to many reports, antibiotic residues in milk have resulted in problems of concern to the dairy industry. Antibiotic residues bring about retardation and complete absence of acid production by bacterial starter cultures employed in many of the manufactured products, including cheese. Because of this, economic loss to the offending dairymen, increase in the cost of milk marketing, and potential health problems for consumers occur. Some of the antibiotics used in the treatment of mastitis are penicillin, streptomycin, neomycin, and polymyxin, used singly or in combination. In cases where proper instructions for the discard of milk are not followed, there is always a possibility that antibiotics given to lactating animals are either excreted in milk or are retained in the animal tissues and thus pass on to consumers (Booth, 1986; Kaneene and Alwynelle, 1987; Marteniuk et al., 1988; Seymour et al., 1988).

C. Effects of Antibiotics on Intestinal Bacterial Flora

As a result of prolonged use of antibiotics, growth of undesirable organisms in the gut may lead to gastrointestinal problems in people and animals. For example, in some cases the use of neomycin by oral route may lead to overgrowth of yeast in the intestine. The tetracyclines produce gastrointestinal irritation in some individuals and induce changes in intestinal flora, and drug-induced diarrhea may be caused by active infection of bowel following their use. In some cases, pseudomembranous colitis has also been reported.

D. Effects of Antibiotics on Environment

Some orally administered antibiotics, e.g., tetracycline, are incompletely absorbed, and large proportions are excreted intact. The effect of such residues on organisms in the environment including *E. coli* microorganisms is largely unknown, but includes the possible development of drug-resistant bacteria (Anonymous, 1978; Bartlett, 1979).

E. Effects of Antibiotics on Immune Response

Various studies reported in the literature have demonstrated that antibiotics may not only act as antimicrobial agents but may also modulate the function of immunocompetent cells. The effect of antibiotics on immune response may occur either by direct effects on immunocompetent cells or indirectly by changes in structure or metabolites of organisms induced by subminimal inhibitory concentrations (subMICs). The direct effects on immune response parameters have been elucidated on phagocytic activity, humoral and cellular immunity, production of interleukin-1 and -2, and/or prostaglandins. On the other hand, the indirect effects reported are concerned with influence of subMICs of antibiotics on microorganisms, on their antigenicity, or on their enzyme and toxin production (Bartlett, 1979; Hauser and Remington, 1982; Gillissen, 1988). It has been reported that tetracycline, in concentrations common during therapy, markedly depressed migration of human leukocytes in vitro (Alexander, 1975). Detailed discussion on this topic is beyond the scope of this paper, and readers are referred to the excellent reviews of Gillissen (1988), Alexander (1975), and Martin et al. (1974).

F. Toxic Effects of Antibiotics

Hepatic injury in several cases where amoxicillin was given in combination with clavulanic acid and necrotic lesions and abscesses at the site of injection in slaughtered cattle following their injection with oxytetracycline by intramuscular route have been reported (Stricker et al., 1989; Petzer et al., 1984). Antibiotic-associated colitis and diarrhea in acne patients treated with topical antibiotics and low doses of oral antibiotics have also been observed (Facklam et al., 1990). Experimental studies in rabbits by Joly et al. (1989) showed immediate nephrotoxicity following their exposure to amphotericin. It has been reported that Epirubicin and Sparso-mycin used to treat cancer cases has caused cardiotoxicity and retinotoxicity, respectively (Neri et al., 1989; Zylicz et al., 1989). A number of antimicrobial agents may have undesirable interactions with cyclosporine. Concurrent use of ketoconazole or erythromycin results in increased serum cyclosporine levels, with associated potential nephrotoxicity or neurotoxicity (Sands and Brown, 1989). It was shown in another study (O'Hanley et al., 1989) that excessive antibiotic usage and multiple antibiotic changes among adult leukemic patients undergoing chemotherapy appear to increase the risks of adverse hepatic and renal effects and death.

VI. ADVERSE REACTIONS AFTER EXPOSURE TO SPECIFIC ANTIBIOTICS

A. Untoward Reactions to Penicillins

Adverse responses to antibiotics are usually related to hypersensitivity and allergic reactions resulting from repeated treatment (Adams, 1975). Further studies suggest that several commonly used antibiotics may cause cardiovascular depression, respiratory difficulties, or alter the metabolic breakdown of other drugs. Hypersensitive reactions are probably the most common cause of drug allergy, which may occur in the form of urticaria, fever, bronchospasm, serum sickness, angioedema, and anaphylaxis, which leads to occasional death (Mandell and Sande, 1985b). There are many documented cases in humans with demonstrated immunopathological reactions as a result of exposure to antibiotic residues in foods. Although under certain conditions, many drugs can serve as antigen, penicillin has been on the top of the list of antibiotics in terms of its allergenic characteristics, in both veterinary and human clinical medicine. Immediate hypersensitive reactions have been reported with consumption of foods of animal origin like milk and meat containing antibiotic residues (Zimmerman, 1959; Nickas, 1975; Livingston, 1985; Okolo, 1986; Van Dresser and Wilcke, 1989).

Penicillins and cephalosporins are commonly associated with hypersensitive reactions. In addition, cephalosporins have been found to cause diarrhea and be nephrotoxic (Petz, 1978; Wade et al., 1978). Aminoglycosides, such as neomycin, may cause toxic and hypersensitivity reactions in some patients when used on the skin. Hypersensitivity reactions by tetracycline rarely occur in the form of urticaria, rashes, and generalized exfoliative dermatitis (Chopra and Howe, 1978). Chloramphenicol, however, may cause vesicular skin rashes and angioedema. Further, it leads to alterations in normal flora as do tetracyclines and causes nausea, vomiting, and diarrhea. Erythromycin produces allergic reactions as well as fever, eosinophilia, and skin eruptions. Prolonged use of this antibiotic sometimes results in development of superinfections caused by bacteria or yeast (Mandell and Sande, 1985b).

B. Untoward Reactions to Aminoglycosides

The antibiotics gentamicin, tobramycin, amikacin, netilmicin, kanamycin, streptomycin, and neomycin are included in this group. All of these drugs contain amino sugars in glycosidic linkage and act by their interference with protein synthesis in susceptible gram-negative bacteria. Although some hypersensitivity reactions have been documented in the literature, all aminoglycosides are capable of producing reversible as well as irreversible vestibular effects and renal toxicity. Numerous studies have demonstrated that aminoglycosides may cause toxic reactions leading to muscular paralysis. Streptomycin, for example, may produce dysfunction of the optic nerve as well as peripheral neuritis (Pittinger et al., 1970; Mandell and Sande, 1985b). High peak concentrations of aminoglycosides following once-daily regimens may maximize bactericidal rates, but the problem of toxicity remains. It has been suggested that the risk factors for nephrotoxicity and ototoxicity should be assessed in the evaluation of clinical trials (Mattie et al., 1989). Further, the nephrotoxic potential of aminoglycoside antibiotics may be associated with the degree of membrane binding and subsequent membrane damage in the renal tubules as it relates to renal damage (Amacher et al., 1989). The readers are referred to other reports on the adverse effects of various members of aminoglycosides (Reiner et al., 1978; Lietman and Smith, 1983; Mandell and Sande, 1985). Davies (1990) has investigated the mechanism of bacterial resistance to the aminoglycosides, and his studies of streptomyces have led to the development of several useful cloning systems and their application to yield-improved methods for antibiotic production in natural isolates. Studies of the biochemical and molecular genetic biosynthesis of an antibiotic-herbicide produced by a streptomycete have revealed that the majority of the biosynthesis genes for this antibiotic are linked in a single multitranscription unit on the chromosome. Following are some of the important aminoglycosides and other antibiotics which have been reported to exhibit specific untoward reactions.

1. *Gentamicin*

The untoward effects of gentamicin are similar to those of other aminoglycosides. However, the most important and serious side effect of this drug is irreversible ototoxicity. Also, gentamicin may produce greater nephrotoxicity when compared with other aminoglycosides.

2. *Tobramycin*

Like other aminoglycosides, this drug causes both nephrotoxicity and ototoxicity. The same is true of amikacin and netilmicin.

3. *Neomycin*

Other important side effects of neomycin as reported by Mandell and Sande (1985b) are renal damage and nerve deafness. The oral use of neomycin sometimes produces a spruelike syndrome with diarrhea, steatorrhea, and azotorrhea and intestinal crypt-cell necrosis.

4. *Tetracyclines*

Toxic effects such as phototoxic reactions have been reported following use of various derivatives of tetracyclines. Hepatic toxicity, jaundice, and irreversible shock may occur as a result of its use. The intravenous administration may cause thrombophlebitis, and prolonged use has reportedly been observed to have led to leukocytosis (Kuzucu, 1970; Martin et al., 1974; Sande and Mandell, 1985b).

5. *Chloramphenicol*

Chloramphenicol causes blurring of vision, optic neuritis and digital paresthesias (Sande and Mandell, 1985b). Prolonged use of this antibiotic has reportedly produced changes in peripheral blood include leukopenia, thrombocytopenia, and aplasia of the marrow with fatal pancytopenia. In the presence of hepatic disease, the use of chloramphenicol in patients, may result in depression of erythropoiesis (Polak et al., 1972; Wallerstein et al., 1969; Suhrland and Weisberger, 1963). The toxicity in neonates and premature babies may lead to death known as "gray syndrome" (Craft et al., 1974). Also in some cases its use has resulted in encephalopathic changes and cardiomyopathy have been reported (Biancaniello et al., 1981).

6. *Erythromycin*

Intramuscular injection of erythromycin produces severe pain at the site of injection and intravenous injection may be followed by thrombophlebitis. This antibiotic produces transient auditory impairment is a rare complication of intravenous treatment (Karmody and Weinstein, 1977). However, cholestatic hepatitis is the most striking side effect (Biancaniello et al., 1981). Detailed discussion on the subject has been presented by Sande and Mandell (1985b) which will serve as a good source of further information.

VII. PROBLEMS OF DRUG RESIDUES IN FOOD ANIMALS

The presence of antimicrobial residues in milk, dairy products, meat, and meat products, and other products of animal origin poses serious problems to the dairy and meat industry because of the public health implications. Confirmed cases of allergic reactions occurring in human consumers of foods of animal origin due to presence of penicillin and other antibiotics are given in Table 1. In addition to other untoward effects, the antibiotic residues in milk may result in economic losses when such milk is used for preparation of dairy products involving bacterial cultures. Higher doses of antibiotics in mastitic preparations as well as the vehicle may result in delays of excretion of antibiotics in milk. Also, the presence or absence of antibiotic in milk may very well depend on the assay methods used for detection of antibiotics in milk. However, it is desirable that the antibiotic levels be adequate in order to be effective. The residues of antibiotics in milk may be reduced by following the guidelines on withholding milk as given on the labels of antibiotic preparations used in the treatment of dairy animals (Siddique et al., 1965; Siddique, 1968, 1983). In a study of antibiotic/antimicrobial residues in commercial milk samples in the eastern Pennsylvania, central New Jersey, and the New York City area, 64 milk samples were obtained over a 3-month period. The results of this study indicated that 63% of milk samples contained one or more residues, 27% contained two residues, and 11% contained three or more residues; tetracyclines and sulfonamides were the most predominant residues detected (Brady and Katz, 1988). In similar reports by Marteniuk et al. (1988) on withdrawal requirements, the most common drugs used in violation were found to be oxytetracycline, gentamicin, chloramphenicol, and a combination of lincomycin/spectinomycin. Oxytetracycline, gentamicin, and chloramphenicol accounted for more than half (57%) of all violations, as these antibiotics are commonly used to treat mastitis and metritis in cows.

Sulfamethazine (SMZ) is an important antibacterial drug used in approximately 75% of all hogs marketed in the United States. The tolerance for residues of SMZ in uncooked tissues is 0.1 ppm, and the withdrawal time is 15 days. The rate of illegal residues in swine from the use of SMZ continued to fluctuate between 4 and 5% from 1980 through 1987. This was not acceptable, and efforts are being made to resolve the SMZ residue problem (Augsburg, 1989). Waltno (1987) and Cordle (1988) have discussed the residues in meat extensively.

The U.S. Department of Agriculture's (USDA) Food Safety and Inspection Service (FSIS) is responsible for the monitoring and surveillance of red meat and poultry for residues of drugs and other chemicals. Under this program, each year, FSIS collects approximately 25,000 random samples from all market classes of food-producing animals at the time of slaughter. Out of these collected samples, 4000 to 6000 are analyzed for specific chemical compounds. The sampling has been found to be statistically valid and is quite sophisticated. The Center for Veterinary Medicine (CVM) reviewed 1988 data which included a total of 460 reports and represented all slaughter classes. With the exception of sulfamethazine in market hogs, the major concern was for residues in antibiotics in the bovine, but more specifically culled dairy cows and fancy veal. Violation rates were generally less than 3% of slaughtered swine, cull dairy cows, and veal calves. In all other classes, rates were below 1%. Intramuscular injection accounted for 60% of the residue cases, and cull dairy cows were the largest contributor of residues in this category. Oral administration accounted for 28% of the violations and many of these occurred in the bob veal. Intramammary infusion accounted for 9% of the residue cases, all of which occurred in culled dairy cows (Anonymous, 1990). Also, extra-label use of antimicrobial drugs seems to be more common, which results in residue violations. During the period between 1960 and 1972, the prevalence of antimicrobial residues in swine, lambs, calves, and fat cattle slaughtered in the United States was 30, 21, 18, and 7%, respectively (Huber, 1971).

Van Dresser and Wilcke (1989) studied the problem of drug residues in food animals. The analysis disclosed the following:

1. Antibiotic residues were most often associated with streptomycin, penicillin, oxytetracycline, and neomycin. Sulfamethazine was, by far, the most frequently cited sulfonamide.
2. Residues are being found predominantly in cows, veal calves, and market hogs (barrows and gilts).
3. The cause of drug residue most frequently cited by the field investigators was failure to observe the withholding time for the drug. Almost half of these investigations revealed that the individual responsible for the sale of the animal did not know the proper withholding time for the drug. Failure to maintain adequate records was also a contributing factor.
4. The producer was considered to be the responsible party in over 80% of the cases for which the responsibility was determined.
5. Residues associated with injectable drugs were investigated most frequently. Long-acting and sustained-release products were most often associated with penicillin and oxytetracycline residues.
6. The two most common sources of purchase for the drugs involved in the investigations were the feed/farm supply store and the veterinarian.
7. Unapproved drug use was not a major cause of residues.

VIII. CONCLUSIONS

The problem of sulfonamides and other antibiotic residues in foods of animal origin is of increasing concern because of public health implications. These drugs are administered to animals either subtherapeutically in their feed to improve their production or therapeutically through parenteral means to treat disease conditions. This emphasizes the need for more prudent use of antimicrobials in both people and animals. The adverse effects of residues of sulfonamides and antibiotics are: (1) hypersensitive reactions, (2) acquisition of resistance by enteric bacterial flora, (3) economic loss due to effects on starter cultures in the dairy industry, (4) effects on the environment, (5) toxic effects, and (6) effects on immune responses in people. A surveillance program by the U.S. Food Safety and Inspection Service, which is designed to investigate and control the movement of potentially adulterated products, was put into place to minimize the residual problem of sulfonamides and antibiotics. This program ensures that unacceptable levels of drug residues are not present in foods of animal origin following their exposure to various antimicrobial agents. Also, the FDA has issued some guidelines on recommended drug withdrawal times and on restrictive use of these drugs including the extra-label use of drugs. Therefore, veterinarians who act responsibly by following the guidelines and by assuring that sulfonamides and antibiotics are used appropriately, at the correct dosage and only when indicated, will have a significant impact on safeguarding public health.

REFERENCES

Adams, R. A. (1975). Acute adverse effects of antibiotics. *J. Am. Vet. Med. Assoc. 166*: 983–987.

Alexander, J. W. (1975). Antibiotic agents and the immune mechanisms of defense. *Bull. N.Y. Acad. Med. 51*: 1039–1045.

Amacher, D. E., Schomaker, S. J., and Meyers, L. L. (1989). Selective membrane toxicity of aminoglycoside antibiotics in membrane vesicles isolated from proximal renal tubules of the rat. *Biochem. Pharmacol.* (England) *38*: 3867–3872.

Anderson, G. W., Cunningham, J. D., and Slinger, S. J. (1952). Effect of protein level and penicillin on growth and intestinal flora of chicken. *J. Nutr. 47*: 175-189.

Anonymous (1978). Residue violations in meat and poultry remain constant. *JAMA 172*: 133–136.

Anonymous (1990). *Alabama Veterinary Notes, 2* (1), Auburn, AL.

Augsburg, J. K. (1989). Sulfa residues in pork: An update. *J. Anim. Sci. 67*: 2817–2821.

Bartlett, J. G. (1979). Antibiotic associated pseudomembranous colitis. *Rev. Infect. Dis. 1*: 530–539.

Biancaniello, T., Meyer, R. A., and Kaplan, S. (1981). Chloramphenicol and cardiotoxicity. *J. Pediatr. 98*: 828–830.

Booth, J. M. (1986). Intramammary antibiotic preparations and their withholding times. *Vet. Rec. 118*: 34–35.

Brady, M. S., and Katz, S. E. (1988). Antibiotic/Antimicrobial residues in milk. *J. Food Protect. 51*: 8–11.

Caldwell, J. R., and Cliff, L. E. (1974). Adverse reactions to antimicrobial agents. *JAMA 230*: 77–80.

Chopra, I., and Howe, T. G. B. (1978). Bacterial resistance to tetracycline. *Microbiol. Rev. 42*: 707–724.

Cordle, M. K. (1988). USDA regulations of residues in meat and poultry products. *J. Anim. Sci. 66*: 413–433.

Corpet, D. E. (1987). Antibiotic residues and drug resistance in human intestinal flora. *Antimicrob-Agents Chemother. 31*: 587–593.

Craft, A. W., Brocklebank, J. T., Hey, E. N., and Jackson, R. J. (1974). The "Grey toddler": Chloramphenicol toxicity. *Arch. Dis. Child. 49*: 235–237.

Davies, J. (1990). Microbial immunology to antibiotics. Ann. Meet. J., Am. Soc. Microbiol, May 13–17, Anaheim, California.

Evangelisti, D. B., English, A. R., Girard, A. E., Lynch, J. E., and Solomons, I. A. (1975). Influence of subtherapeutic levels of oxytetracycline *Salmonella typhimurium* in swine, calves, and chickens. *Antimicrob. Agents Chemother. 8*: 664–672.

Facklam, D. P., Gardner, J. S., Neidert, G. L., and Westland, M. M. (1990). An epidemiologic postmarketing surveillance study of prescription acne medications. *Am. J. Publ. Health 80*: 50–53.

FAO/WHO Expert Consultation Report (1984). Residues of veterinary drugs in foods. Food and Agriculture Organization/World Health Organization, Rome, Oct. 29–Nov. 5.

Gillissen, G. (1988). Side effects of antibiotics on immune response parameters and their possible implications in antimicrobial chemotherapy. *Zbl. Bakt. Hyg. A270*: 177–199.

Hauser, W. E., Jr., and Remington, J. S. (1982). Effect of antibiotics on the immune response. *Am. J. Med. 72*: 711–716.

Hinton, M., Lim, S. K., and Linton, A. H. (1987). The influence of antibacterial agents on the complexity of the *Escherichia coli* flora of chickens. *FEMS Microbiol. Lett. 41*: 169–173.

Huber, W. G. (1971). The impact of antibiotic drugs and their residues. *Adv. Vet. Sci. Comp. Med. 15*: 101–132.

Joly, V., Dromer, F., Barge, J., Yeni, P., Sta, N., Molas, M., and Carbon, C. (1989). Incorporation of amphotericin B (AMB) into liposomes alters AMB-induced acute nephrotoxicity in rabbits. *J. Pharmacol. Exp. Ther. 251*: 311–316.

Kaneene, J. V., and Alwynelle, S. (1987). Drug residues in the dairy cattle industry: Epidemiological evaluation of factors influencing their occurrence. *J. Dairy Sci. 70*: 2176–2180.

Karmody, C. S., and Weinstein, L. (1977). Reversible sensorineural hearing loss with intravenous erythromycin lactobionate. *Ann. Otol. Rhinol. Laryngol. 86*: 9–11.

Kuzucu, E. Y. (1970). Methoxyflurane, tetracycline and renal failure. *JAMA 211*: 1162–1164.

Levy, S. B., Fitzgerald, G. B., and Macone, B. S. (1974). Change in intestinal flora of farm personnel after introduction of tetracycline-supplemented feed on a farm. *N. Engl. J. Med. 295*: 583–588.

Lietman, P. S., and Smith, C. R. (1983). Aminoglycoside nephrotoxicity in humans. *J. Infect. Dis. 5* (Suppl. 2): 284–292.

Livingston, R. C. (1985). Antibiotic residues in animal-derived food. *J. Assoc. Off. Anal. Chem. 68*: 966–967.

Loken, K. I., Wagner, L. W., and Henke, C. L. (1971). Transmissible drug resistance in enterobacteriaceae isolated from calves given antibiotics. *Am. J. Vet. Res. 32*: 1207–1212.

Mandell, G. L., and Sande, M. A. (1985a). Antimicrobial agents—sulfonamides, trimethoprim-sulfamethoxazole, and agents for urinary tract infections. In *Goodman and Gilman's, The Pharmacological Basis of Therapeutics*, 7th ed. Macmillan Publishing Co., New York, pp. 1095–1114.

Mandell, G. L., and Sande, M. A. (1985b). Antimicrobial agents. In *Goodman and Gillman's The Pharmacological Basis of Therapeutics*. Macmillan Publishing Co., New York, pp. 1134–1137.

Marteniuk, J. V., Ahl, A. S., and Bartlett, P. C. (1988). Compliance with recommended drug withdrawal requirements for dairy cows sent to market in Michigan. *JAVMA 193*: 404–407.

Martin, R. R., Warr, G. A., Couch, R. B., Yeager, H., and Knight, V. (1974). Effects of tetracycline on Leukotaxis. *J. Infect. Dis. 129*: 110–116.

Mattie, H., Craig, W. A., and Pechere, J. C. (1989). Determinants of efficacy and toxicity of aminoglycosides. *J. Antimicrob. Chemother.* (England) *24*: 281–293.

Neri, B., Pacini, P., Bartalucci, S., Moroni, F., Menchi, L., and Cappellini, M. (1989). Epirubicin high dose therapy in advanced breast cancer: Preliminary clinical data. *Int. J. Clin. Pharmacol. Ther. Toxicol.* (Germany, West), *27*: 388–391.

Neu, H. C., Cherubin, C. E., Longo, E. D., Flouton, B., and Winter, J. (1975). Antimicrobial resistance and R-factor transfer among isolates of Salmonella in northeastern United States: A comparison of human and animal isolates. *J. Infect. Dis. 132*: 617–622.

Nichols, D. R., and Keys, T. F. (1984). Historical overview of antibiotics and sulfonamides. In *Society in Handbook Series in Zoonoses*, vol. 1, J. S. Steele and G. W. Beran, eds. CRC Press, Inc., Boca Raton, FL, pp. 35–43.

Nickas, G. M. (1975). Antibiotic agents and the immune mechanisms of defense. *Bull. N.Y. Acad. Med. 51*: 1039–1045.

O'Hanley, P., Easaw, J., Rugo, H., and Easaw, S. (1989). Infectious disease management of adult leukemia patients undergoing chemotherapy: 1982 to 1986 experience at Stanford University Hospital. *Am. J. Med. 87*: 605–613.

Okolo, M. I. (1986). Bacterial drug resistance in meat animals: A review. *Int. J. Zoonoses, 13*: 143–152.

Petz, L. D. (1978). Immunologic cross-reactivity between penicillins and cephalosporins: A review. *J. Infect. Dis. 137*: S74–S79.

Petzer, I. M., van-Staden, J. J., and Giesecke, W. H. (1984). Tissue reaction and residues in slaughter cattle after administration of long-acting oxytetracycline formulations. *J. S. Afr. Vet. Assoc. 55*: 107–111.

Pittinger, C. B., Eryasa, Y., and Adamson, R. (1970). Antibiotic-induced parallysis. *Anesth. Analg. 49*: 487–501.

Polak, B. C. P., Wesseling, H., Herxheimer, A., and Meyler, L. (1972). Blood dyscrasias attributed to chloramphenicol. *Acta Med. Scand. 192*: 409–414.

Reiner, N. E., Bloxham, D. D., and Thomson, W. L. (1978). Nephrotoxicity of gentamicin and tobramycin given once daily or continuously in dogs. *J. Antimicrob. Chemother. 4(Suppl. A)*: 85–101.

Sande, M. E., and Mandell, G. L. (1985b). Antimicrobial agents, tetracyclines, chloramphenicol, erythromycin, and miscellaneous antibacterial agents. In *Goodman and Gilman's The Pharmacological Basis of Therapeutics*, 7th ed. Macmillan, New York, pp. 1181–1186.

Sands, M., and Brown, R. B. (1989). Interactions of cyclosporine with antimicrobial agents. *Rev. Infect. Dis. 11*: 691–697.

Schuman, J. D., Zottola, E. A., and Harlander, S. K. (1989). Preliminary characterization of a food-borne multiple-antibiotic-resistant *Salmonella typhimurium* strain. *Appl. Environ. Microbiol. 55*: 2344–2348.

Seymour, E. H., Jones, G. M., and McGilliard, M. L. (1988). Persistence of residues in milk following antibiotic treatment of dairy cattle. *J. Dairy Sci. 71*: 1691–1699.

Siddique, I. H. (1968). Antibiotic residues in foods. In *The Safety of Foods*, Avi, Westport, CT, pp. 358–360.

Siddique, I. H. (1983). Food contaminants: Animal growth promoters (antibiotic residues). In *Handbook of Naturally Occurring Food Toxins*, M. Rechcigl, Jr., ed. CRC Press, Boca Raton, FL, pp. 277–286.

Siddique, I. H., Loken, K. I., and Hoyt, H. H. (1965). Concentrations of neomycin, dihydrostreptomycin, and polymyxin in milk after intramuscular or intramammary administration. *J. Am. Vet. Med. Assoc. 146*: 594–599.

Steele, J. H., and Beran, G. W. (1984). Perspectives in the uses of antibiotics and sulfonamides. In *Handbook Series in Zoonoses*. CRC Press, Boca Raton, FL, pp. 3–34.

Stricker, B. H., VaBroek, J. W., Keuning, J., Eberhardt, W., Houben, H. G., Johnson, M., and Blok, A. P. (1989). Cholestatic hepatitis due to antibacterial combination of amoxicillin and clavulanic acid (augmentin). *Dig. Dis. Sci. 34*: 1576–1580.

Suhrland, L. F., and Weisberger, A. S. (1963). Chloramphenicol toxicity in liver and renal disease. *Arch. Intern. Med. 112*: 747–754.

Sunalof, S. E. (1989). Drug and chemical residues in livestock. In *The Veterinary Clinics of North America*, vol. 5. Food Animal Practice. W. B. Saunders, Philadelphia.

Van Dresser, W. R., and Wilcke, J. R. (1989). Drug residues in food animals. *JAVMA 194*: 1700–1710.

Vecht, U., Wisselink, H. J., and Vette, H. M. C. (1989). Susceptibility of *Staphylococcus aureus* isolated from bovine quarter milk to antimicrobial drugs. *TIJDSCHR DIERGENEESKD 114*: 260–268.

Venkateswaran, K., Nakano, H., Hawakami, H., and Hashimoto, H. (1988). Microbiological aspects and recovery of Salmonella in retained foods. *J. Fac. Appl. Biol. Sci. 27*: 33–39.

Wade, J. C., Smith, C. R., Petty, B. G., Lipsky, J. J., Conrad, J., Ellner, J., and Leitman, P. S. (1978). Cephalothin plus an aminoglycoside is more nephrotoxic than methicillin plus an aminoglycoside. *Lancet 2*: 604–606.

Wallerstein, R. O., Condit, P. K., Kasper, C. K., Brown, J. W., and Morrison, F. R. (1969). Statewide study of chloramphenicol therapy and fatal aplastic anemia. *JAMA 208*: 2045–2050.

Waltno, J. R. Antibiotic residues in meat. (1987). *Brit. Vet. J. 143*: 485–486.

Weinstein, L., Madoff, M. A., and Samet, C. A. (1960). The sulfonamides. *N. Engl. J. Med. 263*: 793–800, 842–849, 900–907.

Zimmerman, M. C. (1959). Chronic penicillin urticaria from dairy products, proved by penicillinase cures. *Am. Med. Assoc. Arch. Dermatol. 79*: 1–6.

Zylicz, Z., De Grip, W. J., Wagener, D. J., Rennes, H. Van., Van Der Kleijn, E., and Van Den Broek, L. A. (1989). Studies on retinotoxic potential of a novel antitumor antibiotic sparsomycin in rats. *Anticancer Res.* (Greece) *9*: 923–927.

IX

OTHERS

20

Nitrosamines and Food Poisoning

Nrisinha P. Sen

Health Protection Branch, Health and Welfare Canada, Ottawa, Ontario, Canada

I. INTRODUCTION

A variety of undesirable compounds can be present in foods consumed by man. These may range from the naturally occurring cyanogenic glycosides to contaminants such as pesticide residues or nonessential trace elements (e.g., Pb, Cd). The presence of mycotoxins (produced by molds), marine toxins (produced by marine organisms), and polynuclear aromatic hydrocarbons (produced as a result of food processing; e.g., roasting) can be cited as further examples of potentially harmful substances that have been shown to be present in certain foods of both animal and plant origin (Concon, 1988). *N*-Nitroso compounds (NOCs), commonly known as nitrosamines, are one of the latest group of such chemicals that have received a great deal of attention during the past 15–20 years. There have been two reasons for concern. First, a majority of these compounds are potent carcinogens in laboratory animals. Second, many of the NOCs occur at trace levels in a wide variety of foods and beverages. It should be emphasized, however, that although nitrosamines are considered as poisonous and toxic substances, there is no evidence to suggest that their presence in foods at trace levels has caused any harmful effects in humans. Nevertheless, there is a potential danger, and hence the reason for concern.

Nitrosamines are formed by the interaction of secondary or tertiary amines with nitrite or other nitrosating agents. This explains why the majority of the foods that have been found to contain nitrosamines are those that are rich in amines and have been preserved with nitrite (e.g., cured meats, smoked cured fish) or have been dried using hot flue gases containing traces of nitrogen oxides. Furthermore, there is the added possibility of formation of these compounds in vivo in humans due to the interaction of ingested amines in the food and salivary or ingested nitrite. However, a great deal of uncertainty exists in this area (see Sec. VI).

An attempt will be made in this review to briefly discuss various facets of the nitrosamine problem, emphasizing their occurrence and formation in foods. A brief discussion of the biological properties of nitrosamines and of the significance of their presence in foods will also be presented. The reader is advised to consult other recent reviews for additional details (Preussmann and Stewart, 1984; Hotchkiss, 1987; Walker, 1990; Bartsch, 1991).

II. CHEMISTRY AND FORMATION OF NITROSAMINES

A. Introduction

NOCs can be described by the general formula:

$$\begin{matrix} R_1 \\ R_2 \end{matrix} \!\!>\! N\text{-}N{=}O$$

These compounds are divided into two main groups, namely nitrosamines and nitrosamides. In nitrosamines, R_1 and R_2 can be either alkyl of aryl groups or may form part of a cyclic ring. These groups may also contain other substituents such as hydroxyl and carboxylic acid functional groups. Chemical formulas and abbreviations of some nitrosamines commonly detected in foods are shown in Figure 1. In nitrosamides, the groups may be alkyl or aryl, one of which contains an acyl functional group. Hence the proper generic name for these should be *N*-acyl-*N*-nitroso compounds. An example of an nitrosamide is *N*-nitroso-*N*-methylurea (NMU) (Fig. 1). Thus far, no nitrosamides have been detected in foods, but they might be formed in vivo in the stomach due to the interaction of foodborne amides and ingested or salivary nitrite (Challis et al., 1982).

B. Formation

Nitrosamines are formed by the reaction of secondary or tertiary amines with suitable nitrosating species. Nitrite ion by itself or nitrous acid are poor nitrosating agents (Douglass, 1978). However, under acidic conditions the above two species are converted to nitrous anhydride, as shown below, which then reacts with a secondary amine to produce a nitrosamine:

$$NO_2^- + H^+ \rightleftharpoons HNO_2$$

$$2\,HNO_2 \rightleftharpoons N_2O_3 + H_2O$$

$$\begin{matrix} R_1 \\ R_2 \end{matrix} \!\!>\! NH + N_2O_3 \rightleftharpoons \begin{matrix} R_1 \\ R_2 \end{matrix} \!\!>\! N\text{-}N{=}O + HNO_2$$

$$\text{rate} = K_1[R_1R_2NH]\,[HNO_2]^2$$

The above reaction rate is first order with respect to the concentration of the unprotonated secondary amine and second order with respect to the concentration of nitrite, as two molecules are needed to form one molecule of N_2O_3. Since the concentration of the unprotonated amine depends on its basicity (pKa), the higher the basicity, the lower the concentration of the unprotonated amine and the lower the rate of nitrosation. For the commonly occurring foodborne secondary amines, most of which are highly basic (e.g., dimethylamine, pyrrolidine, piperidine), the optimum pH for nitrosation lies between 3–3.5 (Mirvish, 1975). Tertiary amines, such as trimethylamine, which occurs in fish in fairly high levels, can also form nitrosamines, but their nitrosation rate is much slower than that of the secondary amines (Fiddler et al., 1972).

On the other hand, the amides do not have a pH optimum for nitrosation. Between pH 1 to 3, the rate of nitrosation of amides seems to increase by 10-fold for a drop of one pH unit and is proportional to the concentration of nitrite and not its square (Mirvish, 1972). In general, the nitrosation rates for various amines and amides increase in the following order (strongly basic amines having the slowest rates): strongly basic amines (e.g., dimethylamine,

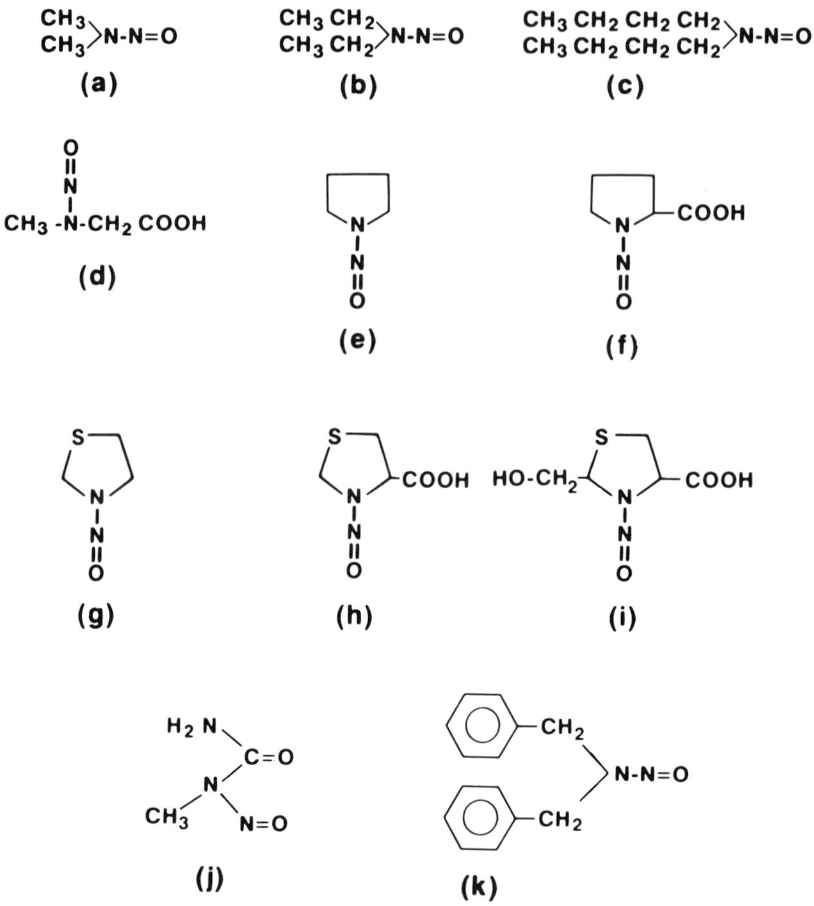

Figure 1 Structural formulas of some common *N*-nitroso compounds: (a) *N*-nitrosodimethylamine (NDMA), (b) *N*-nitrosodiethylamine (NDEA), (c) *N*-nitrosodi-*N*-butylamine (NDBA), (d) *N*-nitrososarcosine (NSAR), (e) *N*-nitrosopyrrolidine (NPYR), (f) *N*-nitrosoproline (NPRO), (g) *N*-nitrosothiazolidine (NTHZ), (h) *N*-nitrosothiazolidine-4-carboxylic acid (NTCA), (i) 2-hydroxmethyl-*N*-nitrosothiazolidine-4-carboxylic acid (HMNTCA), (j) *N*-nitroso-*N*-methylurea (NMU), and (k) *N*-nitrosodibenzylamine (NDBzA).

piperidine), *N*-alkylamides, *N*-alkylguanidines < weakly basic amines (e.g., morpholine, dibenzylamine), certain amino acids (sarcosine, hydroxyproline) < *N*-alkylcarbamates (e.g., ethyl-*N*-methylcarbamate) < *N*-alkylureas (e.g., *N*-methylurea) < alicyclic ureas (e.g., ethylene ureas) (Mirvish, 1972; Douglass, 1978). Within the same series of compounds (e.g., amines or amides), these nitrosation rates can vary over several orders of magnitudes. For example, *N*-methylaniline and morpholine, respectively, nitrosate approximately 147,000 and 250 times faster than dimethylamine. Therefore, the extent of nitrosamine formation in foods or in vivo will depend on the nature of the amines involved as well as other conditions such as pH, concentration of the reactants (both the amines and nitrite), and the presence of catalysts or inhibitors.

C. Catalysis and Inhibition

The nitrosation of secondary amines in acidic aqueous solution is strongly catalyzed by various nucleophilic anions (e.g., SCN^-, I^-, Br^-, Cl^-). Under acidic conditions these anions (X^-) form active nitrosating species that are stronger nitrosating agents than N_2O_3 (Douglass, 1978):

$$HONO + X^- + H^+ \rightleftharpoons X\text{-}NO + H_2O$$

Studies by Roller and Keefer (1974) suggest that electrophilic species such as formaldehyde and chloral can also catalyze nitrosation. In the presence of formaldehyde, the nitrosation of secondary amines by nitrite ion can proceed even at an alkaline pH. It is thought that initial formation of a positively charged imminium ion, produced by the reaction of HCHO and the secondary amine, induces an attack by the negatively charged NO_2^- ion, which is otherwise inactive as a nitrosating agent under acidic conditions (see Sec. II.B). Since many of the above-mentioned nucleophilic anions and HCHO are present in foods as well as in human saliva, they should have a significant influence on the formation of nitrosamines in foods and in vivo in the acidic environment of the human stomach.

On the other hand, phenols can have a catalytic or inhibitory effect on nitrosation of secondary amines depending on the nature of the compound and relative molar ratios of nitrite and the phenol (Davies and McWeeny, 1977; Pignatelli et al., 1980, 1982). For example, when the ratio is very low (e.g., 0.1), most of the nitrite is used up for *C*-nitrosation of the phenol, and very little is available for *N*-nitrosation of the secondary amine. Hence, an inhibitory effect is observed. When the above ratio is considerably higher (e.g., 4 or 5), a strong catalytic effect is observed. Nitrosophenols formed as a result of *C*-nitrosation is believed to be the catalyst but the presence of excess nitrite is necessary (Pignatelli et al., 1980, 1982). However, all naturally occurring phenolic compounds in foods do not elicit this catalytic effect on nitrosation. Of the various phenolic compounds tested, kaempferol, quercetin, catechin, phenol, resorcinol, and phloroglucinol have significant catalytic effect on such nitrosation, whereas chlorogenic acid, caffeic acid, and ferulic acid are devoid of such effects (Pignatelli et al., 1980). Some of these naturally occurring plant phenols or those present in smoked foods may have an influence on nitrosamine formation in vivo as well as during processing and storage of foods.

Other effective inhibitors (e.g., ascorbic acid, α-tocopherol) of *N*-nitrosation are naturally occurring in foods (Mirvish et al., 1972; Newmark and Mergens, 1981). Both ascorbic acid and α-tocopherol (vitamin E) work as inhibitors of nitrosation by reducing nitrous acid to nitric oxide, which is not a nitrosating agent by itself. However, in the presence of oxygen, nitric oxide can be converted to NO_2 and then to N_2O_3, which is a strong nitrosating agent. Therefore, to be effective, excess ascorbic acid should be present to prevent this from happening. Both ascorbic acid (mainly as its Na salt) and α-tocopherol have been proposed or are being used as inhibitors of nitrosamine formation in various cured meat products, especially bacon. Being more lipophilic, α-tocopherol is superior to ascorbic acid as an inhibitor of nitrosamine formation in bacon (Gray et al., 1982).

III. PRECURSOR OF NITROSAMINES IN FOODS

The two main types of precursors for NOCs are the secondary amines or amides and nitrite. These precursors might be naturally occurring in foods, used as an additive, or come in contact with the foods during that processing or packaging. Appreciable levels of nitrosamines are expected to be found in foods that contain nitrite and amines in fairly high concentrations and are processed at an elevated temperature. The first reported finding of *N*-nitrosodimethylamine (NDMA) in fish meal, although an animal feed, can be cited as an example of this (Ender et al., 1964; Sakshaug et al., 1965). Fairly high levels (up to 100 ppm) of NDMA were detected in some of these products. It was subsequently shown that NDMA was formed by the reaction of dimethylamine (DMA) and trimethylamine (TMA) in the fish with nitrite, which was used as a preservative. The highest concentration of NDMA was found in the samples that were processed at 115–130°C immediately after the addition of nitrite.

Although the above is an extreme example, it is not entirely impossible to find similar circumstances with human foods. In fact, extremely high levels (0.85–25 ppm) of *N*-nitrosopiperidine (NPIP), *N*-nitrosopyrrolidine (NPYR), and NDMA have been detected in spice-nitrite premixes that were used until 1973 for processing cured meat products (Sen et al., 1973, 1974; Scanlan, 1975). Apparently, various amines in the spices reacted with the nitrite and produced these high levels of nitrosamines (Sen et al., 1974; Gough and Goodhead, 1975). The finished cured meat products, processed with these premixes, contained varying levels (up to 300 ppb) of nitrosamines. Legislation promulgated in or around 1974 in Canada, the United States, and the United Kingdom banned the use of such premixes for the processing of cured meat products.

DMA, TMA, and trimethylamine oxide occur widely in various foods, especially in fish and seafoods (Maga, 1978; Smith, 1980). DMA and TMA have also been detected in a wide variety of foods including cured meats, cheese, malt, beer, tea, and coffee. Spices, especially black and white pepper and paprika, contain high levels of piperidine, pyrrolidine, and DMA (Gough and Goodhead, 1975). Details of the above findings have been reviewed elsewhere (Maga, 1978; Smith, 1980). Data on the occurrence of secondary amides in foods, however, are limited (Kawabata, 1980). Although methylguanidine and creatinine do occur in some foods (reviewed by Mirvish, 1972), the yield of the corresponding NOCs (e.g., methylnitrosocyanamide, *N*-nitrososarcosine (NSAR), NMU is extremely low, and, therefore, their presence in foods is not of major concern (Mirvish, 1972).

Nitrite in foods can originate in two ways. First, it is present naturally in trace levels in certain vegetables and drinking water (WHO, 1978; Walker, 1990). Traces of nitrite have also been detected in many dried foods (e.g., milk powder, dried cheese, wheat flour) (Walker, 1990). Second, nitrite is used as an additive in cured meats and fish. Nitrite is added to these foods mainly to inhibit the outgrowth of *Clostridium botulinum* spores. In addition, it also imparts the characteristic flavor and color of cured meat products. Until 1973, most countries allowed the addition of 500–1000 ppm nitrate (as Na or K salt) and 200 ppm nitrite (as Na or K salt) in cured meat products (Meester, 1974). Because of the concern about possible formation of NOCs in nitrite-treated foods, their use has been seriously questioned, and action has been taken to reduce the permitted levels of both nitrate and nitrite. Canada was one of the first countries to restrict their use in cured meats. The use of nitrite in curing fish products was prohibited in Canada in 1959, long before the nitrosamine problem became an issue, because its use was considered unnecessary. In 1975, almost all permitted uses of nitrate in curing of meats were stopped; the remaining uses (mainly for the processing of slow-cured products) were restricted to a maximum level of 200 ppm. The level of nitrite was limited to 150 ppm in bacon and to 200 ppm in other cured meats. More recently, the permitted level of nitrite in bacon has been further reduced to 120 ppm (Canadian Food and Drug Regulations, 1987). Other countries, including the United States and the United Kingdom, have passed similar legislation limiting the use of nitrate and nitrite for processing cured meats (USDA, 1986, 1989; Ministry of Agriculture, Fisheries, and Food, 1987).

Furthermore, the increasing use of ascorbate or erythorbate (iso-ascorbate) and α-tocopherol in the processing of cured meat products, and approval of the so-called "Wisconsin" process for processing bacon have significantly reduced the risk of nitrosamine formation in such products. In the "Wisconsin" process, a lower level (40–80 ppm) of nitrite is used in conjunction with an acid-forming bacterial culture (mainly lactic acid–producing bacteria) thus providing adequate protection against botulism (USDA, 1986).

The other major exposure to nitrite by humans arises from salivary nitrite, which is produced by microbial reduction of nitrate in the salivary glands (Tannenbaum et al., 1976). Since most vegetables contain high levels of nitrate (Walker, 1990), the salivary nitrite levels increase significantly (up to 155 ppm) after consumption of vegetables or vegetable juices (Spielgelhalder et al., 1976; Tannenbaum et al., 1976). This, in turn, may increase in vivo intragastric nitrosation due to the interaction of salivary nitrite and ingested amines. Nitrate per se is relatively nontoxic. The two main concerns regarding exposure to nitrate are (1) the possibility of increased in vivo nitrosation as mentioned above, and (2) conversion to nitrite under achlorhydric condition of the stomach in infants leading to methemoglobinemia and possibly death. Walker (1990) has reviewed the literature regarding toxic effects of both nitrate and nitrite.

According to White (1976), the average per capita daily consumption of nitrate and nitrite by an average U.S. resident is 99.8 mg and 11.23 mg, respectively. Of this, approximately 86% of the ingested nitrate originates from vegetables. On the other hand, 77% of the ingested nitrite originates from salivary nitrite and about 21% from cured meats. Various researchers have measured the actual levels of nitrate and nitrite in prepared meals as consumed by an average person. Table 1 presents such data from four countries.

Table 1 Estimated Dietary Intake of Nitrates and Nitrites by the Duplicate Diet Analysis Technique

	Daily intake (range)	
Country	Nitrate (mg/day)	Nitrite (mg/day)
Federal Republic of Germany[a]	59 (12–104)	3.6 (1.5–6.9)
Federal Republic of Germany[b]	97 (30–178)	3.5 (2.5–5.9)
Holland[c]	180 (25–786)	7.7 (2.0–60.3)
Holland[d]	150	4.2
Italy	160	2.8
Sweden	65 (35–110)	4.5 (0.8–8.9)

[a]Normal diet.
[b]Normal diet incorporating home garden produce.
[c]Summer diet for white-collar workers.
[d]Summer plus winter diets for white-collar workers.
Source: Walker (1990), *Food Additiv. Contam.* Reprinted with permission from Taylor & Francis, Ltd.

No such data, however, are available from the United States or Canada. As can be seen from the limited data, the average consumption levels for these two chemicals are well below the accepted guidelines, which are 25 mg/kg body weight/day for nitrate and 0.1 mg/kg body weight/day for nitrite (Walker, 1990).

Various studies have shown that mammals excrete more nitrate in the urine than they ingest (Green et al., 1981; Wagner et al., 1984). It has also been shown that the excess nitrate excretion in mammals is due to biosynthesis and is not produced as a result of intestinal microbial synthesis (Wagner et al., 1984). Conversion of the ^{15}N-labeled ammonia to $^{15}NO_3^-$, as evidenced by excretion of the latter in urine and feces, has been demonstrated in germ-free laboratory animals (Dull and Hotchkiss, 1984; Wagner et al., 1984). Furthermore, experimentally induced fever and inflammatory reaction in laboratory animals or the onset of such conditions in humans are associated with increased excretion of nitrate in the urine (reviewed by Walker, 1990). Macrophages were shown to be involved in the biosynthesis of nitrate, nitrite, as well as nitrosamines. Thus, the biosynthesis of nitrate is a complex process, but its exact mechanism of formation is yet to be elucidated. Contrary to an earlier hypothesis, it appears that a functional membrane-associated superoxide–generating system is not required for the synthesis of NO_3^-/NO_2^- by macrophages, and the oxygen burst is not involved in the process (Stuehr and Marletta, 1987).

IV. OCCURRENCE OF NITROSAMINES IN FOODS AND BEVERAGES

As mentioned earlier, the first conclusive evidence of the occurrence of nitrosamines in food or animal feed came from the analysis of nitrite-preserved herring meal used for animal consumption. The fact that enough NDMA could be formed in such products to cause acute hepatotoxic and sometimes lethal effects in the animals consuming these fish meals caused a great deal of concern. This led to a worldwide search for nitrosamines in human foods, especially those preserved with nitrate/nitrite. The scope of the article does not permit a discussion of the vast amount of data that exist on this topic. Therefore, only a summary of the major findings is presented. Further details can be obtained from other recent reviews (Gray, 1981; Pensabene and Fiddler, 1983; Sen, 1986, 1990; Hotchkiss, 1987; Tricker and Kubacki, 1991).

NOCs can occur in foods in three different ways: (1) formation as a result of the use of nitrate/nitrite additives, (2) formation during processing, and (3) contamination from secondary sources such as packaging materials or other ingredients (e.g., waxes). Table 2 summarizes the major findings in each of these areas. Data on fish and seafoods and several miscellaneous foods are also included in Table 2. The nature of the nitrosating agent(s) in these foods is yet to be established.

A. Occurrences of NOC in Nitrate/Nitrite-Treated Foods

Approximately 18 NOCs have been detected in cured meat products and fried bacon (Table 2). Of these, 9 are carcinogenic in laboratory animals, an additional 2 are genotoxic in in vitro assays, and the remainder are either noncarcinogenic or have not been tested for their carcinogenicity. It should be emphasized, however, that because of improved processing conditions adopted during the past 15–20 years, the levels of these compounds in such products have decreased significantly during this period. Only traces (as indicated in Table 2) of some of these compounds are present in recently produced products. Lowering of permissible levels of nitrate and nitrite, banning the use of nitrite-spice premixes, and increasing use of nitrosation inhibitors (e.g., ascorbate, isoascorbate, α-tocopherol) for the preparation of such products can be cited as examples of the changes introduced that have been responsible for this improvement. In spite of the banning of nitrite-spice premixes, traces of NPIP and NPYR still might be formed in products in which nitrite and spices are added separately. This may explain the occasional finding of the two compounds in heavily spiced cured meat products (Sen et al., 1979; Nitrite Safety Council, 1980; Poirier et al., 1987).

Considerable research has been carried out to elucidate the mechanism of formation of NPYR in fried bacon. The topic has been reviewed by Gray (1981) and Sen (1986). Raw bacon is free of NPYR, which is formed during frying (Pensabene et al., 1974), and its concentration in the cooked-out fat is approximately twice that present in the cooked lean bacon. Also, larger amounts of nitrosamines (both NPYR and NDMA) are found in the fumes than are formed in the cooked-out fat and cooked lean. Initially, it was thought that NPYR was formed by heat-induced decarboxylation of preformed NPRO in the raw bacon, but further research suggested that raw bacon did not contain enough NPRO to account for the high concentrations of NPYR detected in the fried product.

Bharucha et al. (1979) reported that the decarboxylation of NPRO was more facile than that of proline (PRO), and that free PRO was present in the raw

Table 2 Summary of International Surveys on Occurrence of NOCs in Foods and Beverages

Type of foods analyzed	Major NOC detected: NOC	Range of concentration (μg/kg)	Average current level in U.S. and Canadian products (μg/kg)	Minor NOCs detected
Nitrate/nitrite-treated foods				
Fried bacon	NPYR	1–320	10	NPIP, NMOR,
	NDMA	N-44	1	NDEA, NThZ,
	NTCA	5–13,700	100	NHPYR, NHPRO,
	HMNTCA	N-2,100	50	HMNTHZ, NPRO
Cooked-out bacon fat	NPYR	N-207	20	NThZ, NHPYR
	NDMA	N-33	2	
Other cured meat products including those smoked and spiced (sausages, salami, frankfurters, pepperoni, meat loaf, bologna, smoked meat, ham, etc.)	NDMA	N-84	<1	NDEA, NMOR,
	NPYR	N-149	<1	NPRO, NHPYR,
	NPIP	N-300	<1	NHPRO, NSAR
	NTCA	N-6,760	100	
	HMNTCA	N-475	50	
Cured pork products packaged in elastic rubber nettings	NDBA	N-56	<5	NDEA
	NDBzA	N-112	<30	
Smoked, nitrate/nitrite treated fish	NDMA	N-9	?	

Dried foods				
Malt	NDMA	1–600	1	NPYR, NPRO
Beer and ale	NDMA	N-68	0.1	NPYR, NPRO
Whiskey	NDMA	N-2	?	
Skim milk powder	NDMA	N-4.9	0.5	NPYR, NPIP
Whey powder	NDMA	N-4.9	2	NPYR, NPIP
Instant and roasted coffee	NPYR	N-1.4	0.1	
Soy flour and other soy products	NDMA	N-0.6	0.1	
Pancake mix	NDMA	N-0.6	?	
Dried cheeses	NDMA	N-0.3	0.1	
Contamination from secondary sources				
Margarine	NMOR	N-3.8	?	
Fruit drinks	NDMA	N-5.5	N	
Miscellaneous foods including fish and seafoods				
Various canned fish	NDMA	N-1	?	
Miscellaneous smoked fish	NDMA	N-74	<1	NTCA
	NPRO	N-344	?	
Salted/dried fish	NDMA	N-133	<1	NDEA, NDPA, NPRO
Dried squid	NDMA	N-364	?	
Chinese fermented/pickled vegetables	NDMA	N-15	?	
	NDEA	?	?	
	NMBzA	?	?	
Soy sauce	NDMA	N-7	?	
Cheeses	NDMA	N-20	<1	
Sun-dried vegetables (spinach, pumpkin, turnip, etc.)	NDMA	N-10	?	NPYR, NPIP

N = negative (detection limit, 0.1–5 ppb depending on the NOC); ? = either no current data are available or insufficient data; NPIP = *N*-nitrosopiperidine; NMOR = *N*-nitrosomorpholine; NHPRO = *N*-nitroso-4-hydroxyproline; HMNTHZ = 2-hydroxymethyl-*N*-nitrosothiazolidine; NHPYR = *N*-nitroso-4-hydroxypyrrolidine.
See Figure 1 for other abbreviations.
Source: Adapted from Sen (1990). Reprinted with permission from Omega Scientific Publishers.

bacon in much higher concentration than required to account for the NPYR formed in the corresponding fried bacon. This suggested that NPRO might be formed concurrently during frying and then undergo decarboxylation to yield NPYR. The above researchers argued that since NPYR formation was preferred in the fat phase, which would reach a higher temperature faster (the higher the cooking temperature, the higher the yield of NPYR), a free radical mechanism for its formation is a more likely possibility (Bharucha et al., 1979).

The nitrosating agent might be N_2O_3, formed from nitrite ion, or nitric oxide radical formed by dissociation of N_2O_3. Since the nitrosation of pyrrolidine occurs very rapidly in the lipid phase, a lower concentration of pyrrolidine, formed from PRO, could also account for most of the NPYR in the fried bacon (Dennis et al., 1982). This suggests that a variety of pathways might be involved in the formation of NPYR in fried bacon.

Similarly, NDMA in fried bacon might be formed by nitrosation of various precursors such as DMA, TMA, and choline (Gray et al., 1978). Alternatively, creatinine, which is present in bacon in high concentrations, might be nitrosated first to produce sarcosine, which could then decarboxylate to yield NDMA (Archer et al., 1971; Gray et al., 1978).

B. Nitrosamines in Directly Dried Foods

Among the foods in this group, the formation of NDMA in malt and skim milk powder has received the most attention. Although traces of NDMA had been detected in beer earlier (International Agency for Research on Cancer, 1977), the discovery was hardly noticed until 1979, when German researchers (Spiegelhalder et al., 1980) reported their results on NDMA contents of 215 German beers and ales. Sixty-six percent of the samples contained ≥ 0.5 ppb NDMA, and the average level was 2.5 ppb (range, 0.5–68 ppb). Beers with a high gravity (e.g., strong beer) or those undergoing a special treatment, such as high kilning and curing temperatures for the malt (e.g., dark ales and dark lager beers), usually contained higher levels of NDMA. Beers from smoked malt contained the highest levels (up to 68 ppb). The above researchers also demonstrated that nitrogen oxides present in the hot flue gases, often used for direct drying of malt, reacted with the amines in the malt to produce NDMA. Malts produced by indirect drying, where the hot air did not come in contact with the flue gas or the air was heated using electric heat, produced very little NDMA. In addition to NDMA, traces of NPYR and NPRO have also been detected in malt and beer.

After the above important discovery, maltsters in most Western countries switched to indirect drying of the malt. Canada was one of the first such countries to adopt this practice as early as 1981. This resulted in a significant drop in the NDMA contents of Canadian beers and ales, as noted in a 1982 survey (Sen et al., 1982). More recently, Scanlan et al. (1990) carried out an extensive survey of U.S. and Canadian beers for their NDMA contents. The average levels and the ranges of concentration of NDMA in the respective products were found to be 0.067 ppb (negative to 0.59 ppb) and 0.095 ppb (negative to 0.59 ppb). These results indicated an approximately 20-fold decrease in the concentration of NDMA in U.S. and Canadian beers and ales over those produced a decade ago.

In a recent survey of German beers (514 samples), Frommberger (1989) detected an average of 0.16 ppb NDMA (range, negative to 3.2 ppb). Although the average daily consumption of beer in West Germany is 619.4 g for men and 185.08 g for women, in reality, such consumption figures range from 0 to several L/day/person. Based on this assumption, Frommberger (1989) estimated that for heavy drinkers in Germany the average NDMA intake through these beverages might reach as high as 10 μg/person/day. The above researchers recommended adoption of further preventive measures to lower NDMA levels in beers and ales produced in Germany.

Traces of NDMA in skim milk powder (Table 2) were first detected by Sen et al. (1980) and Hotchkiss et al. (1980) in the United States. Further surveys have confirmed these initial findings and indicated occurrences of NDMA, NPYR, NPIP, and NMOR in several other direct dried foods such as dried soup bases, dried cheese and soy flour, and instant coffee (Libbey et al., 1980; Sen and Seaman, 1981; Fazio and Havery, 1982). As in the case of the malt, NDMA in skim milk powder appears to be formed as a result of direct drying (Scanlan, personal communication).

C. Formation of Nitrosamines in Foods from Secondary Sources

Foods can be contaminated with nitrosamines as a result of migration from food contact materials. Migration of NMOR from waxed paper to margarine and butter (Sen and Baddoo, 1986) or of several volatile nitrosamines from baby bottle rubber nipples to sterilizing milk in contact with the nipple (Havery and Fazio, 1982; Sen, 1988) can be cited as examples. Low ppb levels of NDEA *N*-nitrosodi-*n*-butylamine (NBDA), *N*-nitrosodibenzylamine (NDBzA) can also form in cured pork products packaged in elastic rubber nettings due to the interaction of nitrite in the meat and amine additives in the rubber (Sen et al., 1987, 1988).

More recently, traces (0.8–5.5 ppb) of NDMA contamination of some reconstituted fruit drinks produced by a particular company in Canada have been reported, but the exact source of the contamination is unclear (Sen, unpublished). Similar fruit drinks from other manufacturers were negative (<0.03 ppb).

D. Nitrosamines in Miscellaneous Food Including Fish and Seafoods

Of the various foods listed in Table 2 under this category, the occurrence of nitrosamines in Chinese pickled vegetables and salted/dried fish and seafoods deserves special mention (Gao et al., 1991). Significant levels of NDMA, NDEA, and NMBzA in some Chinese pickled vegetables have been detected, but the data are limited (Lu et al., 1991). Further research is desirable in this area. There are a large number of reports on the occurrence of nitrosamines in fish and seafoods. However, the levels of nitrosamines (mainly NDMA) detected in such products vary widely in different countries (reviewed by Hotchkiss, 1987; Walker, 1990). Chinese salted/dried fish seem to contain fairly high levels of

NDMA. Recent studies by Sen et al. (1985) suggest that fresh and canned fish are negative, and only traces (1–4 ppb) of NDMA are present in dried and salted fish available for sale to Canadian consumers. More recently, Polish (Karlowski and Bojewski, 1988) and Russian (Tutelyan et al., 1990) workers reported the occurrence of 1–74 ppb NDMA in various fish and seafoods (including the dried and smoked fish).

Broiling of fish and seafoods (e.g., squid) on a gas flame can lead to increased NDMA formation due to the interaction of amines in such products and nitrogen oxides produced during burning of the natural gas (Kawabata et al., 1980). Up to 313 ppb NDMA has been detected in some squid when broiled on a gas flame. On the other hand, Key et al. (1982) in England failed to observe any significant increase in NDMA contents of fish after cooking over a gas range. The above discrepancy may be due to different types of fish and seafoods used in the two studies.

Siddiqi et al. (1988, 1991) reported widespread occurrence of several nitrosamines (mainly NDMA, NPYR, and NPIP) in various foodstuffs from Kashmir, India. The above researchers also discussed the role these compounds may play in the etiology of esophageal and gastric cancer that are prevalent among the people in the region. Of particular interest is a recent observation (Kumar et al., 1990) that nitrosation of one of the dried vegetables, leaves from the plant *Brassica oleracea*, produced high levels of NMU—a direct-acting carcinogenic nitrosamide. Low ppb levels (10–22 ppb) of preformed NDMA and NPYR were also detected in the unnitrosated dried as well as boiled leave of the above plant, which is frequently consumed by local people. These researchers, however, used an indirect method for determining NMU in the samples. It would be advisable to verify these results by another method that measures NMU concentration directly, and to confirm its identity by mass spectrometry. If confirmed to be true, this will be the first reported finding of a nitrosamide in foods.

V. DAILY INTAKE OF NOC THROUGH FOODS AND BEVERAGES

Various researchers have attempted to estimate per capita daily intake of volatile nitrosamines for humans through diets. A summary of the data reported for different countries is presented in Table 3. It appears that, prior to 1981, beer and ale were the major contributors of nitrosamines in most of the Western diets. The apparent higher NDMA intake in 1987 compared to that in 1978 in the U.K. diets can be explained by the fact that beer was not included in the 1978 data. Among the countries listed in Table 3, people in Japan seem to have the highest nitrosamine intake. This is mainly because of relatively high nitrosamine contents of several typical Japanese foods (e.g., fish and seafoods). Beer and ale play only a minor role in this respect in Japanese diet. Limited data available from China suggest that some commonly consumed Chinese foods (e.g., pickled vegetables, salted and dried fish) contain fairly high levels of nitrosamines. Therefore, the average daily intake of nitrosamines through diet for the Chinese population might be comparable to that for the Japanese, but no data in this regard has been published. It should be emphasized, however, that the above data relate only to volatile nitrosamines; the figures do not include nonvolatile NOCs, nitrosamides, or bound NOCs (e.g., protein bound). The actual amounts of total NOCs ingested through foods and beverages may be much higher than indicated in Table 3.

In addition to diet, humans are exposed to NOCs through a variety of sources. In fact, diet is only a minor contributor to humans' total body burden of nitrosamines. The major exposure to preformed NOCs originates from cigarette and other tobacco products, automobile interiors, and cosmetics (Fine et al., 1980; Hotchkiss, 1987). A National Academy of Sciences report (1981) estimated that cigarette smoking may result in a total nitrosamine intake of about 17 μg/person/day. In addition, humans are also exposed to NOCs formed endogenously in the body, as discussed in Section VI.

VI. IN VIVO FORMATION OF NITROSAMINES

There is some evidence to support the theory that traces of nitrosamines and nitrosamides are formed in vivo in humans (reviewed by Fine, 1982). Fine et al. (1977) were the first to present evidence of in vivo formation of NDMA and NDEA in human volunteers after consumption of meals containing beer, nitrate-rich vegetables (e.g., spinach), and cured meats (e.g., fried bacon). The levels of both NDMA and NDEA in the blood increased after such a meal, and this was taken as an evidence of in vivo synthesis of nitrosamines. The two nitrosamines were thought to have been formed due to the interaction of ingested or salivary nitrite and amines in the meal. Other researchers, however, have either observed only a marginal increase in blood nitrosamine levels or failed to detect any NDMA or NDEA in the blood of human volunteers after consumption of such meals (Garland et al., 1982; Sen, 1986). Further research is obviously needed to resolve the discrepancies in the above sets of results.

The main difficulty in measuring in vivo nitrosamine formation lies in the fact that most NOCs are metabolized rapidly by the liver, and very little is left to be detected in the blood or the urine. The problem can be solved in two ways: (1) by partially or completely blocking hepatic metabolism of the compound or (2) by measuring the formation of a NOC which is not metabolized by the liver and is excreted quantitatively in the urine. Perciballi and Hotchkiss (1989) used the first approach, and pretreated laboratory animals with 4-methylpyrazole, an inhibitor of nitrosamine metabolism. Administration of the drug in the drinking water inhibited NDMA metabolism so that up to 13% of administered NDMA could be detected in the urine. Without the drug, no NDMA could be detected in the urine of NDMA-dosed rats. The above researchers used the model to investigate in vivo NDMA formation in ferrets maintained on various diets (cured meats, fried bacon, malt, fish, dried milk). Except for one sample, a sample of nitrite-treated chopped meat, no significant evidence of in vivo NDMA formation could be demonstrated. However, 4-methylpyrazole–treated ferrets that were fed only cured meats excreted 10-fold higher levels of NDMA in the urine during 24 h than the corresponding control ferrets did. The control ferrets were also treated with the drug but were

Table 3 Average per Capita Daily Intake of Volatile Nitrosamines Through Foods and Beverages

Country	Year study conducted	Nitrosamines[a] ingested through various commodities (μg)		Total intake (%)	Ref.
Federal Republic of Germany	1978–79	Beer and ale	0.7	64	Preussmann et al., 1979
		Cured meats	0.21	10	
		Cheese	0.01	0	
		Other foods and beverages	0.23	25	
		Total	1.15		
Federal Republic of Germany	1983	Total as above	0.6[b]		Preussmann et al., 1984
The Netherlands	1976–78	Beer	0.99	90	Stephany and Schuller, 1980
		Other foods	0.11	10	
		Total	1.10		
The Netherlands	1984–85	Total	<0.1		Ellen et al., 1990
Sweden	1988	Beer and whiskey	0.04	14	Österdahl, 1988
		Cured meats and bacon	0.23	80	
		Dried foods	0.014	5	
		Total	0.28		

Japan	1980	Beer	0.05	2	Maki et al., 1980
		Fish and seafoods	2.37	79	
		Dairy products	0.53	18	
		Others including cured meats	0.03	1	
		Total	2.98		
Japan	1984	Total as above	0.66[c]		Yamamoto et al., 1984
U.K.	1978	Cured meats	0.43	81	Gough et al., 1978
		Fish	<0.01	<2	
		Cheese	<0.01	<2	
		All other foods	0.08	15	
		Total	0.5		
U.K.		All above plus beer and ale	0.7		MAFF, 1987

[a]Mainly NDMA and NYPR.
[b]After NDMA levels in beer and ales have decreased to present levels.
[c]Revised data for fish and seafoods.

fed a semisynthetic diet. Since the data are very limited, further research along these lines should be carried out before reaching a definite conclusion.

Ohshima and Bartsch (1981) used the second approach to study in vivo nitrosation. The method is based on measuring the increase in urinary NPRO output after an oral dose of PRO. Since NPRO is noncarcinogenic in laboratory animals and since it is excreted nearly completely in the urine, the compound appears to be an ideal choice for such a purpose. The method is quantitative, easy to perform, and shows a clear dose-response relationship with ingested nitrate/nitrite. Also, after a single dose of PRO and nitrite to rats, the amount of NPRO excreted in the urine was proportional to the dose of PRO and to the square of the nitrite dose thus bearing the same relationship as that observed in in vitro experiments (see Sec. II.B). Various researchers have used the technique to study in vivo nitrosation in humans and attempted to correlate the results with the incidence of cancers in humans (reviewed by Bartsch et al., 1989; Knight et al., 1991). While the technique can be taken as a general indicator of in vivo nitrosation, its main drawback is that it measures only in vivo nitrosation of PRO but not of other amines (e.g., DMA) or amides (e.g., *N*-methylurea). It is entirely possible that other NOCs (e.g., NDMA, NMU) might not be formed at all because the corresponding amine or amide precursors might not be present in the diets in high enough concentrations.

In view of the above methodology problems, there is a great deal of uncertainty as to the extent of endogenous nitrosation in humans. Some believe that the majority of the total body burden of nitrosamines arise through endogenous nitrosation occurring in the environment of the human stomach (Wagner and Tannenbaum, 1985). Licht and Deen (1988), on the other hand, predicted that even for a DMA-rich diet, the endogenous formation of NDMA would be $\sim 10^2$–10^3 lower than published estimates of NDMA exposure through diet. It appears that further research is needed to gain a clearer understanding of the extent of endogenous nitrosation that can occur under realistic conditions.

VII. BIOLOGICAL ACTIVITY

A. Introduction

While investigating an accident in a laboratory, Freund (1937) reported the first evidence of toxicity of a nitrosamine in humans. Two chemists working in that laboratory with NDMA suffered acute liver poisoning, and one of them eventually died due to severe liver necrosis. The incident was forgotten until the mid-1950s when Barnes and Magee (1954) reported on similar hepatotoxic effects of NDMA in a number of laboratory animals. A dose of 20–40 mg/kg produced severe liver damage (centrilobular necrosis) in mice, rats, guinea pigs, rabbits, and dogs. The dose also proved fatal to all the animals. Soon after, Magee and Barnes (1956) demonstrated that NDMA is also a potent carcinogen in rats. This important discovery led Magee and his co-workers and others, notably Druckrey et al. (1967) in Germany and Lijinsky (1987a) in the United States, to test a wide variety of NOCs for their carcinogenicity in laboratory

Table 4 Types of Various NOCs Tested for Carcinogenicity

Types of compounds	Number tested	Number found carcinogenic
Symmetrical nitrosamines	55	47
Unsymmetrical nitrosamines	95	81
Dinitrosamines	4	4
Cyclic nitrosamines	78	67
Total Nitrosamines	232	199 (86%)
Nitrosoureas	60	57
Nitrosoguanidines	11	7
Nitrosourethanes	17	17
Other nitrosamides	12	10
Total Nitrosamides	100	91 (91%)

Source: Preussmann and Stewart (1984). Reprinted with permission from *Chemical Carcinogens*, 2nd edition, Vol. 2, Copyright © (1984), American Chemical Society..

animals. Of more than 300 NOCs tested thus far, approximately 90% have been found to be carcinogenic (Preussmann and Stewart, 1984) (Table 4). For details the reader should consult the following authoritative reviews on the subject (Okada, 1984; Preussmann and Stewart, 1984; Lijinsky, 1987a).

B. Acute Toxicity and Carcinogenicity

Of all the nitrosamines, NDEA has been tested most widely. It has been shown to induce cancer in 44 species of animals including the primates. Moreover, no animal species tested has been found to be resistant to its carcinogenic action. Other NOCs are also carcinogenic to a large number of animal species. Therefore, it is highly unlikely that humans would be resistant to the carcinogenic action of NOCs although no direct evidence of this has been reported. Table 5 presents a brief list of NOCs that are of interest to food scientists; the table also presents some relevant toxicity and carcinogenicity data for these compounds. There does not appear to be any relationship between the LD_{50} values and carcinogenic potencies of these compounds. For example, NDMA is more toxic than NDEA, but the latter is equally active as a carcinogen.

As a class of chemical carcinogens, NOCs are unique in the sense that there are very few classes of chemicals, if any, that can induce cancer in so many organs of so many animal species. The target organ may vary depending on many factors, predominant among which are the chemical structure of the compound (structure-activity relationship) and the animal species. Other factors such as nutritional status of the animal, its age and sex, route of administration of the compound and its dosing schedule, and the presence of other modifying factors (discussed in Sec. VII.C) also play important roles in this regard. Although there might be some discrepancies, the following generalizations can be made with regard to structure-activity

Table 5 Acute Toxicity (LD_{50}) and Carcinogenicity of Selected NOCs Formed or Detected in Foods

NOC	LD_{50} values in rats (mg/kg, po)	Carcinogenic response		
		Relative potency	Species/Strain	Target organs
NDMA	40	*****	Mouse, rat, hamster, guinea pig, and 10 other species	Liver, kidney, lung, nasal cavity
NDEA	280	*****	Mouse, rat, hamster, monkey, dog, and 39 other species	Liver, lung, esophagus, forestomach, kidney, trachea
NDBA	1,200	****	Mouse, rat, hamster, guinea pig, rabbit	Forestomach, liver, esophagus, urinary bladder, lung, mammary gland
NMBzA	18	****	Mouse, rat	Esophagus, forestomach
NPIP	200	****	Mouse, rat, hamster, monkey	Esophagus, liver, nasal cavity, pharynx, forestomach
NMOR	320	*****	Mouse, rat hamster	Liver, lung, kidney, nasal cavity
NPYR	900	****	Mouse, rat, hamster	Lung, liver, nasal cavity, vagina, testis
NSAR	5,000	*[a]	Mouse, rat	Nasal cavity, lung, liver, small intestine
NTHZ	not available	negative	Rat	
NPRO	4,500	negative	Mouse, rat	
N-Nitrosos-*N*-methyl-acetamide	20	*****	Rat	Forestomach, oral cavity
NMU	110	*****	Mouse, rat, hamster, guinea pig, monkey, and 40 other species	Skin tumors, hematopoietic system, lymphatic tissue, lung, stomach, forestomach, brain, liver, nervous system, spinal cord, mammary gland, colon, rectum, anus, pancreas, and many other organs

[a]Being least potent.
Source: Druckrey et al., 1967; Preussmann and Stewart, 1984; Shephard et al., 1987; Lijinsky, 1987a.

relationships of these compounds in inducing cancer in laboratory animals (Lijinsky, 1987a,b):

1. In rats, the most predominant site after treatment with nitrosamines appears to be esophagus followed by the liver, forestomach, and nasal mucosa. On the other hand, no nitrosamides induce tumors of the esophagus in rats.
2. No NOCs induce tumors of the esophagus in Syrian golden hamsters.
3. Only nitrosoalkylureas (nitrosamides), but no nitrosamines, induce tumors of the central nervous system.
4. Nitrosamides rarely produce liver tumors in rats and hamsters.
5. Nitrosamines containing a β-oxygenated propyl group (e.g., nitrosomethyl-2-hydroxy propylamine) produce pancreatic cancer in hamsters but not in rats.
6. Nitrosomethyl-*n*-alkylamines with an even-numbered carbon chain containing >6 C atoms (e.g., *N*-nitroso-*N*-methyl-*N*-octylamine) give rise to bladder tumors.

C. Metabolism and Mode of Action

Biochemical studies suggest that most nitrosamines require metabolic activation before effecting their toxic and biological properties (reviewed by Magee et al., 1976; Preussmann and Stewart, 1984; Lijinsky, 1987a; Lawley, 1990). The first step in this metabolic activation process is believed to be the hydroxylation of the α-C atom (with respect to the N-N=O group). This implies that to be biologically active, the nitrosamine must have an H atom at the α-C atom. After enzymatic α-hydroxylation, which mostly takes place in the liver, the compounds are converted to carbonium ions or diazoalkanes which alkylate DNA and other macromolecules. Alkylation of DNA is thought to be the initial step causing mutations in target cells eventually leading to the development of malignant tumors. Nitrosamides, on the other hand, do not require any metabolic activation; they spontaneously convert to the alkylating agents. Because of this, nitrosamides can induce tumors both at the site of application (e.g., on skin, in the colon if given intrarectally) as well as at distant sites such as the brain and the central nervous system. Although the above-mentioned DNA alkylation process is widely believed to play a major role in NOC-induced carcinogenesis in experimental animals, there are many observations that cannot be accounted for in terms of alkylation reactions (Lijinsky, 1987a,b).

Of various factors affecting carcinogenicity of NOCs, the role of metabolic modifiers deserves a special mention. Ethanol in alcoholic beverages, dithiocarbamates as fungicide residues or as residues from rubber-based food contact materials, and the naturally occurring isothiocyanates in certain vegetables can significantly inhibit metabolism of nitrosamines by the liver (Swann, 1984; Chung et al., 1984). This removes the protection that the liver offers, and prevention of this first-pass clearance makes the nitrosamines available to other organs (e.g., esophagus) that are particularly susceptible to their carcinogenic effect. Ethanol at a dose equivalent to a man drinking a glass of beer was found to markedly inhibit hepatic metabolism of both NDMA and NDEA in the rat and to increase their residual concentrations as well as rate of DNA alkylation in other organs such as the kidney and the esophagus (Swann, 1984). These data seem to support previously published reports indicating effect of ethanol on the carcinogenicity of nitrosamines in extrahepatic organs of the test animals (Gibel, 1967; Griciute et al., 1981; Anderson, 1988). In all these studies, concurrent administration of ethanol with NDMA or NDEA increased the incidence of lung and esophageal tumors in experimental animals. Similarly, concurrent administration of disulfiram, a dithiocarbamate, and NDEA or NMBzA increased the incidence of tumors in the esophagus and the trachea in the rat (Schmähl et al., 1976).

D. Mutagenicity and Genotoxicity

Many nitrosamines are also potent mutagens, but they need metabolic activation to effect this activity in bacteria, yeast, or fungal assay systems (Preussmann and Stewart, 1984). This metabolic activation is usually carried out by preincubating the nitrosamines with rat liver or hamster liver microsomal enzyme preparations. On the other hand, most nitrosamides are active without metabolic activation. In general, there appears to be a good correlation between carcinogenicity and mutagenicity of NOCs in the modified Ames test, although of 37 carcinogenic nitrosamines tested 2 gave negative results in the mutagenicity testing (Bartsch et al., 1980). Lijinsky (1987b) concluded that the Salmonella reversal assay of Ames is a reasonable qualitative, but not quantitative, predictor of carcinogenesis by NOCs. There are, however, still many gaps in our knowledge that require further research.

Recent findings of NDBzA in cured pork products packaged in elastic rubber nettings and in baby bottle rubber nipples have aroused a great deal of interest in this compound (Sen, 1991). In an earlier study, NDBzA was reported to be noncarcinogenic to rats (Druckrey et al., 1967). The negative result was rationalized by the suggestion that either the compound could not easily form a carbonium ion or, even if it did, the carbonium ion would be too bulky to react at the active sites of DNA (Fig. 2). It is, however, mutagenic to Salmonella (Pool et al., 1986), and it induces single-strand breaks in the DNA of rat and hamster hepatocytes (Schmezer et al., 1987). Furthermore, α-hydroxyl NDBzA (see Fig. 2) is a direct-acting carcinogen in laboratory animals (Wiessler et al., 1983). Other benzylating species such as benzylnitrosourea are also carcinogenic to rodents (Ivankovic, 1978).

In their latest studies, Schmezer et al. (1990) found NDBzA to be inactive in both the rat and mouse bone marrow micronucleus assay as well as the rat liver assay for unscheduled DNA synthesis. It was, however, active as a micronucleus-inducing agent and mitogen in the rat liver, and it induced single-strand breaks in the DNA in rat hepatocytes. The researchers concluded that NDBzA is genotoxic. Boyes et al. (1990) have concluded that NDBzA is weakly mutagenic to both Salmonella and Chinese hamster V79 cells.

These conflicting results regarding noncarcinogenicity of NDBzA to rats, but positive genotoxicity of NDBzA in some in vitro bioassay systems and carcinogenicity of α-acetoxy NDBzA and other benzylating species are puzzling and require further studies.

E. Transplacental Carcinogenesis

Many NOC have been shown to display strong transplacental carcinogenic effects in rat, mouse, golden hamster, and pig (reviewed by Magee et al., 1976). The most critical factor seems to be the time of the treatment. In rat, the maximum transplacental effect is observed when pregnant animals are dosed with NOCs after 12 days of gestation. NMU and *N*-nitroso-*N*-ethylurea (NEU) have been found to be the most potent transplacental carcinogens known. For example, the transplacental carcinogenic effect of NMU has been observed in the rats even at F_3 generation, though only the parent at F_0 generation received a single dose of NMU on the 18th day of pregnancy. The F_1-generation rats were exposed in utero to the compound, but those in F_2 and F_3 generations had no direct contact with NMU. The tumors observed in the rats of all these three daughter (F_1 to F_3) generations were mainly in the mammary gland, kidney, and the nervous system, whereas only tumors in the mammary gland were observed among the rats at F_0 (the parent) generation (Tomatis et al., 1975). NDMA and NDEA have also been shown to induce transplacental carcinogenic effects in laboratory animals.

F. Dose-Response Relationship

Various dose-response studies carried out suggest that nitrosamines are carcinogenic to laboratory animals not only at relatively high doses, but also at extremely low doses. Data from these low-level studies are very useful in assessing risk to humans arising from exposure to trace levels of nitrosamines present in foods and beverages. The pioneering study of Druckrey et al. (1967) in which the researchers investigated carcinogenicity of NDEA in rats at nine dose levels (0.075–14.2 mg/kg body weight/day) over the whole lifetime of the animals is a good example. Even the lowest dose proved carcinogenic, and there appeared to be no no-effect level. Moreover, the total amount of NDEA needed to produce tumors decreased, instead of increasing, with a decrease in the daily dose level, suggesting an acceleration process. The above researchers concluded that a carcinogenic effect at a lower dose would be observed if the animals survived long enough.

More recently, Peto et al. (1984) reported the results of an extensive study on dose and time relationships for nitrosamine carcinogenesis in 4080 rats. Four different nitrosamines (NDMA, NDEA, NPYR, and NPIP) each at 16 dose levels (0.033 to 16.896 ppm) were given in the drinking water to both sexes of Colworth rats. The target organs mainly affected were the liver (for all four compounds) and the esophagus (for NDEA and NPIP only). Since the experiment was extended to an extreme old age, the effects were measurable to a dose as low as 0.01 mg/kg body weight/day. NDEA was the most potent of the four nitrosamines tested. The TD_{50} doses needed to halve the tumorless survivors were estimated to be 0.06 mg/kg body weight/day for NDEA and about 0.12 mg/kg body weight/day for NDMA. NPYR and NPIP were less potent because the corresponding TD_{50} dose values for these compounds were found to be 0.4 (males) and 0.6 (females) mg/kg body weight/day for each compound. Because of the extensive and thorough nature of two studies (Druckrey et al.,

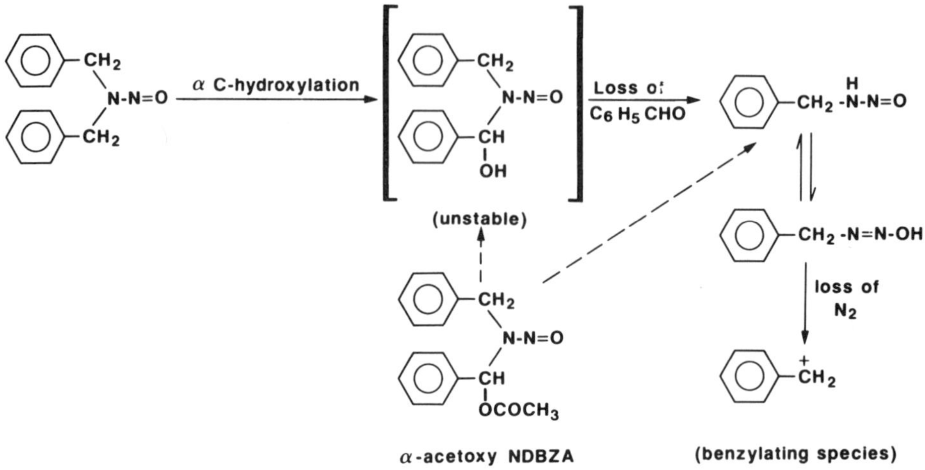

Figure 2 Postulated metabolism of NDBzA and α-acetoxy NDBzA leading to the formation of benzylating species. Source: Schmerzer et al. (1990). Reprinted by permission of *Environ. Mol. Mutagen*, Copyright © (1990), John Wiley & Sons, Inc.

1967; Peto et al., 1984), data obtained in these studies have been or are being widely used in estimating risk to human health due to exposure to nitrosamines.

Furthermore, many foods contain more than one nitrosamine (see Table 2). Therefore, in assessing risk one should consider the possibility of an additive effect of the various nitrosamines present. Berger et al. (1990) investigated the carcinogenic effect of single as well as combined doses of three nitrosamines, NDMA, NDEA, and *N*-nitrosodiethanolamine (NDELA), in rat. A linear relationship was found between exposure to nitrosamine and time to death with liver tumor even at very low exposure levels. The combination effect of the three nitrosamines indicated a mere additivity in liver tumor occurrence at a very low dose. However, when the nitrosamines were administered singly at these low dose levels, the treatment did not induce any significant carcinogenic effect in the rats. The above researchers concluded that the elimination of carcinogens from the environment would contribute to reduced tumor incidence even if no firm relationship to a particular cancer in human had been established, since this would reduce the additive effect of various carcinogens to which humans are exposed.

In view of the extreme carcinogenic potency of many of the NOCs in laboratory animals, it is difficult to decide upon a safe level of nitrosamine in foods. For this reason, most countries as well as the WHO have not set a figure for acceptable daily intake (ADI) for nitrosamines in foods. The most prudent approach would be to treat the presence of these chemicals in foods very seriously, and take every measure to minimize their formation.

VIII. EPIDEMIOLOGICAL STUDIES

Various researchers have attempted to correlate human exposure to nitrosamines with the incidence of specific cancer in human population. If one assumes humans are also susceptible to the carcinogenic action of nitrosamines, one would expect to find such an epidemiological link in situations where exposure level is the highest, i.e., through cigarette and other tobacco products (e.g., chewing tobacco, snuff) but not through food and beverages, which constitute only a minor source of exposure to nitrosamines. In fact, strong evidence of a connection between nitrosamine exposure and cancer in humans appears to emerge from studies relating to tobacco products (both smoke and smokeless) and to consumption of areca nut (betel nut) (Bhide et al., 1979; Hoffmann et al., 1984; IARC, 1985, 1986). Both the above-mentioned products, especially the tobacco-related ones, are associated with high incidence of characteristic oral, nasal, and respiratory tract tumors in humans and contain several carcinogenic nitrosamines in high concentrations or produce them after nitrosation in the oral cavity. Further studies are, however, needed to clearly establish whether nitrosamines in these products are the actual causative agents.

Forman (1987, 1991) and Preston-Martin (1987) have reviewed the literature dealing with dietary exposure to NOCs and the risk of human cancer. Various epidemiological studies that are underway or have been concluded in this area include: (1) studies on the possible correlation between consumption of smoked fish and cured smoked meats and cancer of the upper gastrointestinal tract among certain populations in Canada and the United States, (2) consumption of salted fish and salt-pickled vegetable and its relation to the high gastric cancer mortality among the inhabitants of Japan, (3) the role of nitrosamines in the local diets (pickled/fermented vegetables) on the induction of esophageal cancer among the population of Lin-Xian county of northern China, and (4) a possible link between consumption of salted/dried fish containing high levels of nitrosamines and the high incidence of nasopharyngeal carcinoma among the population in southern China. In reviewing the various studies Preston-Martin (1987) concluded that although evidence presented in support of some of these cases appeared to be quite strong, alternative etiological hypotheses for the cancer in the respective cases could not be ruled out. At present, there does not appear to be any strong evidence to suggest that nitrosamines in the diet are responsible for any specific cancer in humans.

Forman (1987) reached similar conclusion while investigating a possible link between human cancer and ingestion of precursors (amines, amides, nitrate, nitrite) of NOCs through diets. Although it has been well established that concurrent administration of high levels of weakly basic secondary amines or amides and nitrite to laboratory animals induce cancer at various organs, it is not clear how these findings can be extrapolated to the human situation. Consumption of nitrate through cured meats may lead to a higher rate of in vivo nitrosation (due to higher salivary nitrite levels), but, as mentioned earlier, most of our nitrate intakes come from vegetables that also contain high levels of natural inhibitors (e.g., ascorbic acid, phenolic acids, α-tocopherol) of

N-nitrosation. Therefore, ingestion of vegetables would increase salivary nitrite levels but would not necessarily increase in vivo intragastric *N*-nitrosation. This may explain why epidemiologists obtained negative correlation between nitrate intake through vegetables and fruits and the stomach cancer incidence in man. Even if intragastric *N*-nitrosation were found to be a key factor in the etiology of gastric cancer in man, the best way to minimize this nitrosation would be to recommend increased consumption of fruits and vegetables.

IX. CONCLUSION

In reviewing the subject one will conclude that considerable knowledge has been gained in our understanding of both the mechanisms of formation of NOCs and their occurrence in foods and beverages. As a result, it has been possible to modify or change food-processing conditions that have significantly reduced the levels of these compounds in our food supply. However, some problem areas still remain that require further improvement. For example, it would be desirable to minimize formation of nitrosamines in certain Chinese foods, heavily spiced cured meats, some cured smoked meats including bacon, sun-dried vegetables, and possibly beer and ale (if not already reduced to <0.1 ppb). Further research is also needed to determine the nature of unknown nitrosaminelike compounds present in cured meats, Chinese and Japanese pickled vegetables, and beer and ale. If the formation of NMU in nitrosated dried leafy vegetables (*Brassica oleracea*) is confirmed, similar studies with other foods in areas of the world where the incidence of stomach and esophagial cancer is quite prevalent would be desirable. There is also a need for an improved method for studying in vivo nitrosation in humans that will give a more accurate estimate of such formation. It is hoped that future research will be helpful in resolving these problems and in minimizing the total exposure by man to foodborne NOCs.

REFERENCES

Anderson, L. M. (1988). Increased numbers of *N*-nitrosodimethylamine-initiated lung tumors in mice by chronic co-administration of ethanol. *Carcinogenesis 9*: 1717–1719.

Archer, M. C., Clarke, S. D., Thilly, J. E., and Tannenbaum, S. R. (1971). Environmental nitroso compounds: Reaction of nitrite with creatine and creatinine. *Science 174*: 1341–1343.

Barnes, J. M., and Magee, P. N. (1954). Some toxic properties of dimethylnitrosamine. *Brit. J. Ind. Med. 11*: 167–174.

Bartsch, H. (1991). *N*-Nitroso compounds and human cancer: Where do we stand? *IARC Sci. Publ. No. 105*: 1–10.

Bartsch, H., Malaveille, C., Camus, A. M., Martel-Planche, G., Brun, G., Hautefeuille, A., Sabadie, N., and Barbin, A. (1980). Validation and comparative studies on 180 chemicals with *S. typhimurium* strains and V79 Chinese hamster cells in the presence of various metabolizing systems. *Mutat. Res. 76*(1): 1–50.

Bartsch, H., Ohshima, H., Pignatelli, B., and Calmels, S. (1989). Human exposure to endogenous *N*-nitroso compounds: quantitative estimates in subjects at high risk for cancer of the oral cavity, esophagus, stomach and urinary bladder. *Cancer Surv. 8*: 335–362.

Berger, M. R., Schmähl, D., and Edler, L. (1990). Implications on the carcinogenic hazard of low doses of three hepatocarcinogenic *N*-nitrosamines. *Jpn. J. Cancer Res. 81*: 598–606.

Bharucha, K. R., Cross, C. K., and Rubin, L. J. (1979). Mechanism of *N*-nitrosopyrrolidine formation in bacon. *J. Agric. Food Chem. 27*: 63–69.

Bhide, S. V., Shivapurkar, N. M., Gothoskar, S. V., and Ranadive, K. J. (1979). Carcinogenicity of betel quid ingredients: Feeding mice with aqueous extract and the polyphenol fraction of betel nut. *Br. J. Cancer 40*: 922–926.

Boyes, B. G., Rogers, C. G., Matula, T. I., Stapley, R., and Sen, N. P. (1990). Evaluation of genotoxicity of *N*-nitrosodibenzylamine in Chinese hamster V79 cells and in Salmonella. *Mutat. Res. 241*: 379–385.

Canadian Food and Drug Regulations (1987). Food additives that may be used as class I preservatives, item S-5, Table XI, Part I, Div. 16, pp. 67–39 to 67–40B, Health and Welfare Canada, Ministry of Supply and Services, Ottawa, Ontario, Canada.

Challis, B. C., Lomas, S. J., Rzepa, H. S., Bavin, P. M. G., Barkin, D. W., Viney, N. J., and Moore, P. J. (1982). A kinetic model for the formation of gastric *N*-nitroso compounds. In *Nitrosamines and Human Cancer*, P. N. Magee, ed. *Banbury Report No. 12*, Cold Spring Harbor Laboratory, New York, pp. 243–256.

Chung, F.-L., Juchatz, A., Vitarius, J., Reiss, B., and Hecht, S. S. (1984). Inhibition of target tissue activation of *N'*-nitrosonornicotine and *N*-nitrosopyrrolidine by dietary components. *IARC Sci. Publ. No. 57*: 797–804.

Concon, J. M. (1988). *Food Toxicology* (in two parts, A and B). Marcel Dekker, Inc., New York, 1988.

Davies, R., and McWeeny, D. J. (1977). Catalytic effect of nitrosophenols on *N*-nitrosamine formation. *Nature* (London) *266*: 657–658.

Dennis, M. J., Massey, R. C., and McWeeny, D. J. (1982). The effect of oxygen on nitrosamine formation. *Z. Lebensm. Unters. Forsch. 174*: 114–116.

Douglass, M. L. (1978). The chemistry of nitrosamine formation, inhibition and destruction. *J. Soc. Cosmet. Chem. 29*: 581–606.

Druckrey, H., Preussmann, R., Ivankovic, S., and Schmähl, D. (1967). Organotrope Carcinogene Wirkungen bei 65 verschiedenen *N*-nitroso-Verbindungen an BD-Ratten. *Z. Krebsforsch. 69*: 103–201.

Dull, B. J., and Hotchkiss, J. H. (1984). Activated oxygen and mammalian nitrate biosynthesis. *Carcinogenesis 8*: 1161–1164.

Ellen, G., Egmond, E., VanLoon, J. W., Sahertian, E. T., and Tolsma, K. (1990). Dietary intakes of some essential and nonessential trace elements, nitrate, nitrite and *N*-nitrosamines, by Dutch adults: Estimated via 24-hour duplicate portion study. *Food Additiv. Contamin. 7*: 207–221.

Ender, F., Havre, G., Helgebostad, A., Koppang, N., Madsen, R., and Ceh, L. (1964). Isolation and identification of a hepatotoxic factor in herring meal produced from sodium nitrite preserved herring. *Naturwissenschaffen 51*: 637–638.

Fazio, T., and Havery, D. C. (1982). Volatile *N*-nitrosamines in direct flame dried processed foods. *IARC Sci. Publ. No. 41*: 277–286.

Fiddler, W., Pensabene, J. W., Doerr, R. C., and Wasserman, A. E. (1972). Formation of *N*-nitrosodimethylamine from naturally occurring quaternary ammonium compounds and tertiary amines. *Nature* (London) *236*: 307.

Fine, D. H. (1982). Presence of nitrosamines in human beings. In *Nitrosamines and Human Cancer*, P. N. Magee, ed. *Banbury Report No. 12*, Cold Spring Harbor Laboratory, New York, pp. 271–281.

Fine, D. H., Ross, R., Rounbehler, D. P., Silvergleid, A., and Song, L. (1977). Formation *in vivo* of volatile *N*-nitrosamines in man after ingestion of cooked bacon and spinach. *Nature* (London) *265*: 753–755.

Fine, D. H., Reisch, J., and Rounbehler, D. P. (1980). Nitrosamines in new automobiles. *IARC Sci. Publ.* No. 31: 541–551.

Forman, D. (1987). Dietary exposure to *N*-nitroso compounds and the risk of human cancer. *Cancer Surv. 6*(4): 719–738.

Forman, D. (1991). The etiology of gastric cancer. *IARC Sci. Publ.* No. 105: 22–32.

Freund, H. A. (1937). Clinical manifestations and studies in parenchymatous hepatitis. *Ann. Intern. Med. 10*: 1144–1155.

Frommberger, R. (1989). *N*-Nitrosodimethylamine in German beer. *Food Chem. Toxicol. 27*: 27–29.

Gao, J., Hotchkiss, J. H., and Chen, J. (1991). Regional differences in *N*-nitrosamine content of traditional Chinese foods. *IARC Sci. Publ. No. 105*: 219–222.

Garland, W. A., Holowaschenko, H., Kuenzig, W., Norkus, E. P., and Conney, A. H. (1982). A high resolution mass spectrometry assay for *N*-nitrosodimethylamine in human plasma. In *Nitrosamines and Human Cancer*, P. N. Magee, ed. *Banbury Report No. 12*, Cold Spring Harbor Laboratory, New York, pp. 183–196.

Gibel, W. (1967). Experimentelle Unterschungen zur Synkarzinogenese beim Oesophaguskarzinom. *Arch. Geschwulstforsch. 30*: 181–189.

Gough, T. A., and Goodhead, K. (1975). Occurrence of volatile nitrosamines in spice premixes. *J. Sci. Food Agric. 26*: 1473–1478.

Gough, T. A., Webb, K. S., and Coleman, R. F. (1978). Estimate of the volatile nitrosamine content of U.K. food. *Nature* (London) *272*: 161–163.

Gray, J. I. (1981). Formation of *N*-nitroso compounds in foods. In *N-Nitroso Compounds in Foods*, R. A. Scanlan and S. R. Tannenbaum, eds. *ACS Symposium Series 174*, American Chemical Society, Washington, DC, pp. 165–180.

Gray, J. I., Collins, M. E., and MacDonald, B. (1978). Precursors of dimethylnitrosamine in fried bacon. *J. Food Protect. 41*: 31–35.

Gray, J. I., Reddy, S. K., Price, J. F., Mandagere, A., and Wilkens, W. F. (1982). Inhibition of *N*-nitrosamines in bacon. *Food Technol. 36*(6): 39–45.

Green, L. C., Ruiz De Luzuriaga, K., Wagner, D. A., Rand, W., Isfan, N., Young, V. R., and Tannenbaum, S. R. (1981). Nitrate biosynthesis in man. *Proc. Natl. Acad. Sci. USA 78*: 7764–7768.

Griciute, L., Castegnaro, M., and Béréziat, J.-C. (1981). Influence of ethyl alcohol on carcinogenesis with *N*-nitrosodimethylamine. *Cancer Lett. 13*: 345–352.

Havery, D. C., and Fazio, T. (1982). Estimation of volatile *N*-nitrosamines in rubber nipples for babies' bottles. *Food Chem. Toxicol. 20*: 939–944.

Hoffmann, D., Brunnemann, K. D., Adams, J. D., and Hecht, S. S. (1984). Formation and analysis of *N*-nitrosamines in tobacco products and their endogenous formation in consumers. *IARC Sci. Pub.* No. 57: 743–762.

Hotchkiss, J. H. (1987). A review of current literature on *N*-nitroso compounds in foods. *Adv. Food Res. 31*: 53–115.

Hotchkiss, J. H., Libbey, L. M., Barbour, J. F., and Scanlan, R. A. (1980). Combination of a GC-TEA and a GC-MS data system for the μg/kg estimation and confirmation of volatile *N*-nitrosamines in foods. *IARC Sci. Publ.* No. 31: 361–376.

IARC (1985). *IARC Monographs on the Evaluation of the Carcinogenic Risk of Chemicals to Humans: Tobacco Habits Other Than Smoking: Betel Quid and Areca-Nut Chewing; and Some Related Nitrosamines*. Vol. 37. International Agency for Research on Cancer, Lyon, France.

IARC (1986). *IARC Monographs on the Evaluation of the Carcinogenic Risk of Chemicals to Humans: Tobacco Smoking*, Vol. 38. International Agency for Research on Cancer, Lyon, France.

IARC (1977). Carcinogens in alcoholic beverages. In *Annual Report of the IARC*. International Agency for Research on Cancer, Lyon, France, pp. 56–57.

Ivankovic, S. (1978). Carcinogene Wirkung von *N*-Benzyl-*N*-Nitrosoharnstoff (BZNH) an BD-Ratten. *Z. Krebsforch. 91*: 63–86.

Karlowski, K., and Bojewski, J. (1988). Presence of volatile *N*-nitrosamines in fish and fish products. *Rocz. Panstw. Zakl. Hig. 39*: 355–360.

Kawabata, T., Uibu, J., and Ohshima, H. (1980). Occurrence, formation and precursors of *N*-nitroso compounds in the Japanese diet. *IARC Sci. Publ.* No. 31: 481–492.

Key, P. E., Baylor, J. M., Massey, R. C., and McWeeny, D. J. (1982). Nitrosodimethylamine levels in fish cooked by natural gas and by electricity. *J. Food Technol. 17*: 703–708.

Knight, T., Forman, D., Leach, S. A., Packer, P., Cocco, G., Palli, D.,and Pirastu, R. (1991). The *N*-nitrosoproline test as a measure of cancer risk in geographical comparison studies: Results from Italy and an overall comparison. *IARC Sci. Publ.* No. 105: 146–151.

Kumar, R., Mende, P., Tricker, A. R., Siddiqi, M., and Preussmann, R. (1990). *N*-Nitroso compounds and their precursors in *Brassica oleracea*. *Cancer Lett. 54*: 61–65.

Lawley, P. D. (1990). *N*-Nitroso compounds. In *Chemical Carcinogenesis and Mutagenesis*, C. S. Cooper and P. L. Grover, eds. Springer-Verlag, Berlin, pp. 409–469.

Libbey, L. M., Scanlan, R. A., and Barbour, J. F. (1980). *N*-Nitrosodimethylamine in dried dairy products. *Food Cosmet. Toxicol. 18*: 459–461.

Licht, W. R., and Deen, W. M. (1988). Theoretical model for predicting rates of nitrosamine and nitrosamide formation in the human stomach. *Carcinogenesis 9*: 2227–2237.

Lijinsky, W. (1987a). Structure-activity relations in carcinogenesis by *N*-nitroso compounds. *Cancer and Metastasis Rev. 6*: 301–356.

Lijinsky, W. (1987b). Structural relations and dose response studies in nitrosamine carcinogenesis. *Adv. Modern Environ. Toxicol. 10*: 215–241.

Lu, S. H., Chui, S. X., Yang, W. X., Hu, X. N., Guo, L. P., and Li, F. M. (1991). Relevance of *N*-nitrosamines to oesophageal cancer in China. *IARC Sci. Publ.* No. 105: 11–17.

Maga, J. A. (1978). Amines in foods. *Crit. Rev. Food Sci. Nutr. 10* (Part 4): 373–403.

Magee, P. N., and Barnes, J. M. (1956). The production of malignant primary hepatic tumours in the rat by feeding dimethylnitrosamine. *Brit. J. Cancer 10*: 114–122.

Magee, P. N., Montesano, R., and Preussmann, R. (1976). *N*-Nitroso compounds and related carcinogens. In *Chemical Carcinogens*, ACS Symp. Series 173, C. E. Searle, ed. American Chemical Society, Washington, DC, pp. 491–625.

Maki, T., Tamura, Y., Shimamura, Y., and Naoi, Y. (1980). Estimate of the volatile nitrosamine content of Japanese food. *Bull. Environ. Contam. Toxicol. 25*: 257–261.

MAFF (1987). *Nitrate, Nitrite and N-Nitroso-Compounds in Food, Food Surveillance Paper No. 20*, Her Majesty's Stationery Office, London, U.K., pp. 34–35.

Meester, J. (1974). Nitrate and nitrite allowances in meat products. In *Proc. Int. Symp. on Nitrite in Meat Products*, B. Krol and B. J. Tinbergen, eds. Pudoc, Wageningen, pp. 265–268.

Mirvish, S. S. (1972). Studies on *N*-nitrosation reactions: Kinetics of nitrosation, correlation with mouse feeding experiments, and natural occurrence of nitrosatable compounds (ureides and guanidines). In *Topics on Chemical Carcinogenesis*, W. Nakahara, S. Takayama, S. Sugimura, and S. Odashima, eds. University of Tokyo Press, Tokyo, pp. 279–295.

Mirvish, S. S. (1975). Formation of N-nitroso compounds: chemistry, kinetics, and in vivo occurrence. *Toxicol. Appl. Pharmacol. 31*: 325–351.

National Academy of Sciences–National Research Council (1981). *The Health Effects of Nitrate, Nitrite, and N-Nitroso Compounds*. National Academy Press, Washington, DC.

Newmark, H. L., and Mergens, W. J. (1981). Blocking nitrosamine formation using ascorbic acid and α-tocopherol. In *Gastrointestinal Cancer: Endogenous Factors*, Banbury Report No. 7, W. R. Bruce, P. Correa, M. Lipkin, S. R. Tannenbaum, and T. Wilkins, eds. Cold Spring Harbor Laboratory, New York, pp. 285–298.

Nitrite Safety Council, U.S. (1980). A survey of nitrosamines in sausages and dry-cured meat products. *Food Technol. 34*: 45–52.

Ohshima, H., and Bartsch, H. (1981). Quantitative estimation of endogenous nitrosation in humans by monitoring *N*-nitrosoproline excreted in the urine. *Cancer Res. 41*: 3658–3662.

Okada, M. (1984). Comparative metabolism of *N*-nitrosamines in relation to their organ and species specificity. *IARC Sci. Publ.* No. 57: 401–409.

Österdahl, B.-G. (1988). Volatile nitrosamines in foods on the Swedish market and estimation of their daily intake. *Food Additiv. Contam. 5*: 587–595.

Pensabene, J. W., and Fiddler, W. (1983). *N*-Nitrosothiazolidine in cured meat products. *J. Food Sci. 48*: 1870–1874.

Pensabene, J. W., Fiddler, W., Gates, R. A., Fagan, J. C., and Wassermann, A. E. (1974). Effect of frying and other cooking conditions on nitrosopyrrolidine formation in bacon. *J. Food Sci. 39*: 314–316.

Perciballi, M., and Hotchkiss, J. H. (1989). *In vivo* inhibition of *N*-nitrosodimethylamine metabolism by 4-methylpyrazole: A model for endogenous nitrosation. *Carcinogenesis 10*: 2303–2309.

Peto, R., Gray, R., Brantom, P., and Grasso, P. (1984). Nitrosamine carcinogenesis in 5120 rodents: chronic administration of sixteen different concentrations of NDEA, NDMA, NPYR and NPIP in the water of 4440 inbred rats, with parallel studies on NDEA alone of the effect of age of starting (3, 6 or 20 weeks) and of species (rats, mice or hamsters). *IARC Sci. Publ.* No. 57: 627–665.

Pignatelli, B., Friesen, M., and Walker, E. A. (1980). The role of phenols in catalysis of nitrosamine formation. *IARC Sci. Publ.* No. 31: 95–109.

Pignatelli, B., Bereziat, J. C., O'Neill, I. K., and Bartsch, H. (1982). Catalytic role of some phenolic substances in endogenous formation of *N*-nitroso compounds. *IARC Sci. Publ.* No. 41: 413–423.

Poirier, S., Hubert, A., de-Thé, G., Ohshima, H., Bourgade, M.-C., and Bartsch, H. (1987). Occurrence of volatile nitrosamines in food samples collected in three high-risk areas for nasopharyngeal carcinoma. *IARC Sci. Publ.* No. 84: 415–419.

Pool, B. L., Eisenbrand, G., Preussmann, R., Schlehofer, J. R., Schmezer, P., Weber, H., and Wiessler, M. (1986). Detection of mutations in bacteria and of DNA damage and amplified DNA sequences in mammalian cells as a systematic test strategy for elucidating biological activities of chemical carcinogens. *Food Chem. Toxicol. 24*: 685–691.

Preston-Martin, S. (1987). *N*-Nitroso compounds as a cause of human cancer. *IARC Sci. Publ.* No. 84: 477–484.

Preussmann, R. (1984). Occurrence and exposure to *N*-nitroso compounds and precursors. *IARC Sci. Publ.* No. 57: 3–15.

Preussmann, R., and Stewart, B. W. (1984). *N*-Nitroso carcinogens. In *Chemical Carcinogens*, 2nd ed. C. E. Searle, ed. ACS Monograph 182, Vol. 2. American Chemical Society, Washington, DC, pp. 643–828.

Preussmann, R., Eisenbrand, G., and Spiegelhalder, B. (1979). Occurrence and formation of *N*-nitroso compounds in the environment and in vivo. In *Environmental Carcinogens*, P. Emmelot and E. Krieg, eds. Elsevier/North Holland, Amsterdam, pp. 51–72.

Roller, P. P., and Keefer, L. K. (1974). Catalysis of nitrosation reactions by electrophilic species. *IARC Sci. Publ.* No. 9: 86–89.

Sakshaug, J., Soegnen, E., Aas Hansen, M., and Koppang, N. (1965). Dimethylnitrosamine; its hepatotoxic effect in sheep and its occurrence in toxic batches of herring meal. *Nature* (London) *206*: 1261–1262.

Scanlan, R. A. (1975). *N*-Nitrosamines in foods. *CRC Crit. Rev. Food Technol. 5*: 357–402.

Scanlan, R. A., Barbour, J. F., and Chappel, C. I. (1990). A survey of *N*-nitrosodimethylamine in U.S. and Canadian beers. *J. Agric. Food Chem. 38*: 442–443.

Schmähl, D., Krüger, F. W., Habs, M., and Diehl, B. (1976). Influence of disulfiram on the organotrophy of the carcinogenic effect of dimethylnitrosamine and diethylnitrosamine in rats. *Z. Krebsforsch. 85*: 271–276.

Schmezer, P., Pool, B. L., Preussmann, R., and Schmähl, D. (1987). Analysis of *N*-nitrosamines for genotoxicity in primary hepatocytes derived from various species. *IARC Sci. Publ.* No. 84: 270–273.

Schmezer, P., Pool, B. L., Lefevre, P. A., Callander, R. D., Ratpan, F., Tinwell, H., and Ashby, J. (1990). Assay-specific genotoxicity of *N*-nitrosodibenzylamine to the rat liver *in vivo*. *Environ. Mol. Mutagen. 15*: 190–197.

Sen, N. P. (1986). Formation and occurrence of nitrosamines in food. In *Diet, Nutrition, and Cancer: A Critical Evaluation. Vol. II, Micronutrients, Nonnutritive Dietary Factors, and Cancer*, B. S. Reddy, and L. A. Cohen, eds. CRC Press, Inc., Boca Raton, FL, pp. 135–160.

Sen, N. P. (1988). Migration and formation of *N*-nitrosamines from food contact materials. In *Food and Packaging Interactions, ACS Symposium Series 365*, J. H. Hotchkiss, ed. American Chemical Society, Washington, DC, pp. 146–158.

Sen, N. P. (1990). Analysis and occurrence of *N*-nitroso compounds in foods. In *N-Nitroso Compounds: Biology and Chemistry*, S. V. Bhide and K. V. K. Rao, eds. Omega Scientific Publishers, New Delhi, pp. 3–18.

Sen, N. P. (1991). Recent studies in Canada on the occurrence and formation of *N*-nitroso compounds in foods and food contact materials. *IARC Sci. Publ.* No. 105: 232–234.

Sen, N. P., and Baddoo, P. A.(1986). Origin of *N*-nitrosomorpholine contamination in margarine. *J. Food Sci. 51*: 216–217, 232.

Sen, N. P., and Seaman, S. (1981). Volatile nitrosamines in dried foods. *J. Assoc. Off. Anal. Chem. 64*: 1238–1242.

Sen, N. P., Miles, W. F., Donaldson, B., Panalaks, T., and Iyengar, J. R. (1973). Formation of nitrosamines in a meat curing mixture. *Nature* (London) *245*: 104–105.

Sen, N. P., Donaldson, B., Charbonneau, C., and Miles, W. F. (1974). Effect of additives on the formation of nitrosamines in meat curing mixtures containing spices and nitrite. *J. Agric. Food Chem. 22*: 1125–1130.

Sen, N. P., Seaman, S., and Miles, W. F. (1979). Volatile nitrosamines in various cured meat products: Effect of cooking and recent trends. *J. Agric. Food Chem. 27*: 1354–1357.

Sen, N. P., Seaman, S., and McPherson, M. (1980). Further studies on the occurrence of volatile and nonvolatile nitrosamines in foods. *IARC Sci. Publ.* No. 31: 457–465.

Sen, N. P., Seaman, S. W., and Tessier, L. (1982). Comparison of two analytical methods for the determination of dimethylnitrosamine in beer and ale, and some recent results. *J. Food Safety 4*: 243–250.

Sen, N. P., Tessier, L., Seaman, S. W., and Baddoo, P. A. (1985). Volatile and nonvolatile nitrosamines in fish and the effect of deliberate nitrosation under simulated gastric conditions. *J. Agric. Food Chem. 33*: 264–268.

Sen, N. P., Baddoo, P. A., and Seaman, S. W. (1987). Volatile nitrosamines in cured meats packaged in elastic rubber nettings. *J. Agric. Food Chem. 35*: 346–350.

Sen, N. P., Seaman, S. W., Baddoo, P. A., and Weber, D. (1988). Further studies on the formation of nitrosamines in cured pork products packaged in elastic rubber nettings. *J. Food Sci. 53*: 731–734 and 738.

Shephard, S. E., Schlatter, C., and Lutz, W. K. (1987). Assessment of the risk of formation of carcinogenic *N*-nitroso compounds from dietary precursors in the stomach. *Food Chem. Toxicol. 25*: 91–108.

Siddiqi, M., Tricker, A. R., and Preussmann, R. (1988). The occurrence of preformed *N*-nitroso compounds in food samples from a high risk area of esophageal cancer in Kashmir, India. *Cancer Lett. 39*: 37–43.

Siddiqi, M. A., Tricker, A. R., Kumar, R., Fazili, Z., and Preussmann, R. (1991). *IARC Sci. Publ.* No. 105: 210–213.

Smith, T. A. (1980). Amines in food. *Food Chem. 6*: 169–200.

Spiegelhalder, B., Eisenbrand, G., and Preussmann, R. (1976). Influence of dietary nitrate on nitrite content of human saliva: Possible relevance to *in vivo* formation of *N*-nitroso compounds. *Food Cosmet. Toxicol. 14*: 545–548.

Spiegelhalder, B., Eisenbrand, G., and Preussmann, R. (1980). Occurrence of volatile nitrosamines in food: a survey of the West German market, *IARC Sci. Publ.* No. 31: 467–477.

Stephany, R. W., and Schuller, P. L. (1980). Daily dietary intakes of nitrate, nitrite, and volatile *N*-nitrosamines in the Netherlands using the duplicate portion sampling technique. *Oncology 37*: 203–210.

Stuehr, D. J., and Marletta, M. A. (1987). Further studies on murine macrophage synthesis of nitrite and nitrate. *IARC Sci. Publ.* No. 84: 335–339.

Swann, P. F. (1984). Effect of ethanol on nitrosamine metabolism and distribution, implications for the role of nitrosamines in human cancer and for the influence of alcohol consumption of cancer incidence. *IARC Sci. Publ.* No. 57: 501–512.

Tannenbaum, S. R., Weisman, M., and Fett, D. (1976). The effect of nitrate intake on nitrite formation in human saliva. *Food & Cosmet. Toxicol. 14*: 549–552.

Tomatis, L., and Hilfrich, J., Turusov, V. (1975). The occurrence of tumours in F_1, F_2 and F_3 descendants of BD rats exposed to *N*-nitrosomethylurea during pregnancy. *Int. J. Cancer 15*: 385–390.

Tricker, A. R., and Kubacki, S. J. (1991). Review of the occurrence and formation of nonvolatile *N*-nitroso compounds in foods. *Food Additiv. Contam. 8*: (in press).

Tutelyan, V. A., Zhukova, G. F., and Pimenova, V. V. (1990). Assay of *N*-nitrosamines in foodstuffs produced in the USSR by gas-liquid chromatography with a thermal energy analyser. *Food Additiv. Contam. 7*: 43–49.

USDA (1986). Nitrite levels in bacon. *Fed. Register 51*(115): 21731–21736.

USDA (1989). Immersion cured and dry cured bacon (re: nitrite regulation). *Fed. Register 54*(9): 1371–1374.

Wagner, D. A., and Tannenbaum, S. R. (1985). *In-vivo* formation of *N*-nitroso compounds. *Food Technol. 39*(1): 89–90.

Wagner, D. A., Young, V. R., Tannenbaum, S. R., Schultz, D. S., and Deen, W. M. (1984). Mammalian nitrate biochemistry: Metabolism and endogenous synthesis. *IARC Sci. Publ.* No. 57: 247–253.

Walker, R. (1990). Nitrates, nitrites, and *N*-nitroso compounds: A review of the occurrence in food and diet and the toxicological implications. *Food Additiv. Contam. 7*: 717–768.

White, J. W. (1976). Relative significance of dietary sources of nitrate and nitrite. *J. Agric. Food Chem. 24*: 202.

Wiessler, M., Romkuen, K., and Pool, B. L. (1983). Biological activity of benzylating *N*-nitroso compounds. Models of activated *N*-nitrosomethylbenzylamine. *Carcinogenesis 4*: 867–871.

WHO (1978). *Nitrates, Nitrites and N-Nitroso Compounds, Environmental Health Criteria, 5*, World Health Organization, Geneva.

Yamamoto, M., Iwata, R., Ishiwa, H., Yamada, T., and Tanimura, A. (1984). Determination of volatile nitrosamine levels in foods and estimation of their daily intake in Japan. *Food and Chemical Toxicol. 22*: 61–64.

Index

B

C

G

M

Q

R

S